Core Curriculum for Maternal-Newborn Nursing

Core Curriculum for Maternal-Newborn Nursing

Edited by:

Susan Mattson, Ph.D., R.N.,C., C.T.N.
Associate Professor
California State University, Long Beach
Long Beach, California

Judy E. Smith, Ph.D., R.N.,C.
Professor
California State University, Long Beach
Long Beach, California

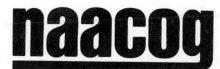

The Organization for Obstetric, Gynecologic, & Neonatal Nurses

W. B. SAUNDERS COMPANY
Harcourt Brace Jovanovich, Inc.
Philadelphia London Toronto Montreal Sydney Tokyo

W. B. SAUNDERS COMPANY
Harcourt Brace Jovanovich, Inc.

The Curtis Center
Independence Square West
Philadelphia, Pennsylvania 19106

Library of Congress Cataloging-in-Publication Data

NAACOG core curriculum for maternal-newborn nursing / edited by Susan
   Mattson, Judy E. Smith.
        p.   cm.
     ISBN 0-7216-3122-3
     1. Maternity nursing.   I. Mattson, Susan.   II. Smith, Judy E.
   III. NAACOG (Organization)
     [DNLM: 1. Curriculum.   2. Education, Nursing.   3. Maternal-Child
   Nursing—education.   WY 18 N11]
     RG951N33   1992
   610.73'678—dc20
   DNLM/DLC   91-45824

Core Curriculm for Maternal-Newborn Nursing   ISBN 0-7216-3122-3

Printed in Mexico.

Last digit is the print number: 9   8   7   6   5   4   3   2   1

Contributors

Dorothy A. Austin, M.S., R.N. • Clinical Nurse Specialist, Women's Hospital, Long Beach Memorial Medical Center, Long Beach, California • *Labor and Delivery at Risk*

Arlene Gray Blix, Dr. P.H., R.N. • Associate Professor, California State University, Fullerton; Childbirth Educator, Circle City Hospital, Corona, California • *Environmental Hazards*

Linda Bond, Ph.D., R.N.,C. • Associate Professor, Kirkhof School of Nursing, Grand Valley State University, Allendale, Michigan • *Physiology of Pregnancy; Physiological Changes*

Bonnie C. Christoff, M.S., C.R.N.P. • University of Pennsylvania, Philadelphia; Osteopathic College of Medicine, Philadelphia; Neonatal Nurse Practitioner, Osteopathic Medical Center of Philadelphia; Neonatal Nurse Practitioner, Abington Memorial Hospital, Abington, Pennsylvania • *Risks Associated with Gestational Age and Birth Weight; Hyperbilirubinemia; Infant of a Diabetic Mother; Congenital Abnormalities*

Kathryn V. Deitch, Ph.D., R.N.,C. • Associate Professor of Nursing, California State University, San Bernardino; Women's Health Care Nurse Practitioner, Private Practice, Newport Beach, California • *Reproductive Anatomy and Physiology; Endocrinology and Pregnancy; Family Planning*

Nancy Donaldson, D.N.Sc., R.N. • Assistant Clinical Professor, School of Nursing, University of California, Los Angeles, Los Angeles; Volunteer Associate Clinical Professor, College of Medicine, University of California; Associate Director of Nursing and Director of Nursing Research, Irvine Medical Center, University of California, Irvine, Orange, California • *Research and Ethical Issues*

Karen Foster-Anderson, M.S., R.N.,C., O.G.N.P. • Private Practice, Centreville, Virginia • *Surgery in Pregnancy*

Harriet Gillerman, M.S., R.N.,C. • Associate Nursing Administrator, Professional Development and Research Services, Long Beach Memorial Medical Center, Long Beach, California • *Other Medical Complications*

Judith Noble Halle, M.S.N., R.N.,C. • Assistant Clinical Professor, Lecturer, School of Nursing, University of California, Los Angeles; Maternal-Child Educator, Methodist Hospital, Arcadia, California • *Diagnostic Evaluation of High-Risk Pregnancies*

Mary Katherine Bourgeois Harris, M.S.N., R.N., C.F.N.P. • Certified Lactation Consultant, Kaiser Permanente Medical Group, Huntington Beach, California • *Breastfeeding*

Patricia Higgins, Ph.D., R.N. • Associate Professor of Parent–Child Nursing, College of Nursing, University of New Mexico, Albuquerque, New Mexico • *Postpartum Complications*

Linda Howard-Glenn, M.N., R.N.,C. • Clinical Nurse Specialist, Memorial Miller Children's Hospital, Long Beach, California • *Adaptation to Extrauterine Life; Biological and Behavioral Characteristics; Immediate Nursing Care; Psychosocial Adaptations*

Leayn Hutchinson Johnson, Ph.D., R.N., C.N.S. • Assistant Professor, California State University, Long Beach, California • *Perinatal Loss and Grief*

Linda C. Johnson, Ph.D., R.N. • Assistant Professor of Pediatric Nursing, School of Nursing, Loma Linda University, Loma Linda; Administrative Director, Parent–Child Nursing, Loma Linda University Medical Center, Loma Linda, California • *Psychological Changes*

Kathleen A. Kalb, Ph.D. • Assistant Professor of Nursing, College of St. Catherine, St. Paul, Minnesota • *Endocrine and Metabolic Disorders*

Bonnie Kellogg, M.S., R.N. • Associate Professor, California State University, Long Beach, California • *Genetics; Fetal Development; Placental Development and Functioning*

Lillian S. Lew, M.Ed., R.D. • Director, Southeast Asian Health Project, St. Mary Medical Center, Long Beach, Long Beach, California • *Nutrition*

Susan Mattson, Ph.D., R.N.,C., C.T.N. • Associate Professor, California State University, Long Beach, California • *Ethnocultural Considerations in the Childbearing Period; Hypertensive States in Pregnancy; Risks Associated with Gestational Age and Birth Weight*

Barbara A. Moran, M.S., R.N.,C. • Perinatal Education Coordinator, Fairfax Hospital, Falls Church, Virginia • *Maternal Infections; Substance Abuse in Pregnancy*

Phyllis Ann Muchmore R.N.,C., M.H.A. • Coordinator, Orange County Regional Perinatal Program, Irvine Medical Center, University of California, Irvine, California • *Respiratory Distress; Sepsis in the Newborn*

Leith Merrow Mullaly, M.S.N., R.N.,C., A.C.C.E. • Director, Women's and Children's Education and Information Services, Alexandria Hospital, Alexandria, Virginia • *Psychology of Pregnancy; Preparation for Childbirth*

Barbara J. Petree, M.A., R.N. • Clinical Instructor, Obstetrics, University of San Francisco; Guest Lecturer, San Jose State University, Evergreen College; Senior Staff Nurse, Labor and Delivery, Stanford Unversity Hospital, Stanford; Instructor, Stanford University Medical School for Electronic Fetal Monitoring, Stanford, California • *Hypertensive States in Pregnancy*

Judy Schmidt, Ed.D., R.N.,C. • Assistant Clinical Professor, University of California, San Francisco; Clinical Nurse Specialist, Sutter Memorial Hospital, Sacramento, California • *Fetal Assessment; Hemorrhagic Disorders*

Sheila Sanning Shea, M.S.N., R.N., C.E.N. • Clinical Nurse Specialist, Department of Emergency Medicine, St. Mary Medical Center, Long Beach, California • *Trauma in Pregnancy*

Gary Sparger, M.S.N., R.N., C.E.N., M.I.C.N. • Late Associate Professor of Nursing, California State University, Long Beach, California • *Trauma in Pregnancy*

Judy E. Smith, Ph.D., R.N.,C. • Professor of Maternal–Child Nursing, California State University, Long Beach, Long Beach, California • *Age-Related Concerns; Hyperbilirubinemia; The Drug-Dependent Neonate; Congenital Abnormalities*

Kathleen V. Smith, M.S.N., R.N.,C. • Assistant Professor, Bishop Clarkson College, Omaha, Nebraska; Casual Staff, Beautiful Beginnings, Mercy Hospital, Council Bluffs, Iowa • *Normal Childbirth*

Gail M. Turley, M.S.N., R.N.,C. • Director, Maternal Child/Ambulatory Nursing, Crozer-Chester Medical Center, Upland, Pennsylvania • *Essential Forces and Factors in Labor*

Ksenia Zukowsky, M.S.N., C.R.N.P. • Lecturer, School of Nursing, University of Pennsylvania, Philadelphia; Neonatal Nurse Practitioner, Thomas Jefferson University Hospital, Philadelphia, Pennsylvania • *Risks Associated with Gestational Age and Birth Weight; Hyperbilirubinemia; Infant of a Diabetic Mother; Congenital Abnormalities*

Preface

This book is intended to be used by practicing nurses for several purposes. Primarily, it is designed as a study guide for those wishing to sit for certification examinations in maternal-newborn nursing. Basic and complex information is presented and accompanied by an extensive reference list to augment the knowledge base.

Secondarily, the text may be used by staff development personnel and educators as orientation for new staff, a source of information for nurses entering or returning to maternal-newborn nursing, and a reference for nurses on those units. With this goal in mind, the complications associated with maternal-newborn nursing are separated from the normally occurring events, allowing ease of retrieval of information.

For both of these audiences, the complications relating to neonates are presented from the perspective of the nurse caring for them in the delivery room, normal newborn nursery, and/or mother-baby care units. Thus, the section is not directed at intensive care, but rather, points out screening techniques and observations necessary to identify the high-risk infant and the care required until the baby can be transferred if necessary. Additionally, theoretical information about the continued care of high-risk neonates with selected conditions is briefly presented. This information is included to provide a basis from which the maternal-newborn nurse may generate answers to parents' questions and to give anticipatory guidance to new parents of sick neonates.

Although nursing diagnoses have been used throughout the book, we do wish to remind the reader that all nursing diagnoses are fluid, designed to be tested in practice and refined. Thus, wording may differ from some NANDA publications or other authorities in the field. This is not to imply that one is right and another wrong, but simply that certain terminology fits more appropriately in some settings than in others and is used to express the need of a particular client at that time.

We hope this text will be helpful to those of you using it, for all purposes. Editing it has been an educational and character-building experience for us both.

SUSAN MATTSON
JUDY E. SMITH

Contents

HUMAN REPRODUCTION

Kathryn V. Deitch

Reproductive Anatomy and Physiology

Objectives

1. Identify and describe the female organs of reproduction

2. Identify and briefly describe the male organs of reproduction

3. Describe the physiological functioning of the female reproductive system

4. Briefly describe the physiological functioning of the male reproductive system

5. Describe deviations from normal anatomy that affect reproduction

6. Describe deviations from normal physiology that affect reproduction

7. Analyze the data from a reproductive history and physical examination to determine overt and covert anatomical and physiological factors that could affect pregnancy

8. Prepare a set of nursing interventions for teaching pertinent concepts of anatomy and physiology to clients

Introduction

FEMALE ORGANS OF REPRODUCTION

A. External genitals: vulva (Fig. 1–1)

1. Mons pubis or veneris
   a. Is a rounded pad of subcutaneous fatty tissue over the symphysis pubis; covered with pubic hair
   b. Function is the protection of the symphysis pubis during intercourse
2. Labia majora
   a. Are two rounded folds of fatty and connective tissue, covered with pubic hair, that extend from the mons pubis to the perineum
   b. Function is the protection of the vaginal introitus
3. Labia minora
   a. Are narrow folds of hairless skin located within the labia majora; begin beneath the clitoris and extend to the fourchette
   b. Are highly vascular and rich in nerve supply; glands lubricate the vulva
   c. Function is erotic; swell in response to stimulation and are highly sensitive
4. Prepuce of clitoris is a hoodlike covering over the clitoris

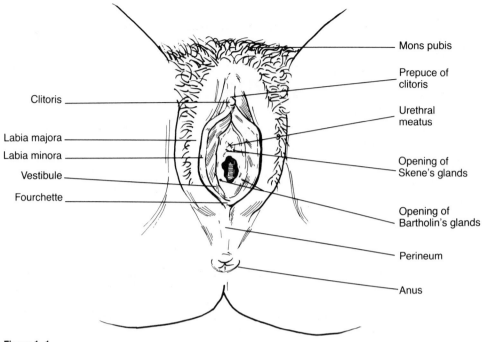

Figure 1–1
Female external genitals.

5. Clitoris
    a. Is an erectile organ located beneath the pubic arch and consists of shaft and glans
    b. Secretes smegma, a pheromone (olfactory erotic stimulant)
    c. Is extremely sensitive to touch, pressure, and temperature
    d. Function is sexual stimulation
6. Vestibule
    a. Is an oval-shaped area whose boundaries are the clitoris, fourchette, and labia minora; contains the following
        (1) Urethral meatus
            (a) Is the terminal portion of the urethra, with puckered or slitted appearance
            (b) Is located 2.5 cm (1 in) below the clitoris
        (2) Skene's glands
            (a) Are located inside the urethral meatus
            (b) Produce mucus for lubrication
        (3) Hymen
            (a) Is tough, elastic, perforated, mucosa-covered tissue across the vaginal introitus
            (b) Hymenal opening may be absent or small, impeding menstrual flow and intercourse
            (c) Characteristics of hymen vary widely among women; size of opening is an unreliable indicator of sexual experience
        (4) Bartholin's glands
            (a) Are located at the base of each of the labia minora, just inside the vaginal orifice
            (b) During coitus, secrete mucus that is hospitable to sperm
7. Fourchette is located in the midline below the vaginal opening where the labia majora and labia minora merge

8. Perineum
   a. Is skin-covered muscular tissue located between the vaginal opening and the anus
   b. Is the area of a midline episiotomy
   c. May be lacerated during childbirth

B. **Internal organs (Fig. 1–2)**

1. Vagina
   a. Is a tubular structure located behind the bladder and in front of the rectum; it extends from the introitus to the cervix
   b. Is thin walled, composed of smooth muscle, capable of great distension as well as collapse
   c. Is lined with a glandular mucous membrane that is arranged in folds called rugae
   d. Is highly vascular and relatively insensitive; it adds little sensation during coitus
   e. Functions as the birth canal and the organ for coitus
2. Uterus
   a. Is located behind the symphysis pubis between the bladder and the rectum
   b. Is muscular, hollow, smooth, mobile, nontender, firm, and symmetrical
   c. In a woman who has not been pregnant, uterine size ranges from 5.5 to 8 cm (2.2 to 3.2 in) in length, 3.5 to 4.0 cm (1.4 to 1.6 in) in width, and 2.0 to 2.5 cm (0.8 to 1.0 in) in depth; size increases after childbirth
   d. Is similar in shape to a light bulb or pear
   e. Is composed of four parts
      (1) Fundus
         (a) Is the upper, rounded portion above the insertion of the fallopian tubes

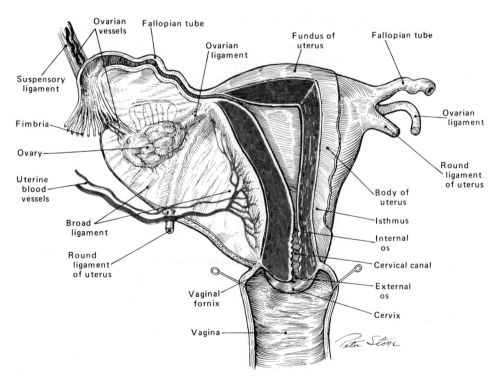

Figure 1–2
Female reproductive organs. Front uterine wall has been removed so that the fallopian tube, uterus, cervical canal, and vagina are seen as a continuous channel. (From Langley, L.L., Telford, I.R., & Christensen, J.B. [1980]. *Dynamic anatomy and physiology.* New York: McGraw-Hill. Copyrighted by The C.V. Mosby Company.)

(b) Uterine size during pregnancy is measured in centimeters from the fundus to the symphysis pubis

(2) Corpus or body is the main portion of the uterus located between the cervix and the fundus

(3) Isthmus

    (a) Is called the lower uterine segment during pregnancy

    (b) Joins the corpus to the cervix

(4) Cervix or neck

    (a) Is divided into two portions: the portion above the site of attachment of the cervix to the vaginal vault is called the supravaginal portion; the portion below the attachment site that protrudes into the vagina is called the vaginal portion

    (b) Is composed of fibrous connective tissue

    (c) Diameter varies from 2 to 5 cm (0.80 to 2.0 in), depending on childbearing history

    (d) Length is usually 2.5 to 3.0 cm (1 to 1.2 in) in the nonpregnant woman

    (e) Vaginal portion is smooth, firm, and doughnut shaped, with visible central opening called the external os

    (f) External os is round before the first childbirth and is often slitlike in shape after childbirth

    (g) Internal os is the opening in the cervix to the uterine cavity

    (h) Cervical canal connects the vagina with the uterine cavity

    (i) Functions include a passage for menstrual products and sperm; its major feature is its ability to stretch to a diameter large enough to allow passage of an infant's head and then to return to a closed position

    (j) Produces mucus in response to cyclic hormones; mucus is an important factor in fertility; observation of changes in mucus is important in fertility awareness methods of family planning

    (k) Vaginal surface is covered with squamous epithelium; cervical canal is lined with columnar epithelium

        (i) Area where two types of epithelium meet is called the squamocolumnar junction

        (ii) This area of rapid cellular growth is the most frequent site of cervical cancer and of precancerous changes assessed with the Papanicolaou (Pap) test

f. Uterine position (Fig. 1–3)

  (1) Five positions are possible

    (a) Anteflexed

    (b) Anterior or anteverted

    (c) Midposition

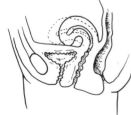
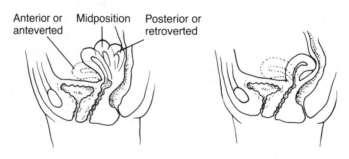

A   Anteflexed   B   C   Retroflexed

Figure 1–3
Uterine positions.

           (d) Posterior or retroverted

           (e) Retroflexed

  g. Uterine support

     (1) Anterior ligament extends from the anterior cervix to the bladder

     (2) Cardinal or transverse ligaments

           (a) Are a portion of the broad ligament

           (b) Contain uterine blood vessels and ureters

           (c) Are connected to the lateral margins of the uterus

     (3) Posterior ligament extends from the posterior cervix to the rectum

     (4) Uterosacral ligaments

           (a) Extend from the cervix over the rectum to the sacral vertebrae

           (b) Maintain traction on the cervix to hold the uterus in position

  h. Uterine wall

     (1) Is composed of three layers

           (a) Endometrium is a highly vascular mucous membrane that responds to hormone stimulation first by hypertrophy and then by secretion to prepare to receive the developing ovum; sloughs if pregnancy does not occur, resulting in menstruation; if pregnancy occurs, sloughs after delivery

           (b) Myometrium is composed of smooth muscle in layers

               (i) Outer layer is composed of longitudinal fibers, which predominate in the fundus and provide power to expel the fetus

              (ii) Middle layer is composed of fibers interlaced with blood vessels in a figure-eight pattern; is called a living ligature because its contraction after childbirth helps control blood loss

             (iii) Inner layer is composed of circular fibers concentrated around the internal cervical os; provides sphincter action to help keep the cervix closed during pregnancy

           (c) Parietal peritoneum covers most of the uterus, except for the cervix and a portion of the anterior corpus

3. Fallopian tubes or oviducts (see Fig. 1–2)

  a. Are attached to the uterine fundus and curve around each ovary

  b. Provide a passageway for the ovum into the uterus

  c. Size is 10 cm (4 in) in length and 0.6 cm (0.25 in) in diameter

  d. Comprises four parts

     (1) Infundibulum is the most distal portion with a funnel shape, and is covered with fimbriae that pull the ovum into the tube by creating a wavelike motion

     (2) Ampulla is the next most distal portion and site of fertilization

     (3) Isthmus is the narrowed part of the tube, closer to the uterus

     (4) Interstitial is the narrowest portion, which passes through the uterine myometrium and opens into the uterine cavity

  e. Functions include

     (1) Capture of the ovum

     (2) Movement of the ovum into the uterus by peristaltic activity and the wavelike movements of the cilia

     (3) Secretion of the nutrients to support the ovum during the transport

4. Ovaries or female gonads (see Fig. 1–2)

  a. Are comparable to the testes in the male

  b. Are located on either side of the uterus, below and behind the fimbriated ends of the oviducts

  c. Are supported by the ovarian ligaments and the mesovarian portion of the broad ligament

  d. Are similar to almonds in size and shape

  e. Are smooth, mobile, slightly tender, firm

  f. Functions include ovulation and production of the hormones estrogen, progesterone, and androgens

C. Support for organs of reproduction

1. Circulation
   a. Blood is supplied to the pelvis by arteries branching from the hypogastric artery (which branches from an iliac artery, a division of the aorta)
   b. Major pelvic arteries include the uterine, the vaginal, the pudendal, and the perineal arteries
   c. Ovarian arteries branch directly from the aorta
   d. Lymphatic drainage is accomplished from the uterus, ovaries, and fallopian tubes to nodes around the aorta, with some use of the femoral, iliac, and hypogastric nodes
2. Pelvic floor and perineum
   a. Functions include
      (1) Support of the suspended internal organs of reproduction
      (2) Support for sphincter control, allowing for expansion of the vagina with expulsion of the fetus, and closure of the vagina after delivery
   b. Pelvic diaphragm (Fig. 1–4)
      (1) Levator ani muscles
         (a) Puborectalis
         (b) Iliococcygeus
         (c) Pubococcygeus
      (2) Coccygeal muscles
   c. Urogenital diaphragm (see Fig. 1–4): transverse perineal muscles
   d. Perineum (see Fig. 1–4)
      (1) Bulbocavernous muscle
      (2) Ischiocavernous muscle
      (3) Anal sphincter muscles
      (4) Perineal strength can be increased through Kegel's exercises
   e. Perineal body
      (1) Is a wedge-shaped area between the vagina and the rectum
      (2) Is an anchor point for muscles, ligaments, and fascia of the pelvis

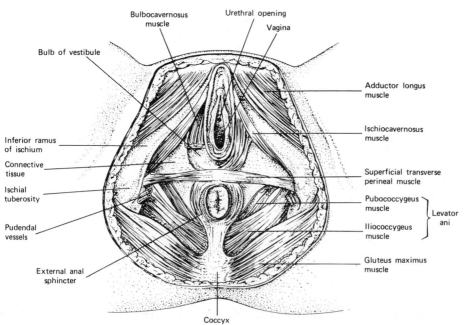

Figure 1–4
Muscles of the pelvic floor, from below. (Reproduced by permission from *Biology of women* [2nd ed., p. 53] by Ethel Sloane. Albany, NY: Delmar Publishers Inc., Copyright 1985.)

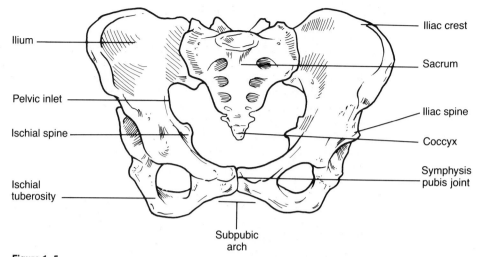

Figure 1–5
The female bony pelvis.

3. Bony pelvis (Fig. 1–5)
   a. Functions include support and protection of pelvic structures, and support for a growing fetus during the birth process
   b. Components include
      (1) Ilium
         (a) Iliac crest
         (b) Anterior, superior iliac spines
      (2) Ischium
         (a) Ischial spine
         (b) Ischial tuberosities
      (3) Pubic bone
         (a) Symphysis pubis joint
         (b) Subpubic arch
      (4) Sacrum; sacral promontory
      (5) Coccyx
   c. Ilium, ischium, and pubic bones fuse after puberty; the pelvic bone then is called the right or left innominate bone
   d. False pelvis (Fig. 1–6)
      (1) Is the area of the pelvis above the anterior, superior iliac spines
      (2) Provides no useful data for estimating the size of the birth canal
   c. True pelvis (see Fig. 1–6)
      (1) Comprises three pelvic planes
         (a) Pelvic inlet is bordered by anterior, superior iliac spines and the sacral promontory
         (b) Midpelvis is the area between the inlet and the outlet
         (c) Pelvic outlet is bordered by ischial tuberosities and the coccyx
4. Nervous innervation
   a. Motor nerves
      (1) Parasympathetic fibers from the sacral nerves cause pelvic vasodilation and inhibit uterine contractions
      (2) Sympathetic motor nerves from ganglia between T-5 and T-10 cause pelvic vasoconstriction and uterine contractions
   b. Sensory nerves
      (1) Fibers from ovaries and uterus carry pain sensations to the spinal cord at T-11 to L-1
      (2) Pain in ovaries, oviducts, and uterus is difficult to differentiate; may be felt in flank, inguinal, vulvar, or suprapubic area

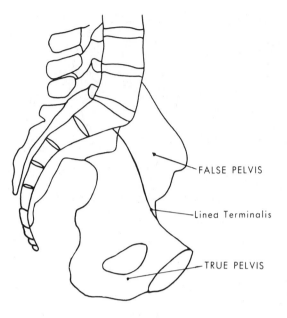

Figure 1–6
True pelvis and false pelvis divided by the linea terminalis. (Reprinted with permission of Ross Laboratories, Columbus, OH 43216, from Clinical Education Aid No. 18, © Ross Laboratories.)

MALE ORGANS OF REPRODUCTION (Fig. 1–7)

A. **External genitals**

1. Mons pubis is covered with long, dense pubic hair forming a diamond-shaped pattern from the umbilicus to the anus
2. Penis
   a. Is the organ of copulation and urination
   b. Consists of
      (1) Shaft or body
         (a) Corpora cavernosa (two)
         (b) Corpus spongiosum
         (c) Erectile tissue
      (2) Glans penis
         (a) Is similar in function to clitoris

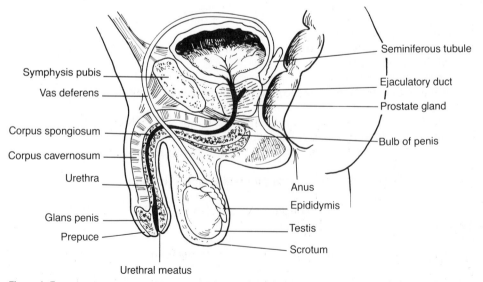

Figure 1–7
Male lower genitourinary tract.

        (b) Is smooth, sensitive to touch, pressure, and temperature

    (3) Urethra

        (a) Is a passageway for both urine and semen

        (b) Consists of four segments

            (i) Prostatic; contains ejaculatory ducts from seminal vesicles

            (ii) Membranous; contains Cowper's glands, which secrete mucus and nutrients to support sperm

            (iii) Bulbous; at the bulb of the urethra

            (iv) Penile; longest portion; extending from the bulb to the glans

    (4) Prepuce or foreskin

        (a) Is a fold of skin that covers the glans in uncircumcised men

        (b) Is retractable in adolescent and adult men

  c. Is loosely covered with skin to permit enlargement during erection

3. Scrotum

  a. Has wrinkled, pouchlike folds of skin

  b. Is divided internally by a septum; each side contains

    (1) Testis

    (2) Epididymis

    (3) Vas deferens

  c. Cremaster fascia and muscle layer

    (1) Protect testes from trauma and temperature change

    (2) Contract during exposure to cold to draw testes closer to the body

    (3) Relax during exposure to heat to move testes away from the body

B. Internal organs

1. Testes (singular, testis) or male gonads

  a. Are similar to ovaries in origin

  b. Are smooth, mobile, slightly tender

  c. Are suspended by the spermatic cord within the scrotum

  d. Length is 4 to 5 cm (1.6 to 2.0 in)

  e. Contain

    (1) Seminiferous tubules; spermatids attach here and become sperm

    (2) Interstitial cells, which produce testosterone

  f. Functions include sperm production and hormone production

  g. Primitive cells are present at birth; maturation process into sperm begins at puberty and continues throughout life

2. Ducts of testes

  a. Sperm move from seminiferous tubules through

    (1) Epididymides (singular, epididymis)

        (a) Provide storage of maturing sperm

        (b) Are located above testes

    (2) Vasa deferentia (singular, vas deferens)

        (a) Carry sperm from the scrotum to the seminal vesicles

        (b) Are located above the prostate

    (3) Ejaculatory ducts allow sperm to enter urethra and then exit the body

  b. Sperm movement occurs during the two phases of orgasm

    (1) Emission: contraction of the vasa deferentia, prostate, seminal vesicles, and ejaculatory ducts

    (2) Ejaculation: propulsion of spurts of semen outward from the penis

Clinical Practice

Assessment

Examples of deviations from normal anatomical structure or physiological functioning that can affect conception or pregnancy follow.

A. Reproductive history

1. Puberty is characterized by developmental milestones that provide evidence that ovaries and uterus are present, for example, the following
   a. Secondary sex characteristics, including breast development and axillary and pubic hair
   b. Menarche occurring before the age of 16 years
2. Congenital abnormalities
   a. Vagina
      (1) Absent
      (2) Imperforate hymen
   b. Uterus
      (1) Bicornuate, septated
      (2) May interfere with conception
   c. Cervix
      (1) Diethystilbestrol (DES) exposure: may be small, flat, and interfere with conception
      (2) Incompetent cervix: unable to remain closed during pregnancy
   d. Ovaries
      (1) "Streak" ovaries result from a chromosomal defect; ovaries are nonfunctional and will never produce the ova or hormones necessary for the changes of puberty
      (2) Menopausal ovaries are seen when ovulation has stopped
3. Disease
   a. Pelvic infection
      (1) Interferes with conception through the formation of scar tissue in response to inflammation
      (2) May be asymptomatic
      (3) Infection of the fallopian tubes, which leaves the oviducts blocked, is a major cause of infertility
   b. Endometriosis
      (1) Interferes with conception
      (2) Scar tissue is formed in response to extrauterine bleeding or inflammation
   c. Uterine fibroids
      (1) Benign tumors that alter the shape of the uterus and its ability to expand; also cause preterm labor
      (2) Common in pregnant women older than 35 years
4. Surgery
   a. Repetitive dilatation and curettage procedures for diagnosis or pregnancy termination
      (1) Asherman's syndrome
         (a) Uterine scar tissue forms
         (b) Scar tissue interferes with the normal cyclical changes in the uterine lining
      (2) Incompetent cervix
         (a) Repetitive dilatation of the cervix
         (b) Cervix is unable to remain closed during pregnancy, which leads to spontaneous abortion
   b. Cone biopsy/cryosurgery or laser surgery to cervix
      (1) Risk of scarring, which prevents conception
      (2) Risk of incompetent cervix
   c. Pelvic surgery (i.e., ovarian cystectomy or uterine myomectomy) increases risk of formation of adhesions that interfere with conception
5. Reproductive functioning
   a. Pregnancy history
      (1) Difficulty in conceiving
      (2) Number and causes of pregnancy losses

(3) Problems in perinatal period
    (a) Labor
        (i) Preterm or prolonged
        (ii) May be due to uterine, cervical, or bony pelvis abnormalities
    (b) Delivery: cephalopelvic disproportion
    (c) Postpartum period: problems of pelvic support
        (i) Uterine prolapse is the relaxation of vaginal support, with the uterus in the vagina
        (ii) Rectocele or cystocele is the herniation of the vaginal wall with the rectum or the bladder protruding into the vagina
        (iii) Difficulty with healing of lacerations or episiotomy (e.g., fistula formation)
        (iv) Increased risk of further problems with succeeding pregnancies
6. Sexual practices that can lead to increased risk of pelvic infection and affect fertility
  a. Multiple partners
  b. Change in sexual partners
  c. Use of an intrauterine device

B. Physical examination

1. General survey
2. Secondary sex characteristics: their presence indicates that sex hormones are functioning
3. Pelvic examination
  a. External genitalia
    (1) Structural abnormalities
    (2) Evidence of infection, as signaled by discharge from glands
  b. Internal organs
    (1) Vagina
        (a) Opening in hymen
        (b) Evidence of infection
    (2) Cervix
        (a) Structural abnormalities
        (b) Patency
        (c) Evidence of infection
    (3) Uterus
        (a) Size, shape, consistency, mobility
        (b) Position
    (4) Adnexa
        (a) Size, shape, consistency, mobility of ovaries
        (b) Oviducts usually not palpable
    (5) Bony pelvis
        (a) Estimate of anterior-posterior diameter of the pelvic inlet, i.e., the distance between sacral promontory and subpubic arch (12.5 to 13 cm)
        (b) Prominence of ischial spines and bispinous diameter (11 cm)
        (c) Prominence of coccyx

C. Psychosocial responses

1. Concerns
2. Meaning of examination for client

Nursing Diagnoses

A. Knowledge deficit related to normal anatomy and physiology of the female reproductive system

B. Alteration in functioning related to deviation from normal anatomical or physiological status of the female reproductive system

Interventions/Evaluations

A. Knowledge deficit related to normal anatomy and physiology of the female reproductive system

1. Interventions
   a. Assess current level of understanding
   b. Identify inaccuracies or gaps in knowledge
   c. Identify the woman's interest in increasing her knowledge
   d. Formulate a teaching plan
   e. Evaluate the effectiveness of the implemented plan
2. Evaluations
   a. The woman will be able to explain anatomical and/or physiological functioning in the areas in which previous inaccuracies or gaps were identified
   b. The woman will state that her learning needs were met

B. Alteration in functioning related to deviation from normal anatomical or physiological status of the female reproductive system

1. Interventions
   a. Identify the specific alteration in functioning
   b. Identify the management plan
   c. Assess the woman's level of understanding of both the problem and plan of management
   d. Add to the management plan
   e. Formulate a teaching plan to increase understanding
   f. Implement the teaching plan
   g. Evaluate the effectiveness of the implemented plan
   h. Communicate the effectiveness to other members of the health care team
2. Evaluations
   a. The woman will repeat an accurate description of the specific problem of alteration in functioning
   b. The woman will describe the proposed management plan accurately
   c. The woman will state that her learning needs were met

Health Education

A teaching plan for reproductive anatomy and physiology follows.

A. Identify the purpose of the instruction

B. Identify the characteristics of the learners
1. Assess the current level of understanding
2. Identify the learning needs
3. Identify the level of comfort with the subject matter
4. Identify the level of comfort of members of the group with each other

C. Choose an instructional method appropriate to the learning needs and comfort level of the participants

D. Develop a teaching plan

E. Implement the teaching plan

F. Evaluate the effectiveness of the teaching plan in terms of meeting the learning needs of the participants

G. Alter the teaching plan

H. Implement the alterations

I. Re-evaluate the teaching plan

CASE STUDY AND STUDY QUESTIONS

An 18-year-old girl has decided to see a health care provider to find out "why I'm so slow in developing." Her last physical examination was 5 years ago; she reports no serious illnesses and no operations. Her chief complaints are lack of breast development and delayed onset of menstruation. She is 156 cm (5 ft, 1 in) tall and weighs 48 kg (105 lb). She states that she has never had a menstrual period, does not have to shave her underarms and legs, and has never had acne. Pertinent physical findings include an absence of secondary sex characteristics, including a lack of breast development and of axillary hair and pubic hair. A vaginal examination was attempted but not completed because of an imperforate hymen. The primary diagnosis is delayed puberty.

1. Further assessment and intervention for this client
   a. Should be delayed, because there is a wide variation in the onset of menses and breast development among young girls.
   b. Are necessary because the development of secondary sex characteristics and the onset of menstruation normally occur by the age of 16 years.
   c. Are not essential because breast development normally precedes menstruation by several years.
   d. Should focus on treatment of her imperforate hymen.

2. Further studies reveal a chromosomal karyotype of XX, the presence of a very small uterus, and streak ovaries. Exogenous sources of estrogen and progesterone are recommended for this young woman to trigger the onset of puberty. She will need to take these hormones
   a. Only until her own ovaries are stimulated to begin producing hormones.
   b. Only until she decides to become pregnant.
   c. Until well past the normal time for menopause because streak ovaries are nonfunctioning and will never produce the necessary hormones.
   d. She will not need to take these hormones because her ovaries will begin functioning soon.

3. The imperforate hymen
   a. Must be treated because menstrual flow started by the use of hormone therapy can be trapped and prevented from exiting the vagina.
   b. Should be treated when she decides to become sexually active.
   c. Should be treated when she decides to become pregnant.
   d. Does not require treatment because it will be broken when she has sexual intercourse.

4. This girl wants to know about her childbearing capabilities. She will
   a. Be able to have as many children as she wishes as long as she takes the necessary hormones.
   b. Need to use birth control to prevent unwanted pregnancies.
   c. Not be able to become pregnant without donor eggs because streak ovaries are non-functioning and do not contain ova.
   d. Not be able to become pregnant because of her imperforate hymen.

ADDITIONAL STUDY QUESTIONS

5. All of the following are components of the external female genitalia except the
   a. Vulva
   b. Vestibule
   c. Fourchette
   d. Vagina

6. In the male, sperm production and the manufacture of the hormone testosterone are functions of the
   a. Seminiferous tubules
   b. Epididymides
   c. Corpora cavernosa
   d. Testes

7. The middle layer of the uterine myometrium is composed of smooth muscle fibers in figure-eight patterns around major blood vessels. This is called a living ligature because
   a. Contraction of these fibers after childbirth or an abortion helps prevent massive blood loss.
   b. These fibers provide support for the major blood vessels that innervate the uterus.

c. These fibers contract before the placenta detaches from the uterine wall, thus preventing blood loss from the umbilical cord.

d. This configuration of smooth muscle fibers provides the optimal amount of force necessary to expel the fetus.

8. Which of the following statements is untrue for the ovaries?
   a. Normally are the size of large almonds in women during the reproductive years.
   b. Are comparable to the testes in the male.
   c. On examination, should be fixed and nonmobile.
   d. Are responsible for the production of estrogen, progesterone, and the androgens.

9. Which of the following uterine positions is considered abnormal?
   a. Anteflexed
   b. Anterior
   c. Posterior
   d. Retroflexed
   e. None of the above

10. Blocked oviducts are a major cause of infertility. They are most often the result of
   a. Pelvic inflammatory disease
   b. Congenital abnormality
   c. Exposure to diethylstilbestrol (or DES)
   d. Cone biopsy

Answers to Study Questions

1. b	2. c	3. a
4. c	5. d	6. d
7. a	8. c	9. e
10. a		

REFERENCES

Anthony, C., & Thibodeau, G. (1983). *Textbook of anatomy and physiology* (11th ed.). St. Louis: Mosby.

Bates, B. (1987). *A guide to physical examination and history taking* (4th ed.). Philadelphia: Lippincott.

Bobak, I., Jensen, M., & Zalar, M. (1989). *Maternity and gynecologic care: The nurse and the family* (4th ed.). St. Louis: Mosby.

Cunningham, F.G., MacDonald, P.C., & Gant, N.F. (1989). *Williams obstetrics* (18th ed.). Norwalk, CT: Appleton & Lange.

Griffith-Kenney, J. (1986). *Contemporary women's health: A nursing advocacy approach*. Menlo Park, CA: Addison-Wesley.

uckmann, J., & Sorensen, K. (1987). *Medical-surgical nursing: A psychophysiologic approach* (3rd ed.). Philadelphia: Saunders.

Willson, J., Carrington, R., & Ledger, W. (1988). *Obstetrics and gynecology* (8th ed.). St. Louis: Mosby.

Kathryn V. Deitch

Endocrinology and Pregnancy

Objectives

1. Identify the paramaters of normal length, duration, flow, and age at the onset and cessation of menstruation

2. Describe the physiological changes in the ovaries, uterus, and cervix that occur during the menstrual cycle

3. Describe the hypothalamic–pituitary–ovarian axis and its effect on the normal menstrual cycle

4. Describe the effect of conception on the menstrual cycle

5. Identify the endocrine changes during pregnancy and the postpartum period

6. Identify the common deviations from normal parameters in the menstrual cycle

7. Identify the common reproductive endocrine problems that affect pregnancy

Introduction

A. Menstruation

1. Menarche, the onset of the first menstrual period, normally occurs between the ages of 9 and 16 years, with a mean age of 12.8 years in the United States
2. Cycles in the first years tend to be irregular and are accompanied by irregular ovulation
3. Cycle length ranges normally from 21 to 36 days; 95% of women have a cycle of between 25 and 32 days
4. Cycles are timed from the first day of menstrual bleeding: the first day of bleeding is marked as day 1 of the cycle
5. Duration of bleeding ranges from 1 to 8 days; most women report a menstrual flow that lasts from 3 to 5 days
6. Amount of blood lost averages 30 ml (1 oz) per menstrual period; a normal range is between 20 and 80 ml (⅔ and 2 ⅔ oz)
7. Cessation of menses, or menopause, occurs normally between the ages of 35 and 60 years, with an average age of 51 years, in the United States
8. Cycle is divided into two phases
   a. Follicular phase

(1) Starts with day 1 of menses

(2) Multiple follicles are maturing in the ovary; the term primary is given to the follicle selected for maturation during this cycle

(3) Maturing follicle is called graafian follicle

(4) Estrogen is produced

(5) Follicular phase ends with the release of the egg from the mature follicle (ovulation)

(6) Normal variation in length of this phase is 7 to 22 days (e.g., it would be 14 days in a 28-day cycle)

(7) Endometrium is in the proliferative phase and thickens during this period of rapid growth

(8) At the end of this phase, the external cervical os opens to admit sperm; the cervix becomes softer

(9) Cervix produces mucus that is thin, clear, slippery, stretchy, copious in quantity, and designed to aid sperm in passage through the cervix; the stretching property is called spinnbarkeit

(10) Ovulation usually occurs within 24 hours before, during, or after the last day of this slippery, copious discharge

b. Luteal phase

(1) Starts with ovulation

(2) Remaining follicle is now called the corpus luteum

(3) Corpus luteum produces both estrogen and progesterone

(4) Lasts 14 days if conception does not occur

(5) Endometrium is in the secretory phase, is increasingly vascular, and is filled with glandular secretions, ready to support the fertilized ovum

(6) If no conception occurs, the corpus luteum deteriorates and levels of estrogen and progesterone decrease

(7) Menstruation begins, signaling the start of a new cycle

9. Common deviations from the normal in the menstrual cycle

a. Amenorrhea

(1) Is defined as an absence of menstrual periods

(2) Pregnancy is a common cause

(3) Delay in the onset of menstruation, or the cessation of menses

(a) Is common in women who are competitive athletes, have eating disorders such as anorexia nervosa, or participate in activities in which extreme thinness is valued, such as ballet and gymnastics

(b) Menarche usually requires a minimum height of 152.4 cm (5 ft) and a minimum weight of 47.5 kg (105 lb), with a fat-to-lean ratio of 1 : 3; women with body fat levels below 16% seldom menstruate

(c) May lead to the development of osteoporosis if estrogen levels are consistently low

b. Anovulatory cycles

(1) Are common in both the early years of menstruation and the late years close to menopause

(2) A graafian follicle matures and estrogen is produced, but ovulation does not occur

(a) Progesterone is not available

(b) Uterine lining thickens in response to estrogen

(c) Progesterone-induced signal to start and stop the menstrual flow is absent

(3) May result in light, irregular menses and difficulty in conceiving

(4) May result in frequent, prolonged, heavy menstrual flow that is debilitating and causes anemia if uterine lining build-up is excessive

c. Inadequate or short luteal phase

(1) Corpus luteum stops producing hormones prematurely or produces inadequate levels of estrogen and, especially, of progesterone

(2) Can lead to infertility

    (3) Can cause early pregnancy losses when progesterone levels are too low to support the pregnancy until the placental formation is complete

    (4) Is diagnosed by analysis of serum progesterone levels and treated with progesterone

B. The hypothalamic–pituitary–ovarian axis

1. Is responsible for the control of the hormones that affect reproduction
2. Sphenoidal sinus in the brain houses the pituitary gland and the hypothalamus is located directly above the pituitary gland
3. Pituitary gland is divided into two parts: the anterior and the posterior; control of the two halves is totally different
4. Hypothalamus releases hormones (called releasing factors) into the hypophysial portal system that supplies the anterior pituitary; these hormones provide instructions to the anterior pituitary
5. Releasing factors signal the anterior pituitary to produce hormones, which stimulate certain target organs to produce hormones
6. Releasing factors are produced by the hypothalamus in response to the decreasing levels of hormones being produced by the target organs; when the levels of hormones from the target organs increase, the hypothalamus responds by decreasing the releasing factors hormones sent to the anterior pituitary
7. This type of system is called a feedback loop; when rising levels of target organ hormones result in a decrease in the releasing factor and stimulating hormones, the system is called a negative feedback loop
8. Target organs include the ovaries, the thyroid, and the adrenal cortex
9. Feedback loop functioning for the ovary
    a. During menstruation, a message is sent through the central nervous system to the hypothalamus that circulating levels of estrogen are low
    b. Hypothalamus responds by sending gonadotropin-releasing hormone to the anterior pituitary
    c. Anterior pituitary responds by sending first follicle-stimulating hormone (FSH) and then luteinizing hormone (LH) to the ovary
    d. Ovary responds to FSH by selecting a follicle for maturation and choosing from among several follicles that are undergoing early development and producing estrogen; the chosen follicle that begins to mature is called the graafian follicle
    e. LH stimulates the graafian follicle to release the egg and ovulation occurs; the graafian follicle becomes a corpus luteum, which produces both estrogen and progesterone
    f. There are now high circulating levels of both estrogen and progesterone
        (1) If conception does not occur, circulating levels of both estrogen and progesterone gradually decrease as the corpus luteum disintegrates
        (2) When estrogen levels are again low, menstruation begins, another message is sent to the hypothalamus, and the cycle begins again

C. Conception and the menstrual cycle

1. If conception occurs
    a. Circulating levels of both estrogen and progesterone continue to increase
    b. A message is sent to the hypothalamus that estrogen levels are high
    c. The hypothalamus stops sending gonadotropin-releasing hormone to the anterior pituitary
    d. The anterior pituitary stops sending FSH and LH to the ovary
    e. The ovary does not select another follicle for ripening
    f. Menstrual periods stop
    g. High levels of circulating estrogen and progesterone for the duration of pregnancy prevent the resumption of the menstrual cycle

D. The postpartum period and the menstrual cycle

1. After delivery, circulating levels of estrogen and progesterone decrease precipitously after the removal of the placenta; a message is sent through the central nervous system to the hypothalamus that circulating levels of estrogen are low, and the cycle begins again
2. Menstrual periods resume in nonlactating women within 4 to 6 weeks after delivery

E. Endocrine changes during pregnancy

1. Thyroid gland
   a. Slight enlargement occurs
   b. Changes occur in the levels of some thyroid hormones
   c. Oxygen consumption increases
   d. Basal metabolic rate increases
   e. Women with an existing thyroid disease, either hyperthyroidism or hypothyroidism, need periodic monitoring of thyroid functioning to evaluate the effectiveness of current medication
2. Parathyroid gland
   a. Parathyroid hormone production increases due to an increased requirement for calcium and vitamin D
   b. A state of hyperparathyroidism exists during pregnancy
   c. Increased demands are greatest in the last half of pregnancy, corresponding to the demands of the developing fetal skeleton for calcium and vitamin D
3. Pancreas
   a. In early pregnancy, maternal insulin production decreases because of the heavy fetal demand for maternal glucose; maternal glucose levels and insulin production decrease
   b. After the first trimester, there is an increased need for insulin production because of the insulin antagonist properties of the steadily increasing levels of estrogen, progesterone, and cortisol
      (1) Normal beta cells of the islets of Langerhans can easily meet this increased need for insulin
      (2) Insulin does not cross the placental barrier
   c. Women with diabetes mellitus need less insulin during the early stages of pregnancy and greatly increased insulin during the middle and late stages of pregnancy
      (1) Non–insulin-dependent diabetics may require insulin during pregnancy
      (2) Women with inadequate numbers of beta cells may develop diabetes during pregnancy
      (3) All pregnant women should be screened for diabetes at approximately 28 weeks' gestation; high-risk women should be screened in the early weeks of pregnancy and again at 28 weeks
4. Pituitary gland
   a. FSH and LH
      (1) Decrease markedly until after delivery and then increase to the early follicular phase during the third week after childbirth, which explains the 6-week delay in the resumption of menses after childbirth in the nonlactating mother
   b. Prolactin
      (1) Is produced by the anterior pituitary
      (2) Is responsible for milk production, which begins after delivery of the placenta; levels are high during pregnancy, but milk production does not occur because of the prolactin antagonist properties of estrogen
   c. Melanocyte-stimulating hormone
      (1) Is produced by the anterior pituitary
      (2) Is responsible for pigment changes such as darkening of the areola, chloasma, and linea nigra

   d. Oxytocin
      (1) Is produced by the posterior pituitary
      (2) Is suppressed by progesterone until late in pregnancy, when the levels of oxytocin surpass the levels of progesterone; this change in the oxytocin/progesterone ratio is believed to be one of the initiators of labor
      (3) Is responsible for uterine contractions
      (4) Is responsible for milk ejection during breastfeeding
      (5) Is responsible for the uterine contractions after delivery (called after pains)
         (a) Are stronger in multiparas
         (b) Occur during breastfeeding
         (c) Purpose is to speed the process of involution
5. Ovary and corpus luteum
   a. Are major sources of the hormones estrogen and progesterone until maturation of the placenta at about 12 weeks
   b. Relaxin
      (1) Promotes the softening of the cervix
      (2) Alters collagen to promote the softening of the articulation of the bones of the pelvis to allow for increased space for the developing fetus and contributes to maternal joint instability
6. Placental-fetal unit
   a. Human chorionic gonadotropin
      (1) Is the biochemical basis for pregnancy tests
      (2) Is produced by the developing placenta to help maintain the corpus luteum
      (3) Inhibits maternal foreign body response to the fetal side of the placenta
      (4) May contribute to hyperemesis gravidarum
      (5) Level climbs rapidly after conception, peaks at about 8 weeks (120 to 130 IU/ml) and decreases to extremely low levels after 16 weeks (20 to 30 IU/ml)
         (a) Low levels or levels that do not rise rapidly during early pregnancy indicate the threat of abortion
         (b) Higher levels are found in multiple pregnancies and in gestational trophoblastic disease
         (c) Pregnancy tests performed after 16 weeks' gestation may be negative
   b. Estrogen
      (1) As the placenta develops, it gradually takes over production from the corpus luteum; the transfer of production is complete after about 12 weeks
      (2) Levels rise steadily throughout pregnancy, eventually increasing to 30 times that of prepregnant levels
      (3) Growth hormone properties
         (a) Uterine enlargement
         (b) Breast enlargement
         (c) Fat deposition
      (4) Promotes sodium and water retention by the kidneys
      (5) Increases the coagulability of blood to decrease the risk of hemorrhage; increases the risk of thrombosis
      (6) Increases available body proteins to maintain a positive nitrogen balance and ensure adequate protein for fetal growth
      (7) Interferes with folic acid metabolism
   c. Progesterone
      (1) Is produced by the corpus luteum; production is taken over by the placenta after about 12 weeks; levels rise steadily throughout pregnancy; production reaches a maximum of 250 mg/day during late pregnancy
      (2) Promotes the relaxation of smooth muscles
         (a) Inhibits uterine contractions, protects the pregnancy
         (b) Reduces gastrointestinal peristalsis

              (i) Promotes constipation and bloating
              (ii) Promotes heartburn
           (c) Promotes vascular dilation and stasis in lower limbs, with formation of edema and varicosities
           (d) Decreases motility in the gallbladder and increases the incidence of gallbladder disease
        (3) Raises body temperature by 0.5°C (0.9°F)
        (4) Promotes fat deposition
        (5) Promotes secretory development in the breasts and the endometrium
    d. Human placental lactogen
        (1) Is produced by the placenta; levels rise steadily throughout pregnancy
        (2) Is similar in effect to the pituitary growth hormone
        (3) Glucose metabolism
           (a) Increases the amount of glucose available for fetal use by increasing the maternal use of fatty acids for energy
           (b) Causes blood glucose levels to rise by increasing tissue resistance to insulin (inhibiting glyconeogenesis)
              (i) May cause problems if the maternal pancreas is unable to increase the supply of insulin as required
              (ii) May cause diabetes mellitus or increase the insulin needs of pregnant diabetics
        (4) Protein metabolism
           (a) Decreases the utilization of protein for energy
           (b) Increases the synthesis of protein, creating a source of amino acids for transport to the fetus
           (c) Results in increased levels of protein available for fetal growth
        (5) Aids in breast preparation for lactation

Clinical Practice

A. Assessment

1. Menstrual history
    a. Age at menarche
    b. Date of the last menstrual period and determination of whether or not the last menstrual period was a normal one for the client
        (1) Note the usual cycle length and the cycle length for this period
        (2) Note the usual duration of bleeding and the duration of bleeding for this cycle
        (3) Note the usual amount of bleeding and the amount of bleeding this cycle
    c. Length of cycle
        (1) Is timed from the first day of menses of one cycle to the first day of menses of the next cycle
        (2) The first day of bleeding is marked as day 1
    d. Duration of menses
    e. Amount of bleeding
        (1) Number of days of heavy bleeding
        (2) Number of hours between pad or tampon changes on the heaviest days
    f. Cramps
        (1) Present or absent
        (2) Degree of interference with normal activities
    g. Clots
        (1) Present or absent
        (2) Number and size
    h. Presence of a change in the cycle
2. Gynecological history related to the menstrual cycle

     a. Moliminal symptoms

       (1) Are defined as cyclical symptoms associated with menses

       (2) Examples include premenstrual bloating, breast tenderness, and irritability

       (3) Presence is due to estrogen and progesterone

     b. Moliminal symptoms plus regular and normal menses imply a pattern of normal ovulation

3. Obstetrical history

     a. Previous fertility or infertility

     b. Previous spontaneous pregnancy losses during the first trimester

     c. Previous gestational diabetes

4. Medical history, including previous or current endocrine disorders

     a. Hypothyroidism or hyperthyroidism

     b. Diabetes mellitus

     c. Parathyroidism

     d. Adrenal disorders

5. Sociocultural history

     a. Attitudes and values toward menstruation

     b. Common cultural attitudes include menstruation as illness, as a state of uncleanliness, a time of decreased competence, and as causing fear of contamination

       (1) Some Native American cultures isolate the menstruating woman

       (2) Orthodox Judaism requires a ritual bath after menstruation

       (3) In post-World War II Japan, a policy of menstrual leave for "incapacitated" women was enacted

       (4) In the United States and Great Britain, criminal court cases have been tried with defenses of diminished capacity from premenstrual syndrome pleaded for women accused of acts of violence

6. Physical examination

     a. General survey

     b. Pelvic examination

7. Diagnostic procedures

     a. Menstrual calendar

     b. Blood chemistry

       (1) Complete blood count

         (a) Anemia may result from excessive menstrual blood loss

         (b) Anemia is the diagnosis when hemoglobin levels are below 12 g/dl and hematocrit levels are below 37%

       (2) FSH and LH levels

         (a) Are elevated when ovaries are not functioning normally with cyclical ovulation

         (b) FSH levels higher than 40 mIU/ml and LH levels higher than 25 mIU/ml are diagnostic for anovulation

         (c) Normal levels of FSH are 5 to 30 mIU/ml and normal LH levels are 5 to 20 mIU/ml in women

       (3) Prolactin

         (a) Elevated levels block the action of estrogen

         (b) Normal levels are 0 to 23 mg/dl

       (4) Thyroid function tests

         (a) Identify hyperthyroidism and hypothyroidism

         (b) Normal nonpregnant values are

           (i) Serum thyroxine (T_4), 5 to 12 μg/dl

           (ii) Serum triiodothyronine (T_3), 80 to 200 mg/dl

           (iii) Thyroid-stimulating hormone (TSH), 2 to 5.4 mIU/ml

       (5) Serum estradiol

         (a) Provides an indication of ovarian function

         (b) Is highest at midcycle and again at days 21 to 23

(c) Levels fluctuate greatly from day to day

(d) FSH levels are better indicators of hormone production by the ovaries

(6) Progesterone

(a) Level is tested on menstrual days 21 to 23 (28-day cycle)

(b) Provides evidence of ovulation

(c) Low levels after conception may lead to a spontaneous abortion

(7) Testosterone and dehydroisoandrosterone sulfate (DHEAS)

(a) Androgens are produced by the normal ovary

(b) High levels usually are associated with anovulation

c. Endometrial biopsy

(1) Evaluates the influences of hormones on the uterine lining

(2) Is performed on days 21 to 23 of a 28-day cycle

(3) Estrogen and progesterone, which are present after ovulation, produce the characteristic changes in the microscopic lining of the uterus

B. Nursing Diagnoses

1. High risk for carbohydrate intolerance related to a change in insulin requirements during pregnancy
2. Knowledge deficit related to self-care requirements during early pregnancy with a history of repeated, spontaneous early abortions secondary to the luteal phase defect
3. Knowledge deficit related to difficulty in conceiving and the presence of irregular, infrequent menses
4. Knowledge deficit related to a lack of understanding of the physical changes that occur during the normal menstrual cycle

C. Interventions/Evaluations

1. High risk for carbohydrate intolerance related to a change in insulin requirements during normal pregnancy

a. Interventions

(1) Identify pregnant women who have a family history of diabetes mellitus, both insulin-dependent and adult-onset

(2) Identify women with a personal history of diabetes mellitus, both insulin-dependent and adult-onset as well as gestational

(3) Identify women at high risk for developing gestational diabetes

(4) Screen high-risk women early in pregnancy and again at 28 weeks' gestation

(5) Screen low-risk women at 28 weeks' gestation

(6) Instruct women in the proper preparation required for the screening test

(7) Provide dietary counseling, particularly for high-risk women, to decrease the consumption of simple carbohydrates and to increase the consumption of complex carbohydrates to prevent an increased strain on the pancreas

(8) Teach the signs, symptoms, and management of hypoglycemia, which is common during the first trimester of pregnancy because of the fetus's need for maternal glucose

b. Evaluations

(1) Women with a family history of diabetes mellitus will be identified during the first trimester

(2) Women with a history of gestational diabetes will be identified during the first trimester

(3) Women with a history of diabetes mellitus will be identified during the first trimester

(4) High-risk women will be screened during the first trimester

(5) All women will be screened at 25 to 26 weeks' gestation

    (6) Women will be instructed in the proper preparation for the screening test

    (7) Women will explain why it is necessary to avoid simple carbohydrates during pregnancy

    (8) Women will give examples of both simple and complex carbohydrates

    (9) Women will be able to identify symptoms of hypoglycemia during early pregnancy and will explain their personal management plan for these symptoms

2. Knowledge deficit related to self-care requirements during early pregnancy with history of repeated, spontaneous early abortions secondary to luteal phase defect

  a. Interventions

    (1) Explain the importance of keeping a complete menstrual calendar so that conception can be dated precisely

    (2) Explain the importance of immediate pregnancy testing as soon as pregnancy is suspected

    (3) Explain the need to obtain serial serum progesterone levels early to evaluate the adequacy of the corpus luteum during pregnancy

    (4) Evaluate understanding of the proper use of supplemental progesterone therapy to support the corpus luteum until maturation of the placenta

  b. Evaluations

    (1) The woman will keep a menstrual calendar, including a record of moliminal symptoms and of intercourse

    (2) The woman will obtain a pregnancy test as soon as pregnancy is suspected

    (3) The woman will participate in testing for serum progesterone levels

    (4) The woman will explain the proper use of supplemental progesterone

3. Knowledge deficit related to difficulty in conceiving and the presence of irregular, infrequent menses

  a. Interventions

    (1) Identify the woman's level of understanding of her own menstrual calendar

    (2) Assess the current level of knowledge of the menstrual cycle

    (3) Provide necessary instruction about the menstrual cycle

    (4) Explain the moliminal symptoms and their importance

    (5) Describe the type of menstrual cycle necessary to conceive

    (6) Explain the link between irregular, infrequent periods and irregular, infrequent ovulation

  b. Evaluations

    (1) The woman will explain her own menstrual calendar

    (2) The woman will describe the type of menstrual cycle that is compatible with conception

    (3) The woman will identify any moliminal symptoms that she experiences

    (4) The woman will explain that irregular, infrequent menstrual periods without moliminal symptoms occur because of infrequent ovulation; because ovulation must occur in order for conception to be possible, this type of menstrual cycle is associated with difficulty in conceiving

4. Knowledge deficit related to a lack of understanding of the physical changes that occur during the normal menstrual cycle

  a. Interventions

    (1) Assess the current level of knowledge of the cyclical physical changes that occur because of the menstrual cycle

    (2) Provide necessary instruction for learning gaps that have been identified

    (3) Reassess the level of knowledge of physical changes attributed to the menstrual cycle after instruction

  b. Evaluations

(1) The woman will describe the timing of the physical changes that commonly occur during her own menstrual cycle
(2) The woman will identify whether or not those changes are within the normal range
(3) The woman will identify potential changes in her menstrual cycle that require medical attention

Health Education

Health education about the menstrual cycle and the normal variations in endocrine functioning that occur during pregnancy should be based on an assessment of the current level of knowledge of the woman as well as on her level of interest in the subject. The teaching plan should use the particular concerns of the woman or the particular details of her diagnosis to help her understand both her own situation and the parameters of normal functioning.

CASE STUDIES AND STUDY QUESTIONS

Alice, 25 years old and married, wants to use the techniques of natural family planning to help her to conceive. She had her first menstrual period at the age of 12 years. Her periods are regular, occur every 28 days, and last 4 to 5 days. She has no trouble with cramping or excessive flow. She has noticed breast tenderness, feelings of heaviness and bloating, and irritability in the few days before each period. She also notices an increase in her vaginal discharge in the middle of her cycle; the discharge is thin, slippery, stretchy, and clear.

1. Alice is probably experiencing
   a. Regular ovulation because her periods are regular and she is experiencing normal moliminal symptoms.
   b. A vaginal infection because of the repetitive discharge.
   c. Anovulatory cycles because she is not having trouble with cramps or clots.
   d. Some anovulatory cycles because her cycle length varies by a few days and is not always consistent.

2. The breast tenderness, bloating, and irritability are due to
   a. The effects of falling levels of estrogen during this phase of the cycle.
   b. The effects of progesterone produced by the corpus luteum after ovulation occurs.
   c. The effects of rising levels of testosterone during this phase of the cycle.
   d. These symptoms have no relationship to the levels of hormones in the body.

3. Clear, slippery cervical mucus that occurs at midcycle has a quality of stretchiness called spinnbarkeit. This quality is associated with cervical changes including
   a. The opening of the cervical os to aid the sperm in moving into the uterus.
   b. The closing of the cervical os to become more hostile to sperm.
   c. The shortening of the cervix to prepare for cervical dilation in labor.
   d. A maturation of the cervix that occurs after puberty.

Barbara, a 35-year-old woman pregnant with her third child, is beginning prenatal care after she missed her second period. Her last child weighed 4.5 kg (10 lb) but was delivered vaginally without difficulty. She is 160 cm (5 ft 3 in) tall and weighs 74.8 kg (165 lb). She tells you that her mother has adult-onset diabetes and that her sister had gestational diabetes during her last pregnancy. It has been recommended to Barbara that she be screened for diabetes now as well as later in her pregnancy. Barbara states that she does not understand why she could develop diabetes during pregnancy.

4. You explain to Barbara that
   a. Her body will be required to produce greatly increased amounts of insulin throughout pregnancy to support the developing fetus, and her pancreas might not be able to keep up with the demands.
   b. Diabetes develops during pregnancy in women who eat too much sugar and can be prevented by controlling sugar intake.
   c. After the first trimester, there is an increased need for maternal insulin because the fetus does not produce enough insulin and replaces fetal insulin stores from the maternal circulation.

d. After the first trimester, there is a need for increased levels of insulin in the mother. Because Barbara has a strong family history of diabetes, her beta cells in the pancreatic islets may not be able to meet this increased demand for insulin.

5. Insulin needs increase during pregnancy because
   a. Estrogen, progesterone, and cortisol levels steadily increase and these hormones are all insulin antagonists.
   b. Human placental lactogen, produced by the placenta, increases blood glucose levels by inhibiting glyconeogenesis.
   c. Basal metabolic rate increases, thus increasing the need for glucose for metabolism.
   d. All of the above.

ADDITIONAL STUDY QUESTIONS

6. Which of the following describes a menstrual cycle that is within the normal parameters?
   a. Age at menarche: 11 years; cycle length: 42 days; duration of menses: 3 days; blood loss: light.
   b. Age at menarche: 8 years; cycle length: 28 days; duration of menses: 4 days; blood loss: heavy.
   c. Age at menarche: 12 years; cycle length: 26 to 28 days; duration of menses: 5 days; blood loss: moderate.
   d. Age at menarche: 12 years; cycle length: 14 days; duration of menses: 8 days; blood loss: heavy.

7. During the menstrual cycle, the hormone progesterone is produced
   a. Throughout the cycle.
   b. From days 1 to 14 by the graafian follicle.
   c. From days 14 to 28 by the graafian follicle.
   d. Beginning just after ovulation by the corpus luteum.

8. Menstrual periods do not occur during pregnancy because
   a. High levels of circulating estrogen signal the hypothalamus to stop producing the releasing hormones; therefore, the anterior pituitary stops producing ovarian-stimulating hormones.
   b. High levels of circulating estrogen signal the hypothalamus to begin producing the releasing hormones; therefore, the anterior pituitary stops producing ovarian-stimulating hormones.
   c. High levels of circulating estrogen directly signal the ovary that no further ovulation is needed.
   d. Ovarian-stimulating hormones continue to be produced by the anterior pituitary, but high levels of estrogen block the action of the stimulating hormones on the ovary.

9. The smooth muscle relaxation effects of progesterone are responsible for all of the following during pregnancy except
   a. Cramping in the calf muscles of the legs.
   b. Heartburn.
   c. Constipation.
   d. Urinary retention.

10. Susie, age 15 years, goes to a clinic for a pregnancy test. She states that she wants an abortion if she is pregnant. She has regular sexual intercourse without using contraception, and she is unsure how long it has been since her last period. A urine pregnancy test is negative. Relieved, Susie decides to leave without an examination because she is not pregnant. You recommend to Susie that she
    a. Return in a few weeks for an examination since she needs advice on contraception if she does not want a pregnancy.
    b. Go ahead and leave because her main concern was whether or not she was pregnant, and she now knows that she is not.
    c. Stay for an examination since she does not know the date of her last menstrual period and pregnancy tests revert to negative after 16 weeks' gestation because of the decrease in levels of human chorionic gonadotropin.
    d. Obtain a blood pregnancy test because urine tests are not reliable.

Answers to Study Questions

1. a	2. b	3. a
4. d	5. d	6. c
7. d	8. a	9. a
10. c		

REFERENCES

Anthony, C., & Thibodeau, G. (1983). *Textbook of anatomy and physiology* (11th ed.). St. Louis: Mosby.

Bobak, I., Jensen, M., & Zalar, M. (1989). *Maternity and gynecologic care: The nurse and the family* (4th ed.). St. Louis: Mosby.

Cunningham, F.G., MacDonald, P.C., & Gant, N.F. (1989). *Williams obstetrics* (18th ed.). Norwalk, CT: Appleton & Lange.

Droegemueller, W., Herbst, A., Mishell, D., & Stenchever, M. (1987). *Comprehensive gynecology*. St. Louis: Mosby.

Griffith-Kenney, J. (Ed.). (1986). *Contemporary women's health: A nursing advocacy approach*. Menlo Park, CA: Addison-Wesley.

Speroff, L., Glass, R., & Kase, N. (1989). *Clinical gynecologic endocrinology and infertility*. Baltimore: Williams & Wilkins.

Willson, J., Carrington, E., & Ledger, W. (1988). *Obstetrics and gynecology* (8th ed.). St. Louis: Mosby.

FETAL GROWTH AND DEVELOPMENT

Bonnie Kellogg

Genetics

Objectives

1. Define the terms commonly used in genetic diseases

2. Describe the implications of an increased amount of chromosome material, of a deletion, and translocation process in chromosomal disorders

3. Explain the basic mendelian modes of inheritance

4. Identify client situations that indicate the need for a chromosomal analysis

5. Assess the emotional impact on couples of the birth of a baby with a genetic disorder

Introduction

A. **Definition: genetics is a medical science concerned with the transmission of characteristics from parent to child**

B. **Foundation of inheritance**

1. Cell division: all beings begin life as a single cell (zygote). The single cell continues to reproduce itself by the process of either mitosis or of meiosis
   a. Mitosis is the process of cell division in which new cells are made. The new cells have the same number and pattern of chromosomes as the parent cell (46 chromosomes comprising 44 autosomes and 2 sex chromosomes); mitosis occurs in five stages: interphase, prophase, metaphase, anaphase, and telophase (Fig. 3–1)
      (1) Interphase: before cell division, the deoxyribonucleic acid (DNA) replicates itself so that the genes will double
      (2) Prophase: the strands of chromatin shorten and thicken; the chromosomes reproduce; spindles appear and the centrioles migrate to the opposite poles of the cell; the membrane separating the nucleus from the cytoplasm disappears
      (3) Metaphase: the chromosomes line up along the poles of the spindle
      (4) Anaphase: the two chromatids in each chromosome separate and move to the opposite ends of the spindle
      (5) Telophase: a nuclear membrane forms, the spindles disappear, and the centrioles relocate to the outside of the new nucleus; toward the end of this phase, the cells divide into two new cells, each with its own nucleus and each having the same number of chromosomes as the parent cell

Interphase (1)

Prophase

Metaphase

Anaphase

Telophase

Interphase (2)

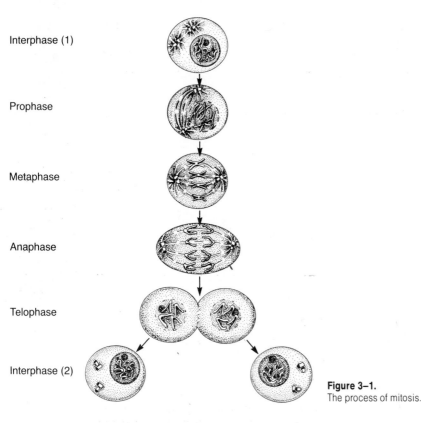

Figure 3–1.
The process of mitosis.

   b. Meiosis is a process of cell division that occurs in the maturation process of the sperm and ova and is known as gametogenesis; this process decreases the number of chromosomes by one-half (from 46 to 23 per cell) and occurs in two successive cell divisions (Fig. 3–2)
      (1) The first division consists of four phases
         (a) Prophase: the chromosomes move close together
            (i) A crossover of genetic material can take place at this time
            (ii) The crossover accounts for the wide variation of features seen within same-parent siblings
         (b) Metaphase: spindle fibers attach to separate chromosomes
         (c) Anaphase: intact chromosome pairs migrate to opposite ends of the cell (the distribution of maternal and paternal chromosomes is random)
         (d) Telophase: the cell divides into two cells, each with one-half (23) of the usual number of chromosomes (22 autosomes and 1 sex chromosome)
      (2) Second division
         (a) The chromatids of each chromosome separate and move to the opposite poles of each of the daughter cells
         (b) This is followed by each of the cells dividing into two cells, which results in four cells (spermatogenesis and oogenesis)
            (i) Spermatogenesis is continuous from puberty to senescence
            (ii) Oogenesis is noncontinuous
               • Begins in utero, and by the fifth intrauterine month a full complement of primary oocytes has been produced
               • Primary oocytes are dormant until puberty, at which time one or two will complete the meiotic cycle each month during a woman's reproductive years

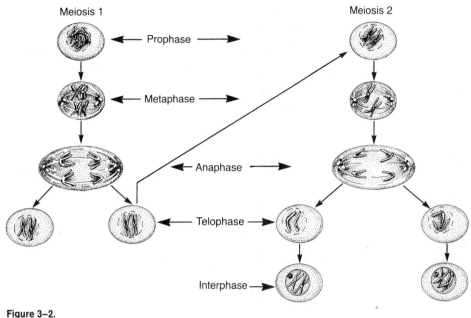

Meiosis 1

Meiosis 2

←— Prophase —→

←— Metaphase —→

←— Anaphase —→

←— Telophase —→

Interphase —→

Figure 3–2.
The process of meiosis.

(c) During the meiotic division, two of the chromatids may not move apart when the cell divides; this lack of separation is referred to as autosomal nondisjunction; this is also the stage at which breakage can occur, resulting in abnormalities of chromosomal structure such as that producing cri du chat syndrome

2. Genetic information is present on the chromosomes
   a. Chromosomes are composed of DNA, a complex protein that carries the genetic information
   b. DNA is a macromolecule made up of
      (1) Five-carbon sugars
      (2) A phosphate group
      (3) A nitrogen base of purine and pyrimidines
   c. DNA occurs as a double-stranded helix found in the cell nucleus
      (1) Two long strands of DNA molecules are wound around each other
      (2) The strands are linked by chemical bonds
      (3) The strands are complementary
      (4) The chains are made up of four nitrogen base subunits
         (a) Adenine
         (b) Guanine
         (c) Thymine
         (d) Cytosine
   d. Genes are the smallest known unit of heredity
      (1) Genes are present on the chromosomes
      (2) Each gene codes for a particular cellular function
      (3) Genes occur in pairs derived from the mother and father during reproduction
      (4) Each gene has a specific location on the chromosomes
      (5) Genetic errors can occur when there are changes in the gene's location or in the gene's products

3. Chromosomes form a genetic blueprint that is made up of tightly coiled structures
   a. Are threadlike structures, within the nucleus of the cell, that carry the genes

b. Humans have 46 chromosomes in each body cell (22 pairs of autosomes and 1 pair of sex chromosomes [diploid])
c. The sex cells contain 23 chromosomes (haploid)
d. Abnormalities of chromosome number are as follows
  (1) Paired chromosomes fail to separate during cell division (nondisjunction)
  (2) If nondisjunction occurs during meiosis (before fertilization), the fetus usually will have abnormal chromosomes in every cell (trisomy or monosomy)
    (a) Trisomy is a product of the union between a normal gamete (egg or sperm) and a gamete that contains an extra chromosome
      (i) The individual will have 47 chromosomes; one "pair" will have three chromosomes instead of two
      (ii) Examples of trisomies are Down's syndrome (47, XY + 21 [the extra chromosome is in the 21st pair]); trisomy 18 (47, XX + 18); and trisomy 13 (47, XY + 13).
    (b) Monosomy is the product of a union between a normal gamete and a gamete with a missing chromosome
      (i) The individual will have 45 chromosomes instead of 46
      (ii) Monosomy of an entire autosome is incompatible with life
      (iii) Complete monosomy of a sex chromosome is compatible with life; an example is a female with only one X chromosome (45, XO), that is, Turner's syndrome
  (3) If nondisjunction occurs after fertilization, the fetus may have two or more chromosomes that evolve into more than one cell line (mosaicism), each with a different number of chromosomes
    (a) Different body tissues may have different chromosome numbers or a mixture of cells, depending on when the nondisjunction occurred
    (b) Clinical signs and symptoms may vary in mosaicism; they may be severe or not apparent, depending on the number and location of the abnormal cell line
e. Abnormalities in chromosome structure are as follows
  (1) There are abnormalities of the chromosomes that involve only a part of the chromosome
  (2) Chromosomes have a primary constriction called the centromere (Fig. 3–3)

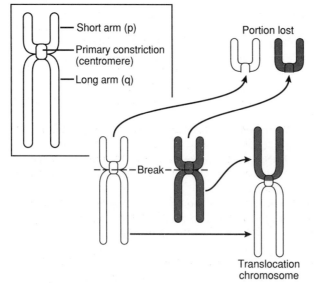

Short arm (p)

Primary constriction (centromere)

Long arm (q)

Portion lost

Break

Translocation chromosome

Figure 3–3
The process of translocation. Detail shows chromosomal representation. (Adapted from Genetics Screening and Counseling Service, Texas Department of Mental Health and Mental Retardation.)

(a) The portion above the centromere is referred to by the letter p
(b) The portion below the centromere is referred to by the letter q
(3) Abnormalities can occur in one of two forms: by translocation and by deletions or additions
    (a) Translocation occurs when the individual has 45 chromosomes, with one of the chromosomes fused to another chromosome (usually number 21 fused to number 14) (see Fig. 3–3)
        (i) The person has the correct amount of chromosomal material (45, t(14q21q)), but it has been rearranged: this individual is known as a balanced translocation carrier
        (ii) When such an individual and a structurally normal mate have a child, there is a possibility that the offspring
           • Will receive the carrier parent's abnormal 21/14 chromosome and a normal 14 and 21 from the other parent; thus, the child will be a carrier
           • Will receive the abnormal chromosome, plus a normal 21 from the carrier parent; this will result in an extra amount of chromosomal material for the 21 pair (unbalanced translocation), and the child will have Down's syndrome (46, −14, +t(14q21q))
    (b) Additions and/or deletions: a portion of a chromosome may be added or lost, which will result in adverse effects on the infant
        (i) Deletions and additions result from a small breakage in the chromosomal structure during early cell division
        (ii) An example of the consequences of a deletion is the cri du chat syndrome, in which a small amount of chromosomal material is missing from the upper portion (short arm) of chromosome 5 (5p−)

C. Modes of inheritance

1. Many diseases are caused by an abnormality of a single gene or a pair of genes; in these cases, the chromosomes are grossly normal
2. Autosomal dominant inheritance: autosomal dominant disorders occur when an individual has a gene that produces an effect whenever it is present (homozygous or heterozygous); this gene overshadows the other gene of the pair
    a. Mode of transmission (Fig. 3–4)
    b. Characteristics
        (1) Affected individuals generally have an affected parent; the family tree (genogram) usually shows multiple generations of individuals with the condition
        (2) The affected individual has a one in two (50%) chance with each pregnancy of passing the abnormal gene on to his or her child
        (3) Males and females are equally affected
        (4) An unaffected individual cannot transmit the disorder to his or her children
        (5) A mutation (a normal gene that has been spontaneously altered) can result in a new case
        (6) Autosomal dominant disorders have great variation in the degree of characteristics that are seen within a family (e.g., in Marfan's syndrome, the parent may have only elongated extremities but the child may have a more involved condition, including dislocation of the lens of the eye and severe cardiovascular abnormalities)
3. Autosomal recessive inheritance: an individual has an autosomal recessive disorder if he or she has a gene that produces its effects only when there are two genes on the same chromosome pair (homozygous trait)
    a. A carrier state can occur
        (1) An individual who is heterozygous for the abnormal gene does not manifest obvious symptoms

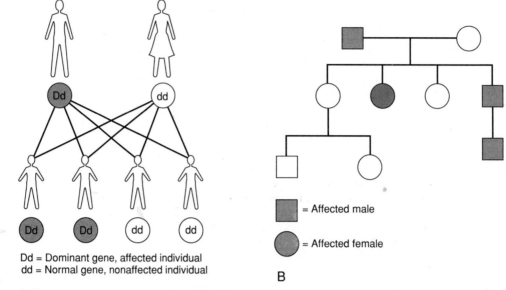

Figure 3–4.
Dominant inheritance. *A,* Autosomal dominant inheritance. One parent is affected. Statistically, the offspring have a one in two chance of being affected, regardless of sex. *B,* Autosomal dominant genogram.

      (2) It is not until two individuals mate and pass on the same abnormal gene that the condition may appear
    b. Mode of transmission (Fig. 3–5)
    c. Characteristics
      (1) An affected individual has clinically normal parents, but they are both carriers for the abnormal gene
      (2) If both parents are carriers for the abnormal gene, they have a one in four

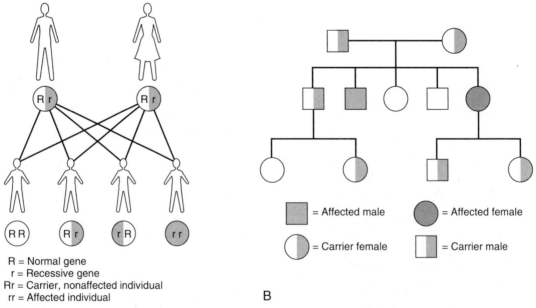

Figure 3–5.
Recessive inheritance. *A,* Autosomal recessive inheritance. Both parents are the carriers. Statistically, the offspring have a one in four chance of being affected, regardless of sex. *B,* Autosomal recessive genogram.

(25%) chance with each pregnancy of passing the abnormal gene on to their offspring; in this case, the child will have the disorder

(3) If the offspring of two carrier parents is clinically normal, there is a one in two (50%) chance with each pregnancy that he or she will be a carrier, like the parents

(4) Males and females are affected equally

(5) The family genogram usually shows siblings affected in a horizontal pattern

(6) There is an increased risk for autosomal recessive conditions if intermarriage occurs (consanguineous matings); individuals who are closely related are more likely to have the same genes in common

(7) Recessive disorders tend to be more severe in their clinical manifestations

(8) The presence of certain autosomal recessive genes can be detected in the normal carrier parent; examples of diseases for which carrier screening is available are sickle cell anemia, Tay-Sachs disease, and cystic fibrosis

4. Sex-linked recessive inheritance

  a. Sex-linked or X-linked disorders are those for which the gene is carried on the X chromosome

  b. A female may be heterozygous or homozygous for a trait carried on the X chromosome because she has two X chromosomes

  c. A male has only one X chromosome, and there are some traits for which no comparable genes are located on the Y chromosome; in this case, the gene will be expressed

  d. The X-linked disorders are manifested only in the male who carries the gene

  e. Mode of transmission (Fig. 3–6)

  f. Characteristics

    (1) There is no male-to-male transmission; fathers pass on their Y chromosome to their sons and their X chromosome to their daughters

    (2) Affected males are related through the female line

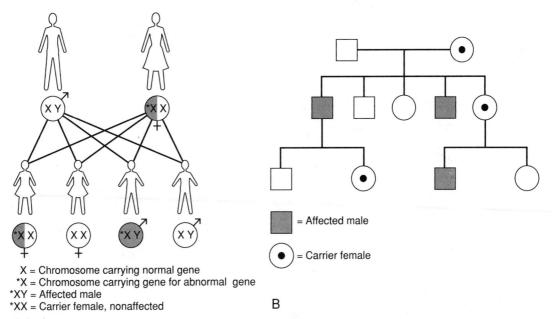

X = Chromosome carrying normal gene
*X = Chromosome carrying gene for abnormal gene
*XY = Affected male
*XX = Carrier female, nonaffected

A   B

■ = Affected male

● = Carrier female

Figure 3–6.
Recessive inheritance. A, X-Linked recessive inheritance. The mother is the carrier. Statistically, the male offspring have a one in two chance of being affected and none of the females will be affected. The female offspring have a one in two chance of being a carrier. B, X-Linked genogram.

(3) There is a one in two (50%) chance with each pregnancy that a carrier mother will pass the abnormal gene on to her sons, who will then be affected

(4) There is a one in two (50%) chance with each pregnancy that a mother will pass the abnormal gene to her daughter, who will then be a carrier like herself

(5) A father affected with an X-linked condition cannot pass the disorder on to his sons, but all of his daughters will be carriers

(6) Occasionally, a female carrier will demonstrate the symptoms of an X-linked disorder; this situation is probably due to the random inactivation of the second X chromosome

D. Polygenic or multifactorial disorders

1. Many common congenital malformations are caused by the interaction of many genes and environmental factors, such as the health status and age of the parents and exposure to pollutants and viruses
2. Characteristics
   a. Malformations may vary from mild to severe
   b. The more severe the defect, the greater the number of genes present for that defect
   c. There is often a sex bias in occurrence rates for a malformation
      (1) Congenital hip dysplasia occurs in females
      (2) Pyloric stenosis occurs in males
      (3) When a member of the less commonly affected sex manifests the condition, a greater number of genes must be present to cause the defect
   d. In the presence of environmental influences, it may take fewer genes to manifest the disease in the offspring
   e. In contrast to single-gene disorders, there is an additive effect in multifactorial inheritance that occurs
      (1) When more than one family member is affected
      (2) In proportion to the severity of the condition in the child
   f. Risk factors are determined by the distribution of cases found in the general population
   g. The risk of recurrence is usually 2 to 5% for all first-degree relatives but is higher (10 to 15%) if more than one member is affected

Clinical Practice

A. Assessment

1. Family history: take a thorough family history going back at least three generations (genogram) (Fig. 3–7)
2. Physical findings: evaluate all systems; chromosomal disorders affect multiple body systems, and many gene disorders have subtle signs that will be detected only through careful assessment of, for example, skin pigmentation, color of sclera, fingernail patterns, texture of the hair, and neurological responses
3. Diagnostic tests that may be performed are
   a. Maternal serum alpha-fetoprotein to screen for neural tube defects (elevated) or Down's syndrome (low) in the fetus
   b. Chromosomal analysis via chorionic villi sampling or amniocentesis
   c. Developmental assessment of parents or siblings as indicated by possible risk status established by a family history, such as for fragile X syndrome
   d. Fetal ultrasonography for suspected structural disorders, such as omphaloceles or renal agenesis
   e. Newborn screening test (for example, phenylketonuria [PKU], galactosemia, hypothyroidism, and sickle cell anemia)
   f. Other laboratory tests as indicated by physical signs and symptoms

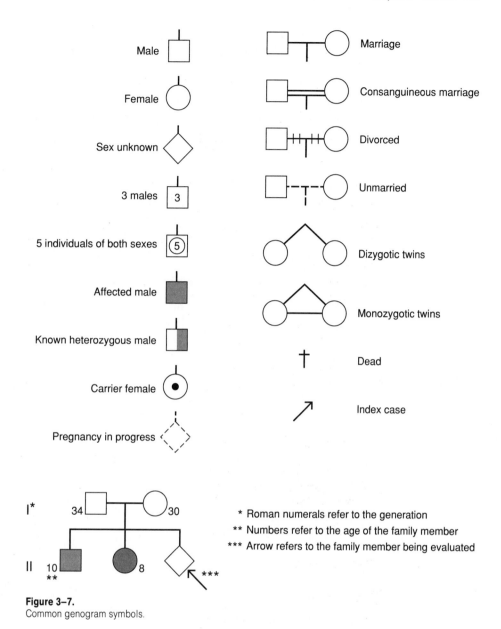

Figure 3–7.
Common genogram symbols.

B. Nursing Diagnoses

1. Knowledge deficit related to factors of heredity, infant potential, and community resources
2. High risk for ineffective family coping related to physical and/or mental handicap of a family member
3. High risk for alteration in the family process related to diagnosis of a genetic disorder in the fetus or newborn
4. High risk for alteration in parenting related to the diagnosis of a genetic disorder in the fetus or newborn
5. Grief related to loss of a normal child
6. High risk for social isolation of the family and the infant related to embarrassment about child's appearance and/or behavior and lack of knowledge

C. Interventions/Evaluations

1. Knowledge deficit related to factors of heredity, infant potential, and community resources
   a. Interventions
      (1) Explain appropriate genetic information to the family
      (2) Discuss implications of the condition for the parent, the infant, and the siblings
      (3) Provide written educational material or refer the family to the appropriate agency (such as the March of Dimes National Foundation) for educational materials
      (4) Refer the family to a genetics center for a complete evaluation
      (5) Maintain a supportive attitude toward the family's questions, need for clarification, and final decision about actions to be taken
      (6) Explain diagnostic procedures before the test and emphasize the purpose, findings anticipated, and possible side effects
   b. Evaluations
      (1) The family demonstrates an understanding of the information provided through feedback and appropriate questions
      (2) The family has obtained the appropriate diagnostic tests
2. High risk for ineffective family coping related to physical and/or mental handicap of a family member
   a. Interventions
      (1) Assure family members that they do not need to rush into a decision
      (2) Provide the necessary information and resources for the family to make an informed decision
      (3) Encourage family members to verbalize their feelings
      (4) Interact with family members to encourage individual feelings of self-worth
      (5) Recognize that grief is appropriate during a difficult decision-making process
   b. Evaluation: the family is able to make appropriate decisions
3. High risk for alteration in the family process related to diagnosis of a genetic disorder in the fetus or newborn
   a. Interventions
      (1) Recognize that grief is appropriate during a difficult decision-making process
      (2) Encourage family members to verbalize their feelings
      (3) Interact with family members to encourage individual feelings of self-worth
      (4) Refer family members to appropriate resources to deal with current crises
   b. Evaluations
      (1) The family is able to make appropriate decisions
      (2) Family members are able to provide each other with the necessary emotional and physical support and care
4. High risk for alteration in parenting related to diagnosis of a genetic disorder in the fetus or newborn
   a. Interventions
      (1) Explain appropriate genetic information to the family
      (2) Discuss implications of the condition
      (3) Interact with the family to encourage feelings of self-worth
      (4) Recognize that grief is appropriate during a difficult decision-making process
      (5) Refer the family to the appropriate resources or agency to assist in the parenting of an affected child
   b. Evaluations
      (1) Family members have obtained needed services

(2) Family members are able to make appropriate decisions
5. Grief related to the loss of a normal child (see Chapter 25 for a complete discussion of grief and loss)
   a. Interventions
      (1) Assure family members that they do not need to rush into a decision
      (2) Encourage family members to verbalize their feelings
      (3) Recognize that grief is a normal response
      (4) Provide the necessary information and resources
   b. Evaluations
      (1) Family members verbalize grief and feelings of loss
      (2) Family members make the appropriate decisions
6. High risk for social isolation of the family and the infant related to embarrassment about the child's appearance and/or behavior and lack of knowledge
   a. Interventions
      (1) Explain appropriate genetic information to the family
      (2) Discuss the implications of the condition and the resources available for the family to deal with the condition
      (3) Maintain a supportive attitude toward the family
      (4) Encourage family members to verbalize their feelings
      (5) Refer family members to appropriate agencies to deal with their concerns
   b. Evaluations
      (1) The family is able to provide necessary care for the affected individual
      (2) The family has obtained services from referral agencies
      (3) The family is able to make the appropriate decisions

Health Education

A. Explain the known causes for the condition (the genetics of the disorder)

B. Describe the referral agencies that are available for the follow-up and support

C. Explain the reproductive options and recurrence risks

D. Discuss available treatment options

E. Discuss the prognosis of condition

F. Discuss the measures to be taken to prevent the condition in future offspring

CASE STUDIES AND STUDY QUESTIONS

Mrs. C. is a 43-year-old, gravida 3, para 2(G3, P2) and is at 16 weeks' gestation. She underwent a prenatal diagnostic test for chromosomal abnormalities. She received the result of the test, which was 47,XY +21 (male with Down's syndrome). Otherwise, the pregnancy has been normal with no complications to date.

1. What information would you need to know to assist Mr. and Mrs. C. in understanding the cause of chromosomal abnormalities?
   a. A history of maternal substance use during pregnancy.
   b. The level and quality of prenatal care received to date.
   c. The family history of chromosomal abnormalities.
   e. The birth history of previous children.

2. Mr. and Mrs. C. do not understand what 47,XY +21 means. What is the correct interpretation?
   a. The 47th chromosome has 21 extra genes and XY refers to gender.
   b. There is an extra chromosome in the 21st pair and XY refers to gender.
   c. The 21st chromosome has additional genetic material and XY refers to location on the gene.

d. The number 47 refers to the type of test and +21 refers to the number of abnormal cells identified.

3. Mr. and Mrs. C. believe that they must have done something that caused this abnormality in their fetus. You can tell them
   a. They are not responsible because this was an accident that occurred in early cell division before fertilization.
   b. Mrs. C. may have had a viral infection in the first few days after conception.
   c. Mr. C. may have been exposed to an environmental toxin during adolescence, thus altering his ability to produce normal sperm.
   d. Mrs. C. may have exposed the embryo to an environmental toxin that altered the basic cell structure.

4. Mr. and Mrs. C. are concerned about the potential risks to their future grandchildren. What is an appropriate response?
   a. With each occurrence of a chromosomal abnormality, there is an increased risk of recurrence of 2 to 5%.
   b. Recommend that their children receive regular chromosomal monitoring to rule out a future translocation.
   c. Recommend that only male children should consider future pregnancies because they would not be at risk.
   d. The recurrence risk should not be higher than that for the general population.

Mrs. K. is a 29-year-old white woman. She is a G1P1, and has been delivered of a baby boy. The child was diagnosed as having achondroplasia (a type of dwarfism that is inherited via the autosomal dominant mode). The child weighs 2722 g (6 lb) and is in no apparent distress. Upon further questioning, you learn that Mr. K. is 45 years old and also has achondroplasia. Mrs. K. has three sisters with no health problems, and her parents are living and well. Mr. K. has one brother and one sister; both are normal. Mr. K.'s mother is living and well; Mr. K.'s father is dead and he, too, had achondroplasia. Both Mr. and Mrs. K. are interested in future pregnancies.

5. The couple does not understand what autosomal dominant means. You tell the couple that an autosomal dominant condition is
   a. A disorder that is caused by a single gene that overshadows a gene that is at the same location on the other chromosome pair.
   b. A condition that occurs when each parent contributes a gene for the particular disorder.
   c. A condition that produces a result that is severe and usually is not correctable.
   d. A condition that is caused by a combination of many genes and an environmental factor.

6. Because they would like to have other children, they are interested in knowing the recurrence risk for this condition. The estimated risk is
   a. Quite small
   b. 10 to 15%
   c. 25%
   d. 50%

7. Mr. and Mrs. K. note that two individuals with achondroplasia in their family were males, and they would like to know if boys are at a greater risk. You advise them that this dominant condition
   a. Has a 25% increased risk for males.
   b. Occurs in both males and females.
   c. Occurs more frequently when the woman is older than 35 years old.
   d. Has a 50% increased risk for males.

Mr. and Mrs. Y. were contacted by their pediatrician because their newborn son's screening PKU test results were abnormal (the PKU level was elevated). The baby is now 5 days old and appears normal although a little col-

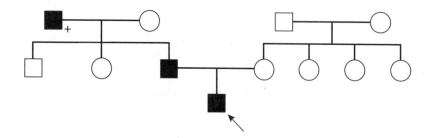

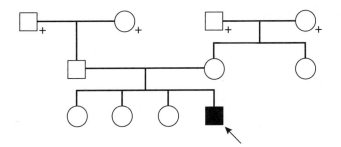

icky. Further testing verified the diagnosis of PKU. Mr. and Mrs. Y. are in their late 20s; they have three normal daughters, and Mr. Y. is convinced that if their next child is a girl, she will be normal. Mrs. Y. has one sister who has three normal children. Her parents died in an automobile accident when she was small. Mr. Y. is an only child and his parents died when he was a young child.

8. The couple does not understand what autosomal recessive means. You could tell them that an autosomal recessive condition is
   a. A disorder that is caused by a single gene that overshadows a gene that is at the same location on the other chromosome pair.
   b. A condition that occurs when each parent contributes a gene for the particular disorder.
   c. A condition that produces a result that is not severe and usually is correctable.

9. Because they would like to have other children, they are interested in knowing that the recurrence risk for this condition is
   a. Extremely small
   b. 10 to 15%
   c. 25%
   d. 50%

10. Mr. and Mrs. Y. do not understand why the girls were normal and the boy was not; they would like to know if only a boy would be at risk. You advise them that this recessive condition
    a. Has a 25% increased risk for males.
    b. Occurs in both males and females.
    c. Occurs more frequently in women older than 35 years old.
    d. Has a 50% increased risk for males.

11. The couple have difficulty believing that the condition is inheritable in their family, because no one else has a similar problem. You can explain to them that recessive disorders
    a. Occur among siblings versus occuring from generation to generation.
    b. Occur in a random pattern in the first two or three generations.
    c. Have a high frequency of mutations in the original case.
    d. Usually skips a generation before it manifests itself.

Answers to Study Questions

1. c	2. b	3. a
4. d	5. a	6. d
7. b	8. b	9. c
10. b	11. a	

REFERENCES

Auvenshine, M., & Enriquez, M. (1990). *Comprehensive maternity nursing: Perinatal and women's health* (2nd ed.). Boston: Jones & Bartlett.

Carpenito, L.J. (1984). *Handbook of nursing diagnosis.* Philadelphia: Lippincott.

Creasy, R.K., & Resnik, R. (1989). *Maternal-fetal medicine: Principle and practice* (2nd ed.). Philadelphia: Saunders.

Lodewig, P., London, M., & Olds, S. (1990). *Essentials of maternal-newborn nursing* (2nd ed.). Redwood City, CA: Addison-Wesley Nursing.

Ince, S. (Ed.). (1987). *Genetic counseling.* White Plains, NY: March of Dimes, Birth Defect Foundation.

May, K., & Mahlmeister, L.R. (1990). *Comprehensive maternity nursing* (2nd ed.). Philadelphia: Lippincott.

Pritchard, J., MacDonald, P., & Grant, M. (1985). *Williams obstetrics* (17th ed.). New York: Appleton-Century-Crofts.

Rauch, J. (1988, September/October). Social work and the genetic revolution: Genetic services. *Social Work*, 389–395.

Roberts, A. (1983, July 20). Setting up the system—3. *Nursing Times, 79*(29), 57–60.

Roberts, A. (1983, October 5). Setting up the system—6. *Nursing Times, 79*(40), 49–52.

Roberts, A. (1983, November 2). Setting up the system—7. *Nursing Times, 79*(44), 61–64.

Roberts, A. (1984, January 11). Setting up the system—9. *Nursing Times, 80*(2), 57–60.

Roberts, A. (1984, February 15). Setting up the system—10. *Nursing Times, 80*(7), 1–4.

Thompson, J., & Thompson M. (1986). *Genetics in medicine* (4th ed.). Philadelphia: Saunders.

Bonnie Kellogg

Fetal Development

Objectives

1. Describe the process of fertilization

2. Explain the major developmental phenomena that take place during the pre-embryonic stage

3. Identify the important milestones for the development of fetal organs, such as the heart, lungs, kidney, and brain

4. Develop teaching strategies to assist families in making appropriate reproductive decisions

5. Identify the periods when the developing body systems of the fetus are most susceptible to teratogenic influences

Introduction

A. Conception

1. Fertilization usually occurs in the ampulla of the fallopian tube
2. High estrogen levels during ovulation
   a. Thin the cervical mucus, which allows the sperm to enter the uterus
   b. Increase the ability of the ovum to travel down the fallopian tube
3. The ovum membrane is surrounded by two layers of tissue
   a. The layer closest to the cell membrane is called the zona pellucida
   b. Surrounding this layer is a ring of elongated follicular cells called the corona radiata (Fig. 4–1)
4. The mature ovum and spermatozoon have only a short time to unite
   a. Ova are considered fertile for about 24 hours after ovulation
   b. Sperm are viable for up to 72 hours but are believed to be fertile for only 24 hours
   c. In a single ejaculation, the penis deposits approximately 400 million spermatozoa in the vagina
      (1) The sperm propel themselves by the flagellar movements of the long tail
      (2) Following ejaculation, the first sperm reach the cervical mucus within 90 seconds
      (3) Within 5 minutes, sperm can be found in the fallopian tubes

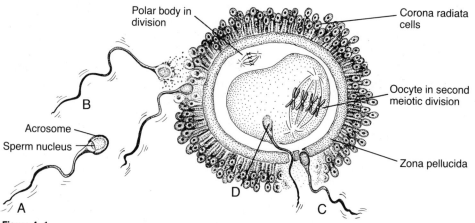

Figure 4–1
Process of fertilization. *A*, Sperm moves toward ovum using movement of the flagellum; *B*, acrosomal reaction; *C*, sperm penetrates corona radiata and zona; *D*, once sperm penetrates the ovum, fusion of the oocyte and sperm cell membranes occurs.

      (4) Less than 200 sperm actually reach the fallopian tubes
  d. A sperm undergoes two processes of change before it is able to penetrate the ovum
      (1) Capacitation: structural alteration of the sperm once it enters the female genital tract
      (2) Acrosomal reaction: the head of the sperm releases enzymes (see Fig. 4–1)
        (a) Hyaluronidase causes sloughing and separation of the corona radiata
        (b) Acrosin and neuraminidase facilitate the passage of the sperm through the zona pellucida
  e. Cellular change occurs at the moment of penetration, preventing other sperm from penetrating the ovum (zona reaction)
  f. At the moment of penetration, the oocyte completes the second meiotic division (see Fig. 4–1)
 5. With fertilization, the diploid number (46) of chromosomes is restored and cell division begins
  a. The sex of the new individual is established
  b. Within the cell, the nuclei of the spermatozoon and oocyte unite and their nuclear membranes disappear
  c. The chromosomes pair up and a new cell, the zygote, is formed
      (1) The zygote contains a new combination of genetic material
      (2) This process creates an individual who is different from both parents

B. **Pre-embryonic and embryonic stages**

 1. Pre-embryonic stage
  a. First week (Fig. 4–2)
      (1) Characterized by extremely rapid cell division, cell differentiation, and the development of embryonic membranes and germ layers
      (2) Division of the zygote occurs within the first 30 hours and continues for the next 3 days
      (3) The conceptus travels toward the uterus
      (4) During this time, the zygote divides into a solid ball of cells (the morula)
      (5) The morula floats inside of the uterus for 2 or 3 days
        (a) It obtains nourishment from the mucous lining of the uterus and the fluid in the uterine cavity
        (b) Zona pellucida begins to thin, and fluid enters between the cells
        (c) The fluid hollows out the morula, which is now called the blastocyst

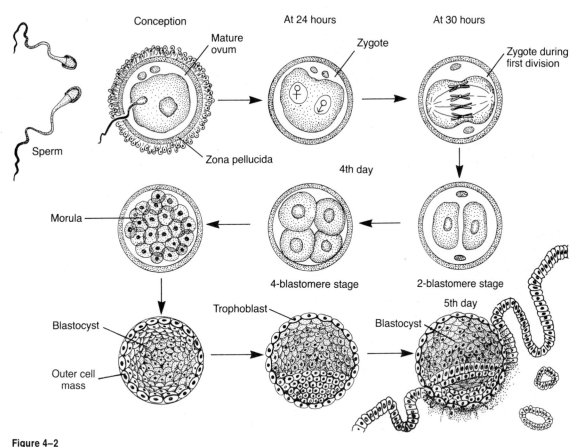

Figure 4–2
Process of implantation.

    (6) Two distinct layers of cells develop
        (a) The inner cell mass (blastocyst) will eventually become the embryo,
            the amnion, and the yolk sac membrane
        (b) The outer cell layer (trophoblast) will become the fetal side of the
            placenta and chorion
    (7) Zona pellucida disappears at about 5 days
        (a) The blastocyst enlarges
        (b) The trophoblast attaches to the endometrial epithelium and begins
            the process of implantation
        (c) The attached portion of the trophoblast develops into two layers
            (i) The internal cellular layer is called the cytotrophoblast
           (ii) The outer layer is called the syncytiotrophoblast, which invades
              the endometrial epithelium and connective tissue by the end of
              the seventh day
          (iii) Invasion and embedding occur and are completed by the
              11th day
  b. Second week
    (1) The inner cell mass differentiates into two cell layers: the endoderm (the
      inside of the embryo) and the ectoderm (the outside of the embryo)
        (a) The amniotic cavity appears as a space between the inner cell mass
            and the trophoblast
        (b) When the embryo becomes a cylinder, the amnion surrounds it and
            becomes the amniotic sac
    (2) By the end of the second week, the embryonic cells and the associated

amniotic and yolk sacs are attached to the chorionic sac by a slender band, which becomes the umbilical cord

(3) Malformations that occur during the pre-embryonic stage development seldom result in a viable fetus

2. Embryonic stage
   a. Third week
      (1) Gastrulation
         (a) The embryonic disc converts into a trilaminar embryonic disc composed of three germ layers: ectoderm (will become the epidermis and the nervous system), mesoderm (will become the smooth muscle), and endoderm (will become the epithelial lining of the respiratory and digestive tracts)
            (i) Begins in the first week with the appearance of the hypoblast (primitive endoderm)
            (ii) Continues in the second week with the formation of the epiblast
            (iii) Is completed in the third week with the formation of intraembryonic mesoderm by the primitive streak
         (b) This process gives rise to the future development of tissue and organs
         (c) Primitive streak (Fig. 4–3A)
            (i) Thick band of epiblast develops at the end of the dorsal aspect of the embryonic disc
            (ii) Proliferation and migration of cells from the primitive streak give rise to mesenchyme

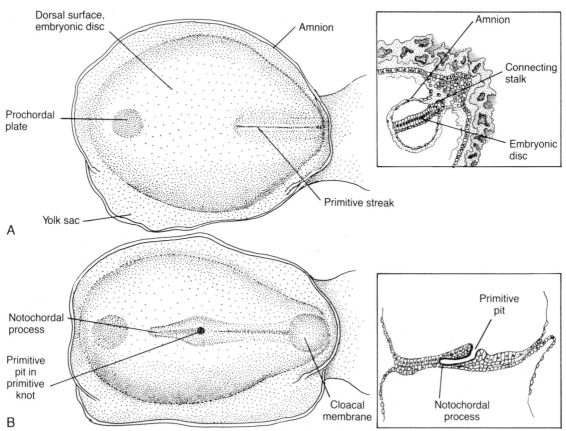

Figure 4–3
Schematic of embryonic disc and extraembryonic membranes. *A*, Embryonic disc; *B*, extraembryonic membranes.

- Cells spread cranially and caudally
- These cells begin to form the embryonic endoderm, which will give rise to the lining of the digestive and respiratory tracts
- The cells that remain on the surface of the embryonic disc form the layer of cells called the embryonic ectoderm, which will develop into the nervous system, i.e., the sensory epithelium of the eye, ear, and nose

(2) Notochordal process (Fig. 4–3B)
  (a) The mesenchymal cells migrate cranially under the embryonic ectoderm and form the midline cellular cord, which is called the notochordal process
  (b) These cells grow until they reach the prochordal plate, the future site of the mouth
  (c) Caudal to the primitive streak is a circular area called the cloacal membrane, which becomes the anus
  (d) The primitive streak continues to form mesoderm until the end of the fourth week

(3) The notochord develops by transformation of the notochordal process
  (a) Defines the primitive axis of the embryo
  (b) Gives the embryo some rigidity
  (c) By the end of the third week, it is almost completely formed

(4) Neurulation is the process of developing the neural plate, neural folds, and neural tube
  (a) Neural plate (Fig. 4–4)
    (i) Embryonic ectoderm lying over the notochord thickens to form the neural plate
    (ii) It first appears near the primitive knot but as it enlarges it forms a neural groove, which becomes bounded by the neural folds on each side
  (b) Neural tube
    (i) By the end of the third week, the neural folds begin to fuse
    (ii) This fusion converts the neural plate into a neural tube
    (iii) This fusion occurs near the middle of the embryo and progresses toward the cranial and caudal ends
  (c) Neural crest (Fig. 4–5)
    (i) Cells lying along the neural fold migrate ventrolaterally on each side of the neural tube

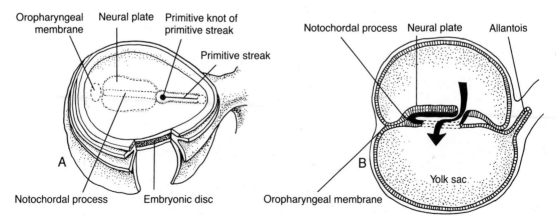

Figure 4–4
Embryonic disc at approximately 3 weeks. Neural plate. *A*, Horizontal section showing notochordal process and associated mesenchyme stimulating ectoderm to form the neural plate; *B*, vertical section showing the notochordal process beginning to degenerate. (Adapted from Moore K.L. [1988]. *Essentials of human embryology* [p. 19]. Philadelphia: Decker.)

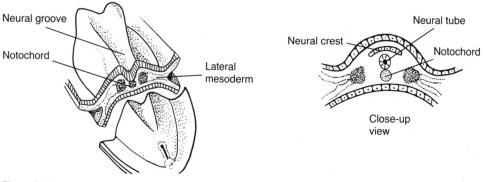

Figure 4–5
Transverse section of developing embryo at 3½ weeks. (Adapted from Moore K.L. [1988]. *Essentials of human embryology* [p. 20]. Philadelphia: Decker.)

(ii) They form an irregular mass called the neural crest
(iii) These cells migrate widely throughout the embryo and give rise to the spinal ganglia
(iv) The neural crest cells also form the meninges of the brain and spinal cord and give rise to the adrenal medulla and several components of the skeletal and muscular parts of the head
(5) Somite development (Fig. 4–6A)
    (a) Some of the mesoderm begins to form long columns, called the paraxial mesoderm
    (b) These columns divide into paired cuboidal bodies, called somites
    (c) Subsequent pairs form in a craniocaudal sequence
    (d) The somites form distinct surface elevations
    (e) Mesenchymal cells from the somites give rise to the vertebral column, the ribs, the sternum, the skull, and associated muscles
(6) Intraembryonic coelom
    (a) First appears as cavities in the lateral mesoderm
    (b) These spaces form a horseshoe-shaped cavity called the intraembryonic coelom (Fig. 4–6B)
    (c) The intraembryonic coelom divides the lateral mesoderm into two layers
        (i) Somatic layer is continuous with the extraembryonic mesoderm covering the amnion

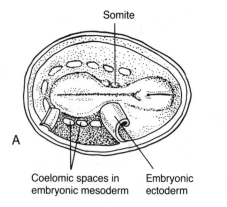

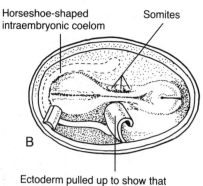

Figure 4–6
Dorsal view of the developing embryo. (Adapted from Moore K.L. [1988]. *Essentials of human embryology* [p. 23]. Philadelphia: Decker.)

(ii) Visceral layer is continuous with the extraembryonic mesoderm covering the yolk sac

(d) During the second month, the intraembryonic coelom will become the pericardial, the pleural, and the peritoneal cavities

(7) Primitive cardiovascular system (Fig. 4–7)

(a) Blood vessels start forming in the extraembryonic mesoderm of the yolk sac, connecting stalk and chorion at the end of the third week

(b) Mesenchymal cells (angioblasts) aggregate to form blood islands

(c) Cavities appear in the islands

(d) Mesenchymal cells arrange around cavities to form the endothelium of primitive blood vessels

(e) Primitive blood vessels fuse to form a series of networks

(f) Vessels begin to extend into adjacent areas

(g) Primitive blood cells develop from the endothelial cells of the vessels in the walls of the yolk sac; blood formation does not begin in the embryo until the fifth week

(h) Primitive heart is a tubular structure that is formed from the mesenchymal cells in the cardiogenic area

(i) Paired endocardial heart tubes develop

(ii) These fuse and form a primitive heart

(iii) The heart tubes join blood vessels in the embryo, connective stalk, chorion, and yolk sac, forming a primitive cardiovascular system

(iv) The primitive blood cells begin to circulate at the end of the third week as the tubular heart begins to beat

(8) Malformations that may occur during this stage of development follow

(a) Anencephaly as a result of a defect in the closure of the anterior neural tube, which results in the degeneration of the forebrain

(b) Cyclopia occurs as a result of an alteration in the prechordal mesodermal development and produces secondary defects of the midface and forebrain

(c) Ectromelia (congenital absence of a limb)

(d) Ectopia cordis (heart remains outside of the thoracic cavity)

b. Fourth week

(1) Embryo is almost straight (Fig. 4–8A)

(2) Somites produce obvious surface elevations

(3) The neural tube is formed near the middle of the embryo

(4) The neural tube is open at the rostral and caudal neuropores (Fig. 4–8B)

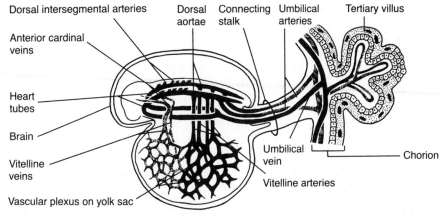

Figure 4–7
Primitive cardiovascular system (at about 20 days). (Adapted from Moore K.L. [1988]. *Essentials of human embryology* [p. 61]. Philadelphia: Decker.)

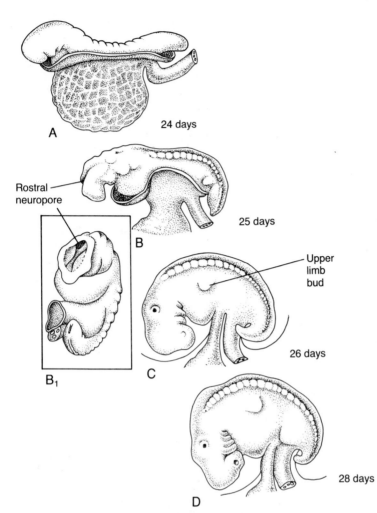

A   24 days

Rostral neuropore

B   25 days

B₁

Upper limb bud

C   26 days

Figure 4–8
Development of head and tail regions (fourth week). (Adapted from Moore K.L. [1988]. *Essentials of human embryology* [p. 29]. Philadelphia: Decker.)

28 days

D

(5) The first and second pairs of the branchial arches (become the future head and neck) are visible
(6) The otic placodes (primordia of the internal ears) are developed
(7) By the middle of the fourth week, the embryo is cylindrical and curved because of the folding of the median and horizontal planes
   (a) The rostral neuropore closes
   (b) The upper limb buds appear as small swellings on the lateral wall (Fig. 4–8C)
   (c) Three pairs of branchial arches are visible
   (d) The heart forms a distinct prominence on the surface of the embryo
   (e) The otic pits are formed
(8) By the end of the fourth week, the embryo is C shaped
   (a) The neuropore has closed
   (b) The oral cavity begins
   (c) The esophagotracheal septum begins to divide into the esophagus and the trachea
   (d) The stomach, the pancreas, and the liver begin to form
   (e) Upper limb buds have a flipper shape (Fig. 4–8D)
   (f) Lower limb buds appear as small swellings (Fig. 4–9A)
   (g) Four pairs of branchial arches and lens placodes (the lens of the eye) have developed
   (h) A tail is prominent at this time

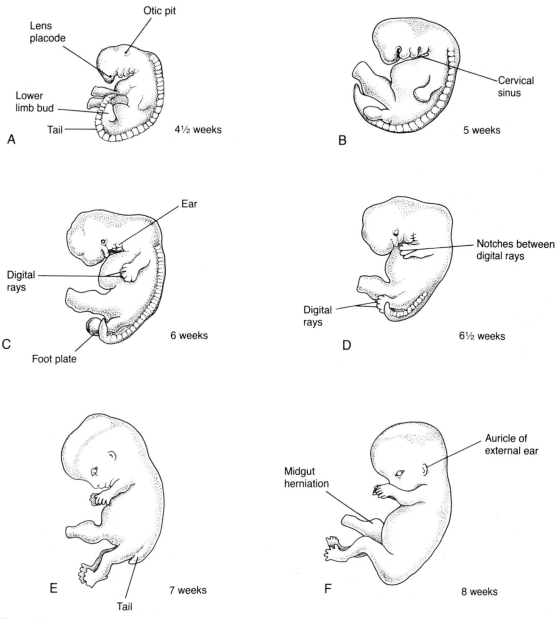

Figure 4–9
Embryo from 4½ weeks to 8 weeks. (Adapted from Moore K.L. [1988]. *Essentials of human embryology* [p. 37]. Philadelphia: Decker.)

  (9) Malformations that may occur during this stage of development follow
    (a) Meningomyelocele occurs as the result of a defect in the closure of the posterior neural tube
    (b) Esophageal atresia and tracheoesophageal fistulas may occur as a result of the lateral septation of the foregut
    (c) Extravasation of the bladder occurs if the infraumbilical mesenchyme does not migrate effectively
  c. Fifth week (Fig. 4–9B)
    (1) The embryo is approximately 8 mm (⅓ in) in length
    (2) Growth of the head is obvious because of the rapid development of the brain
    (3) The brain differentiates

        (4) The cranial nerves have developed

        (5) Atrial division in the heart has begun

        (6) Upper limbs become shaped like paddles

        (7) Cervical sinuses are visible as a result of the growth of the second branchial arch over the third and fourth pairs

        (8) Malformations that may occur during this stage of development follow

            (a) Cleft lip and other facial clefts result from a defect in the closure of the lip

            (b) Transposition of the great vessels can occur if the aorticopulmonary septum fails to spiral

            (c) Nuclear cataracts

            (d) Microphthalmia (small eyeballs)

            (e) Carpal and pedal ablation

  d. Sixth week (Fig. 4–9, C and D)

        (1) The embryo is 12 mm (½ in) long

        (2) Brain and neurological system

            (a) Flexures of the brain are obvious

            (b) The head structures are more highly developed

        (3) Heart and circulatory systems

            (a) The heart begins to divide into chambers

            (b) The liver begins to form red blood cells

        (4) Respiratory system

            (a) The trachea and lung buds appear

            (b) The oral and nasal cavities are formed

        (5) Gastrointestinal systems

            (a) The upper and lower jaw is forming

            (b) The upper lip is formed

            (c) The palate is developing

        (6) Genitourinary system: embryonic sex glands appear

        (7) Skeletal and muscular system

            (a) Bone rudiments are present

            (b) Ossification of the jaw and skull begins

            (b) The wrist and elbow are identifiable

            (d) Ridges form on the paddle-shaped hands and are called digital rays (future fingers and thumb)

            (e) Muscle begins to develop

        (8) Eyes, ears, skin, and hair

            (a) The primordia of the external acoustic meatus and external ear are present

            (b) The external, middle, and inner ears continue to form

        (9) Malformations that may occur during this period of development follow

            (a) Rectal atresia with fistula occurs if there is a defect in the lateral septation of the cloaca into the rectum and urogenital sinuses

            (b) Diaphragmatic hernia occurs when there is a defect in the closure of the pleuroperitoneal canal

            (c) Ventricular septal defect results during the closure of the ventricular septum

  e. Seventh week (Fig. 4–9E)

        (1) The embryo is approximately 18 mm (¾ in) in length

        (2) Brain and neurological systems

            (a) There is a disproportion in size between the head and spinal cord

            (b) The tail begins to recede

        (3) Heart and circulatory system

            (a) Fetal heartbeat can be heard

            (b) The heart has most of its definitive characteristics

            (c) Fetal circulation begins

        (4) Gastrointestinal system

        (a) The tongue separates
        (b) The palate begins to fold inward
        (c) Midgut herniation is visible
        (d) The stomach assumes its final shape
        (e) The diaphragm separates the abdominal and thoracic cavities
    (5) Genitourinary system
        (a) The bladder and the urethra separate from the rectum
        (b) The sex glands begin to differentiate into testes or ovaries
    (6) Skeletal and muscular systems
        (a) Notches develop between the digital rays of the hand
        (b) Digital rays appear in the developing feet
        (c) By the end of the seventh week, the following have occurred
           (i) Upper limbs are bent at the elbow
          (ii) Finger and thumb are distinct but are still webbed
         (iii) Notches appear between the digital rays of the feet
    (7) Eyes, ears, skin, and hair
        (a) The optic nerve forms
        (b) Eyelids appear
        (c) Eye lenses begin to thicken
    (8) Malformations that may occur during this stage of development follow
        (a) Duodenal atresia may result from an error in the recanalization of the duodenum
        (b) Pulmonary stenosis
        (c) Brachycephalism (shortening of the head)
        (d) Alteration in sexual characteristics
        (e) Cleft plate
f. Eighth week (Fig. 4–9F)
    (1) The embryo is 2.5 to 3 cm (1 to 1½ in) in length and weighs 8 g (0.25 oz)
    (2) Brain and neurological system
        (a) Sensory and motor neurons have functional connections
        (b) Embryo is able to contract large muscles
    (3) Heart and circulatory system
        (a) Development of the heart is complete
        (b) The circulatory system through the umbilical cord is established
    (4) Gastrointestinal system
        (a) Abdomen protrudes because the intestines are in the proximal part of the umbilical cord
        (b) Midgut rotates
        (c) Anal membrane perforates and rectal passage opens
        (d) Lips are fused
    (5) Genitourinary system
        (a) External genitalia begin to differentiate
        (b) Genitalia still appear similar
    (6) Skeletal and muscular systems
        (a) Distinct notches are present between the toes
        (b) By the end of the eighth week, the fingers and toes are distinct and separated
        (c) Differentiation of the cells occur in the primitive skeleton
        (d) Cartilaginous bones begin to ossify
        (e) Muscle development begins to occur in the trunk, limbs, and head
    (7) Eyes, ears, skin, and hair
        (a) Embryo has human characteristics
        (b) Eyes are open but fuse at the end of the eighth week
        (c) Auricles of the external ear begin to assume their final appearance
    (8) Malformations that may occur during this stage of development follow
        (a) Persistent opening of the atrial septum
        (b) Digital stunting

3. Fetal stage: every organ system and external structure is present, and the remainder of gestation is devoted to refining the function of the organs
   a. At 9 to 12 weeks
      (1) By the 10th week, the fetus is 5 cm (2 in) in length and weighs about 14 g (0.5 oz); by 12 weeks, the fetus is 8 cm (3 in) in length and weighs about 45 g (1.6 oz)
      (2) Brain and neurological system
         (a) Divisions of the brain begin to develop
         (b) The head is large and constitutes almost half of the fetus's size
         (c) The neck is distinct from the head and body
         (d) Neurons appear at the caudal end of the spinal cord
         (e) By the 12th week, spontaneous movements of the fetus occur; lip movements indicate the development of the sucking reflex
      (3) Heart and circulatory system
         (a) Red blood cells are produced in the liver by the ninth week
         (b) By end of 12th week, the spleen begins to produce red blood cells
      (4) Gastrointestinal system
         (a) The buccopharyngeal and anal membranes open (the intestinal system from mouth to anus is patent)
         (b) Intestinal loops are visible in the proximal end of the umbilical cord and re-enter the abdomen during the 11th week
         (c) By the 12th week, the face is well formed and broad
            (i) The nose begins to protrude
            (ii) The chin is small and receding
            (iii) Tooth buds appear
            (iv) The palate is complete
         (d) Bile secretions begin
      (5) Genitourinary system
         (a) The kidneys begin to produce urine (amniotic fluid volume begins to increase)
         (b) Well-differentiated genitals appear
         (c) Urogenital tract is developed
      (6) Skeletal and muscular systems
         (a) The limbs are long and slender
         (b) The digits are well formed, and the fetus can curl the fingers and make a tiny fist
         (c) The legs are still shorter and less well developed than the arms
         (d) Primary ossification centers appear, and ossification begins in the skull and long bones
         (e) Involuntary muscles in the viscera begin to appear
      (7) Eyes, ears, skin, and hair
         (a) Eyes are widely spaced and fused
         (b) Ears are set low and beginning to acquire an adult shape
      (8) Endocrine and immunological systems
         (a) The thyroid begins to secrete hormones
         (b) Lymphoid tissue develops in the fetal thymus
      (9) Malformations that can occur during this stage of development follow
         (a) Cleft palate
         (b) Malrotation of the gut
         (c) Omphalocele
         (d) Meckel's diverticulum
   b. Between 13 and 16 weeks there is a period of rapid growth
      (1) At 13 weeks, the fetus is about 9 cm (3.6 in) in length and weighs between 55 and 60 g (2 oz)
      (2) Brain and neurological system
         (a) Fetal movements are present
         (b) Thumbsucking can be detected by ultrasonography

    (3) Respiratory system
        (a) Bronchial tubes are branching out in the primitive lungs
        (b) Lungs are fully shaped
    (4) Gastrointestinal system
        (a) Hard and soft palates are developed
        (b) Fetus begins to swallow amniotic fluid
        (c) Fetus is able to produce meconium in the intestinal tract
        (d) Liver and pancreas begin to produce the appropriate secretions
        (e) Gastric and intestinal glands begin to form
    (5) Genitourinary system
        (a) The ovaries have differentiated
        (b) Primordial follicles containing primitive oocytes and ova (oogonia) are
            visible
        (c) External genitalia are formed
        (d) Kidneys assume the normal shape
    (6) Skeletal and muscular systems
        (a) More muscle tissue has developed
        (b) Ossification of the skeleton is occurring
        (c) By the 16th week, skeletal structure is identifiable
        (d) Lower limbs are longer than the upper limbs
        (e) Hard tissue in the jaw begins to form (this will develop into the central
            incisors)
    (7) Eyes, ears, skin, and hair
        (a) Downy lanugo hair begins to develop
        (b) Fetal skin is transparent and the blood vessels are clearly visible
        (c) Eyes have moved to the front of the face
        (d) Ears migrate upward to the side of the head and are fully formed
c. At 17 to 20 weeks
    (1) At 20 weeks, the fetus measures 19 cm (8 in) and weighs between 435 and
        465 g (1 lb, 0.5 oz)
    (2) Brain and neurological system: myelination of the spinal cord begins
    (3) Heart and circulatory system: fetal heart tones may be audible with a
        fetoscope
    (4) Respiratory system
        (a) Lung development continues
        (b) Gas exchange does not occur at this stage
        (c) Bronchial branching is complete and pulmonary capillary beds are
            forming
        (d) Terminal sacs (alveoli) are developing
        (e) Primitive respiratory-type movements begin
    (5) Gastrointestinal system
        (a) Fetus is able to suck and swallow amniotic fluid
        (b) Peristaltic movements begin
    (6) Eyes, ears, skin, and hair
        (a) Subcutaneous deposits of brown fat make the skin less transparent
        (b) Nipples begin to develop over the mammary glands
        (c) The head has woollike hair, and the eyebrows and eyelashes are
            beginning to form
        (d) Nails are present on both fingers and toes
        (e) Muscles are well developed and fetal movements can be felt by the
            mother
        (f) The sebaceous glands become active and produce a greasy substance
            called vernix caseosa
            (i) Vernix caseosa covers the fetal skin
            (ii) It protects the fetus from the effects of the amniotic fluid
            (iii) It prevents the skin from becoming chapped and hardened
    (7) Endocrine and immunological system

(a) Detectable levels of fetal antibodies are present

(b) The fetus is able to store iron, and the bone marrow begins to function

d. At 21 to 24 weeks

(1) At 24 weeks the fetus is 28 cm (11.2 in) long and weighs approximately 780 g (1 lb, 10 oz)

(2) Brain and neurological system

(a) The fetus has a reflex hand grip

(b) By the sixth month, the fetus will exhibit a startle reflex

(c) The brain structure is mature

(3) Heart and circulatory system

(a) The fetal heartbeat is audible through a stethoscope

(b) The blood in the capillaries is visible

(4) Respiratory system

(a) The alveoli of the lungs are beginning to form

(b) Secretory epithelial cells in the interalveolar walls begin to secrete surfactant

(i) Surfactant facilitates expansion of the alveoli, but not in a quantity sufficient to prevent respiratory distress syndrome (RDS)

(ii) A fetus born at this stage may survive

(c) Lecithin can be detected in the amniotic fluid

(d) Respiratory movements may occur

(e) Gas exchange is possible

(f) The nostrils reopen

(5) Genitourinary system: the testes descend to the inguinal ring

(6) Skeletal and muscular systems: the muscles are developed and the fetus is active

(7) Eyes, ears, skin, and hair

(a) The eyes are fully developed and will open

(b) The hair is growing longer

(c) Eyebrows and eyelashes have formed

(d) The ears are flat and shapeless but the fetus is able to hear

(e) The skin is red and wrinkled, with little subcutaneous fat

(f) Skin ridges on the palms and soles of the feet are forming footprints and fingerprints

(g) The skin is less transparent because of deposits of subcutaneous brown fat

(h) Vernix caseosa covers the entire body

(i) Fingernails are well developed and toenails are starting to develop

(8) Endocrine and immunological systems: immunoglobulin G (IgG) levels in the fetus reach maternal levels

e. At 25 to 29 weeks

(1) The fetus is now between 35 and 38 cm (14 to 15 in) in length and weighs about 1200 g (2 lb, 10.5 oz)

(2) Brain and neurological system

(a) The brain continues to mature and grow in size

(b) The nervous system is complete enough to provide some regulation of the body functions and body temperature

(3) Heart and circulatory system: erythropoiesis ends in the spleen and begins in the bone marrow

(4) Respiratory system

(a) Respiratory system is sufficiently developed to provide gaseous exchange

(b) Lungs are capable of breathing air, but the fetus will need intensive care to survive

(c) Surfactant forms on the alveolar surfaces

(5) Genitourinary system

(a) In the male, the testes descend into the scrotal sac

  (b) In the female, the clitoris is prominent and the labia majora are small and do not cover the labia minora
  (6) Eyes, ears, skin, and hair
    (a) Adipose tissue begins to accumulate
    (b) Eyebrows and eyelashes develop
f. At 30 to 34 weeks
  (1) The fetus is gaining weight from an increase in muscle and fat
  (2) The fetus now weighs about 2000 g (4 lb, 6.5 oz) and has a length of about 40 cm (16 in)
  (3) Brain and neurological system
    (a) The central nervous system has matured enough to direct breathing movements and partially control body temperature
    (b) Reflexes are present
  (4) Respiratory systems
    (a) The lungs are not fully developed, but the fetus is able to survive if born
    (b) The lecithin/sphingomyelin (L/S) ratio is approximately 1.2:1
  (5) Genitourinary system
    (a) The testes descend into the scrotum
    (b) The scrotal sac has few rugae
  (6) Eyes, ears, skin, and hair
    (a) Pinna is still folded and soft
    (b) Skin is less wrinkled and the fetus is more filled out
    (c) Fingernails extend to the ends of the finger tips: the fetus can scratch itself at this time
g. At 35 to 38 weeks
  (1) The fetus is 46 cm (17.5 in) in length and weighs approximately 2600 g (6 lb)
  (2) A fetus born at this time has a fairly good chance of surviving
  (3) Respiratory system: the L/S ratio is greater than 2:1 by 38 weeks
  (4) Genitourinary system
    (a) Scrotum is small and rugae are present anteriorly
    (b) Clitoris is covered and labia majora increase in size
  (5) Skeletal and muscular systems: distal femoral ossification centers develop
  (6) Eyes, ears, skin, and hair
    (a) The body and extremities are filling out
    (b) The fetus is less wrinkled
    (c) Lanugo is disappearing
    (d) The fetus has a firm grasp and begins to orient to light
h. At 39 to 40 weeks, the fetus is considered full-term
  (1) The fetus is approximately 50 cm (20 in) in length and weighs between 3000 and 3600 g (6 lb, 10 oz and 7 lb, 15 oz)
  (2) Genitourinary system
    (a) The testes should be in the scrotum and be palpable in the inguinal canals
    (b) The labia majora are well developed
  (3) Eyes, ears, skin, and hair
    (a) The skin is smooth and has a polished look
    (b) Vernix caseosa is still present, with the heaviest deposits in the creases and folds of the skin
    (c) The chest is prominent and slightly smaller than the head
    (d) The mammary glands protrude in both sexes
    (e) The fetal body fills most of the uterine cavity, and the amniotic fluid volume diminishes to about 500 ml
    (f) Lanugo remains on shoulders and upper back only
    (g) Fingernails extend beyond the tips of digits
    (h) Ear lobes become firm as the cartilage thickens

   (4) Malformations that may occur during this stage of development follow
    (a) Patent ductus arteriosus
    (b) Cryptorchidism (failure of the testes to descend into the scrotum)
  i. Post-term (42 weeks and beyond)
   (1) Some fetuses continue to gain weight, increasing the difficulty of labor
   (2) Some fetuses lose weight because the placenta fails to function efficiently
   (3) The fetus may pass meconium as a result of hypoxia from placental insufficiency
   (4) Nails and hair continue to grow
 j. Congenital malformations
  (1) Approximately 3 to 4% of all live-born infants have obvious malformations
  (2) Genetic factors are involved in over one-third of all congenital malformations
  (3) Environmental factors cause approximately 7% of malformations
   (a) Organs and parts of the embryo affected will be determined by the time of ingestion or exposure to the teratogen (an environmental agent that causes malformations) (Fig. 4–10) (see Chapter 13 for a complete discussion of environmental hazards)
   (b) The organs and fetal system are most sensitive to teratogens during their periods of rapid growth during the first trimester

Clinical Practice

A. Assessment

1. History
 a. Knowing the date of day 1 of the last menstrual period is important for monitoring fetal development
 b. Knowing the dates of immunizations for rubella, rubeola, and mumps is important
 c. Knowledge of any infections during pregnancy is important because viruses are known to cross the placental barrier and the timing of viral infections may determine the type and extent of fetal injury
 d. A thorough family history is needed to detect potential inheritable diseases
 e. A complete medical history can identify maternal high-risk conditions, such as diabetes mellitus, that may adversely affect fetal development
 f. A comprehensive assessment of drug intake should include prescription, over-the-counter, and illicit drugs; teratogenic effects of chemical substances will be determined by the stage of fetal development at the time of drug consumption
2. Physical findings
 a. Excessive weight gain or lack of weight gain during pregnancy
 b. Delayed or accelerated uterine growth related to gestational age may indicate serious problems with fetal development
 c. Diagnostic procedures
  (1) Monitoring of uterine growth by measuring fundal heights
  (2) Ultrasonography
   (a) Monitors fetal growth and development
   (b) Can identify major congenital malformations such as hydrocephalus, renal agenesis, and anencephaly
  (3) Maternal serum alpha-fetoprotein (msAFP)
   (a) Lower-than-normal results may indicate a chromosomal abnormality such as trisomy 21 (Down's syndrome)
   (b) Elevated maternal alpha-fetoprotein levels may indicate a neural tube defect

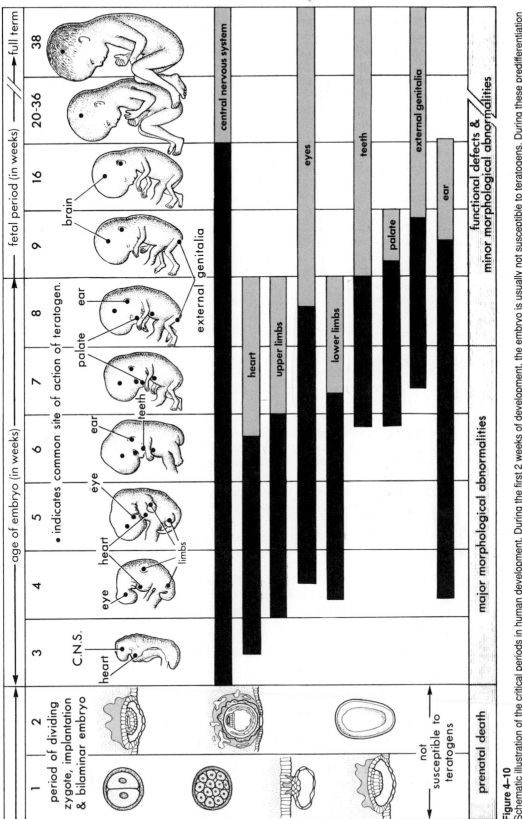

Figure 4–10

Schematic illustration of the critical periods in human development. During the first 2 weeks of development, the embryo is usually not susceptible to teratogens. During these predifferentiation stages, a substance either damages all or most of the cells of the embryo, resulting in its death, or damages only a few cells, allowing the embryo to recover without developing defects. Black denotes highly sensitive periods; gray indicates stages that are less sensitive to teratogens. Severe mental retardation may result from the exposure of the embryo/fetus to certain teratogenic agents (e.g., high levels of radiation during the 8- to 16-week period). (From Moore K.L. [1988]. *The developing human: Clinically oriented embryology* [4th ed.] [p. 143]. Philadelphia: Saunders.)

(4) Amniocentesis is the withdrawal of fluid from the amniotic cavity
   (a) Identifies chromosomal abnormalities
   (b) Assesses the fluid for alpha-fetoprotein levels to rule out open–neural tube defects
(5) Chorionic villi sampling is performed for chromosome analysis and selected metabolic tests on the fetus (see Chapter 11 for a complete discussion of antenatal testing)

B. Nursing Diagnoses

1. High risk for congenital malformation related to exposure to teratogens
2. High risk for altered growth/development related to inadequate maternal nutrition
3. High risk for altered development related to genetic disorder

C. Interventions/Evaluations

1. High risk for congenital malformation related to exposure to teratogens
  a. Interventions
    (1) Assess for exposure to infection and to chemical or environmental factors
    (2) Identify at what stage of fetal development exposure occurred
    (3) Provide parents with the information they need to understand risks and make appropriate medical and health decisions about the pregnancy
    (4) Refer parents to appropriate resources to assess the effects of exposure, for example, to a genetic center or tertiary high-risk obstetrical services
    (5) Maintain an accepting and supportive approach toward the parents
    (6) Listen to their fears and concerns and provide health information that is appropriate to their level of understanding
  b. Evaluations
    (1) Parents are able to express an understanding of the risks from exposure
    (2) Parents have obtained appropriate services from referral agencies
    (3) Parents have made an appropriate decision regarding the outcome of the pregnancy that is based on their values and needs
2. High risk for altered growth/development related to inadequate maternal nutrition
  a. Interventions
    (1) Assess maternal nutritional intake to identify deficiencies
    (2) Assess maternal understanding of nutritional needs for fetal development
    (3) Educate the mother about healthy nutritional intake
    (4) Provide supplements for nutritional deficiencies, as indicated
      (a) Supplement the mother's diet with vitamins and iron
      (b) Refer the parents to a nutritionist for further counseling or to Women, Infants, and Children (WIC) nutritional supplement program, if eligible (see Chapter 12 for a complete discussion of nutrition)
  b. Evaluations
    (1) Maternal nutritional intake improves
    (2) Fetus continues to grow
    (3) Mother obtains services from referral sources
3. High risk for altered development related to genetic disorder
  a. Interventions
    (1) Assess parents for a genetic history
    (2) Interpret risks, as indicated
    (3) Refer the parents for genetic counseling, as indicated
    (4) Provide appropriate information to assist the couple in making decisions about the outcome of pregnancy

(5) Maintain a nonjudgmental attitude toward the couple and allow the couple to discuss fears and concerns

b. Evaluations

(1) Parents have made an appropriate decision about the outcome of the pregnancy, based on their values and needs

(2) Parents have obtained the necessary services from referral sources

Health Education

A. Nutritional needs for adequate fetal development

1. Calories: 2300 to 2400 per day
2. Protein: 74 to 76 g/day
3. Carbohydrates: an increased requirement is needed to allow for protein uptake for fetal development
4. Fat: provides energy, and fat deposits increase in the fetus from 2% at midpregnancy to 12% at term
5. Vitamins and minerals: a slight increase in intake is needed to provide for the growth of new tissue in the fetus

B. Effects of chemical use (smoking, alcohol, and drugs) on the fetus

1. Timing of ingestion
2. Effect on fetus (teratogenic)
   a. Intrauterine growth retardation
   b. Premature birth
   c. Congenital malformations, as determined by the effects on developing fetal systems
   d. Newborn withdrawal
3. Importance of eliminating chemical use during pregnancy

STUDY QUESTIONS

1. The most critical stage of physical development for the unborn child occurs
   a. During the pre-embryonic stage.
   b. From the third to the eighth week of development.
   c. From the 9th to the 20th week of development.
   d. From the 20th week to delivery.

2. Every organ system and external structure is present in the unborn child by the
   a. Pre-embryonic stage.
   b. Embryonic stage.
   c. Early fetal stage.
   d. Midfetal stage.

3. The major function of vernix caseosa is to
   a. Protect fetal skin from the amniotic fluid.
   b. Prevent adhesions to the amniotic sac.
   c. Enhance the nutrient balance of the amniotic fluid.
   d. Prevent the excessive shedding of fetal tissue.

4. Once a sperm has penetrated the ovum, what prevents other sperm from entering the ovum?
   a. The process of capacitation, which alters the sperm.
   b. The process of acrosomal reaction of the sperm.
   c. The sloughing of the zona pellucida layer.
   d. The zona reaction, which results in cellular changes in the ovum.

5. During which weeks of development is the fetus first able to provide some regulation of its own body functions and body temperature?
   a. At 17 to 20 weeks.
   b. At 21 to 24 weeks.
   c. At 25 to 29 weeks.
   d. At 30 to 34 weeks.

Answers to Study Questions

1. b   2. c   3. a
4. d   5. c

REFERENCES

Auvenshine, M., & Enriquez, M. (1990). *Comprehensive maternity nursing: Perinatal and women's health* (2nd ed.). Boston: Jones & Bartlett.

Bethea, D.C. (1989). *Introductory maternity nursing* (5th ed.). Philadelphia: Lippincott.

Carpenito, L.J. (1984). *Handbook of nursing diagnosis.* Philadelphia: Lippincott.

Creasy, R.K., & Resnik, R. (1989). *Maternal-fetal medicine: Principle and practice* (2nd ed.). Philadelphia: Saunders.

Ladewig, P., London, M., & Olds, S. (1990). *Essentials of maternal-newborn nursing* (2nd ed.). Redwood City, CA: Addison-Wesley Nursing.

Moore, K.L. (1988). *Essentials of human embryology.* Philadelphia: Decker.

Pritchard, J., MacDonald, P., & Grant, M. (1985). *Williams obstetrics* (17th ed.). New York: Appleton-Century-Crofts.

Roberts, A. (1984, April 18). Setting up the system—3. *Nursing Times, 80*(16), 1–4.

Roberts, A. (1984, May 16). Setting up the system—6. *Nursing Times, 80*(20), 1–4.

Roberts, A. (1984, June 20). Setting up the system—9. *Nursing Times, 80*(25), 1–4.

Roberts, A. (1984, July 18). Setting up the system—10. *Nursing Times, 80*(29), 1–4.

Roberts, A. (1984, August 22). Setting up the system—10. *Nursing Times, 80*(34), 1–4.

Roberts, A. (1984, December 19). Setting up the system—10. *Nursing Times, 80*(51), 1–4.

Roberts, A. (1985, January 9). Setting up the system—10. *Nursing Times, 81*(2), 1–4.

Smith, D.W. (1982). *Recognizable patterns of human malformation. Genetic, embryologic and clinical aspects* (3rd ed.). Philadelphia: Saunders.

Spence, A., & Mason, E. (1987). *Human anatomy and physiology* (3rd ed.). Menlo Park, CA: Benjamin/Cummings.

Bonnie Kellogg

Placental Development and Functioning

Objectives

1. Discuss the stages of placental development

2. Describe the functions of the placenta

3. Identify the basic structure of the placenta and cord

4. Explain the implications of ineffective placental development on fetal development

5. Describe the functions of the amniotic fluid

Introduction

A. Placenta

1. Description: the placenta is the temporary organ that provides for fetal respiration and maintains the metabolic and nutrient exchange between the maternal and fetal circulations
2. Development
   a. Endometrium
      (1) Preparation of the endometrium for implantation follows
         (a) Initial preparation occurs during the proliferation phase of the menstrual cycle
         (b) The endometrium becomes thick and increases in vascularity
         (c) Endometrial glands become elongated, and there is an increase in nutrients, such as glycogen, progesterone, and human chorionic gonadotropin (HCG)
      (2) The fertilized egg travels along the fallopian tube toward the uterus
      (3) The egg enters the uterine cavity as a blastocyst; it is nourished by the uterine glands, which produce a fluid in the uterine cavity
      (4) The trophoblast (the outer cell layer of the blastocyst) attaches to the surface of the endometrium
         (a) Approximately 5 to 6 days after fertilization, the blastocyst adheres to the uterine lining
         (b) The site of attachment is usually the upper part of the posterior uterine wall, but it can also be anywhere within the uterine cavity and, occasionally, outside of the uterine cavity

(c) Blastocyst penetrates toward the maternal capillaries by eroding the uterine epithelium

(d) The erosion process continues until the blastocyst is completely embedded in the uterine wall

    (i) The blastocyst collapses

    (ii) Fibrin and coagulum are released at the site of penetration

    (iii) Engulfment of the trophoblast by endometrium occurs

b. Decidua: the portion of the endometrium enveloping the developing fertilized ovum (Fig. 5–1)

(1) On approximately the 14th day, the endometrium begins to change at the site of implantation and is then called the decidua

(2) Implantation causes the adjacent decidual cells to engorge with glycogen and lipids (decidual reaction)

(3) The swollen decidual cells release their contents during the erosion process to provide nourishment to the embryo

(4) The portion of the decidua that covers the embryoblast is called the decidua capsularis

(5) The section below the embryoblast is called the decidua basalis

    (a) This section becomes the maternal portion of the placenta

    (b) It contributes to the vascular supply that nourishes the intervillous spaces

(6) The portion that lines the remainder of the uterine cavity is called the decidua parietalis

c. Placenta

(1) When the embryoblast is partially embedded in the decidua, two distinct layers of cells can be seen in the trophoblast

    (a) Inner layer (cytotrophoblast) is composed of mononucleated cells

        (i) It is the functional layer because it provides the process of nutrient and waste exchange in early fetal development

        (ii) It thins out and disappears at approximately 20 to 24 weeks

    (b) Outer layer (syncytiotrophoblast) consists of multinucleated cells and is responsible for the erosive ability of the trophoblast

(2) The cytotrophoblast and the syncytiotrophoblast separate the maternal and fetal circulations; this barrier is referred to as the placental barrier

(3) On approximately the ninth day, spaces (vacuoles) appear in the syncytium

    (a) These fuse together to form lacunae

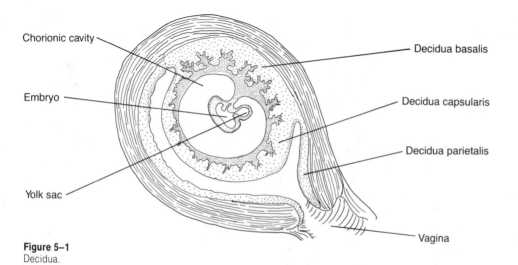

Figure 5–1
Decidua.

Chorionic cavity

Embryo

Yolk sac

Decidua basalis

Decidua capsularis

Decidua parietalis

Vagina

        (b) The lacunae eventually develop into an interconnecting system
        (c) Intervillous spaces are derived from this system
  (4) On approximately the 11th day
        (a) Invading syncytium encounters the congested capillaries of the decidua
        (b) Syncytium enzymes break down the vessel walls, releasing blood into the lacunae
        (c) Eventually, the syncytium encounters the larger arteries and veins and establishes a directional flow of blood
        (d) Blood enters the lacunae
           (i) The embryo experiences rapid growth because of a high concentration of nutrients
          (ii) This growth results in an increase in the distance that nutrients must travel by diffusion to reach the embryo
  (5) Chorionic villi develop between the 9th and 25th days (Fig. 5–2)
        (a) The chorion (trophoblastic cells) is the first placental membrane to form
           (i) It encloses the embryo, amnion, and yolk sac
          (ii) It grows outward, forming fingerlike projections
         (iii) The projections take on a fine, villous appearance
         (iv) Blood vessels develop within the villi
        (b) Initially, the chorion covers the whole chorionic surface
           (i) As the fetus grows and fills the uterus, the intraluminal villi become compressed
          (ii) The compressed villi degenerate
         (iii) Villi located below the embryo continue to grow, forming a large surface for exchange
        (c) The villi develop multiple branches
           (i) The villi that contact the decidua basalis become anchoring villi
             • Decidual septa form between anchoring villi, which results in 15 to 20 lobes (cotyledons)
             • Exchange of gases and nutrients occurs in this vascular system
             • Exchange is limited in the first trimester of development because the placenta has limited permeability
          (ii) Other villi float free and conduct most of the exchange between mother and developing fetus
         (iii) No further villi are formed after the 12th week

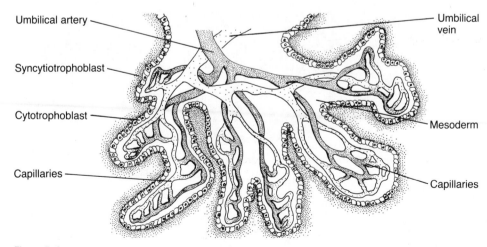

Figure 5–2
Chorionic villi.

(6) Placental growth continues until the 20th week
 (a) At this time, it covers half of the uterine surface
 (b) After 20 weeks, the placenta increases in thickness only
(7) At term
 (a) Placenta is round and flat
 (b) Placenta is approximately 15 to 20 cm (6 to 8 in) in diameter and 2.5 cm (1 in) thick
 (c) Placenta weighs approximately one-sixth of the weight of the baby
 (d) Maternal surface
  (i) Arises from the decidua basalis
  (ii) Has multiple lobules (cotyledons)
  (iii) Is red and blue
 (e) Fetal surface
  (i) Develops from the chorionic villi
  (ii) Is smooth, white, and shiny
  (iii) Contains branches of umbilical veins and arteries
  (iv) Is covered with the chorionic and the amniochorionic membranes
3. Circulation (Fig. 5–3)
 a. Maternal placental circulation
  (1) Oxygenated blood enters the intervillous spaces from the decidua basalis
  (2) Maternal blood pressure directs the blood toward the chorionic villi
  (3) Deoxygenated blood leaves the intervillous spaces through openings in the cytotrophophoblast and enters the endometrial veins

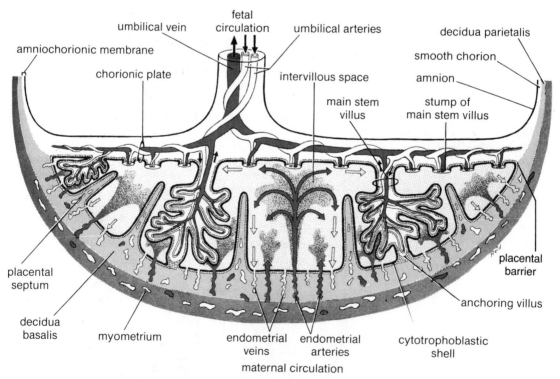

Figure 5–3
Placental circulation. Arrangement of the placental blood vessels. Blood of the fetus flows through the umbilical arteries into the fetal capillaries in the villi and then back to the fetal circulation through the umbilical vein. Maternal blood is transported by the uterine arteries to the intervillous space and leaves by the uterine veins to go back to the maternal circulation. (From Moore, K.L. [1988]. *The developing human* [p. 109]. Philadelphia: Saunders.)

(4) Uterine contractions compress intervillous spaces, forcing the blood into the uterine veins

b. Fetal placental circulation

    (1) Deoxygenated blood leaves the fetus through the two umbilical arteries

    (2) Umbilical arteries divide into multiple branches as they enter the chorionic villi

    (3) Oxygenated blood returns via venules and veins in the chorionic villi

    (4) The veins in the chorionic villi join to form the umbilical vein

4. Mechanism of placental transfer (Table 5–1)

a. Active transport

    (1) Is the passage of substances from mother to fetus against a concentration gradient

    (2) Requires expenditure of energy by the cells

    (3) Can be inhibited by substances that interfere with energy production

    (4) Amino acids, iron, calcium, iodine, and water-soluble vitamins are transported by this process

b. Breaks in the placental membrane

    (1) Defects or breaks allow for the transfer of large cells, such as red blood cells

    (2) This process is responsible for Rh sensitization

        (a) Only when the mother is Rh negative and the fetus is Rh positive

        (b) Rh-positive fetal cells enter the maternal system through a break or defect in the placenta

        (c) Maternal system develops antibodies to the Rh-positive fetal cells

        (d) Process occurs most frequently during delivery

c. Bulk flow

    (1) Transfers substances by osmosis through micropores in the membrane

    (2) This process maintains the maternal-fetal exchange of water

d. Diffusion

    (1) Is the passage of a substance on the basis of its concentration

    (2) The speed of diffusion depends on

        (a) Level of concentration: molecules in higher levels of concentration move more rapidly toward lower concentrations

        (b) Size of the molecule: larger molecules move at a different rate

        (c) Temperature: the higher the temperature, the greater the activity

Table 5–1
PLACENTAL TRANSFER

Type of Transfer	Products Transferred
Active transport	Amino acids Iron Calcium Iodine Water-soluble vitamins
Breaks in membrane	Rh factors which result in isoimmunization
Bulk flow	Water
Diffusion	Oxygen Carbon dioxide Electrolytes Lipid-soluble vitamins
Facilitated diffusion	D-Glucose
Pinocytosis	Some immunoglobulins

(3) Provides the mechanism for the transfer of respiratory gases (oxygen and carbon dioxide) electrolytes, and some lipid-soluble vitamins

(4) Limitations in diffusion are a major factor in placental failure

e. Facilitated diffusion

(1) Occurs when the concentration of material on the maternal side is greater than the concentration levels on the fetal side

(2) Occurs without an expenditure of energy

(3) Occurs at a rate greater than that of simple diffusion

(4) D-Glucose, galactose, and some oxygen are transported by this process

(5) Substances that are highly soluble cross the placenta at a faster rate

   (a) Uncharged particles, such as dissolved carbon dioxide, pass rapidly

   (b) Explains the rapid effect that maternal respiratory acidosis or alkalosis has on the fetus, versus the effect of maternal metabolic acidosis

f. Pinocytosis

(1) Is the transfer by invagination into the cell membrane of a molecule, which then crosses to the opposite side

(2) Microdrops of plasma are taken up by the trophoblasts

(3) Trophoblasts transport immunoglobulins from the plasma to the fetus

5. Transfer disorders

a. Separation of the placenta from the uterine wall

(1) Placenta previa

(2) Placental infarcts

(3) Abruptio placentae

b. Intervillous coagulation and ischemic necrosis

c. Alterations in the membrane as a result of calcifications, thickening, and degeneration may alter permeability

d. Usually result from a problem in maternal circulation

(1) Hypertensive disorders in pregnancy

(2) Diabetes mellitus

(3) Severe maternal malnutrition

e. For placental insufficiency to occur, a major portion of the placenta must be involved

6. Function

a. Respiration

(1) Oxygen in the maternal blood crosses the placental membrane and enters the fetal blood supply by diffusion

(2) Carbon dioxide returns to the maternal system across the placental membrane

(3) Actual fetal pulmonary respiration does not take place in utero

b. Nutrition

(1) Water, inorganic salts, carbohydrates, fats, proteins, and vitamins pass from the maternal blood through the placental membrane into the fetal system via enzymatic carriers

(2) The placenta metabolizes glucose and stores it in the form of glycogen until the fetal liver is able to function

c. Excretion

(1) Waste products cross the placental membrane and enter the maternal blood

(2) Waste products produced by the fetus are minimal

   (a) Fetal metabolism is mainly anabolic (the process of building)

   (b) Waste products are produced through catabolic actions (the breaking down of tissue)

d. Protection

(1) Placental barrier prevents the transfer of many harmful substances from the maternal blood system

(2) Maternal immunity is transferred to the fetus across the placenta

e. Storage: placenta stores carbohydrates, proteins, calcium, and iron until needed

f. Hormonal production
   (1) Placenta secretes and synthesizes hormones necessary for the maintenance of the pregnancy and for fetal development
   (2) These hormones are the steroid hormones estrogen and progesterone and the protein hormones human chorionic gonadotropin, human chorionic somatomammotropin (HCS) (also known as human placental lactogen [HPL]), and thyrotropin

7. Risks
  a. Placenta previa: placenta is implanted in the lower uterus and in some cases, the placenta is over the cervical os
    (1) Cause is unknown but women with a previous history of placenta previa appear to be at increased risk for recurrence
    (2) Types are low lying, partial, and complete
      (a) Low lying placenta previa: attached close to but not over the cervical os
      (b) Partial placenta previa: a small portion of the placenta lies over the cervical os
      (c) Complete placenta previa: the placenta covers the entire cervical os (see Chapter 28 for a complete discussion of placenta previa)
  b. Abruptio placentae: premature separation of the placenta from the maternal surface, resulting in hemorrhage
    (1) Is associated with
      (a) Severe maternal trauma
      (b) Hypertension
      (c) Cigarette smoking
      (d) Alcohol consumption
      (e) Short umbilical cord
      (f) Previous precipitous labor
      (g) Uterine abnormalities
    (2) Three types are central, marginal, and complete
      (a) Central: separation occurs centrally and blood is trapped and, therefore, concealed
      (b) Marginal: blood passes between uterine wall and membrane and escapes out through the vagina
      (c) Complete: total separation results in massive bleeding
    (3) Results for fetus
      (a) If diagnosed early, there may not be any adverse effects on fetus
      (b) If undiagnosed, abruptio placentae may result in fetal death (see Chapter 28 for complete discussion of abruptio placentae)
  c. Infarction of the placenta
    (1) Common placental finding
    (2) Results from an interference in the blood supply to the placental region
    (3) May be associated with maternal disease, such as pre-eclampsia, chronic hypertension, or collagen-vascular disease
  d. Extrachorial placentas
    (1) Membrane rises 1 cm or more central to the margin of the chorionic plate
    (2) May be the result of lateral placental growth or of an implantation that was too deep, causing an undermining of the membranes
    (3) Hemorrhage and separation with resealing may be a cause
    (4) Are frequently seen in the placentas of extramembranous pregnancies
      (a) Rare occurrence: amniotic fluid may leak throughout the pregnancy because of rupture of the membranes
      (b) The ruptured membrane may retract to such an extent that the pregnancy is extramembranous and the fetus is no longer contained within the amniotic sac
      (c) The newborn may have pulmonary hypoplasia because of a lack of amniotic fluid and a resultant inability to inspire in utero
    (5) May be present in 20% of placentas

(a) Are more common in multigravid pregnancies
(b) Familial occurrence has been noted
(c) Are not related to maternal age
(6) Are usually of no major fetal consequence but, if severe, can result in
(a) Prematurity
(b) Hemorrhage
(c) Fetal growth retardation
e. Amnionic bands (Table 5–2)
(1) Believed to arise from ruptures in the amnion, resulting in floating strands and cords of the amnion
(2) Etiology of these ruptures is unknown but ruptures are usually seen near the cord insertion site
(a) Inflammation and trauma have been suggested as possible causes
(b) Amnionic bands have been seen in some pregnancies after amniocentesis has been performed
(c) Oligohydramnios may be present
(3) The floating amnionic strands are sticky and may adhere to the fetus
(a) The bands may restrict embryonic development; facial defects, such as clefts and encephaloceles, and thoracic and abdominal defects, such as scoliosis and gastroschisis, may result
(b) If the bands constrict the extremities, amputation and constriction bands on limbs and digits may result

B. Cord

1. Description: the cord is the connecting link between the fetus and the placenta; it usually contains one large vein and two smaller arteries
2. Development
   a. Formed from the union of the amnion, yolk, and connecting stalk
   b. First trimester
      (1) The body stalk, which attaches the embryo to the yolk sac, contains blood vessels that extend into the chorionic villi
      (2) The body sac fuses with the embryonic portion of the placenta to provide a circulatory pathway from the chorionic villi to the embryo

Table 5–2
ABNORMALITIES RESULTING FROM AMNIONIC BANDS

Fetal Age	Abnormality Most Likely Seen
3 weeks	Anencephaly Facial distortions Facial clefting Encephaloceles
5 weeks	Cleft lip Choanal atresia Limb reduction Syndactyly Abdominal wall defects Thoracic wall defects Scoliosis
7 weeks and after	Ear deformities Amputations Distal lymphedema Foot deformities Omphaloceles

Adapted from Smith, D.W. (1982). *Recognizable patterns of human malformation: Genetic, embryologic, and clinical aspects* (3rd ed.). Philadelphia: Saunders.

(3) The body stalk elongates and becomes the umbilical cord
  (a) The vessels of the cord decrease to one large vein and two smaller arteries
    (i) The umbilical vein contains placental oxygenated blood that returns to the fetus
    (ii) The arteries carry unoxygenated blood to the placenta
  (b) About 1% of umbilical cords have only two vessels, an artery and a vein; this condition is frequently associated with congenital malformations such as
    (i) Sirenomelia, in which the lower limbs are fused, giving the infant a "mermaid" appearance
    (ii) VATERS syndrome, which may comprise any or all of the following
      • Vertebral and ventricular septal defects
      • Anal atresia
      • Tracheoesophageal fistula
      • Esophageal atresia
      • Radial and renal dysplasia
      • Single umbilical artery
    (iii) Trisomies 13 and 18
  (c) The cord has no nerves
(4) Specialized gelatinous connective tissue, called Wharton's jelly, surrounds the blood vessels
  (a) This tissue and the high blood volume provide pressure through the vessel
  (b) Prevents compression of the umbilical cord in utero
(5) At term, the average cord is about 55 cm (22 in) long
  (a) A cord of less than 32 cm (13 in) may indicate problems with the fetus
    (i) There may be severe fetal abnormalities, such as renal agenesis
    (ii) A short cord is often seen in cases of pulmonary hypoplasia
    (iii) A short cord may predispose to abruptio placentae or cord rupture
  (b) An unusually long cord is associated with cord prolapse and fetal entrapment
(6) The cord can attach itself to the placenta at various sites, but central insertion into the placenta is considered normal; abnormalities include
  (a) Velamentous insertion, in which the cord is implanted at the edge of the placenta and fetal vessels separate in the membranes before reaching the placenta (see Chapter 15, Fig. 15–1)
    (i) Origin is related to an eccentric development of primary vasculation
    (ii) Increased incidence of structural defects in the fetus is seen
      • Congenital hip dislocation
      • Asymmetrical head shape
    (iii) May increase risk for intrauterine growth retardation and preterm birth
  (b) Vasa praevia is associated with velamentous insertion of the cord, in which the vessels lie over the internal os in front of the fetus
    (i) The vessels may be compressed, compromising oxygen exchange in the fetus
    (ii) If the vessels rupture, the fetus may experience severe blood loss, which may occur when membranes rupture
  (c) Marginal insertion (battledore)
    (i) Occurs in 2 to 15% of gestations
    (ii) Is associated with a higher-than-normal frequency of preterm labor and birth
(7) The cord can appear twisted or spiraled

(a) Is most likely caused by fetal movement
(b) A true knot in the cord rarely occurs; when there is a true knot in the cord, the cord is usually longer than normal, allowing the fetus to pass through a loop in the cord
(c) So-called false knots are more common
    (i) False knots are caused by the folding of the cord vessel
    (ii) False knots are not usually a problem for the developing fetus
(8) When the umbilical cord is around the neck of the fetus, it is called a nuchal cord

C. Amniotic fluid

1. Description: amniotic fluid is pale, straw-colored fluid in which the fetus floats
2. Development
  a. Early pregnancy
    (1) Shortly after fertilization, a cleft forms in the morula
    (2) Two membranes form around the developing embryo
      (a) The outer membrane is the chorion
      (b) The inner membrane is the amnion
    (3) As the cleft enlarges, it becomes fused with the surrounding amnion, creating the amniotic sac
    (4) The sac then fills with colorless fluid
    (5) The volume of fluid increases to an average of 50 ml at 12 weeks' gestation
    (6) The fluid is produced by the amnionic membrane covering the placenta
  b. Second trimester to delivery (Fig. 5–4)
    (1) Fetus modifies amniotic fluid through the processes of swallowing and urinating
    (2) The volume can also be modified through movement of fluid through the fetal respiratory tract
3. Volume
  a. There is a wide range of amniotic fluid volume during pregnancy
  b. Normal approximations of volume
    (1) At 12 weeks, there is approximately 50 ml
    (2) At 20 weeks, there is approximately 400 ml
    (3) At 36 to 38 weeks, there is approximately 1 l
    (4) Volume decreases after 38 weeks
4. Function
  a. Provides a medium for fetal movement
  b. Protects the fetus against injury from external causes
  c. Assists in maintaining temperature
  d. Distends the amniotic sac
  e. May be an important factor in dilating the cervical canal
  f. Prevents the amnion from adhering to the developing fetus
5. Composition
  a. Consists of approximately 98% water
  b. Is alkaline in reaction (pH is 7.0 to 7.25)
  c. Early pregnancy
    (1) Similar in composition to maternal plasma
    (2) Contains a lower protein concentration than maternal plasma
    (3) Is nearly devoid of particulate matter
  d. Second trimester to delivery (see Fig. 5–4)
    (1) As pregnancy progresses, phospholipids (from the lung) accumulate in the fluid
    (2) Variable amounts of particulate matter occur from the shedding of fetal cells, lanugo, scalp hair, and vernix caseosa into the fluid
    (3) Osmolality decreases
    (4) Fluid becomes hypotonic as a result of fetal urination

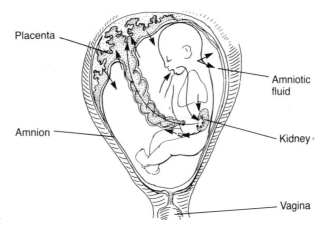

Placenta

Amniotic
fluid

Amnion

Kidney

Figure 5–4
Circulation of amniotic fluid.

Vagina

(5) Fluid contains higher levels of urea, creatinine, and uric acid than the plasma does
6. Abnormalities in volume
    a. Oligohydramnios (decreased amounts of amniotic fluid)
      (1) Less than 500 ml between 32 and 36 weeks
      (2) Common causes
        (a) Amniotic leakage
        (b) Abnormalities of the fetal kidneys (for example, renal agenesis)
      (3) Primary oligohydramnios is associated with fetal abnormalities such as
        (a) Renal agenesis
        (b) Polycystic kidneys
        (c) Urinary tract obstructions
      (4) Oligohydramnios that occurs during or before the second trimester usually results in a poor pregnancy outcome
        (a) Compression of the fetus
        (b) Fetal death is due to respiratory insufficiency and a lack of late development of the lung
    b. Hydramnios (increased amounts of amniotic fluid)
      (1) Exceeds 2 l of fluid between 32 and 36 weeks
      (2) Is often associated with poor fetal outcomes because of
        (a) Preterm delivery
        (b) Fetal malpresentation
        (c) Cord prolapse
      (3) Hydramnios that occurs during or before second trimester spontaneously resolves in 45% of the cases, resulting in normal outcomes
      (4) Pathogenesis is usually unclear
        (a) Is possibly caused by defective regulation of fluid transfer across the amniochorion
        (b) Is seen in Rh-sensitized pregnancies, monozygotic multiple pregnancy, and gestational or insulin-dependent diabetes mellitus
        (c) May be seen with fetal gastrointestinal obstructions or atresias

Clinical Practice

A. Assessment

1. History
    a. Previous pregnancies and outcomes
    b. Known uterine infections
    c. Episodes of bleeding, hypertension, and trauma

2. Physical signs of placental risk
   a. Bleeding
   b. Sudden and severe abdominal pain
   c. Uterine rigidity
   d. Fundal height not appropriate for gestational age
3. Diagnostic tests
   a. Ultrasonography can determine
      (1) Location of the placenta
      (2) Placental grading
      (3) Amniotic volume
      (4) Fetal growth
      (5) Fetal abnormalities
   b. Kleihauer-Betke blood test to determine if of maternal or fetal origin
   c. Amniocentesis for analysis of fluid

B. Nursing Diagnoses

1. High risk for altered fluid volume (deficit or excess) related to impaired placental transport
2. High risk for altered fetal growth related to impaired placental transport of nutrients
3. High risk for impaired fetal gas exchange related to impaired placental transport

C. Interventions/Evaluations

1. High risk for altered fluid volume (deficit or excess) related to impaired placental transport
   a. Interventions
      (1) Explain diagnostic tests (ultrasonography and amniocentesis) to client and family
      (2) Remain with client during procedure, if possible
      (3) Clarify misconceptions and allow client to discuss fears and concerns
      (4) Ensure that the client and her family understand the test results and the test's implications
   b. Evaluations
      (1) Client and family can explain the reason for the diagnostic procedure
      (2) Client reports an understanding of test results
      (3) Client reports decreased anxiety about the test procedure
2. High risk for altered fetal growth related to impaired placental transport of nutrients
   a. Interventions
      (1) Explain the importance of adequate nutritional intake
      (2) Discuss the possible consequences of poor nutritional intake
      (3) Evaluate maternal nutritional intake
   b. Evaluations
      (1) Client complies with proposed nutritional program
      (2) Client can explain the possible negative consequences to the fetus resulting from poor maternal nutritional intake
3. High risk for impaired fetal gas exchange related to impaired placental transport
   a. Interventions
      (1) Explain the possible outcome of poor fetal gas exchange
      (2) Explain the importance of compliance with the testing regimen
      (3) Reinforce the need for the left lateral position to improve uteroplacental circulation when the client is recumbent
   b. Evaluations
      (1) Client is able to explain the possible outcome to fetus of poor gas exchange

(2) Client agrees to comply with recommended antepartal testing

(3) Client agrees to lie in the left lateral position when recumbent during the remainder of the pregnancy

Health Education

A. Thorough explanation of the reasons for and the procedures used in ultrasonography and amniocentesis

B. Importance of prenatal visits for assessing fetal well-being

C. Importance of relating any unusual symptoms to health care provider

D. Implications of any symptoms

E. Review of the stages of fetal development and the role of the placenta and amniotic fluid

---

STUDY QUESTIONS

1. The main function of the placenta is
   a. To provide a nutrient exchange between maternal and fetal circulations.
   b. To ensure that the fetus is protected from trauma.
   c. To provide a mechanism for the direct exchange of oxygen and carbon dioxide.
   d. To allow for the elimination of excess fetal hormones.

2. Which of the following statements best describes placental development?
   a. It develops rapidly, with limited changes after the first month.
   b. It continues to develop and grow throughout pregnancy.
   c. Major growth and development occur in the first trimester.
   d. There are two major stages of development; these are in the first and third trimesters.

3. The cord is formed from
   a. Union of the amnion and the yolk sac.
   b. Maternal tissue.
   c. Combination of Wharton's jelly and chorionic villi.
   d. Compressed endometrium.

4. What is the major reason for monitoring placental growth and function?
   a. To predict fetal positioning at time of birth.
   b. To evaluate fetal well-being.
   c. To predict gestational age at delivery.
   d. To indicate risk factors for chromosomal abnormalities.

5. Which of the following are the major functions of amniotic fluid?
   a. Provides respiratory and nutritional exchange between fetal and maternal circulation.
   b. Is a major component of fetal blood circulation and hormone production.
   c. Protects the fetus from injury by cushioning it from trauma and maintains a constant temperature.
   d. Is an important component in monitoring and altering fetal biochemical status.

6. Which of the following produces the majority of human chorionic gonadotropin?
   a. The uterus.
   b. The ovarian follicles.
   c. The umbilical cord.
   d. The placenta.

Answers to Study Questions

1. a	2. c	3. a
4. b	5. c	6. d

REFERENCES

Auvenshine, M., & Enriquez, M. (1990). *Comprehensive maternity nursing: Perinatal and women's health* (2nd ed.). Boston: Jones & Bartlett.

Carpenito, L.J. (1984). *Handbook of nursing diagnosis*. Philadelphia: Lippincott.

Gabbe, S.G., Niebyl, J.R., & Simpson, J.L. (Eds.) (1986). *Obstetrics: Normal and problem pregnancies.* New York: Churchill Livingstone.

Green, J. (1989). Placental abnormalities: Placenta previa and abruptio placentae. In R. Creasy & R. Resnick (Eds.), *Maternal fetal medicine: Principles and practices.* Philadelphia: Saunders.

Ladewig, P., London, M., & Olds, S. (1990). *Essentials of maternal-newborn nursing* (2nd ed.). Redwood City, CA: Addison-Wesley Nursing.

Lavery, J.P. (1987). *The human placenta.* Rockville, MD: Aspen.

May, K.A., & Mahlmeister, L.R. (1990). *Comprehensive maternity nursing: Nursing process and the childbearing family.* Philadelphia: Lippincott.

Myles, M.F. (1985). *Textbook for midwives with modern concepts of obstetrics and neonatal care* (10th ed.). London: Churchill Livingstone.

Pritchard, J., MacDonald, P., & Grant, M. (1985). *Williams obstetrics* (17th ed.). New York: Appleton-Century-Crofts.

Reeder, S.J., Mastroianni, L., & Martin, L.L. (1983). *Maternity nursing* (15th ed.). Philadelphia: Lippincott.

Roberts, A. (1983, July 20). Setting up the system—3. *Nursing Times, 79*(29), 57–60.

Roberts, A. (1983, October 5). Setting up the system—6. *Nursing Times, 79*(40), 49–52.

Roberts, A. (1983, November 2). Setting up the system—7. *Nursing Times, 79*(44), 61–64.

Roberts, A. (1984, February 15). Setting up the system—10. *Nursing Times, 80*(7), 1–4.

Smith, D.W. (1982). *Recognizable patterns of human malformation: Genetic, embryologic, and clinical aspects* (3rd ed.). Philadelphia: Saunders.

Spence, A., & Mason, E. (1987). *Human anatomy and physiology* (3rd ed.). Menlo Park, CA: Benjamin/Cummings.

Thompson, E.D. (1990). *Introduction to maternity and pediatric nursing.* Philadelphia: Saunders.

NORMAL PREGNANCY

Susan Mattson

Ethnocultural Considerations in the Childbearing Period

Objectives

1. State the need for a cultural assessment of the childbearing family

2. Describe data to be collected through a cultural assessment

3. Perform a cultural assessment of a childbearing family

4. Use data obtained to formulate a care plan for the childbearing family

5. Analyze data obtained from a cultural assessment for potential problem areas

6. Formulate nursing interventions to prevent anticipated problems identified from the assessment

7. Identify barriers to care that are frequently encountered by the culturally diverse client

8. Identify ways to decrease barriers to care encountered by the culturally diverse client

Introduction

A. **According to Boyle and Andrews (1989), the major goal of transcultural nursing is to provide nursing care that is culturally relevant and meets the needs of diverse clients**

1. Applying transcultural concepts to nursing practice includes
   a. Identifying cultural needs
   b. Understanding the cultural context of the client and family
   c. Using culturally sensitive strategies to meet mutually satisfying goals
2. A common problem faced by nurses who want to use cultural data is knowing what data to collect and how to use the data effectively
   a. A major purpose of collecting cultural data is to give the nurse greater insight into and understanding of
      (1) The nature and behavior of clients
      (2) The problems that clients encounter in health promotion and maintenance
      (3) Clients' ways of coping with illness
   b. These data should be relevant to potential or actual nursing problems
   c. Transcultural knowledge is used to augment, clarify, explain, or assist in attaining client-centered goals

B. Kitzinger (1982) believed that any approach to culturally sensitive care for childbearing women and their families must focus on the interaction between cultural meaning and biological functions

1. All cultures recognize pregnancy as a special transitional period
2. Many cultures have particular customs and beliefs that dictate activities and behavior during this time
3. The labor and delivery and postpartum periods may also be governed by unique customs
   a. Cultural factors influencing labor and delivery center on a general attitude toward
      (1) Birth
      (2) Methods of dealing with the pain of labor
      (3) Preferred positions during delivery
      (4) The role of support persons and health practitioners
   b. Many cultures consider the postpartum period to be one of increased vulnerability for both mother and infant
      (1) Dietary and activity proscriptions are very common at this time and may be in conflict with the usual Western methods of obstetrical care
      (2) Infant care also varies from culture to culture in regard to
         (a) Bathing
         (b) Swaddling
         (c) Feeding
         (d) Care of the umbilical cord
         (e) Circumcision

C. The different ways in which a particular society views this transitional period and manages childbirth are dependent on the culture's beliefs about health, medical care, reproduction, and the role and status of women (Fig. 6–1)

1. These beliefs also contribute to an unwillingness on the part of the client to use existing health care services
2. The practice of these beliefs often creates barriers for the nurse, who attempts to deliver care from a U.S. model
3. In addition to the previous concepts, there are others that influence the interaction between a culturally diverse client and U.S. health care
   a. Language
   b. Time orientation
   c. Use of folk practices for healing (including the concept of a hot and cold balance)
   d. Religious beliefs
   e. Family structure and dynamics in decision making
4. One must keep in mind the individual differences that are present *within* cultures as well as those found *between* cultures
5. It is difficult to portray an example of cultural behaviors without seeming to stereotype
6. In the following discussion, try to view the descriptions as general overviews, not as examples of the way that every person from that cultural group acts

Clinical Practice

A. Assessment

1. Introduction
   a. Cultural assessment is defined as assessment of
      (1) Shared beliefs
      (2) Values
      (3) Customs that have relevance to health behaviors (Tripp-Reimer & Brink, 1984)

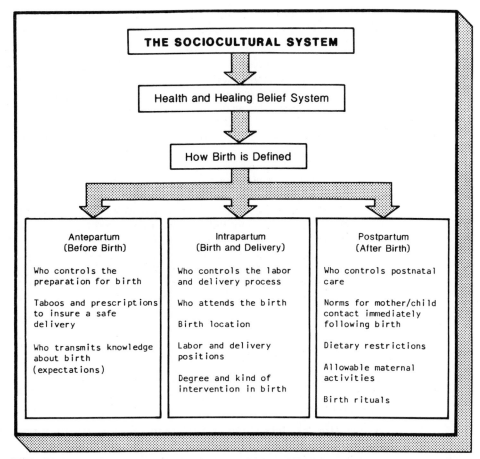

Figure 6–1
Components of the childbearing system. A culturally diverse woman, familiar with her own ethnic group's childbearing system, may feel estranged by the dominant culture's birth practices. (From Mattson, S., Galanti, G., Lettieri, C., & Kellogg, J. [1986]. *Culture and health module 2: The family and life cycle in transcultural perspective* [p. 60]. Carson, CA: Statewide Nursing Program, Consortium of the California State University.)

   b. It is performed to identify patterns that may assist or interfere with a nursing intervention or planned treatment regimen
   c. To understand why birth is managed in a particular way, it is necessary to view the process in terms of the society's
      (1) Social organization
      (2) Political and economic system
      (3) Medical theory
   d. In addition, Kay (1982) delineated specific cultural data for the four periods during childbearing: antepartum, intrapartum, postpartum, and newborn period; this chapter discusses assessment needs during each of these four periods (for specific details about particular cultural groups, see the material referenced in appropriate chapters and sections; see also the appendix at the end of this chapter)
2. History
   a. Antepartum period
      (1) Determinants of the society's acceptance of the pregnancy
         (a) Acceptable age
         (b) Marriage requirements
         (c) Acceptable father
         (d) Pregnancy frequency
      (2) Consideration of pregnancy as a state of illness or of health
      (3) Behavioral expectations

(a) Dietary prescriptions or restrictions
    (i) Adherence to the hot or cold theory of health and diet (especially with Hispanic and Asian clients)
- This theory describes the intrinsic properties of foods, beverages, medicines, and their effects on the body
- Health is maintained through a balance of these forces
- If an imbalance occurs, illness results
- To produce balance (and restore or maintain health), illness and conditions such as pregnancy are treated with substances having the opposite property of the illness (i.e., pregnancy is considered to be a hot state; thus any treatments must be of a cold nature)
  - □ However, temperature and spiciness do not determine classification, which varies among cultural groups
  - □ Generally, warm or hot foods are believed to be easier to digest than cold or cool foods
- These properties of hot and cold are also part of the yin-yang belief system prevalent among Asian approaches to health and diet (Andrews, 1989)

    (ii) Another unfamiliar practice that nurses might encounter is that of pica, or the ingestion of nonfood substances, especially clay or starch
- Pica is often practiced by Afro-American women, usually in the rural southern United States
- There are many explanations for why this occurs
  - □ A result of an iron deficiency that leads to the craving
  - □ A carryover from behaviors practiced in Africa
  - □ For attention

(see Chapter 12 for a further discussion of nutrition)
(b) Activity restrictions or prescriptions, including the use of massage as a treatment for the various ills experienced during pregnancy
(c) Expression of emotions, including anger, fear, and anxiety
(4) People from whom to seek advice, and the appropriate time to do so
    (a) Women from many cultures may refuse to seek early prenatal care because they consider pregnancy a normal and healthy state
    (b) Fear, modesty, and a wish to avoid a physical examination by a male care provider may also prevent some women from seeking care from Western providers (Andrews, 1989)
  b. Intrapartum period
    (1) Appropriate setting for labor and delivery to occur
    (2) Appropriate attendants for support and as a "practitioner"
      (a) Most non-Western cultures see childbearing as being within the woman's domain
        (i) Support during labor and assistance after delivery are usually provided by women relatives or friends
        (ii) It is unusual, and should not be expected, for a father from a non-Western culture to provide this support and caretaking
      (b) Male caregivers may be refused
    (3) Expectations of pain control, including what expressions of discomfort are permitted and expected
    (4) Restrictions and prescriptions for activity, including ambulation and massage
    (5) Dietary recommendations, including the continuation of intake of food and drink; many women prefer herbal teas
    (6) Expected length of labor
      (a) Behaviors that are necessary to ensure the appropriate length, including diet and activity

      (b) Expected interventions if the time is prolonged
- (7) Expected and ideal positions for facilitating pushing and delivery
    - (a) Squatting
    - (b) Sitting
    - (c) Side-lying
- (8) Appropriate disposition of placenta and umbilical cord after delivery
    - (a) Some cultural groups believe that burying the placenta, the umbilical cord, or both in a particular place will bring good fortune to the child and family
    - (b) Others wish to preserve the cord through drying to use it medicinally at a later time
- c. Postpartum period
    - (1) Activity restrictions and prescriptions
        - (a) The postpartum period is viewed by many as one that is fraught with dangers for both mother and infant
            - (i) One way to protect against danger is for the mother to remain quietly in bed, with little activity to disturb her
            - (ii) This includes a restriction on
                - Ambulating
                - Bathing (especially showering)
                - Infant caretaking
                - Other activities seen as normal from a Western medical perspective
        - (b) In some cultures, women are considered to be in a state of impurity during the puerperium, which often coincides with the period of lochial flow; common behaviors include
            - (i) Seclusion and avoidance of contact with others
            - (ii) Avoidance of sexual relations
    - (2) Dietary restrictions and prescriptions
        - (a) Many of the same requirements that are based on a theory of hot and cold also affect postpartum guides
        - (b) The puerperium is a cold time, so foods should be hot in nature; women will avoid fruits and vegetables that are considered cold
    - (3) Appropriateness of therapeutic heat and cold
        - (a) Western practitioners often use cold packs or sitz baths for perineal comfort and healing
        - (b) These practices are not acceptable to women from many cultures
            - (i) Cold air and water are frequently believed to be harmful
            - (ii) They are believed to cause uterine problems and even infertility when they enter the uterus through the vagina (Greener, 1989)
- d. Newborn period
    - (1) Feeding of the infant, including the method and timing of the first feeding
        - (a) Cultures' advocacy of breastfeeding varies, and many influences must be taken into consideration
        - (b) While American women are choosing to breastfeed in increasing numbers, immigrants from developing and poorer countries see bottlefeeding as the modern way to provide nourishment to their infants
        - (c) Hispanic women, in particular, believe that colostrum is bad for the baby and prefer to bottlefeed until their milk comes in
    - (2) Bathing of the baby, including
        - (a) Time of the first bath
        - (b) Appropriate person to perform the bath
        - (c) Measures used to protect the infant during the procedure
            - (i) Traditional Hispanics believe that both the head and feet should be wet

(ii) Water will be placed on the head at the same time that the body is immersed in the bath (Clark, 1978)

(3) Sleeping arrangement provided for the baby and what is done to promote sleeping

(a) Women often keep the baby physically as close as possible, often sharing the same bed

(b) This is particularly true if ritual seclusion and limited activity are enforced

(4) Swaddling practices

(5) Circumcision

(a) Cultures vary greatly in their beliefs about this practice

(b) Ritual circumcision is frequently practiced in traditional Judaism

(6) Caretaking of the baby at home

(a) Appropriate person to do so

(b) Length of time that the baby is allowed to cry before being attended to

(i) Some cultures expect that babies will be picked up and attended to (usually breastfed) immediately

(ii) Others believe that the infant should be allowed to cry for a certain period

(c) Care of the umbilical cord

(i) Hispanic, Filipino, and Afro-American women may use an abdominal binder or "belly band" to protect the umbilical area against dirt, injury, or hernia

(ii) These binders are usually not seen by the Western care provider because they are removed before office or clinic visits

(iii) Oils may also be applied to the umbilical cord stump (Greener, 1989)

(7) Ritual beautification varies according to cultural interpretation and may be done to avoid the evil eye: Navajo babies have their ears pierced and turquoise earrings inserted to provide protection from evil forces (Kay, 1982)

(8) Attachment behaviors toward the infant

(a) Asian and Middle Eastern women, in particular, may be erroneously assessed as demonstrating maladaptive attachment behaviors

(b) Asian women maintain a distance and do not praise their infants because of a fear of evil influences harming the baby if he or she were seen to be joyfully received

(c) Middle Eastern women believe that the mother is the one deserving of praise for her great work in producing the infant (Meleis & Sorrell, 1981)

3. Physical findings (Fig. 6–5)

a. Differences in pelvic shape and size related to race; (see Chapter 14 for further discussion)

b. Differences in infant size related to ethnic influences (see Chapter 22 for further discussion)

4. Psychosocial findings

a. Refusal to accept or use Western medical services

b. Distress occurs when women are forced to do so if care is provided without cultural sensitivity, for example, when

(1) Modesty is not acknowledged and protected

(2) Male caretakers are provided

(3) There are inappropriate expectations of participation by the expectant father or husband and restrictions on other family members' presence

(4) There are inappropriate expectations of caretaking activities of the client in regard to herself and her infant

B. Nursing Diagnoses

Transcultural nursing diagnoses can be adopted that will expand the scope of practice to include the specific cultural needs of clients and reflect cultural sensitivity rather than bias, for example
1. Adherence to traditional beliefs about hot and cold
2. Alteration in communication patterns related to language barrier
3. Adherence to the traditional cultural group's dietary beliefs
4. Adherence to the traditional cultural group's activity practices

In addition, more familiar diagnoses are also appropriate

5. Fear secondary to an unknown environment
6. Anxiety related to culturally unusual expectations for behavior and treatment

C. Interventions/Evaluations

1. Adherence to traditional beliefs about hot and cold
   a. Interventions
      (1) Offer warm drinks immediately post partum
      (2) Offer heat lamps or hot packs rather than sitz baths or ice application to the perineum
      (3) Provide extra blankets for warmth
      (4) Provide a balance between the hot and cold forces by offering medications with warm liquids if requested by client
   b. Evaluation: client successfully balances hot and cold elements in diet, medication, and treatment regimens, as evidenced by her expression of satisfaction
2. Alteration in communication patterns related to language barrier
   a. Interventions
      (1) Provide and use an interpreter, when necessary
      (2) Use the interpreter appropriately
         (a) Most women prefer another woman when discussing intimate matters
         (b) The interpreter should not be a child
            (i) It is not appropriate for a child to have knowledge of childbearing
            (ii) The child will have unusual power over the parent because of the knowledge gained
         (c) Refrain from using slang or medical jargon that may be difficult for the interpreter to translate
      (3) Assess the client's ability to read and write before providing written information in the native language
   b. Evaluation: client experiences an increase in communication with the nurse through the appropriate use of an interpreter
3. Adherence to the traditional cultural group's dietary practices
   a. Interventions
      (1) Assess what foods the client prefers to eat or not to eat
      (2) Encourage preferred dietary practices if they are not shown to cause harm to the mother or fetus
      (3) Permit and encourage family members to bring foods into the hospital, if necessary
   b. Evaluation: client expresses satisfaction with dietary provisions
4. Adherence to traditional cultural group's practices
   a. Interventions
      (1) Assess what practices the mother wishes to follow related to
         (a) Bathing
         (b) Ambulation

(c) Infant caretaking
(2) Modify usual hospital practices to accommodate client preferences
   (a) Explain the rationale for early ambulation
   (b) Encourage the mother to move frequently in bed and perhaps to sit by the bedside rather than to completely ambulate
   (c) Provide an opportunity for bathing in bed with warm water, rather than showering
   (d) Encourage family members or the other support person to assume care of the infant
   b. Evaluation: client expresses satisfaction with activity level and caretaking responsibilities
5. Fear secondary to an unknown environment
   a. Interventions
      (1) Encourage family members to remain with the client if so desired
      (2) Explain procedures and reinforce the explanations given by others
         (a) Use terminology that is understood
         (b) Avoid taboo or inappropriate language or terminology
      (3) Include family members in decision making, particularly the expectant father or husband
      (4) Incorporate traditional practices as expressed by the client into the care plan, when possible
      (5) Avoid practices in conflict with cultural traditions, when possible
   b. Evaluations: client experiences a decrease in fear of the unknown environment
      (1) By describing expected behaviors or treatment
      (2) Through use of a family member for support and decision making
      (3) By using traditional elements of care
      (4) By avoiding practices that conflict with cultural traditions
6. Anxiety related to culturally unusual expectations for behavior and treatment
   a. Interventions
      (1) Assess the level of anxiety through overt and covert manifestations
      (2) Assess the client's expectations for behavior and treatment
      (3) Incorporate culturally traditional expectations into the care plan
         (a) Allow the activity and position of choice during labor and delivery
         (b) Allow the family member of choice to provide support
         (c) Alter Western expectations for activity and hygiene during the postpartum period to allow comfort for the new mother
         (d) Observe mother-infant interactions in the context of cultural expectations
   b. Evaluations: client experiences less anxiety about unexpected behaviors and treatment
      (1) By sharing with the nurse culturally expected behaviors
      (2) By using usual behaviors, when possible
      (3) By expressing an understanding of the need to use unfamiliar behaviors, when necessary

Health Education

A. **Before education can begin with culturally diverse clients, the assessment just described must be performed to establish a valid data base**

1. Strategies that are based on cultural knowledge are more likely to be successful than those not based on such data
2. Unless based on cultural information, nursing interventions may be inappropriate or incomplete, rather than allowing modification to meet the client's cultural needs

B. Approaches may

1. Integrate scientific knowledge and folk practices, if necessary
2. Affect the client's behavior
3. Result in understanding on the nurse's part about why change cannot occur

C. Educational strategies

1. Explain the rationale for a scientific approach to care if it is significantly different from that proposed by the client
2. If proposed practices are not harmful to the mother or fetus, allow them to continue
3. If proposed practices are harmful, attempt to alter behaviors to include more beneficial ones
4. Elicit assistance and support from the established caretaker in the family, e.g., a grandmother or an aunt
5. Obtain approval and consent for treatment from the proper person, e.g., the husband or father
6. Demonstrate how scientific and folk practices can be combined to provide optimum care for the mother and baby
7. Recognize when compromise is not possible without destroying the family's entire cultural belief system

CASE STUDIES AND STUDY QUESTIONS

Mrs. Gonzales, a Mexican-American, has come to your antepartum clinic for the first time. She is a gravida 3, para 2 (G3,P2) and is at 32 weeks' gestation. Through an interpreter, she tells you that she is feeling fine, had no problems with her previous pregnancies, and has only come for prenatal care at the urging of the nurse in the well-child clinic where her two children receive immunizations. She believes it is important to balance the hot and cold humors and eats according to the prescriptions for accomplishing this during pregnancy; she avoids "hot" foods, iron preparations, and milk (because of a lactose intolerance). She is kept active caring for her family (her children are ages 2 and 5 years) and believes that this will ensure a small baby and an easy delivery; she also believes that sleeping flat on her back protects the fetus from harm.

1. Who is the best person to serve as an interpreter for this woman?

   a. A woman 20 to 30 years old.

   b. A man 20 to 30 years old.

   c. A young girl in her early teens.

   d. A young boy 8 to 10 years old.

2. What is an appropriate approach to discussing her possible dietary deficiencies?

   a. Tell her the beliefs in a balance of hot and cold are superstition.

   b. Tell her that it is important that she include milk and an iron preparation in her diet.

   c. Explore with her acceptable alternatives to milk and iron preparations that she can ingest.

   d. Refer her to a nutritionist who will construct a specific diet for her.

3. What is an appropriate question to ask this woman?

   a. Will your husband be with you during labor and delivery?

   b. Who will you want to be with you during labor and delivery?

   c. Are you attending any childbirth preparation classes?

   d. Do you know that sleeping on your back is actually bad for the baby?

4. What is a good approach for the nurse in caring for this woman?

   a. Instruct her in the components of a balanced diet.

   b. Tell her the benefits of regular and early prenatal care.

   c. Enroll her and her husband in a childbirth preparation class.

   d. Ensure female care providers as often as possible.

You are assigned to care for Mrs. Tran, a Vietnamese who gave birth 12 hours previously. When you enter the room, she is lying in bed with the baby in the bassinette beside her. There is a full bottle in the crib. She has not had a shower, and most of her food remains on her breakfast tray: she has eaten only the tea and toast. When you exclaim over the baby, she merely turns her head away and does not comment.

5. What is an appropriate comment or question for her regarding her food intake?

   a. "If you don't eat more you won't have the strength to care for your baby."

   b. "Why didn't you eat your cereal, juice, and fruit?"

   c. "Do you have special food requirements during this time that I could help with or that your family could bring in?"

   d. "Don't you like our food?"

6. What should you assess about her activity and bathing?

   a. Whether there are cultural restrictions on her activity that prohibit her from showering at this time.

   b. When she will take a shower.

   c. When she will get out of bed and ambulate.

   d. Whether she is going to feed the baby soon.

7. What kind of behavior would you expect to see in regard to the baby?

   a. Great joy expressed by the mother about the birth of the baby.

   b. Appreciation for compliments about the baby by the staff.

   c. Willingness to take complete charge of caring for the baby.

   d. Maintaining of a distance toward the baby during the first few days, with caretaking done by others.

8. Who would you expect to be at her bedside helping her to take care of herself and the infant?

   a. No one.

   b. Her mother or grandmother.

   c. Her husband.

   d. Her neighbors.

You are interviewing Ms. Green, a 17-year-old gravida 2, para 1 (G2, P1) Afro-American originally from Georgia, who at 28 weeks of gestation is now attending your prenatal clinic for the first time.

9. Which of the following questions is appropriate for you to ask when taking her history?

   (1) "Do you have any special food requirement or cravings that you need to follow during pregnancy?"

   (2) "Do you believe any special restrictions on your activity are necessary for a safe pregnancy?"

   (3) "Do you consider pregnancy an illness?"

   (4) "Why haven't you come in for prenatal care before? You know you should have done so."

   (5) "Aren't you a little young to be pregnant for the second time?"

   a. 1, 3, 5.

   b. 1, 2, 3.

   c. 2, 3, 5.

   d. 1, 2.

Mrs. Chao, a Laotian, her husband, and her mother come into the labor and delivery area. She is a 20-year-old gravida 1, para 0 (G1, P0) at term. When being examined, she frequently pulls the sheet over her and looks away from her husband, who appears uncomfortable. She is found to be 7 cm dilated, completely effaced, and at −1 station. She sits upright in the bed, only grimacing with contractions. Her mother asks if her daughter may have a cup of hot tea to drink.

10. What is an important component of a care plan for this family?

   (1) Determine which family member(s) the patient would prefer to support her during labor.

   (2) Make sure that the patient has ice chips at the bedside at all times.

(3) Assess the patient frequently for signs and behavior indicative of increasing discomfort.

(4) Provide for as much privacy and modesty as possible.

(5) Insist that the patient lie on one side or the other during the rest of her labor.

a. All of the above.

b. 1, 3, 4.

c. 1, 3.

d. 2, 3, 5.

11. Which of the following is essential to providing effective perinatal care to families of different cultures?

(1) Including cultural and family assessments as part of the routine history.

(2) Insisting that the family adhere to scientific and medical principles of care at all times.

(3) Assessing all culturally different beliefs as harmful.

(4) Providing the services of an interpreter if a language barrier exists.

(5) Fostering an attitude of respect for alternative healing practices.

a. 1, 3, 5.

b. 2, 3, 5.

c. 1, 4, 5.

d. All of the above.

12. Which of the following might prevent culturally diverse families from seeking maternity care in U.S. health care institutions?

a. The presence of interpreters to assist with language differences.

b. Culturally sensitive care provided by health care practitioners.

c. Clinics that are easily accessible and in local neighborhoods.

d. Long clinic waits in urban centers that are structured to accommodate clients as a group, not as individuals.

Answers to Study Questions

1. a	2. c	3. b
4. d	5. c	6. a
7. d	8. b	9. b
10. b	11. c	12. d

REFERENCES

Andrews, M. (1989). Culture and nutrition. In J. Boyle & M. Andrews (Eds.), *Transcultural concepts in nursing care* (pp. 333–355). Glenview, IL: Scott, Foresman/Little, Brown College.

Boyle, J., & Andrews, M. (1989). *Transcultural concepts in nursing care.* Glenview, IL: Scott, Foresman/Little, Brown College.

Brown, M. (1976, September–October). A cross-cultural look at pregnancy, labor and delivery. *Journal of Obstetric, Gynecologic, and Neonatal Nursing, 5,* 35.

Calhoun, M. (1985). The Vietnamese woman: Health/illness attitudes and behavior. *Health Care of Women International, 6,* 61.

Clark, A. (1978). *Culture, childbearing, health professionals.* Philadelphia: Davis.

Dempsey, P., & Gesse, T. (1983). The childbearing Haitian refugee—Cultural applications to clinical nursing. *Public Health Report, 98*(3), 261–267.

Enriquez, M. (1982). Studying maternal-infant attachment: A Mexican-American example. In M. Kay (Ed.), *Anthropology of human birth.* Philadelphia: Davis.

Greener, D. (1989). Transcultural nursing care of the childbearing woman and her family. In J. Boyle & M. Andrews (Eds.), *Transcultural concepts in nursing care* (pp. 95–119). Glenview, IL: Scott, Foresman/Little, Brown College.

Griffith (Mattson), S. (1982, May–June). Childbearing and the concept of culture. *Journal of Obstetric, Gynecologic, and Neonatal Nursing, 11*(3), 181–184.

Grosso, C., Barden, M., Henry, C., & Vieau, G. (1981, May–June). The Vietnamese American family and grandma makes three. *MCN: American Journal of Maternal Child Nursing, 6,* 177–180.

Hollingsworth, A. (1980, November). The refugees and childbearing: What to expect. *RN, 43,*45.

Hook, E. (1978). Dietary craving and aversions during pregnancy. *American Journal of Clinical Nutrition, 31,* 1355–1362.

Horn, B. (1981). Cultural concepts and postpartal care. *Nursing and Health Care, 2*(9), 516–517, 526–527.

Jimenez, M., & Newton, N. (1979). Activity and work during pregnancy and the postpartum period: A cross-cultural study of 202 societies. *American Journal of Obstetrics and Gynecology, 135*(2), 171–176.

Kay, M. (1982). *Anthropology of human birth.* Philadelphia: Davis.

Kitzinger, S. (1982). The social context of birth: Some comparisons between childbirth in Jamaica and Britain. In C.P. MacCormack (Ed.), *Ethnography of fertility and birth.* New York: Academic.

Kulig, J. (1990). Childbearing beliefs among Cambodian refugee women. *Western Journal of Nursing Research, 12*(1), 108–117.

Lee, R. (1989, Spring). Understanding Southeast Asian mothers-to-be. *Childbirth Educator,* 32–39.

Mattson, S., Galanti, G., Lettieri, C., & Kellogg, J. (1986). *Culture and health. Vol. 2: The family and life cycle in transcultural perspective.* Long Beach, CA: The Statewide Nursing Program.

Meleis, A., & Sorrell, L. (1981, May–June). Arab-American women and their birth experiences. *Maternal-Child Nursing Journal, 6,* 171–176.

Messer, E. (1981). Hot-cold classification: Theoretical and practical applications of a Mexican study. *Social Science and Medicine, 15B,* 133.

Miller-Karas, E. (1990, Summer). Ethnicity and perinatal patient care. Mid-Coastal California Perinatal Outreach Program *Newsletter,* 1–3.

Minkler, D. (1983). The role of a community-based satellite clinic in the perinatal care of non–English-speaking immigrants. *Western Journal of Medicine, 139*(6), 905–909.

Murillo-Rhode, I. (1979). Cultural sensitivity in the care of the Hispanic patient. (Special supplement). *Washington State Journal of Nursing,* 5.

Oakley, A. (1977). Cross-cultural practices. In T. Chard & M. Richards (Eds.), *Benefits and hazards of the new obstetrics.* Philadelphia: Lippincott.

Perry, D. (1982). The umbilical cord: Transcultural care and customs. *Journal of Nurse–Midwifery, 27*(4), 25–30.

Poma, P. (1987). Pregnancy in Hispanic women. *Journal of the National Medical Association, 79*(9), 929–935.

Scott, M., & Stern, P. (1985). The ethno market theory: Factors influencing childbearing health practices of northern Louisiana black women. *Health Care of Women International, 6,* 45.

Stern, P. (1981, June). Solving problems of cross-cultural health teaching: The Filipino childbearing family. *Image: The Journal of Nursing Scholarship, XII,* 47–50.

Stern P., Tilden, B., & Maxwell, E. (1985). *Culturally induced stress during childbearing: The Phillipine-American experience.* New York: Hemisphere.

Thiederman, S. (1986, August). Ethnocentrism: A barrier to effective health care. *Nurse Practitioner, 11,* 52.

Tripp-Reimer, T., & Brink, P. (1984). Cultural brokerage. In G. Bulechek & J. McCloskey (Eds.), *Nursing interventions: Treatment for nursing diagnoses.* Philadelphia: Saunders.

Tripp-Reimer, T., Brink, P., & Saunders, J. (1984). Cultural assessment: Content and process. *Nursing Outlook, 32*(2), 78–82.

Appendix: Quick Reference Guide to Ethnocultural Differences

Table 6–1
ANTEPARTUM VARIATIONS

	Native American	Afro-American	Asian	Hispanic	Arab Heritage
Pregnancy normal	Yes	Yes	Yes (must maintain balance between yin/yang)	Yes	Yes, but seek care
Prefer women attendants	Yes	No	Yes	Yes	Yes
Diet	Often have lactose intolerance (especially Eskimos, who are used to high protein, low carbohydrates)	Pica, eat salty (soul) foods, avoid acids, use sassafrass tea; are at risk for overeating of fats and carbohydrates	Often are vegetarian, use herbal teas; often are lactose-intolerant (tofu is a good alternative; also use fish bones for calcium); may not eat eggs, may refuse iron (believe it causes a difficult delivery)	Are clay eating, use herbal teas and remedies; use much fat in cooking; may not consider greens to be vegetables	If Moslem, eat no pork or pork products, caffeine, or alcohol
Activity	Should be active	Should continue sexual activity	Remain moderately active; avoid sexual activity in third trimester	Are active, use massage	Have no restrictions
Emotions	Should be happy	Avoid stress	Should be serene, calm, not sad	Do not quarrel with husband	Have no special needs

Table 6–2
INTRAPARTUM VARIATIONS

	Native American	Afro-American	Asian	Hispanic	Arab Heritage
Prefer women attendants	Yes, some want the whole family (Navajo)	Yes, especially mother or grandmother	Yes	Yes	Yes
Pain	Endure quietly	Usually are taught not to show weakness or call attention to themselves	Should not show pain, shameful to scream; often avoid verbal expression, use no medication (Samoan)	Endure pain with patience, but consider it acceptable to cry out	Are verbally expressive, cry and scream loudly; refuse medication
Positions	Choose various positions, often use birth chair	Choose various positions	Like to move around but must stay warm, to not lose heat; come to hospital in advanced labor; squatting (Laotian, Hmong)	Use massage, would use birth chair; like to move around/walk; come to hospital in advanced labor	Choose various positions
Food/drink	Have no special needs	Have no special needs	Drink herbal teas	Drink manzanilla tea (makes uterine contractions stronger)	Have no special needs

Table 6–3
POSTPARTUM VARIATIONS

	Native American	Afro-American	Asian	Hispanic	Arab Heritage
Hot/cold beliefs	Not applicable	Prevent cold air from entering uterus: wear pad, abdominal binder	Believe that exposure to cold may cause arthritis, asthma; avoid showers, ice packs, ice water; use hot blankets, avoid drafts	Believe that exposure to cold may cause sterility; use abdominal binder	Have no special needs
Diet	Drink hot herbal teas	Use sassafras tea: avoid eggplant, okra, tomatoes, cold drinks, milk (Haitians) avoid chitterlings, liver, and onions (southern Afro-Americans believe that these will affect breast milk)	Drink ginseng tea, eat only "hot" foods: chicken every day, plus other meats and fish for 30 days; may eat warm, dry, salty foods with little liquids (Korean, Vietnamese); avoid green vegetables, fruits	Eat cold food for 1 to 2 months, corn gruel is good; avoid acidic foods: citrus fruits, vegetables, chili, pork	Have no special needs
Activity	Have no special needs	See themselves as sick: avoid bathing, washing hair, heavy work	Need to rest, relatives do all work, including care of infant; avoid contact with others and going out into sun	Remain indoors, stay in bed up to 1 month; avoid strenuous work, bathing; avoid sexual contact for 40 days	Expect a lot of visitors, often request pain medications
Purification?	Take a ritual bath on the fourth post partum day (Navajo)	Not applicable	Avoid sexual contact for 3 to 4 months	Have a ritual bath 2 weeks post partum	Not applicable

Table 6–4
VARIATIONS IN NEWBORN CARE

	Native American	Afro-American	Asian	Hispanic	Arab Heritage
Breastfeeding	Yes; urban dwellers may use bottle	Yes; urban dwellers may use bottle	Yes	Yes, after milk comes in; consider colostrum bad for the baby, use bottle	Varies
Special clothes	Use cradle boards in rural areas	Use belly bands to prevent hernias	Wear old, ragged clothes (Southeast Asians)	Swaddle tightly, abdominal binder is common (infant is susceptible to "bad air")	Do not plan ahead for baby, would tempt evil eye; often have no layette ready
Activity	Consider babies important to family; keep baby close and handle often	Not applicable	Keep baby close by continuously; have no circumcision performed	Believe that baby is vulnerable to the evil eye (if stranger admires baby, believe should touch baby to dispel harm; no circumcision performed	Believe that baby is vulnerable to evil eye, needs protection
Praise of baby	Not applicable	Not applicable	No; believe that praise will call attention of the gods to vulnerable newborn	Yes	No; praise mother instead; if do praise infant, touch wood or mention God's blessing

Table 6–5
BIOLOGICAL VARIATIONS TO CONSIDER

	Native American	Afro-American	Asian	Hispanic	Arab Heritage
Sickle cell trait	Yes	Yes	No	No	Yes
Diabetes	Yes (especially Pima and Papago of Arizona)	No	No	No	No
Abnormal Hemoglobin (other than sickle cell)	No	No	Yes (especially Thais and Cambodians)	No	No
Tuberculosis	No	No	Yes (especially recent refugees)	No	No

Linda Bond

Physiology of Pregnancy

Objectives

1. Describe systemic changes occurring in the woman's body during pregnancy

2. Describe changes in the uterus, cervix, vagina, and vulva during pregnancy

3. Identify the presumptive signs and symptoms of pregnancy

4. Identify the probable signs and symptoms of pregnancy

5. Identify signs that are positively diagnostic of pregnancy

6. Differentiate between normal and abnormal laboratory results observed during pregnancy

7. Design an individualized patient education plan based upon data from history

8. Detect potential complications of pregnancy based on data from a history, a physical examination, and laboratory test results

9. Formulate nursing interventions to prevent anticipated problems identified from the nursing assessment

Introduction

A. **Conception and the 40 weeks of gestation constitute a time of numerous changes within a woman's body; pregnancy, a normal physiological event, signals a time of changes, many of which happen unbeknown to the woman.**

1. Regular health care supervision is necessary to make certain that subtle and untoward changes will not go undetected, ensuring a positive outcome for mother, baby, and the entire family

2. The health care team is responsible for monitoring expected physiological and psychological changes and for providing health teaching for greater understanding of the events of pregnancy as well as preparation for the postpregnancy events

B. **Maternal system changes**

1. Reproductive system
    a. Uterus

(1) Size increases to 20 times that of nonpregnant size
    (a) Hyperplasia and hypertrophy of myometrial cells, including muscle fibers, occur
    (b) Increases are related to estrogen and progesterone, along with mechanical factors of stretching related to the developing fetus
(2) Wall thins to 1.5 cm (.6 in) or less (changes from almost a solid globe to a hollow vessel)
(3) Weight increases from 50 to 1000 g (1.8 oz to 2.2 lb)
(4) Volume (capacity) increases from less than 10 ml to 4 to 8 l (2 tsp to 1 to 2 gal)
(5) Contractions (Braxton Hicks)
    (a) Irregular, painless
    (b) Begin during the first trimester
(6) Shape changes from that of an inverted pear to that of a soft globe that enlarges, rising out of the pelvis by the end of first trimester
(7) Endometrium is referred to as the decidua after implantation
    (a) Decidua vera: all of the uterine lining that is not in contact with the fetus
    (b) Decidua basalis: uterine lining beneath implantation
    (c) Decidua capsularis: portion of the decidua that covers the embryo

b. Cervix
  (1) Softening related to increased vascularity and slight hypertrophy (Goodell's sign)
  (2) Cervical glands
    (a) Mucous plug (operculum)
      (i) Formed from the thick mucus produced by endocervical glands
      (ii) Function is to prevent ascending infections
    (b) Mucorrhea

c. Ovaries and fallopian tubes
  (1) Anovulation results from the suppression of follicle-stimulating hormone (FSH) and luteinizing hormone (LH) related to high levels of estrogen and progesterone
  (2) Corpus luteum remains active for 8 to 10 weeks into pregnancy, producing progesterone and estrogen to maintain pregnancy. After 9 to 10 weeks' gestation, the placenta will produce the progesterone and estrogen to maintain pregnancy

d. Vagina
  (1) Increased vascularity
  (2) Bluish violet discoloration (Chadwick's sign)
  (3) Hypertrophy and hyperplasia of epithelium and elastic tissues
  (4) Leukorrhea, acid pH 3.5 to 6

e. Vulva
  (1) Increased vascularity
  (2) Hypertrophy of structures, along with fat deposits, causes labia majora to close to cover introitus

f. Breasts
  (1) Increased vascularity
  (2) Hypertrophy of mammary alveoli (because of high estrogen and progesterone levels)
    (a) Size increases
    (b) Breasts become nodular
  (3) Areola and nipples
    (a) Pigmentation darkens (begins during the first trimester)
    (b) Montgomery's glands become more prominent
    (c) Secondary areola may develop
    (d) Nipples enlarge and become more erectile (second trimester)
  (4) Colostrum from mammary glands

  (a) Precolostrum secreted in early second trimester
  (b) Colostrum secreted in third trimester
2. Cardiovascular system
  a. Heart
    (1) Slight enlargement, approximately 12%
    (2) Auscultatory changes
      (a) Exaggerated split heard in first sound
      (b) Second and third sounds are more obvious
      (c) Systolic murmurs are common
    (3) Shift in chest contents: heart is displaced upward and to the left in late pregnancy
  b. Hemodynamic changes
    (1) Heart rate increases by 10 to 15 beats per minute
    (2) Cardiac output increases by 30% during first two trimesters
    (3) Blood volume increases 40 to 50% (may be even greater with multiple births) over prepregnant level
    (4) Stroke volume increases by as much as 30% over prepregnancy level
    (5) Vasodilation occurs because of progesterone
    (6) Arterial blood pressure
      (a) Readings, positional variations
        (i) Supine hypotension, which results from uterine pressure on inferior vena cava (supine hypotensive syndrome)
        (ii) Left lateral recumbent position is optimal for cardiac output and uterine perfusion
        (iii) Brachial artery pressure is highest when woman is in the upright position
      (b) Diastolic readings often drop by about 5 mm Hg during the second trimester and rise to the first-trimester level after midpregnancy (26 to 28 weeks)
      (c) Systolic pressures are not significantly changed
    (7) Venous pressure increases; the femoral system accounts for dependent edema, varicose veins, and hemorrhoids
  c. Hematological changes
    (1) Red blood cell (RBC) production escalates
      (a) Total RBC volume increases approximately 30%
      (b) Percentage of increase is influenced by blood iron levels
    (2) White blood cell count (WBC) increases 5000 to 12,000, may normally increase to 25,000 during parturition
      (a) White blood cells in pregnant women are less effective in fighting infection and disease than they are in nonpregnant women
      (b) Infection must be diagnosed by history and physical examination
    (3) Blood volume expansion is made up of increased volume of plasma increased numbers of RBCs (plasma volume increases more rapidly than RBC production and causes hemodilution or physiological anemia of pregnancy)
      (a) Primary function is to offset blood loss at delivery
      (b) Supplies the increased vascular system during pregnancy
    (4) Clotting factors increase
      (a) Plasma fibrin levels increase by approximately 40%
      (b) Fibrinogen levels increase by approximately 50%
      (c) Clotting time remains unchanged
    (5) Hemoglobin and hematocrit decrease (in relation to plasma volume)
      (a) Hemoglobin of < 11 g/dl indicates anemia
      (b) Hematocrit lower than 35% indicates anemia
3. Respiratory system
  a. Respiratory rate and maximal breathing capacity remain unchanged while vital capacity may increase slightly

    b. Tidal volume, minute ventilatory volume, and minute oxygen uptake increase as pregnancy advances, as evidenced by deeper breathing
    c. Carbon dioxide output increases
    d. Increased vascularity is influenced by estrogen
    e. Thoracic circumference increases by 5 to 7 cm (2 to 3 in), and the diaphragm elevates approximately 4 cm (1.5 in)
    f. Basal metabolic rate increases and oxygen requirement increases by 30 to 40 ml/min
    g. Acid-base balance: arterial blood is slightly more alkalotic
4. Urinary system
    a. Renal structure changes
      (1) Influenced by
        (a) Estrogen and progesterone levels
        (b) Uterine pressure
        (c) Increased blood volume
      (2) Collection system changes (physiological hydronephrosis can occur because of the progesterone influence)
        (a) Renal pelvis dilates
        (b) Ureters elongate and become tortuous; the upper one-third of the ureters may dilate (particularly the right ureter)
        (c) Urinary stasis or stagnation occurs and increases the danger of pyelonephritis
      (3) Increased urinary frequency is related to the increasing size of the uterus and its pressure on the bladder
      (4) Bladder is pulled up into the abdominal cavity by the growing uterus, and the bladder tone is decreased
    b. Renal function changes
      (1) Changes in kidney function occur to accommodate a heavier workload while maintaining stable electrolyte balance and blood pressure
        (a) Increased glomerular filtration rate
        (b) Increased renal plasma flow
      (2) Laboratory values
        (a) Glucosuria may occur (may not be abnormal; warrants further evaluation and monitoring)
        (b) Proteinuria is abnormal except in very concentrated urine or in the first-voided specimen on arising (total urine protein of 150 mg in 24 hours is a warning of impaired kidney function and/or pregnancy-induced hypertension)
5. Gastrointestinal system
    a. Mouth and teeth
      (1) Gums become hyperemic, swollen, and soft and have a tendency to bleed (estrogen influence)
      (2) Saliva production remains unchanged (ptyalism is seen in some women and is associated with nausea and decreased swallowing)
      (3) Teeth remain unchanged
    b. Gastrointestinal tract
      (1) Smooth muscle relaxation occurs related to the progesterone influence; this can cause
        (a) Constipation and decreased peristalsis
        (b) Hemorrhoids from the pressure of the gravid uterus
        (c) Heartburn, slowed gastric emptying, and esophageal regurgitation (reflux)
      (2) Positional changes of organs occur because of uterine enlargement
        (a) Upward displacement of the stomach
        (b) Colon shifted and compressed
      (3) Appetite usually increases (nausea and vomiting associated with the first trimester may temporarily decrease appetite)

      c. Liver function undergoes insignificant, minor changes

      d. Gallbladder: emptying time is prolonged, which could lead to formation of gallstones

  6. Musculoskeletal system

      a. Alterations in posture can result in lordosis

      b. Relaxation and increased mobility of joints occur because of the hormone relaxin and steroid sex hormones

      c. Diastasis recti, a separation of the rectus muscles of the abdominal wall, is associated with the enlarging uterus in some women

  7. Integumentary system

      a. Skin undergoes hyperpigmentation

        (1) Melasma (formerly known as chloasma) is the blotchy, brownish "mask of pregnancy"

        (2) Linea nigra (abdomen)

        (3) Nipples, areolae, axillae, vulva, and perineum all darken

        (4) Moles (nevi) and freckles may darken

      b. Hair: some women may note increased growth

      c. Connective tissue fragility can cause striae gravidarum (breasts and abdomen)

      d. Blood vessels have increased permeability, causing

        (1) Edema

        (2) Spider angiomas

        (3) Palmar erythema

      e. Skin disorders and skin problems associated with pregnancy may include noninflammatory pruritis and acne vulgaris (especially in the first trimester)

  8. Metabolic changes

      a. Nutrient metabolism (see Chapter 12 for a complete discussion of nutrition)

        (1) Protein: demands increase

        (2) Carbohydrate: demands increase

          (a) Diabetogenic state occurs because of the influence of placental hormone (human placental lactogen [human chorionic somatomammotropin]), which serves as an insulin antagonist

          (b) Glycosuria may be present

        (3) Mineral: iron needs increase

      b. Water metabolism

        (1) Water requirement is increased to supply fetus, placenta, amniotic fluid, and expanded maternal blood volume

        (2) Minimum fluid intake is 6 to 8 glassfuls (each 240 ml [8 oz]) of liquid daily

        (3) Fluid retention is common because of adrenocorticosteroid influence

      c. Weight gain: 11 to 16 kg (25 to 35 lb)

        (1) Underweight (90% of expected body weight): recommendation is 14 kg (30 lb)

        (2) Overweight (20% over expected body weight): recommended weight gain is 7 to 9 kg (15 to 20 lb) (see Chapter 12 for a further discussion of nutrition)

  9. Endocrine system

      a. Pituitary gland

        (1) Anterior lobe: slight increase in size

          (a) Follicle-stimulating hormone and luteinizing hormone production is suppressed

          (b) Thyrotropin and adrenocorticotropic hormone may increase slightly

          (c) Melanotropin production is increased

          (d) Human placental lactogen production is suppressed

(e) Prolactin (PRL) production is increased
(2) Posterior lobe: oxytocin production gradually increases as the fetus matures
b. Thyroid
(1) Gland enlarges, resulting in increased iodine metabolism
(2) Thyroxine (T_4) level, unbound to plasma proteins, remains unchanged (T_3 [triiodothyronine] and T_4 increase but are bound to thyroxine-binding globulin)
(3) Basal metabolic rate (BMR) increases up to 25% by term
c. Parathyroid gland-activity increases and blood levels of parathyroid hormone are elevated
d. Adrenal glands: little change in function
e. Pancreas: insulin production is increased throughout pregnancy to compensate for placental hormone insulin antagonism
(1) Insulin antagonists (human placental lactogen hormones, estrogen, progesterone, and adrenal cortisol) cause decreased tissue sensitivity
(2) Women with poor pancreatic function may develop true diabetes during pregnancy (see Chapter 29 for complete discussion of diabetes in pregnancy)
f. Ovaries
(1) Estrogen (also from adrenal cortex and later the placenta) is responsible for
(a) Enlargement of breasts, uterus, and genitals
(b) Fat deposit changes
(c) Alterations in thyroid function and nutrient metabolism
(d) Changes in sodium and water retention
(e) Hematological changes
(f) Vascular changes
(g) Stimulation of melanin-stimulating hormones, hyperpigmentation
(2) Progesterone from the corpus luteum (later, the placenta) is responsible for
(a) Facilitating implantation
(b) Decreasing uterine contractility
(c) Development of secretory ducts and lobular-alveolar system of breasts
(d) Fat deposit changes
(e) Reducing smooth muscle tone
(f) Increasing sensitivity of respiratory system to carbon dioxide
(g) Reducing gastric motility
(3) Relaxin from corpus luteum is thought to be responsible for musculoskeletal changes
10. Immunological system
a. Resistance to infection is decreased
(1) Total white blood cell count increased and T-lymphocyte activity is decreased
(2) Cellular immune response is decreased
b. Immunoglobulin (Ig) levels
(1) Maternal IgG levels are decreased because of crossplacental transfer to the fetus near term
(2) Maternal IgA and IgM levels remain unchanged

C. Pregnancy signs and symptoms

1. Presumptive evidence
a. Signs
(1) Amenorrhea
(2) Breast changes
(3) Vaginal mucosa discoloration (Chadwick's sign)

          (4) Skin pigmentation changes (melasma/chloasma, linea nigra, and linea alba)

          (5) Abdominal enlargement and striae

      b. Symptoms

          (1) Nausea and vomiting

          (2) Urinary frequency

          (3) Weight gain

          (4) Constipation

          (5) Fatigue

          (6) Perception of fetal movement (quickening)

          (7) Breast tenderness, tingling, and heaviness

  2. Probable evidence

      a. Signs

          (1) Uterine changes: softening of isthmus (Hegar's sign)

          (2) Cervical softening (Goodell's sign)

          (3) Ballottement

          (4) Laboratory tests for human chorionic gonadotropin (HCG) levels

      b. Symptoms are same as presumptive symptoms

  3. Positive evidence

      a. Fetal heartbeat heard by the examiner

      b. Fetal outline confirmation by ultrasonography

      c. Fetal movement detected by examiner

Clinical Practice

A. **Assessment (comprehensive general health examination at first prenatal visit)**

1. History

    a. Current pregnancy

      (1) Menstrual history

        (a) Last menstrual period (LMP)

        (b) Previous menstrual period (PMP)

        (c) Last normal menstrual period (LNMP)

        (d) Menarche

    b. Signs and symptoms (see the section on pregnancy signs and symptoms)

    c. Risk assessment (at risk for a problem pregnancy)

      (1) Younger than 17 years, older than 35 years (see Chapter 10 for a complete discussion)

      (2) History of induced abortions

      (3) Five or more pregnancies

      (4) Previous stillbirth or neonatal loss

      (5) Infant born prematurely, excessively large, with isoimmunization, or with congenital anomaly

      (6) History of maternal malignancy, genital tract anomaly, or medical indication for termination of previous pregnancy

      (7) Substance use or abuse: tobacco products, alcohol, illicit or prescription drugs (see Chapter 32 for a complete discussion)

2. Obstetrical and gynecological history

    a. Gravida/para system or gravidity, term, preterm, abortions, living children (G/TPAL) system

    b. Sexual history, including sexually transmitted diseases (STD): syphilis, gonorrhea, herpes genitalis, trichomoniasis, condylomata acuminata (genital human papillomavirus [HPV] infection or genital warts), hepatitis B, chlamydia infection, human immunodeficiency virus (HIV) infection (see Chapter 27 for a complete discussion)

    c. Contraceptive history and use

    d. Infertility problems

    e. Description of previous pregnancies (length of gestations, type of delivery, and fetal outcome, including birth weight and maternal complications)

3. Racial or ethnic background

4. Medical history

    a. Childhood diseases (especially infectious diseases)

    b. Other diseases (e.g., diabetes, asthma, urinary tract infections, varicosities, seizures)

    c. Surgery (blood transfusions)

    d. Injuries

    e. Allergies (especially to drugs)

    f. Immunizations (especially rubella)

    g. Current medications

    h. Alcohol, tobacco, and other drug use or abuse

    i. Radiation exposure

5. Nutrition history

6. Family medical history

    a. Health status of parents and siblings

    b. Family incidence of diabetes, cardiovascular disease, and hypertension

    c. Congenital diseases, deformities, or unexplained stillbirths

    d. Multiple births

7. Father's health history

    a. Current health status, including health problems

    b. Blood type and rhesus (Rh) factor

    c. Family medical history

    d. Alcohol and drug use and abuse

8. Social, family, and emotional history

9. Review of physical systems

    a. Skin, hair, and nails

    b. Head, ears, eyes, nose, and throat

    c. Mouth and teeth

    d. Breasts

    e. Respiratory system

    f. Cardiovascular system

    g. Gastrointestinal system

    h. Genitourinary system

    i. Extremities

    j. Back

    k. Central nervous system

    l. Hematopoietic system

    m. Endocrine system

B. **Physical examination**

1. Initial visit

    a. Temperature, pulse, and respiration; blood pressure; height; and weight

    b. Breasts (changes consistent with early pregnancy)

    c. Abdomen (changes consistent with pregnancy)

    d. Pelvic (external genitalia, vagina, uterus, cervix, and adnexa) (see Chapter 1 for a complete discussion of anatomy)

        (1) Bony pelvis, internal

            (a) Diagonal conjugate measurement, 12.5 cm

            (b) Sacral curve and shape (concave)

            (c) Ischial spines (bluntness)

            (d) Coccyx (moveable)

        (2) Pelvic outlet

            (a) Subpubic arch 4 to 5 cm wide and rounded

(b) Distance between ischial tuberosities more than 11 cm
2. Calculation of expected delivery date
   a. Nägele's rule: 1st day of last menstrual period (LMP) + 7 days − 3 months + 1 year
   b. McDonald's rule: fundal height measure corresponds to the week of gestation ± 2 to 4 weeks after 24 weeks
   c. Sonogram method: measurement of gestational sac, crown-to-rump or crown-to-heel length, biparietal diameter
3. Diagnostic procedures
   a. Pregnancy test (HCG levels in serum or urine)
      (1) Radioimmunoassay (RIA)
         (a) Based on antibodies against beta subunit HCG, RIA is accurate as early as 1 week postovulation
         (b) Other bioassay tests are prone to false positives and false negatives because of cross-reaction with luteinizing hormone
      (2) Biological tests are available but are rarely used now (Ashheim-Zondek, Friedman)
      (3) Home pregnancy tests are sensitive and accurate as early as day 1 of the expected menstrual cycle (provided the directions have been carefully followed)
   b. Blood
      (1) Complete blood count (CBC) with differential smear
      (2) Hemoglobin, 12 to 16 g/dl
      (3) Hematocrit, 38 to 47%
      (4) Type and Rh factor
      (5) Antibody screen (Rh, D [Rho], rubeola, hepatitis B, and toxoplasmosis)
      (6) Rubella titer more than 1:10 to confirm immunity
      (7) Sickle cell anemia screen for Afro-American clients
      (8) Syphilis tests (serologic test for syphilis or VDRL)
   c. Urinalysis: urine culture if history suggests a urinary tract infection
   d. Cervical smears
      (1) Papanicolaou
      (2) Gonorrhea culture
      (3) Chlamydia culture
      (4) Herpes simplex (types 1 and 2) if indicated by history or observation
      (5) Tuberculosis: skin test
   e. Periodic revisits: normal pregnancy
      (1) Schedule is usually
         (a) Monthly until 28 weeks' gestation
         (b) Biweekly from 28 to 36 weeks' gestation
         (c) Weekly from 36 weeks until delivery
      (2) Interval history: physical symptoms and maternal well-being, including emotional adjustment
      (3) Blood pressure and weight
      (4) Urinalysis: glucose, protein (dipstick, first morning voided specimen)
      (5) Fetal well-being
         (a) Fundal height (Fig. 7–1)
            (i) Fundus elevates out of pelvic area and can be palpated just above the symphysis pubis at about 12 weeks
            (ii) Fundus rises to the level of the umbilicus at about 20 weeks and to the xiphoid process near term
         (b) Fetal heart rate
         (c) Fetal position determination: Leopold's maneuvers (see Chapter 14 for complete discussion of Leopold's maneuvers)
         (d) Other tests: fetal movements determined by examiner, ultrasonography, nonstress test (NST) for example
      (1) Pelvic examination, if indicated

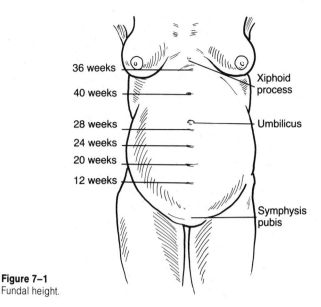

Figure 7–1
Fundal height.

(2) Repeated or additional laboratory examinations
    (a) Hemoglobin or hematocrit at 26 to 28 weeks
    (b) Blood glucose screen at 24 to 28 weeks
    (c) Antibody screen (D [Rho] at 28 weeks for Rh-negative mother and Rh-positive father or father's Rh unknown)
    (d) Maternal serum alpha-fetoprotein (must offer, but remains the client's choice) at 14 to 18 weeks
    (e) Tests for sexually transmitted diseases (STD), if indicated (e.g., gonorrhea)

C. Nursing Diagnoses

1. Knowledge deficit about normal physical responses to pregnancy
2. Alteration in comfort related to advancing pregnancy
3. Alteration in bowel elimination: constipation
4. Activity intolerance related to fatigue associated with physiological changes of pregnancy

D. Interventions/Evaluations

1. Knowledge deficit about normal physical responses to pregnancy
  a. Interventions
    (1) Provide teaching and anticipatory guidance at each prenatal visit
    (2) Provide written instructions and materials to support teaching
    (3) Use pictures and models to illustrate teaching
    (4) Create an environment of trust so that questions may be asked and answered
    (5) Provide a telephone number to call with questions or for information
    (6) Refer to childbirth education classes
    (7) Instruct in danger signs of pregnancy and to call care provider on occurrence of the following
      (a) Vaginal bleeding
      (b) Leaking of fluid from the vagina
      (c) Sudden swelling of the face or fingers
      (d) Headache not relieved by normal measures
      (e) Blurred vision
      (f) Abdominal pain

(g) Chills or fever

(h) Severe or prolonged vomiting

b. Evaluations: appropriate knowledge level indicated by

(1) Client verbalizing trimester appropriate physical changes

(2) Client identifying danger signals of pregnancy (e.g., vaginal bleeding)

(3) Client identifying how she would handle an emergency (e.g., who is to be called, what action is to be taken)

(4) If a positive outcome not indicated, re-evaluate plan of care

2. Alteration in comfort related to advancing pregnancy

a. Interventions

(1) Provide information regarding trimester-specific common discomforts and causes and comfort measures

(2) Encourage adequate nutrition, rest, and activity level to promote optimal health and body function

(3) Teach stress-reduction techniques (e.g., relaxation) as coping strategies

(4) Provide instruction about when to call the doctor, nurse midwife, or nurse practitioner

b. Evaluations

(1) Client can identify discomfort-specific comfort measures

(2) Comfort measures are effective, as indicated by symptom reduction

3. Alteration in bowel elimination: constipation

a. Interventions

(1) Review the importance of maintaining a regular bowel elimination pattern

(2) Review nutrition's effect on the elimination and encourage a balanced diet high in fiber

(3) Review the importance of fluid intake of 6 to 8 glassfuls (each 240 ml [8 oz]) of water per day

(4) Teach the importance of physical activity on bowel regularity

(5) Teach about the role of hormones, of the growing fetus, and of iron supplements on bowel function

(6) Teach about the dangers of taking laxatives during pregnancy

b. Evaluation: bowel elimination is regular with soft, formed stool

4. Activity intolerance related to fatigue associated with physiological changes of pregnancy

a. Interventions

(1) Review body changes of pregnancy, which can lead to previously unexperienced fatigue

(2) Have client keep a log of activities and note times when fatigue was experienced; identify with patient where adjustments might be needed and can be made

(3) Encourage regular rest periods

(4) Encourage adequate nutrition, rest, and activity level to promote optimal health and body function

b. Evaluations

(1) Activity level is adjusted to avoid fatigue

(2) Daily schedule includes rest periods

(3) Intake of food and fluid is adequate

Health Education

A. First trimester

1. Physiological changes of pregnancy with resulting discomforts

a. Pain and tingling in breasts

b. Nausea and vomiting (morning sickness)

c. Urinary frequency

      d. Fatigue
      e. Mood swings
  2. Danger signs that should be reported
      a. Bleeding
      b. Cramping
      c. Severe and prolonged vomiting
  3. Health teaching (use principles of teaching and learning)
      a. Schedule of return visits for routine prenatal care
      b. General hygiene (tub baths and showers are allowed throughout pregnancy)
      c. Comfort measures for trimester-related discomforts (e.g., for morning sickness, eat dry carbohydrates before arising; for fatigue, plan rest periods and a well-balanced diet)
      d. Anticipatory guidance regarding duration of present discomforts
      e. Sexual activity (may need reassurance about safety of sexual activity during pregnancy)
      f. Physical activity, exercise, and rest
      g. Nutritional guidance, weight gain, and diet

B. Second trimester

1. Physiological changes with resulting discomforts
      a. Enlargement of abdomen
      b. Skin pigmentation
      c. Striae gravidarum
      d. Vascular spiders
      e. Constipation
      f. Heartburn
      g. Leg cramps
      h. Groin pain from round ligament stretching
      i. Leukorrhea
2. Danger signs that should be reported
      a. Vaginal bleeding
      b. Burning or painful urination
      c. Fever
      d. Reduction in or absence of fetal movements
      e. Nausea and vomiting
      f. Abdominal pain or cramping
3. Health teaching
      a. Reinforce and reiterate previous teaching
      b. Comfort measures specific to trimester-related discomforts (for heartburn: small frequent meals, milk; for leg cramps: heat, stretching, oral calcium supplement; for round ligament stretching: good posture, knee-to-chest position when recumbent)
      c. Anticipatory guidance regarding duration of present discomforts
      d. Choices of prenatal education classes

C. Third trimester

1. Physiological changes with resulting discomforts
      a. Dyspnea
      b. Leg and feet cramps
      c. Constipation
      d. Indigestion, heartburn
      e. Pedal edema
      f. Fatigue
      g. Vaginal discharge
      h. Urinary frequency
      i. Braxton Hicks contractions
2. Danger signs that should be reported

a. Visual disturbance
b. Headache
c. Facial edema
d. Fever
e. Vaginal bleeding
f. Abdominal pain; uterine contractions
g. Premature rupture of membranes (PROM)
h. Decreased or lack of fetal movement

3. Health teaching
   a. Signs and symptoms of labor
   b. When to call the health care provider, when to go to the hospital or birthing place
   c. Comfort measures for trimester-related discomforts (for leukorrhea: hygiene, perineal pads; for Braxton Hicks contractions: reassurance, rest, and support garments)
   d. Anticipatory guidance regarding duration of present discomforts
   e. Reinforce and reiterate previous teaching

CASE STUDIES AND STUDY QUESTIONS

Ann Lowe is a 26-year-old woman who has registered at the clinic for prenatal care. She reports fatigue, nausea, and constipation. Her last normal menstrual period was 8 weeks ago and the home pregnancy test was positive. This is Ann's first pregnancy.

1. Presumptive signs of pregnancy include
   a. Ballottement.
   b. Braxton Hicks contractions.
   c. Breast changes.
   d. Positive pregnancy tests.

2. The bluish discoloration of the vagina is known as
   a. Chadwick's sign.
   b. Hegar's sign.
   c. Goodell's sign.
   d. Braxton's sign.

3. A normal physiological change associated with the first trimester of pregnancy is
   a. Increased respirations.
   b. Increased peristalsis.
   c. Increased resistance to infection.
   d. Increased cardiac output.

4. Health teaching of particular importance at this early stage of pregnancy includes
   a. Comfort measures for trimester-related discomforts.
   b. Choices of prenatal education classes.
   c. Signs and symptoms of labor.
   d. Infant feeding techniques.

Sara Thompson, at 27 weeks' gestation, Rh negative, comes to the clinic for a routine prenatal visit. This is her fourth pregnancy and she has four living children (one set of twins).

5. Routine laboratory tests that should be repeated at this visit include
   a. HCG level.
   b. Rubella titer.
   c. Antibody screen.
   d. Complete blood count with differential smear

6. Prenatal revisits during weeks 28 to 36 are routinely scheduled
   a. Monthly.
   b. Every 2 weeks.
   c. Weekly.
   d. As needed.

7. Sara reports feeling fatigued and is bothered by constipation. These symptoms are related to the hormone
   a. Estrogen
   b. HCG
   c. Thyroxine
   d. Progesterone

8. Sara's hemoglobin value is 11.7 g/dl. Which factor explains this finding?

   a. The trimester of pregnancy.

   b. Hemodilution of pregnancy.

   c. The presence of iron deficiency anemia.

   d. Greater-than-expected weight gain.

ADDITIONAL STUDY QUESTIONS

9. The increase in uterine size during pregnancy is primarily the result of which of the following factors?

   a. Growth of the fetus.

   b. Formation of new muscle fibers.

   c. Increase in blood circulation to the uterus.

   d. Enlargement of existing muscle fibers.

10. The primary source of the hormones estrogen and progesterone during early pregnancy is the

    a. Placenta.

    b. Anterior lobe of the pituitary gland.

    c. Corpus luteum.

    d. Adrenal cortex.

11. The expected height of the fundus at 20 weeks' gestation is

    a. At the xyphoid process.

    b. At the umbilicus.

    c. Half-way between the symphysis pubis and umbilicus.

    d. At the symphysis pubis.

12. A pregnant woman should immediately report which of the following symptoms to her health care provider?

    a. Leg cramps.

    b. Abdominal pain.

    c. Dyspnea.

    d. Heartburn.

13. Normal physiological responses to pregnancy include

    a. Increased cardiac output.

    b. Increased peristalsis.

    c. Increased respirations.

    d. Increased blood pressure.

Answers to Study Questions

1. c	2. a	3. d
4. a	5. c	6. b
7. d	8. b	9. d
10. c	11. b	12. b
13. a		

REFERENCES

ACOG Committee on Obstetrics: Maternal and Fetal Medicine. (1989, November). *ACOG antepartum record*. Washington, DC: ACOG.

ACOG Committee on Obstetrics: Maternal and Fetal Medicine. (1990, January). *Guidelines for HBV screening and vaccination during pregnancy*, No. 78. Washington, DC: ACOG.

ACOG Committee on Obstetrics: Maternal and Fetal Medicine. (1990, March). *Cocaine abuse: Implications for pregnancy*, No. 81. Washington, DC: ACOG.

ACOG Committee on Obstetrics: Maternal and Fetal Medicine. (1990, January). *Scope of services for uncomplicated obstetric care*. Washington, DC: ACOG.

Alley, N.M. (1984). Morning sickness, the client's perspective. *Journal of Obstetric, Gynecologic, and Neonatal Nursing, 13*(3) 185–189.

Avenshine, M.A., & Enriques, M.G. (1990). *Comprehensive maternity nursing: Perinatal and women's health* (2nd ed.). Boston: Jones & Bartlett.

Beaufoy, A., Goldstone, I., & Riddell, R. (1988). AIDS: What nurses need to know. Part I. HIV disease and AIDS. *Canadian Nurse, 84*(7), 16–22.

Bengtson, J.M., Petrie, R.H., & Shank, J.C. (1987, December 15). Managing the uncomplicated pregnancy. *Patient Care*, 56–60, 73–76.

Bobak, I.M., Jensen, M.D., & Zalar, M.K. (1989). *Maternity and gynecologic care* (4th ed.). St. Louis: Mosby.

Bourcier, K.M., & Seidler, A.J. (1987). Chlamydia and condylomata acumenata: Update for the nurse practitioner. *Journal of Obstetric, Gynecologic, and Neonatal Nursing, 16*(1), 17–22.

Brucker, M.C. (1988). Management of common minor discomforts in pregnancy. Part II: Managing minor pain in pregnancy. *Journal of Nurse Midwifery, 33*(1), 25–30.

Brucker, M.C. (1988). Management of common minor discomforts in pregnancy. Part III: Managing gastrointestinal problems in pregnancy. *Journal of Nurse Midwifery, 33*(2), 67–73.

Brucker, M.C., & Macmullen, N.J. (1985). What's new in pregnancy tests. *Journal of Obstetric, Gynecologic, and Neonatal Nursing, 14*(5) 353–359.

Carpenito, L.J. (1989). *Nursing diagnosis* (3rd ed.). New York: Lippincott.

Doenges, M.E., Kenty, J.R., & Moorhouse, M.F. (1988). *Maternal/newborn care plans*. Philadelphia: Davis.

Dohrmann, K.R., & Ledgerman, S.A. (1986). Weight gain in pregnancy. *Journal of Obstetric, Gynecologic, and Neonatal Nursing 15*(6), 446–453.

Engstrom, J.L. (1988). Measurement of fundal height. *Journal of Obstetric, Gynecologic, and Neonatal Nursing, 17*(3), 172–178.

Ketter, D.E., & Shelton, B.J. (1984). Pregnant and physically fit, too. *MCN: American Journal of Maternal-Child Nursing, 9*(2) 120–122.

Loveman, A., Colburn, V., & Dobin, A. (1986). AIDS in pregnancy. *Journal of Obstetric, Gynecologic, and Neonatal Nursing, 15*(2), 91–93.

Marecki, M.A. (1988). Chlamydia trachomatis: A developing perinatal problem. *Journal of Perinatal and Neonatal Nursing, 1*(4), 1–11.

NAACOG. (1987). *Competencies and program guidelines for nurse providers of childbirth education*. Washington, DC: Author.

OGN Nursing Practice Resource. (1989, December). *Nursing diagnosis*. Washington, DC: NAACOG.

Olds, S.B., London, M.L., & Ladewig, P.A. (1988). *Maternal-newborn nursing* (3rd ed.). Menlo Park, CA: Addison-Wesley.

Poole, C.J. (1986). Fatigue during the first trimester of pregnancy. *Journal of Obstetric, Gynecologic, and Neonatal Nursing, 15*(5), 375–379.

Reich, C.L. (1987). Exercise in pregnancy: A review for nurse practitioners. *Health Care of Women International, 8*(5/6), 349–360.

Sherwin, L.N., Scoloveno, M.A., & Weingarten, C.T. (1991). *Nursing care and the childbearing family*. Norwalk, CT: Appleton & Lange.

Stevens, K.A., & Pavlides, C. (1989). Individualized prenatal nursing care of pregnant adolescents makes a difference. *Journal of Obstetric, Gynecologic, and Neonatal Nursing, 18*(6), 521–522.

Weiner, S.M. (1989). *Clinical manual of maternity and gynecologic nursing*. St. Louis: Mosby.

Woleske, M. (1989). Antenatal HIV screening. *Neonatal Network, 8*(2), 7–13.

Leith Merrow Mullaly

Psychology of Pregnancy

Objectives

1. Describe two or three stages of family development pertinent to pregnancy

2. List the developmental tasks of pregnancy

3. List the general concepts in Rubin's tasks of pregnancy

4. Identify two or three potential characteristics of expectant fathers

5. Discuss two or three psychosocial findings in normal pregnancy

6. List two special considerations of American culture about pregnancy

7. Discuss strategies to minimize self-concept disturbances during pregnancy

8. Describe two or three needs of fathers during labor and delivery

9. Describe changes in sexual feelings and behaviors in pregnancy

10. Discuss the concept of developmental crises in pregnancy

11. Assist families in developing a birth plan

12. Enumerate maternal behaviors exhibited during pregnancy validation

13. Describe maternal behaviors exhibited during fetal embodiment

14. Differentiate maternal behaviors seen during fetal distinction

15. List the most common maternal behaviors observed in role transition

16. Identify appropriate behaviors of safe passage seen in the last trimester of pregnancy

17. Describe critical issues seen in the last trimester involving acceptance of the child by others

18. Identify two or three possible reactions of fathers to pregnancy

Introduction

Pregnancy is a time of increased susceptibility to psychological stress for expectant mothers and fathers. Pregnancy and childbearing are developmental phases in family life that are often characterized by ambivalence and conflicting emotions as expectant parents face significant role and lifestyle changes.

Clinical Practice

A. Assessment

1. History
   a. Family background
      (1) Economic status (poverty/financial well-being)
      (2) Marital status
      (3) Age
      (4) Support system
      (5) Self-esteem
      (6) Role models
      (7) Culture
      (8) Religion
      (9) Stability of living conditions
   b. Obstetrical experience
      (1) Previous pregnancies
      (2) Prior pregnancy outcomes
      (3) Pregnancy experiences of extended family and friends
      (4) Previous experience with neonates
   c. Present pregnancy
      (1) Whether it is wanted or unwanted
      (2) Whether it is planned or unplanned
      (3) Whether the mother was healthy or unhealthy before and during this pregnancy
      (4) The woman's learning capabilities and/or limitations
      (5) Whether the woman has healthy or unhealthy personal relationships
      (6) The status of her pregnancy: whether it is low risk or high risk
2. Duvall's stages of family development
   a. Married couple that is beginning a family
      (1) Attainment of a satisfying relationship
      (2) A dyad: the easiest and first relationship of family development
   b. Expectant family: role preparation
      (1) Need to reorganize the household for the baby
      (2) Need to develop new patterns of making and spending money
      (3) Need to realign their tasks and responsibilities
      (4) Need to adapt their sexual relationship to the pregnancy
      (5) Need to reorient their relationships with relatives
      (6) Need to adapt their relationships with friends and associates
      (7) Need to increase their knowledge about pregnancy, birth, and parenting
      (8) Is a time of accelerated emotional changes
   c. Childbearing family (from the time of the first birth to the time when the last child attains the age of 30 months)
      (1) Must adjust to a changing relationship (e.g., dyad to triad)
      (2) Must encourage the development of the new infant
      (3) Must introduce each new infant to the existing sibling(s)
3. Psychosocial findings
   a. Thoughts and desires
      (1) Food cravings may occur during pregnancy
      (2) Sexual behaviors, desires, and thoughts are variable throughout pregnancy
         (a) May decrease in late pregnancy for some
         (b) May remain unchanged for others
      (3) Dream life is very active in pregnancy
      (4) Chronic fatigue, especially during the first and third trimesters, may influence desires and thoughts

   b. Mood swings
      (1) Ambivalence about becoming a mother marks early pregnancy in most women
      (2) Increased irritability may exist throughout pregnancy and may peak in the ninth month when fatigue is the greatest
      (3) Increased sensitivity may exist throughout the entire pregnancy
      (4) The sense of vulnerability tends to peak during the seventh month
      (5) The woman may experience frustration with her own indecisiveness throughout the pregnancy
      (6) Normal fears may exist (e.g., about the health of the baby and about her ability to give birth safely)
4. Pregnancy as a developmental (maturational) crisis
   a. There is a danger of increased psychological vulnerability at this time
   b. There is an increased opportunity for personal growth
   c. There is increased susceptibility to stress, with potential for increased changes in areas such as work, housing needs, and access to care
   d. There is an alteration in life roles and identity for each parent and for each member of the family
5. Developmental tasks of pregnancy that are progressive over time
   a. Pregnancy validation
      (1) The woman has an initial ambivalence about the pregnancy
      (2) She experiences fantasies and dreams about herself and how pregnancy will change her life
   b. Fetal embodiment
      (1) The woman incorporates the fetus into her body image
      (2) She becomes dependent on her partner or significant others
      (3) She is typically introspective and calm
   c. Fetal distinction
      (1) The woman conceptualizes her fetus as a separate individual
      (2) She accepts her new body image and expresses it as being full of life
      (3) She becomes more dependent on her mother or feels closer to her mother at this time
   d. Role transition
      (1) She prepares to separate from and give up the physical, symbiotic attachment with her fetus
      (2) She becomes anxious about impending labor and delivery
      (3) She exhibits "nesting" behaviors or a need to get all the supplies needed for the baby (preterm labor is a major disruption of the need to nest)
      (4) She becomes impatient with her awkward body and is anxious for pregnancy to end; she states frequently that she is tired of being pregnant
      (5) She feels prepared to mother the infant
6. Rubin's tasks of pregnancy, which occur concurrently with each other
   a. General principles
      (1) Pregnancy progressively becomes a part of the woman's total identity
      (2) The woman is able to share relatively little of her sensory experience with others (feels unique)
      (3) The woman's focus turns progressively inward as the pregnancy advances
      (4) The woman generally becomes overly sensitive
      (5) She seeks the company of other women, especially other pregnant women
      (6) The absence of a female support system during pregnancy is a singular index of a high-risk pregnancy
   b. Acceptance of pregnancy and incorporating the reality of pregnancy into her self-concept ("binding-in")

(1) First trimester: she accepts the idea of pregnancy but not of the child

(2) Second trimester: there is a dramatic change, called quickening; she becomes aware of the child here and now

(3) Third trimester: she wants the child and hates being pregnant

c. Acceptance of the child

(1) First trimester: acceptance by herself and by others of the pregnancy

(2) Acceptance of the child by others is the keystone of a successful adjustment to pregnancy

(3) Second trimester: the family needs to relate to the baby (e.g., as a son or brother)

(4) Third trimester: the critical issue is the unconditional acceptance of the child; conditional acceptance implies rejection

d. Reordering of relationships and learning to give of herself

(1) First trimester: examines what needs to be given up

(a) Trade-offs for having the baby

(b) May grieve the loss of a carefree life

(2) Second trimester: identifies with the child

(3) Third trimester: has decreased confidence in her ability to become a good mother to her child

e. Safe passage: Rubin suggests that this task usually receives most of the woman's attention

(1) First trimester: she has a focus on herself, not on her baby

(2) Second trimester: she develops an attachment of great value to her baby

(3) Third trimester: she has a concern for herself and her baby as a unit

(a) At the seventh month, she is in a state of high vulnerability

(b) She sees labor and delivery as deliverance and as a hope, not as a threat

7. Expectant fathers

a. Psychosocial findings during pregnancy

(1) Couvade: some men actually experience symptoms of pregnancy

(a) Weight gain

(b) Nausea

(c) Other common physical symptoms of pregnancy

(2) Expectant fathers have wide variations in their reactions to pregnancy and to the psychological and physical changes in the woman

(a) Some enjoy the role of nurturer

(b) Some experience alienation, which may lead to extramarital affairs

(c) Some view the pregnancy as a proof of masculinity and assume a dominant role

(d) To some expectant fathers, pregnancy has no meaning and carries no responsibility to the mother or child

b. Paternal tasks of pregnancy

(1) First trimester: announcement phase

(a) The man must cope with his ambivalence about becoming a father

(b) He strives to accept the biological fact of pregnancy

(c) He attempts to take on the expectant father role

(2) Second trimester: moratorium phase

(a) The man often has a delay in binding-in to the pregnancy when compared with the woman

(b) He accepts the woman's changing body

(c) He accepts the reality of the fetus, particularly when he can feel fetal movement

(d) He adapts to the changes in their sexual relationship

(i) He has fears about harming the fetus during sexual intercourse

(ii) He may experience a potential rivalry with a male obstetrician

(e) He experiences confusion when dealing with the woman's intense introspection

(f) He fantasizes about the father-child relationship (with the child not as an infant but as an older child, playing ball, for example)

(3) Third trimester: focusing phase

(a) He negotiates what his role will be during labor and delivery

(b) He prepares for the reality of parenthood

(c) He may change his self-concept and image (e.g., may shave his beard and buy new clothes)

(d) He engages in preparing the nursery

(e) He copes with fears about the mutilation or the death of his partner and child

c. Fathers at labor and birth

(1) Benefits

(a) Dispels his feelings of alienation

(b) Increases his sense of significance and importance

(c) Increases his sense of control

(d) Increases his appreciation for his laboring woman/partner

(e) Develops a closer attachment to his newborn earlier in the father-child relationship

(2) There is a need for a sensitivity to a father's unfamiliarity with such things as

(a) Unfamiliar sights, for example

(i) His woman/partner in pain, grimacing

(ii) Bulging perineum

(b) Unfamiliar sounds, for example

(i) Moans, grunts

(ii) Hospital noises

(c) Unfamiliar smells, for example

(i) Vaginal discharge, amniotic fluid

(ii) Cleaning solutions and medications

(d) The father is not merely a coach; he also has his own needs

(i) Fatigue

(ii) Hunger

(iii) Fears and concerns

(3) Other considerations about expectant fathers at labor and birth

(a) Some cultures bar men from labor (e.g., certain Middle Eastern cultures)

(b) Some men do not want to be present for labor

(c) Some women do not want the father to see them "like that"

8. Other family members' psychosocial reactions to pregnancy and childbirth

a. Expectant siblings

(1) Reaction to pregnancy is age dependent (e.g., 2 years old versus 8 years old)

(2) Siblings may express excitement and anticipation

(3) Siblings may verbalize negative reactions

(4) Siblings may be unaware or noncommittal

(5) Siblings who are present at birth need a caretaker whose major focus is meeting the needs of the sibling(s), i.e., involvement, or withdrawal from the process

(6) Siblings may exhibit ambivalent reactions to a newborn in the home

(a) Affection and excitement

(b) May vacillate, with regressive behavior, anger, or both

b. Expectant grandparents

(1) Often express excitement and anticipation

(2) May express resentment (e.g., "I'm too young to be someone's grandmother!")

           (3) May verbalize anger if the pregnancy was unplanned or if the mother is a teenager or is unwed

           (4) Often express anxiety about the health and well-being of the expectant mother (daughter or daughter-in-law) and fetus

           (5) May be concerned about the expectant parents' age, income, and emotional stability to have a child

  9. Single expectant mother's psychosocial needs

    a. Reason for single status needs to be assessed to better understand the meaning of pregnancy

       (1) Single by choice: pregnancy may have been by artificial insemination

       (2) Single by accident; for example, a woman became a widow after conception or became pregnant through rape

       (3) Single by divorce or separation after conception

       (4) Single and pregnant by a casual acquaintance (unplanned or planned)

    b. Presence or absence of strong support person(s) can significantly influence the woman's adaptation to pregnancy

    c. Future plans for the baby are an important factor influencing the mother's psychological needs (i.e., planning to keep and raise the child or planning to place the child for adoption?)

 10. Ethnocultural considerations

    a. American women are in a transitional culture in which there is a lack of well-established prescriptions for pregnant behavior

    b. Technological culture exists in American society

       (1) Use of technology creates a potential to increase stress and anxiety in the pregnant woman

         (a) Moral and ethical dilemmas frequently are associated with diagnostic tests

         (b) The woman's interpersonal and emotional needs may be missed or ignored in favor of technological information

       (2) There is an increased chance of caregivers' shifting their focus from the woman to the equipment

    c. General principles about different ethnic groups

       (1) Pregnancy is considered to be normal, not a state of illness (e.g., some Native American tribes)

       (2) The culture does not see the need for medical care if pregnancy is a well state of being

       (3) Pregnancy often has many rigid taboos (e.g., some African nations)

       (4) Pregnancy may be viewed as only woman's work (e.g., Middle Eastern cultures)

       (5) Yin-yang: everything in nature is balanced for example, hot/cold (e.g., Korean cultures)

       (6) Strong needs for modesty to be protected (Middle Eastern cultures)

B. **Nursing Diagnoses**

1. High risk for disturbance in body image, role performance, and self-esteem
2. Altered sexuality patterns secondary to changes in libido during pregnancy
3. Alteration in family process related to developmental stressors of pregnancy
4. Anxiety related to fear of the unknown
5. Coping, family, opportunity for growth/mastery
6. Alteration in parenting secondary to lack of knowledge and skills

C. **Interventions/Evaluations**

1. High risk for disturbance in body image, self-esteem, role performance, and personal identity

    a. Interventions

       (1) Use effective listening and nonjudgmental communication skills

       (2) Encourage the woman to seek prenatal care

      (3) Provide resources—books, magazines, videos, and support groups—to assist in role changes of pregnant woman and mother

      (4) Encourage childbirth and baby care classes

      (5) Encourage the family to provide material symbols of role changes

         (a) Maternity clothes

         (b) Baby equipment

      (6) Explain the normal, expected emotional ramifications of pregnancy and role changes

      (7) Assist the couple to set realistic goals and expectations for themselves

      (8) Explore expectations for labor

         (a) Birth plans

         (b) Choice of support persons

         (c) Offer options and opportunities for decision making to increase self-esteem

      (9) Offer realistic concepts of the early parental-infant attachment process

         (a) Provide early infant contact

         (b) Explain normal newborn behaviors

  b. Evaluations

      (1) The woman has received prenatal care

      (2) The couple has attended childbirth and/or baby care classes

      (3) The woman exhibits acceptance of role (e.g., can be concerned about being a good mother, but not ambivalent about becoming a mother)

      (4) The woman has determined how she will feed her baby (by breast or bottle)

      (5) The couple has chosen the infant's name

      (6) The couple has prepared the home for the infant

      (7) The couple negotiates options and desires for labor and birth

      (8) The parents demonstrate an active interest in the newborn at birth

2. Altered sexuality patterns secondary to changes in libido during pregnancy

  a. Interventions

      (1) Explain the wide variety of sexual feelings and behavior

         (a) The couple may enjoy sexual activity more because there is

            (i) No fear of pregnancy

            (ii) No need for contraceptive use (which, depending on the method, can disrupt spontaneity)

            (iii) Increased pelvic congestion with fulminating orgasm; some women experience their first orgasm during pregnancy

            (iv) Increased vaginal lubrication

            (v) A perception of the pregnancy as very sensuous

         (b) The couple may have decreased desires and responses because of

            (i) A negative body image (may be experienced by the man, the woman, or both)

            (ii) A belief in myths about harming the fetus by intercourse

            (iii) Physical symptoms such as fatigue, nausea, and vomiting, which may influence desire and response

            (iv) A psychological restriction some couples feel toward sexual intercourse during pregnancy

            (v) Taboos that some cultural and social groups have against sexual intercourse during pregnancy

      (2) Determine and fulfill informational needs

         (a) There are many ways of expressing affection and intimacy beyond intercourse alone (for example, "necking", massage, and romantic dinner)

         (b) Positions for intercourse may need to change as the uterus grows (e.g., to side-lying or female superior)

         (c) Masturbation or manual stimulation may cause a more intense orgasm than intercourse (and needs to be avoided if intercourse is contraindicated for preterm labor risk)

      (d) Provide accurate information about the safety of intercourse throughout a normal pregnancy

      (e) Pregnancy is a time of vulnerability and couples need to be encouraged to be sensitive to one another's needs for affection and intimacy

      (f) Orgasm causes harmless contractions and does not cause any problems in normal pregnancy

      (g) Blowing into the vagina is contraindicated because of the potential of causing an air embolus

    (3) Contraindications to intercourse

      (a) Ruptured membranes because of potential for infection

      (b) Incompetent cervix because of potential to cause preterm labor

      (c) Spotting or bleeding, especially with a placenta previa

      (d) Preterm labor history because of potential to start premature labor

  b. Evaluations

    (1) Comfort level is established for open dialogue with the health care provider about sexual questions and concerns

    (2) The couple maintains intimacy during pregnancy

    (3) The couple can discuss satisfaction with options for expressing affection

3. Alterations in family process related to developmental stressors of pregnancy

  a. Interventions

    (1) Offer anticipatory guidance about normal developmental stressors of pregnancy, for example

      (a) Ambivalence during early pregnancy

      (b) Vulnerability

      (c) Impatience, irritability

      (d) Active dream/fantasy life

    (2) Encourage parents to ask questions

    (3) Help parents appreciate the normal and universal nature of the emotional changes in pregnancy and identify areas of stress

    (4) Acknowledge the ethical dilemmas and the emotional stress of some prenatal diagnostic testing procedures

    (5) Discuss the common phases through which men progress during pregnancy

      (a) Announcement phase: when the diagnosis is made

      (b) Moratorium phase: occuring during early pregnancy, when there is often little overt interest on the expectant father's part

      (c) Focusing phase: related to the new role as father which occurs during late pregnancy

    (6) Provide encouragement that a couple's adaptive coping strategies are effective (or help the couple alter them if the strategies are not working)

    (7) Assist the couple to identify and use support systems

  b. Evaluations

    (1) The couple can verbalize feelings and concerns to each other and to the health care provider

    (2) The couple discusses available support systems and uses them (family, friends, and other expectant families)

    (3) The couple attends childbirth or baby care classes together

    (4) The couple demonstrates mutual support

    (5) The parents seek help with emotional concerns about prenatal testing

4. Anxiety related to fear of the unknown

  a. Interventions

    (1) Offer education and information on an individual basis and encourage attendance at childbirth classes

    (2) Explain all procedures and rationales before implementing them and keep parents informed of progress

    (3) Help the couple verbalize fears and determine the level of anxiety (from mild anxiety to panic)

(4) If anxiety is related to a specific maternal or fetal complication, refer the couple to an appropriate resource

(5) Do not overburden the couple with too much information at one time

(6) Assist the family to develop a realistic birth plan to better focus on concerns and to gain a sense of control for themselves

    (a) Primipara: help her to focus on alternatives and to transform dreams and fantasies into real choices

    (b) Multipara: assess what went well in her last labor and birth, and what she would like to change this time

b. Evaluations

(1) The couple develops a realistic birth plan with several different alternatives and options

(2) The couple seeks appropriate resources for specific problems

(3) The couple can verbalize fears to health care providers and to each other

(4) The couple demonstrates a calm demeanor with relaxed voices and body language

(5) The couple states a feeling of less anxiety and fearfulness

5. Coping, family, and opportunity for growth/mastery

a. Interventions

(1) Offer the couple the necessary data and information for decision making

(2) Encourage the couple to make decisions based on realistic alternatives

(3) Praise the couple each time the couple demonstrates effective coping (e.g., a written birth plan, breathing in synchrony, and mutual support)

(4) If the couple is not coping effectively, actively assist the couple to regain control

(5) Offer oneself as a role-model to demonstrate skills the couple can learn (e.g., relaxation strategies, breathing techniques, breastfeeding guidance)

(6) Assist the couple to envision changes in plans (e.g., having an unplanned epidural) as an appropriate coping mechanism within the context of a particular situation and not as a failure

b. Evaluations

(1) The couple verbalizes a sense of pride of accomplishment

(2) The couple discusses resources and support systems used during pregnancy and childbirth

(3) The couple seeks to understand any events during labor and birth that were unclear or misinterpreted and to put them into an appropriate context

(4) The couple expresses realistic uncertainities about infant care while expressing confidence in the ability to learn

6. Alterations in parenting secondary to a lack of knowledge and skills

a. Interventions

(1) Assist the parents to develop realistic expectations of themselves as parents

    (a) Primipara: help her to shift the focus from the common myth of a "blissful" newborn parenting to a more realistic view of initial sleep deprivation and disorganization

    (b) Multipara: help her to identify how a new baby will change her present family constellation

    (c) Multipara: assess family plans to incorporate the new baby into the family's daily life

(2) Offer "hands-on" demonstration/return demonstration opportunities for baby care (e.g., bathing or cord care) to increase practical parenting skills

(3) Give the parents community resources to solicit assistance and support, as needed

(4) Send the parents home from the hospital with written materials to reinforce hospital staff teaching about baby care and parenting
b. Evaluations
(1) The couple demonstrates basic baby care skills with confidence
(2) The couple verbalizes a plan for meeting early parenting demands
(3) The couple identifies appropriate resources to offer assistance

Health Education

A. Early pregnancy

1. Developmental tasks of pregnancy
   a. Mother: acceptance of pregnancy integration into her self system
   b. Father: announcement and realization of the pregnancy
   c. Couple: realignment of relationships and roles
2. Psychosocial changes of pregnancy
   a. Ambivalence about pregnancy
   b. Introversion
   c. Passivity and difficulty with decision making
   d. Sexual and emotional changes
   e. Changing self-image
   f. Ethical dilemmas of prenatal testing

B. Midtrimester pregnancy

1. Developmental tasks of pregnancy
   a. Mother: binding-in to the pregnancy, ensuring safe passage, and differentiating the fetus from herself
   b. Father: anticipation of adapting to the role of fatherhood
   c. Couple: realignment of roles and division of tasks
2. Psychosocial changes
   a. Active dream and fantasy life
   b. Concerns with body image
   c. Nesting behaviors
   d. Sexual behavior adjustment
   e. Expanding to a variety of methods of expressing affection and intimacy

C. Last-trimester pregnancy

1. Developmental tasks of pregnancy
   a. Mother: separating herself from the pregnancy and the fetus, trying various caregiving methods
   b. Father: role adaptation; preparation for labor and birth
   c. Couple: preparation of the nursery
2. Psychosocial changes
   a. Hates the pregnancy, loves the baby
   b. Although anxious about childbirth, the mother also sees labor and delivery as a deliverance
   c. The couple experiments with various mothering or fathering roles
   d. Mother is introspective

D. Evaluation

1. The couple can verbalize the educational content
2. The couple seeks assistance and support with psychological concerns
3. The couple demonstrates insight into psychological processes (e.g., increasing introspection and isolation during labor)

CASE STUDY AND STUDY QUESTIONS

Marjorie is a 36-year-old primigravida woman who has deliberately delayed pregnancy because she wanted to establish her career first. She and her husband, David, carefully planned the timing of the pregnancy to coincide with her teaching schedule so that she could take maternity leave over the summer.

When she became pregnant and her expected date of confinement was May 16, she and her huband were thrilled! However, despite the careful planning and successful diagnosis, Marjorie confided to the nurse that she was not sure she really wanted to be pregnant. When her chorionic villi sampling results were normal, she began to really embrace pregnancy. She purposefully stopped and talked to neighbors who were out pushing baby carriages, and she began to call her mother with questions about her own birth.

As the pregnancy progressed, David signed them up for every childbirth class he could find. He also put on weight and complained of stomachaches and various pains.

Last month at the doctor's office, Marjorie was relieved when the nurse asked about her dreams. She had felt so uncomfortable telling anyone about the weird dreams and fantasies that she had been having. For example, she was illogically concerned about David's driving; he had always seemed to be speeding but it had never bothered her before. Now she was dreaming about her abdomen being run over by a truck!

Marjorie and David are now attending Lamaze classes. David seems preoccupied with learning about the role of coach. The teacher has been helping each couple develop a birth plan and encouraging them to explore alternatives in case all does not go according to the ideal. David and Marjorie have found this to be both helpful and calming.

1. When a woman desires to have a baby and receives a positive pregnancy diagnosis, her emotions may include
   a. Ambivalence.
   b. Joy.
   c. Surprise.
   d. All of the above.

2. Men whose partners are pregnant sometimes experience sympathetic feelings and symptoms called
   a. Pseudopregnancy.
   b. Male pregnancy.
   c. Couvade.
   d. Pseudogestation.

3. Pregnant women who tell the nurse about strange dreams should be
   a. Referred to a psychiatrist.
   b. Assured that such dreams are common and normal in pregnancy.
   c. Offered a psychosocial interpretation.
   d. Told to ignore them.

4. The concept of developing a birth plan
   a. Should upset nurses who are the real experts about labor and birth.
   b. Is illegal in some states.
   c. Is acceptable only in home births.
   d. Increases a couple's sense of control and mastery.

5. Many Native American women do not seek prenatal care because
   a. They see tribal healers instead.
   b. They remain in bed throughout pregnancy.
   c. They believe that pregnancy is normal with no necessity for seeing a doctor.
   d. None of the above.

6. The critical third-trimester issue in acceptance of the child is that
   a. The nursery is ready.
   b. The family describes the fetus as a real person.
   c. Acceptance is unconditional.
   d. The father is concerned about the baby's well-being.

7. Nesting behaviors are disrupted by
   a. Baby showers.
   b. Preterm labor.
   c. Father's business plans.
   d. Anxiety about labor.

8. Two third-trimester developmental tasks of expectant fathers include
   a. His changing image and negotiation of his role during labor and delivery.
   b. Taking on the expectant father role and preparing the nursery.
   c. Preparing for parenthood and accepting the woman's changing body.
   d. Dealing with the woman's introspection and accepting the biological fact of pregnancy.

9. A common principle found among many ethnic cultures is that
   a. Pregnant women are sick.
   b. Everything in nature is balanced (e.g., yin-yang)
   c. A pregnant woman must wear a gold necklace in labor.
   d. A pregnant woman's mother must be barred from the birth.

10. If expectant parents tell the labor nurse that they have taken childbirth classes, have chosen a name for their baby, have decided to breastfeed, and have prepared their home for the newborn, the nurse

can surmise they are successfully coping with changes in

a. The expectant couple role.
b. Self-concept as a couple.
c. The developmental stressors of pregnancy.
d. Anxiety.

Answers to Study Questions

1. d	2. c	3. b.
4. d	5. c	6. c
7. b	8. a	9. b
10. b		

REFERENCES

Anderberg, G.J. (1988). Initial acquaintance and attachment behavior of siblings with the newborn. *Journal of Obstetric, Gynecologic, and Neonatal Nursing, 17*(1), 49–54.

Aquilera, D.C., & Messick, J.M. (1974). *Crisis intervention: Theory and methodology* (2nd ed.). St. Louis: Mosby.

Avant, K.C. (1988). Stressors on the childbearing family. *Journal of Obstetric, Gynecologic, and Neonatal Nursing, 17*(3), 179–185.

Brouse, A.J. (1988) Easing the transition to the maternal role. *Journal of Advanced Nursing, 13*(3), 167–172.

Caplan, G. (1957). Psychological aspects of maternity care. *American Journal of Public Health, 47*(25), 11–20.

Carter, J.L. (1981). Promoting maternal attachment through prenatal intervention. *MCN: American Journal of Maternal Child Nursing, 6*(2), 107–112.

Choi, E.C. (1986). Unique aspects of Korean-American mothers. *Journal of Obstetric, Gynecologic, and Neonatal Nursing, 15*(5), 394–400.

Choi, E.S.C., & Hamilton, R.K. (1986). The effects of culture on mother-infant interactions. *Journal of Obstetric, Gynecologic, and Neonatal Nursing, 15*(3), 256–261.

Clark, A. (1978). *Culture, childbearing, health professionals*. Philadelphia: Davis.

Coleman, A., & Coleman, L. (1971). *Pregnancy: The psychological experience*. New York: Seabury.

Connor, G.K. (1990). Expectant fathers' response to pregnancy: Review of literature and implications for research in high-risk pregnancy. *Journal of Perinatal-Neonatal Nursing, 4*(2), 32–42.

Duvall, E. (1977). *Marriage and family development*. Philadelphia: Lippincott.

Ellis, D. (1980). Sexual needs and concerns of expectant parents. *Journal of Obstetric, Gynecologic, and Neonatal Nursing, 9*(5), 306–308.

Fishbein, E.G. (1984). Expectant fathers' stress due to mothers' expectations? *Journal of Obstetric, Gynecologic, and Neonatal Nursing, 13*(5), 325–328.

Green, J.M., Coupland, V.A., Kitzinger, J.U. (1990). Expectations, experiences and psychological outcomes of childbirth: A prospective study of 825 women. *Birth, 17*(1), 15–24.

Green, N.L. (1990). Stressful events related to childbearing in African-American women: A pilot study. *Journal of Nurse-Midwifery, 35*(4), 231–236.

Greenberg, M. (1985). *The birth of a father*. New York: Continuum.

Gruis, M. (1977). Beyond maternity: Postpartum concerns of mothers. *MCN: American Journal of Maternal Child Nursing, 2*(3), 182–188.

Hammer, T.J., & Turner, P.H. (1985). *Parenting in contemporary society*. Englewood Cliffs, NJ: Prentice Hall.

Hames, C. (1980). Sexual needs and interests in postpartum couples. *Journal of Obstetric, Gynecologic, and Neonatal Nursing, 9*(5), 313–315.

Hampson, S.J. (1989). Nursing interventions for the first three postpartum months. *Journal of Obstetric, Gynecologic, and Neonatal Nursing, 18*(2), 116–122.

Harris, K. (1987). Beliefs and practices among Haitian American women in relation to childbearing. *Journal of Nurse-Midwifery, 32*(3), 149–155.

Heise, J. (1975). Toward better preparation for involved fatherhood. *Journal of Obstetric, Gynecologic, and Neonatal Nursing, 4*(5), 32–35.

Jones, C. (1987). *Mind over labor*. New York: Viking.

Jones, C. (1985). *Sharing birth*. New York: Quill.

Jones, K. (1990). Expectant fears . . . psychological self-assessment by pregnant women. *Nursing Times, 86*(15), 36–38.

Jordan, P.L. (1990). Laboring for relevance: Expectant and new fatherhood. *Nursing Research, 39*(1), 11–16.

Kay, M. (1982). *Anthropology of human birth*. Philadelphia: Davis.

May, K. (1978). Active involvement of expectant fathers: Some further considerations. *Journal of Obstetric, Gynecologic, and Neonatal Nursing, 7*(2), 7–12.

May, K.A. (1982). Three phases of father involvement in pregnancy. *Nursing Research, 31*(6), 337–342.

McNall, L. (1976). *Concerns of expectant fathers, current practices in obstetrical and gynecological nursing*. St. Louis: Mosby.

Meleis, A., & Sorrell, L. (1981). Arab-American women and their birth experience. *MCN: American Journal of Maternal Child Nursing, 6*(3), 171–176.

Poole, C. (1986). Fatigue during the first trimester of pregnancy. *Journal of Obstetric, Gynecologic, and Neonatal Nursing, 15*(5), 375–379.

Pruett, K.D. (1987). *The nurturing father.* New York: Warner.

Rubin, R. (1967). Attainment of the maternal role—part I: Processes. *Nursing Research, 16*(3), 237–245.

Rubin, R. (1984). *Maternal identity and the maternal experience.* New York: Springer.

Ruff, C.C. (1987). How well do adolescents mother? *American Journal of Maternal-Child Nursing, 12*(4), 249–253.

Satz, K. (1982). Integrating Navajo tradition into maternal-child nursing. *Image, 14*(3), 89–91.

Shapiro, J.L. (1987). *When men are pregnant.* San Luis Ibispo, CA: Impact.

Sherwen, L.N. (1987). *Psychosocial dimensions of the pregnant family.* New York: Springer.

Spector, R. (1985). Cultural diversity in health and illness. Norwalk, CT: Appleton-Century-Crofts.

Stern, P. (1981). Solving problems of cross-cultural health teaching: The Filipino childbearing family. *Image, 13*(2), 47–50.

Stichler, J., Bowden, M., & Reimer, E. (1978). Pregnancy: A shared emotional experience. *American Journal of Maternal-Child Nursing, 3*(3), 153–157.

Storch, M.L. (1987). Taking a sexual history. *Contemporary OB/GYN 29* (special issue), 111.

Strickland, O.L. (1987). The occurrence of symptoms in expectant fathers. *Nursing Research, 36*(3), 184–189.

Swanson, T. (1980). The marital sexual relationship during pregnancy. *Journal of Obstetric, Gynecologic, and Neonatal Nursing, 9*(4), 267–270.

Wadd, L. (1983). Vietnamese postpartum practices: Implications for nursing in the hospital setting. *Journal of Obstetric, Gynecologic, and Neonatal Nursing, 12*(4), 252–258.

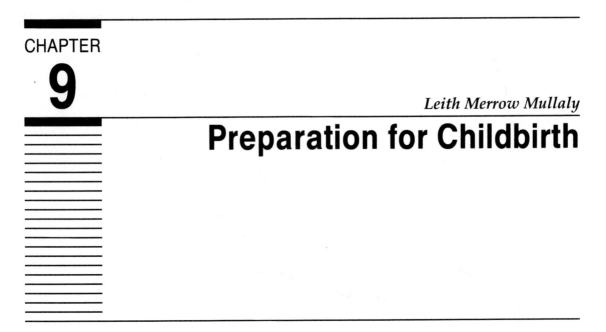

Leith Merrow Mullaly

Preparation for Childbirth

Objectives

1. Compare the fear-tension-pain cycle with the knowledge-and-relaxation cycle and the decreased-pain-perception cycle

2. Discuss the basic concept of the gate theory of pain control

3. Recall three nonpharmacological techniques used to decrease labor pain

4. Identify and discuss the rationale for paced breathing techniques in labor

5. Relate basic principles of touch relaxation

6. List three or four supportive measures taught to the support person to meet emotional changes during the different stages of labor

7. Explain slow-paced, modified-paced, and patterned-paced breathing (Lamaze) and abdominal breathing (Bradley)

8. Describe what expectant couples learn about the basic sequence of cesarean birth procedures

9. Describe two or three emotional reactions that parents may experience immediately after the baby is born

10. Identify specific comfort measures to use in back labor

11. Discuss the benefits of pelvic rock exercises and of tailor sitting

12. Explain how expectant parents can negotiate their birth plans within the context of the hospital setting

13. Describe an environment within the labor and delivery unit that is conducive to relaxation for the laboring woman

14. Discuss the concept of guided imagery to enhance relaxation

15. Identify two or three different positions for pushing and discuss the advantages of different positions

16. Offer anticipatory guidance about the possible emotional ramifications of unexpected outcomes

17. Detect subtle cues from a couple that may precede a loss of appropriate control, panic intimidation, and feelings of failure

Introduction

The broadest goal of childbirth education is to assist individuals and family members to make informed decisions about pregnancy and birth, based on knowledge of their options and choices. This goal is operationalized by providing specific information about the components of a healthy pregnancy, the process of labor and birth with the necessary tools/skills to work with, and the coping strategies to deal successfully with the challenges of early parenting.

Clinical Practice

A. Assessment

1. Target populations
   a. Prospective parents
   b. Expectant parents
   c. Expectant siblings
   d. Expectant grandparents
   e. Expectant adolescents
2. Basic underlying principles of childbirth education are
   a. The concept of the fear-tension-pain cycle
   b. The counter concepts of knowledge and relaxation and of decreased pain perception
   c. Pregnancy, birth, and early parenting all involve adaptation to stressors
   d. Partner participation and support are very important
   e. With practice, relaxation and breathing strategies can be initiated via a conditioned response to the stimulus of a uterine contraction
   f. Relaxation and breathing patterns are aids to cope with labor pain and to enhance labor effectiveness
   g. Knowledge of choices, options, and alternatives can empower a laboring woman and her support person
   h. Practice of relevant coping strategies and support skills by expectant parents affects their experience of birth

B. Nursing Diagnoses

1. Knowledge deficit related to health maintenance needs during pregnancy
2. Knowledge deficit related to the process of labor and birth
3. Anxiety related to a lack of knowledge and fear of the unknown
4. Knowledge deficit related to the needs of the mother, father, and infant during the postpartum period
5. Knowledge deficit related to the special needs of the pregnant adolescent

C. Interventions/Evaluations

1. Knowledge deficit related to health maintenance needs in pregnancy
   a. Interventions
      (1) Preconception classes should discuss
         (a) Nutritional needs of women before conception
         (b) Environmental hazards to avoid periconceptually
         (c) Genetic family history
         (d) Maternal age factors in planning conception
         (e) Benefits of prenatal care in the prevention and detection of complications
      (2) Early pregnancy classes should discuss
         (a) Nutrition information related to early pregnancy needs
         (b) Common physical discomforts of early pregnancy and nonpharmaceutical relief measures

(c) Appropriate exercise
   (i) Avoid jumping and jarring
   (ii) Avoid raising maternal body temperature
(d) Emotional and sexual changes in early pregnancy
(e) Exploration of different birthing options to register appropriately for childbirth preparation classes
   (i) Prepared natural childbirth (e.g., Lamaze, Bradley)
   (ii) Labor and birth using analgesics or anesthesia
   (iii) Settings for birth
       ● Hospital: delivery room (OR)
       ● Hospital: labor/delivery/recovery (LDR) room
       ● Hospital: labor/delivery/recovery/postpartum (L/D/R/P) room
       ● Birthing center: free standing
       ● Home

b. Evaluations (by hospital nurses)
  (1) The woman began prenatal care during the first trimester
  (2) The woman appears well nourished and can relate key nutrients that she has included in her diet throughout the pregnancy
  (3) The woman has abstained from use of alcohol, nontherapeutic drugs, and cigarettes

2. Knowledge deficits related to the process of labor and birth
  a. Interventions: prepared natural childbirth classes
    (1) Concept of psychoprophylaxis: fear is replaced by knowledge, tension is replaced by relaxation, pain is replaced by a decreased perception of pain

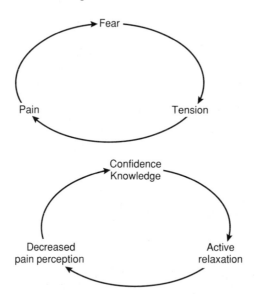

(a) Brief review of the gate theory of pain control
   (i) Pain sensations travel up sensory nerve pathways to brain
   (ii) Only a limited number of sensations or messages can travel through nerve pathways at one time
   (iii) By bombarding sensory nerve pathways with distractors such as touch, music, and imagery, the nerve pathways for pain perception are reduced or completely blocked
(b) Interrupt fear with information
(c) Limit tension with active relaxation strategies
(d) Decrease pain perception by using focusing strategies (e.g., breathing patterns, imagery, music, hydrotherapy, and massage)

(e) Conditioned response concept: contractions trigger relaxation
(f) Presence of a loving family and supportive people
(2) Common childbirth glossary of terms
(3) Conditioning exercises (e.g., Kegel's exercises and the pelvic rock)
(4) Active relaxation strategies to use in the face of pain and discomfort (e.g., touch, guided imagery, hydrotherapy, and music)
(5) Lamaze breathing patterns (any of the techniques can be used at any time during labor)
  (a) Basic breathing awareness that is taught to expectant parents (Fig. 9-1*A*)
    (i) Breathe in comfortably, blow the air out slowly
    (ii) Allow the body to go limp
    (iii) Allow breathing to continue quietly, easily, and rhythmically

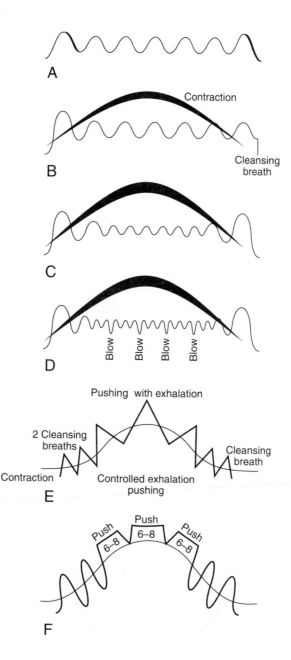

Figure 9–1
Breathing patterns. *A,* Normal breathing awareness; *B,* slow-paced breathing; *C,* modified-paced breathing; *D,* patterned-paced breathing; *E,* breath-holding pattern.

        (iv) Focus on complete relaxation with each outward breath

        (v) Woman may use any breathing technique at any stage of labor, according to her comfort needs

    (b) Cleansing breath

        (i) Rationale

- Signals that a contraction is beginning or ending
- Begins a contraction in relaxed state
- Assists oxygen and carbon dioxide balance

        (ii) Technique that is taught to expectant parents

- Deep inhalation
- Slow exhalation by sighing or blowing

    (c) Slow-paced breathing that is taught to expectant parents (Fig. 9–1*B*)

        (i) Approximately one-half of the normal resting respiratory rate (usually is approximately six to nine breaths per minute, excluding cleansing breaths)

        (ii) Begin and end the contraction with a cleansing breath

        (iii) Breathing is relaxed, slow, and easy

        (iv) Attention focus

- Inhale and exhale through the nose
- Inhale and exhale through the mouth
- Inhale through the nose and exhale through the mouth
- May use rocking, massage, or walking (physical)
- May use timing, counting, or imagery (mental)

    (d) Modified-paced breathing that is taught to expectant parents (Fig. 9–1*C*)

        (i) Increase the rate to twice that of the mother's normal rate (better to keep the rate below 40 breaths per minute, excluding cleansing breaths)

        (ii) May be used any time during labor, by itself or in combination with slow-paced breathing (e.g., slow-paced breathing at the beginning, modified-paced breathing over the peaks, and return to slow-paced breathing)

        (iii) Attention focus, as in slow-paced breathing

        (iv) Breathing should be shallow, with a shallow inhalation followed by a shallow exhalation

    (e) Patterned-paced breathing that is taught to expectant parents (Fig. 9–1*D*)

        (i) Increase the rate to twice that of the mother's normal rate (better to keep at or below 40 breaths per minute, excluding cleansing breaths)

        (ii) May be used any time during labor

        (iii) Movement is relaxed, rhythmical breathing patterned with soft blows that do not change the rate during the contraction (i.e., may range from one breath and one blow to six breaths and one blow)

        (iv) Support person who is counting the pattern may be helpful

        (v) Breathing movement is with face, chest, and abdomen relaxed

        (vi) Emphasis is on the pattern of breathing with the variety of patterns designed by the mother and the support person

    (f) Controlled-exhalation pushing (also known as gentle pushing or physiological pushing) that is taught to expectant parents (Fig. 9–1*E*)

        (i) Mother assumes a comfortable position (e.g., pelvic tilt)

        (ii) Two cleansing breaths (somewhat quicker than before) are taken

        (iii) Take a third breath in and slowly exhale by blowing and hissing through slightly parted lips; continue the slow exhalation until able to feel abdominal muscles contracting completely: push while slowly exhaling

(iv) Concentrate on relaxing the face and pelvic floor muscles: Kegel out; concentrate on the direction of the push

(v) Repeat once or twice until the contraction is over

(vi) End with a deep cleansing breath

(g) Breath-holding pushing that is taught to expectant parents (Fig. 9-1*F*)

(i) Mother assumes a comfortable position

(ii) Two cleansing breaths

(iii) Take a third breath in, raise the back and the shoulders up so that the body is in a curved-back position; release a small amount of air from the throat, relax the mouth and the face: Kegel out and push

(iv) Continue pushing for 6 to 8 seconds, then blow out the air, drop the head back, breathe again with the head down on the chest, hold the breath and push; do not release abdominals while taking the next breath or the effectiveness of pushing will be somewhat diminished

(v) Repeat for the duration of contractions (usually 3 or 4 pushes)

(6) Bradley's breathing that is taught to expectant parents

(a) Diaphragmatic (i.e., from the stomach) breathing is believed to be the most efficient for relaxation, according to the Bradley philosophy

(b) No specific techniques are taught or believed to be necessary

(c) Women are reminded to become aware of their own breathing with the needs of their body determining the rate and depth of breath

(d) Using only diaphragm muscle requires less work and conserves energy

(7) Cognitive strategies that are taught to expectant parents

(a) Auditory stimuli: count breaths; use rhythmic phrases (e.g., "I am relaxed") or music (Lamaze, Bradley)

(b) Visual stimuli: the coach uses fingers to count breaths; use of a focal point or photograph (Lamaze)

(c) Principles of touch and massage relaxation

(i) Touch and warmth aid relaxation

(ii) Touch strokes should be in the direction of hair growth (e.g., stroke down the arm from the elbow to the wrist)

(iii) Touch can be a light, finger-tip effleurage massage

(iv) Touch can be a firm, brisk, whole-hand massage

(v) The laboring woman needs to show the support person where and how touch feels good

(d) Internal visualization to help the woman get in touch with her own body and natural process of birth (Lamaze, Bradley)

(e) Visualization to focus on external factors of distraction (Lamaze)

(8) Stage I labor: couples need to know that there is a wide variety of labor patterns and that few labor patterns proceed like the textbook version

(a) Early phase averages 8 to 10 hours in primiparas and averages 5 to 7 hours in multiparas: coping strategies taught to expectant mothers are

(i) Ambulate

(ii) Take fluids and easily digested foods (gelatin, tea with honey, for example)

(iii) Save the "energy burst" (e.g., do not scrub the floor)

(iv) Sit in a warm bath if membranes are intact or take a warm shower

(v) Remain at home as long as possible

(vi) Listen to music

(vii) Use meditation

(viii) Have a massage (in the direction of hair growth)

(ix) Call the caregiver according to instructions (i.e., when there are regular contractions every 10 minutes for a multipara, [regular contractions every 5 minutes for 1 hour for a primipara]; need to call if there is a rupture of membranes [ROM] or bleeding, regardless of the presence or absence of contractions)

(x) May use slow-paced breathing pattern (Lamaze) or may use abdominal breathing (Bradley)

(b) Active phase averages 3 to 6 hours in primiparas and averages 2 to 3 hours in multiparas; coping strategies taught to expectant parents are

(i) Warm showers, bath (if membranes are intact)

(ii) Touch relaxation to release tension (e.g., jaw, forehead, shoulders, thighs, and feet)

(iii) Use "goodie bag" contents, as needed (e.g., socks for cold feet, talcum for massage, tennis ball or rolling pin for back labor, photograph for focus, lip moisturizer for dry lips, and music tape to enhance relaxation)

(iv) Change positions frequently (e.g., sitting, rocking, walking, side-lying, standing, squatting)

(v) Empty bladder

(vi) Fluids and oral hygiene

(vii) Coach is taught to accept irritability and support the woman's choice of pain relief techniques

(viii) Coach is taught to praise hard work

(ix) Woman may request analgesic medication or epidural anesthesia (note: the specific goal of the Bradley method is an unmedicated delivery)

(x) Effleurage (light stroking, often in figure-eight pattern) may be helpful

(xi) Imagery: "picture the baby pushing the cervix open or the unfurling of a flower"

(xii) Relief from back labor: counter pressure with the heel of the hand or tennis balls, pelvic rocking, tailor sitting, getting on all fours (on hands and knees), heat or ice applied to lower back

(xiii) Active support and coaching: nurse should work through the coach by

- Assessing the support person's role as coach (i.e., is he or she physically close to the patient or withdrawn? Is he or she breathing with the woman, counting off the pattern? Is he or she focused on the patient and not on the personnel or monitor?

- Giving instructions through the coach for him or her to communicate with the patient if the couple is working well together; nurse is available, as needed

- Remaining on the periphery if the couple is working intimately and effectively together, the nurse is available, as needed

- Reinforcing and encouraging the coach's good work and effort

- Actively intervening with specific suggestions of comfort measures and/or breathing techniques if the couple is not working effectively or has temporarily lost a sense of control

(xiv) Use a breathing pattern that is effective in aiding relaxation in the particular woman

(c) Transitional phase averages 30 to 90 minutes in primiparas and averages 15 to 30 minutes in multiparas; coping strategies taught to expectant parents are

    (i) Intense support and encouragement; coaches are instructed not to leave the woman alone at this time

    (ii) Short, crisp directions and low-key verbal support from the nurse and coach are most effective (the woman is internally focused and cannot absorb complex directions)

    (iii) Focus on only one contraction at a time and remind her that this is the shortest phase of labor and that birth is near

    (iv) Coaches usually need to breathe with the woman; the breathing pattern used is usually patterned-paced (Lamaze) or abdominal deep breathing (Bradley) but need not be a specific pattern if the woman is comfortable and in control

    (v) Touch
- Woman may desire and like touch or may push coach away, not wanting touch
- Woman may want intense touch or counter pressure or may prefer light stroking instead
- Woman may be kept fasting (NPO) in some settings; may take fluids or ice chips by mouth in other settings; keep the mouth and lips lubricated with a wet washcloth or glycerine sticks if kept fasting
- Change the woman's position every ½ hour; use pillows to support position
- Remind the woman to empty her bladder every ½ hour
- Focus on relaxation of specific areas of tension (use words such as "let go," "release," "float," "droop"; the coach or nurse can demonstrate tension and relaxation on an area of his or her own body, which may be helpful if the client is more a visual than a verbal learner
- Use a warm wet cloth applied to the perineum to help relax these muscles; may use perineal massage and vitamin E oil, especially if the couple has practiced perineal massage during pregnancy and feels comfortable with it
- Assure the woman that her sensations and feelings are normal
- Use blowing and panting techniques to stop pushing (Lamaze)

(d) Stage II averages 1 to 2 hours for primiparas and averages 30 to 60 minutes for multiparas; strategies taught to expectant parents are

    (i) Positions: physiological advantages of
- Squatting
- Semisitting
- Side-lying

    (ii) Open glottis; short breath-holding for voluntary pushing (preferred physiological method) or closed glottis method (with prolonged breath-holding)

    (iii) Encouragement or cheering on

    (iv) Relaxation of perineum via the Kegel maneuver

    (v) Use of a mirror, as needed, to motivate the woman

    (vi) Explanation of the use of forceps or of a vacuum extractor, if indicated in particular situation

    (vii) Provide individual instruction on videotape to high-risk women restricted to bed rest

b. Evaluations (by hospital nurses)

(1) During labor, the woman and her coach demonstrate the ability to articulate knowledge of the birth process by

    (a) Arriving at the health care facility at the appropriate time, with signs of labor

    (b) Knowing pertinent results of any prenatal testing

    (c) Describing potential genetic problems of this pregnancy

(d) Expressing their own hopes and expectations for this labor and birth, including plans concerning medication

(e) Understanding the various birthing options

(2) The laboring woman demonstrates the various coping strategies to reduce the pain of labor

(a) She uses breathing patterns appropriate to the intensity of labor, resulting in control and comfort

(b) Relaxation strategies are used

(i) Changes positions every 2 hours

(ii) Responds to massage or effleurage

(iii) Responds with relaxation to a warm water bath or shower

(iv) Relaxes the tense area with touch intervention

(v) Uses music effectively

(vi) Is able to focus on a photograph, a picture, or a support person

(vii) Appears relaxed between contractions

(c) Couple verbalizes basic understanding of medication options

(i) Analgesics (e.g., meperidine [Demerol], butorphanol [Stadol]) for pain relief

(ii) Tranquilizers (e.g., vistaril, phenergran) for relaxation

(iii) Barbiturates (e.g., pentobarbital sodium (Nembutal), secobarbital sodium (Seconal) for sleep

(iv) Oxytocins (e.g., Pitocin) may increase pain

(d) Couple expresses a general understanding of anesthetic options

(i) Regional anesthesia using the so-called -caine drugs
- Saddle block
- Spinal block
- Epidural or caudal
- Pudendal
- Local infiltration

(ii) Inhalation anesthesia
- Nitrous oxide
- Penthrane

(iii) General anesthesia: thiopental sodium (Pentothal) (used primarily for emergency cesarean birth)

(e) Couple is able to discuss the possible side effects of medications

(3) Coach or support person interacts positively with the laboring woman

(a) Demonstrates familiarity with specific breathing techniques

(b) Detects tension in the woman and intervenes effectively

(c) Offers encouragement and support via

(i) Verbal communication

(ii) Facial expression

(iii) Touch

(iv) Presence at bedside

(v) Assistance with guided imagery and other individual relaxation responses

(4) Couple discusses alternatives

(a) Woman and coach express goals or concerns for childbirth

(b) Couple lists indications for augmentation or induction

(i) Dystocia or failure to progress

(ii) Postdates

(iii) Medical complications

(c) Various desired choices include

(i) Walking or standing

(ii) Rocking

(iii) Shower or baths

(iv) Sitting

(v) Side-lying

(vi) Effleurage or firm massage

        (vii) Support person's presence if the birth is by cesarean section

       (viii) Breastfeeding soon after birth

        (ix) Bottlefeeding

        (x) Twenty-four hour rooming-in

       (xi) Early hospital discharge

3. Anxiety related to lack of knowledge and fear of the unknown
   a. Interventions
      (1) Replace fear of the unknown with information about the birth process
      (2) Encourage expectant parents to discuss fears and concerns
      (3) Offer assistance in practicing breathing and relaxation techniques to gain mastery of skills
      (4) Encourage couples to discuss myths
      (5) Conduct small group discussions separately for men and women to discuss specific concerns
      (6) Open discussion of unexpected outcomes
         (a) Labor does not progress as planned
         (b) Fetal distress in labor (e.g., a need for oxygen, position change, scalp pH)
         (c) Use of unanticipated medications for analgesia or anesthesia
         (d) Unexpected cesarean birth
         (e) Infant problems: need for intensive care
         (f) Pregnancy loss, stillbirth, or neonatal death
         (g) Anticipatory guidance for grieving process for a variety of losses, including all of the above (for a complete discussion of perinatal grieving, refer to Chapter 25 on loss and grieving)
      (7) Specific symptoms to report immediately
         (a) Vaginal bleeding or change in vaginal discharge
         (b) Sharp pain in abdomen
         (c) Fluid leaking from vagina (rupture of membranes)
         (d) More than four contractions in 1 hour if less than 38 weeks' gestation
         (e) Preterm cramping or backache
         (f) Persistent vomiting or diarrhea
         (g) Temperature elevation
         (h) Persistent headache
         (i) Blurred vision or spots before eyes
      (8) Birth films, videotapes, or slides used to visualize birth in concrete terms
      (9) Role playing to practice alternative types of labors and coping strategies (mock labors)
      (10) Suggestions to create a relaxing, homelike environment within the hospital
         (a) Bring own pillows or pillowcases
         (b) Bring tapes of favorite relaxation music
         (c) Bring a photograph, picture, or painting from home
         (d) Wear one's own nightgown and robe
         (e) Use camera or videotape camera to record events
         (f) Provide snacks for the expectant father and family members
   b. Evaluations (by hospital nurses)
      (1) The woman acts appropriately if she notices specific signs or adverse symptoms, such as persistent headaches, signs of preterm labor, and vaginal bleeding
      (2) The woman brings personal items to the hospital to create a homelike environment: own pillows, photographs, music tapes, own nightgown, for example
      (3) The couple talks about the labor and birth process, using the correct terminology
      (4) The woman and support person work well together; the coach is familiar

with the woman's breathing pattern and preferred techniques for relaxation (e.g., brisk touch and specific guided imagery scene)
- (5) The woman and support person are able to address unexpected situations, such as prolonged labor, fetal distress, or unanticipated cesarean birth, with a sense of control and input into the decision making, when possible or appropriate
- c. Intervention: cesarean birth class: instruct couple about the following
  - (1) Indications for a cesarean birth
    - (a) Placenta abnormalities such as previa or abruption
    - (b) Cephalopelvic disproportion (CPD)
    - (c) Genital herpes and maternal diseases, such as heart disease, cancer, and diabetes (under certain circumstances)
    - (d) Umbilical cord prolapse
    - (e) Abnormal fetal position (e.g., transverse or breech)
    - (f) Fetal distress
  - (2) Procedures associated with a cesarean birth
  - (3) Immediate recovery from surgical birth
    - (a) Lochia
    - (b) Vital signs
    - (c) Pain control
      - (i) Morphine epidural
      - (ii) Patient-controlled analgesia
      - (iii) Analgesia, as needed, administered either intramuscularly or orally
    - (d) Potential maternal-infant separation
    - (e) Flatulence (gas): cause and treatment
    - (f) Exploration of the meaning of and feelings about a cesarean birth
      - (i) Relief after a nonproductive labor
      - (ii) Saved my baby, grateful that the baby is safe
      - (iii) Sad and disappointed because delivery did not go as planned
    - (g) The coach and nurse can assist to "fill in missing pieces" (e.g., aspects not understood or misinterpreted)
- d. Intervention: vaginal birth after cesarean (VBAC) class: instruct the couple about the following
  - (1) Indications for VBAC
    - (a) Nonrecurring cause of the previous cesarean birth (e.g., fetal distress or breech)
    - (b) CPD is relative; many women deliver via VBAC with a baby larger than the one delivered by cesarean section
  - (2) VBAC is not appropriate under the following circumstances
    - (a) Prior classical or vertical uterine incision
    - (b) Fetal position is abnormal (e.g., transverse position)
    - (c) Multiple gestation (relative to position and size)
    - (d) Very large baby (confirmed by ultrasonography)
  - (3) Procedure includes
    - (a) Intravenous line (e.g., heparin lock) in some settings
    - (b) Careful electronic monitoring of fetus and uterine contractions
    - (c) Ability to perform a cesarean section in 15 minutes, if needed
    - (d) Use of prepared childbirth techniques and/or epidural block
    - (e) Possible use of Pitocin
    - (f) Woman should mentally prepare herself for the possibility of either a vaginal or a cesarean birth
    - (g) May be kept NPO in some settings
- e. Evaluations (by hospital nurses)
  - (1) The woman and her support person can recall a particular indication for cesarean birth specific to her labor, such as CPD, placenta previa, or fetal distress

(2) The couple asks appropriate questions about cesarean birth procedures based on an established knowledge base

(3) The couple is able to communicate with the staff regarding feelings about cesarean birth (relieved, grateful, or disappointed)

(4) The woman planning a VBAC articulates the need to prepare for either a vaginal or a cesarean birth

(5) The woman desiring VBAC is able to describe possible procedures that her hospital or physician may require

(6) The couple is able to list important aspects of having a cesarean birth, such as epidural anesthesia, presence of expectant father or other support person, and breastfeeding of the infant

f. Interventions to meet the educational needs of an untrained, unprepared woman in labor

  (1) Explain that the idea or purpose of contractions is to open the cervix

  (2) Use a knitted uterus and charts to demonstrate cervical dilation

  (3) Briefly explain the normal progression of labor

    (a) First phase is long, with rest periods between contractions

    (b) Later phase is faster and more intense

    (c) Project only a few hours ahead

  (4) The woman is highly susceptible to suggestion from the nurse

    (a) Encourage and reinforce relaxation

    (b) Demonstrate slow chest breathing for the labor and re-teach slow chest breathing, as needed, throughout the labor

  (5) Express confidence in the woman's ability to cope with labor

  (6) Explain the physical sensations during childbirth

    (a) Pelvic fullness: baby's descent

    (b) The splitting or tearing sensation is the perineum thinning and opening

  (7) Praise the woman's efforts and hard work: let her know frequently throughout labor that everything is normal

  (8) Support the support person: work through him or her

  (9) Offer information on cesarean, as needed

g. Evaluation (by hospital nurses)

  (1) The woman demonstrates some control in labor under guidance of nurse

  (2) The woman achieves varying levels of relaxation

  (3) The woman expresses feelings of accomplishment when labor is over

h. Intervention: sibling class: sibling preparation classes are designed to assist children and their parents to plan for the introduction and integration of a new baby into the family constellation; children are helped to gain some comfort with the hospital or other birth setting, to anticipate some separation from their mother (in most cases), to see newborns as small and helpless, not as playmates, and to begin to take on the big brother or big sister role

  (1) Divide sibling classes into age-appropriate groups

  (2) Relate mother's pregnancy to when the sibling was a baby

  (3) Use models to explain the birth process briefly

  (4) Incorporate a hospital tour

    (a) Show where the mother will be

    (b) Show what a newborn really looks like (e.g., is not a playmate)

    (c) Incorporate activity centers

      (i) Show handwashing area

      (ii) Diaper anatomically correct dolls

      (iii) Color workbooks on families

  (5) Families are taught strategies to ease the new baby into the family

    (a) Hold a birthday party in the hospital

    (b) Give a sibling his or her own baby doll

(c) Have the newborn send "gifts" to the sibling
(d) Have a sibling's photograph in the newborn's hospital crib
(e) Plan a special time for the sibling and mother in the hospital
(f) Encourage sibling visits in the hospital
(6) For siblings planning to be present at birth, families are taught
(a) Individual family preparation
(b) To use color photographs and slides of birth
(c) Role playing, which emphasizes the hard work of labor
(d) To prepare the child's caretaker (e.g., grandmother or friend)
(i) Caretaker's role during the labor
(ii) Caretaker's role during the birth
(e) Plan activities if the child wishes to leave the labor room
(f) Pack snacks and refreshments for the child
(g) Consider bringing a favorite pillow, blanket, or toy
i. Evaluations (by hospital nurses)
(1) The sibling visits in the hospital with the mother and newborn
(2) The sibling's photograph is in the newborn's crib
(3) The sibling holds a birthday party in the hospital for the newborn
(4) The sibling learns baby care with a doll while the mother reviews infant care in the hospital
(5) The sibling attending birth is chaperoned by a familiar, supportive caretaker with whom the child appears comfortable
(6) The sibling who is present for labor comforts the mother by such actions as massaging her back, and offering fluids
(7) The sibling participates in the labor and withdraws to rest, play games, or watch television as he or she likes
(8) The sibling attending birth may express awe and joy, and a desire to touch or hold the newborn
j. Intervention: grandparenting classes: classes for prospective grandparents are designed to update their information on current birthing options and trends; to examine how they can be most supportive of the emerging new family; and to explore their appropriate role with their new grandchild and the child's parents; they are taught the following
(1) Prospective grandparents are encouraged to recall their own labor and birth experiences and to select the pros and cons of those birthing practices
(2) Prospective grandparents are updated on current birthing choices and practices
(a) Prepared childbirth rationale
(b) Presence and role of partner or other person as a coach
(c) Epidural anesthesia is presented as the current anesthesia of choice, and methodology is briefly explained
(d) Concepts of L/D/R; L/D/R/P and/or birthing centers
(e) Early mother (parent)-infant contact (bonding) explained without making grandparents feel guilty about own experiences (early and prolonged mother-infant separation, for example)
(f) Use of electronic fetal monitors
(g) Increased prevalence of cesarean birth and the relative safety of surgery for mother and infant
(h) Midwifery option (in some settings)
(i) Early discharge programs (in some settings)
(3) Opportunity for grandparent participation during labor and at birth in some settings and anticipatory guidance on what to expect
(4) Changes in infant care philosophies and techniques
(a) Prevalence of breastfeeding
(b) Use of disposable diapers
(c) Demand feedings

(d) Not letting small infants cry for protracted periods

(e) New equipment such as swings, umbrella-strollers, and car seats, for example

(5) Helpful role for grandparents

(a) Support and encourage new parents' parenting methods

(b) Actively encourage breastfeeding mothers, especially during early learning stage

(c) Assist with household chores as the primary focus and allow parents to interact and take care of the newborn

(d) Offer advice only when requested and try not to play the expert role regarding infant care

(6) Rights of grandparents are explored (e.g., babysit when it is convenient for the grandparents)

k. Evaluations (by hospital nurses)

(1) Grandparents who are present during labor and birth appear to have a basic familiarity with electronic monitors, birthing setting, and breathing

(2) Grandparents negotiate a supportive role vis à vis the woman's partner's role

(3) Grandparents encourage the couple's choices and coping patterns in the hospital

(4) Grandparents ask the new parents how they can be more helpful in supporting new parents and baby

(5) Grandparents express to the staff an interest in learning and reviewing infant care, new parenting concepts, and infant feeding methods

4. Knowledge deficit related to the needs of the mother, father, and infant during the postpartum period

a. Intervention: baby care classes: parents are taught

(1) Practical aspects of baby care

(a) Bathing

(b) Umbilical cord care

(c) Diapering

(d) Care of genitals (female or male [circumcised or uncircumcised])

(e) Understanding of infant crying

(f) Infant safety

(g) Infant equipment (e.g., car seat and crib)

(h) Normal newborn's physical characteristics

(i) Bottlefeeding and breastfeeding

(j) Normal voiding and stool patterns

(2) Emotional components of care

(a) Attachment process is gradual, not instantaneous

(b) Sensitive period occurs after birth

(c) En face position is within the 9- to 12-inch focusing distance of newborn sight

(d) Importance of touch

(e) Learning baby's cues

(f) Frustrations of trying to meet the infant's demands

(3) Needs of infant versus needs of parents

(a) Adults are deprived of sleep

(b) Adults need to learn new skills

(c) Parents need uninterrupted adult socialization

(d) Mother's recuperation and rest needs

(e) Anticipatory guidance that postpartum period can be a stressful time

(f) Availability of community resources to help and support new parents

b. Evaluations (by hospital nurses)

(1) Mother will identify practical learning needs about infant care

(2) Mother will demonstrate practical beginning or refresher skills in diapering, cord care, and feeding
(3) Mother will be able to describe a preliminary understanding of infant needs for comfort and safety
(4) Family has a child's car seat properly installed at the time of hospital discharge
(5) Parents articulate the importance of touch and closeness to the infant
(6) Parents can appropriately describe the gradual nature of the attachment process
(7) The couple describes two or three potentially difficult emotional elements of the postpartum period
(8) The couple has a list of available community resources to telephone for guidance and assistance
c. Intervention: breastfeeding class; parents are taught
(1) Advantages of breastfeeding
(a) Is species specific and provides complete nutrition for the newborn
(b) Is nonallergic
(c) Provides immunoglobulin to protect against disease
(d) Provides milk that is the correct temperature and is sterile
(e) Provides skin-to-skin contact
(f) Aids in the involution of the uterus
(g) Decreases uterine bleeding
(h) Aids in maternal weight loss
(2) Physiology of lactation (for a complete discussion of the physiology of lactation refer to Chapter 19 on lactation)
(a) Infant sucking at breast causes milk production
(b) Infant sucking at breast causes milk ejection (let-down)
(c) Breastfeeding is a perfect supply-and-demand relationship (e.g., the more the baby demands, the more the mother produces)
(d) Adequate milk supply requires 8 to 10 feedings per day
(3) Mechanics of breastfeeding (see Chapter 19)
d. Evaluations (by hospital nurses)
(1) The mother articulates two or three benefits of breastfeeding for her and her baby
(2) The mother describes the importance of the infant's sucking at the breast (for production and let-down)
(3) The mother places the baby at the breast at least 8 to 10 times per day during the hospital stay
5. Knowledge deficit related to the special needs of pregnant adolescents (for a complete discussion of pregnant adolescent, refer to Chapter 10 on age-related concerns)
a. Intervention: school-based courses: pregnant adolescents are taught
(1) Process of labor and birth (same as for adults, use audiovisual aids)
(2) Specific problems
(a) Nutritional requirements (for a complete discussion of pregnant adolescent nutritional requirements, refer to Chapter 12 on nutrition)
(i) Anemia
(ii) Junk food does not always meet needs
• Protein: 92 g/day
• Calcium: 1.0 to 1.6 g/day
• Calories: 11 to 14 years old: 2700/day; 15 to 17 years old: 2400/day
(iii) Modify teen-age diet: establish a "contract" and recommend the following
• Pizza
• Salad bar

- Milk, ice cream, yogurt, and grilled cheese
- Cheeseburger

    (iv) Appropriate use of prenatal vitamins

  (b) Lack of early and adequate prenatal care

    (i) Teacher should have an accepting attitude and maintain non-judgmental open communications

    (ii) Access to care can be facilitated by school-based or community-based adolescent clinics

    (iii) Explain the reason for and benefits of prenatal care in the prevention of pregnancy complications

    (iv) Provide education about and support of emotional changes of pregnancy

  (c) Avoid assumptions

    (i) Not all adolescents feel guilty

    (ii) Some adolescents feel positive about pregnancy

    (iii) Some adolescents easily relinquish their newborns

    (iv) Other adolescents find it difficult or impossible to place their infant for adoption

    (v) Adolescents may or may not have strong support at home

    (vi) Encourage adolescents to continue schooling or job training

    (vii) Some pregnant teenagers are married and have either a planned or an unplanned pregnancy

(3) Special needs in labor: anticipatory guidance

  (a) Natural modesty is invaded: forewarn the client and protect her modesty

  (b) Regression in behavior is common (e.g., may need a "security" item, such as a stuffed animal)

  (c) She may have conflicting needs for support by her mother or the expectant father

  (d) She may have difficulty developing trust in caregivers and request that the number of personnel interacting with her be limited

  (e) CPD is more common, especially with younger adolescents, and the possibility of a cesarean section is increased

  (f) Labor and birth can be an opportunity for mastery and increased self-esteem for the adolescent

(4) Special needs in the postpartum period: anticipatory guidance

  (a) Role model the desirable interactions with her infant (e.g., touch and verbalization)

  (b) Elicit the teenager's fantasies about the baby (e.g., "to love me") and offer reality-based advice about the newborn's needs and development

  (c) Help the adolescent develop realistic future goals

b. Intervention: clinic-based or office-based teaching

  (1) Assess the meaning of pregnancy to this adolescent

  (2) Assess individual learning needs and offer guidance

  (3) Assist the teenager with dietary needs, based on her present diet

  (4) Show videotapes, movies, or slides of a birth

  (5) Help the teenager determine whom she wants for support in labor

  (6) Communicate the teenager's needs and desires to the hospital staff

  (7) Point out prior positive coping strategies

c. Evaluations (by hospital nurses)

  (1) When diet is assessed, the adolescent describes appropriate nutritional intake (e.g., pizza, salad bar, and milk)

  (2) The adolescent tells the nurse whom she needs for support

  (3) The adolescent talks about labor and delivery using the correct basic terminology

  (4) The adolescent touches and talks to her infant

(5) The adolescent demonstrates basic, practical baby care skills

(6) The adolescent grieves appropriately if she gives her baby up for adoption

Health Education

In this chapter, Clinical Practice and Health Education are identical.

CASE STUDY

Jane had been in latent labor for hours before finally coming to the hospital. She was fatigued and discouraged on learning that she was only 3 cm dilated. Jane's nurse suggested sitting in the shower to help Jane relax and to solicit her husband, Fred, to help in the activity. The nurse got the couple a cool beverage and asked Jane what her favorite way to relax was. Jane stated that she had practiced imagery and felt that that was the most effective way for her. Fred repeated the details that they had reviewed many times. By the time Jane was out of the shower, she was 7 cm dilated. She and Fred used the breathing patterns together, increasing the pace over the peaks of the contractions as they walked the halls. The nurse stayed nearby, assessing the labor and fetus with periodic monitoring. She noted that this couple was emotionally close, and she made recommendations through Fred to Jane, who was becoming restless and tense. The nurse demonstrated tense muscle groups on herself and suggested how Fred could help relax these same muscles on Jane. Fred used firm massage to release Jane's muscular tension. Jane made moaning sounds, which seemed to help her stay calm as she rocked. Finally, it was time to push. Jane used the squatting bar and at 7:12 am gave birth to a 3232 g (7 lb, 2 oz) boy.

CASE STUDY

Sixteen-year-old Marianne has come into your labor and delivery area with her girl-friend, apprehensive and laughing nervously. Marianne's mother and boyfriend arrive minutes later and ask excitedly where Marianne is. The nurse working with her asks Marianne which people she wants at her bedside at the moment. Marianne asks for her mother but says she wants everyone else to stay in the den next door and visit. The nurse makes every effort to protect Marianne's modesty by carefully draping her for the vaginal examination and suggests that her mother hold her hand. She asks Marianne if she has taken any birth classes. Marianne explains that all pregnant girls take a class in school but says, "I'm still scared and my back hurts so much." Marianne is 4 cm dilated. The nurse shows Marianne how to do the pelvic rock and suggests that she try it to help relieve her back pain. She also shows her mother how to use the frozen rolling pin on the small of her back. The nurse keeps Marianne's friends informed of her progress. Despite position changes, rocking, firm massage, and attempts at relaxation, Marianne says she cannot cope with the pain. Her nurse suggests medication; Marianne receives an epidural and becomes much calmer. Her friends join her and they play cards for a while. When the physician says she is ready to push, she wants only her mother to stay. The nurse clears the room and shows Marianne's mother how to encourage her daughter, supporting her back and holding her legs. Together, the nurse and mother intensely coach Marianne's efforts. After almost 2 hours of pushing, the doctor suggests using a vacuum extractor. The nurse carefully explains the procedure. Marianne says she wants her boyfriend to see the baby born. He comes in just as Marianne delivers a 2948 g (6½ lb) girl.

STUDY QUESTIONS

1. To enhance relaxation, Jane used

   a. Effleurage (light touch and strokes).

   b. Visualization of the opening of the birth canal.

   c. Warm shower.

2. What position did Jane not use in labor?

   a. Sitting

   b. Standing

   c. Squatting

3. The nurse used which three comfort measures with Jane?

   a. Cool beverage, demonstrated tension on self, cheering at pushing stage.

   b. Cool beverage, use of focal point, correcting Jane's moaning sounds.

   c. Shower, cool beverage, pelvic rock.

4. When working with the pregnant adolescent, the nurse should

   a. Suggest that the girl's mother is a more mature support person for her than the expectant father.

   b. Be careful to protect the teenager's modesty.

   c. Recommend that stuffed animals be taken away so that the teenager can assume a more adult role in anticipation of motherhood.

5. For back labor the nurse recommended

   a. Pelvic rock and effleurage.

   b. Hot shower and walking.

   c. Firm massage and frozen rolling pin.

6. The most important element that a supportive person provides the woman in labor is

   a. Help with practical techniques.

   b. Maintaining quiet voices of all staff.

   c. Emotional presence and support.

   d. Directing relaxation of key muscle groups.

7. When the nurse begins working with the laboring woman, she should

   a. Explain all the options available.

   b. Feel the abdomen to assess contractions.

   c. Ask who the childbirth teacher was.

   d. Observe how effectively the woman and her partner are coping with labor.

8. One of the most successful teaching aids that the nurse can use during labor is

   a. Chart showing phases of labor.

   b. Her own body for demonstration.

   c. Breathing pattern poster.

   d. Slide show.

9. Paced breathing is based on

   a. Chart showing phases of labor.

   b. A formula founded in Switzerland.

   c. The woman's own resting respirations.

   d. A 1:5 breathing ratio.

10. A teenager in labor needs

   a. To make choices.

   b. Her mother.

   c. General anesthesia.

   d. To place her baby for adoption.

Answers to Study Questions

1. c	2. b	3. a
4. b	5. c	6. c
7. d	8. b	9. c
10. a		

REFERENCES

Barr, L., & Monserrat, C. (1979). *Teenage pregnancy: A new beginning.* Albuquerque: New Futures.
Bing, E. (1982). *Six practical lessons for an easier childbirth.* New York: Bantam.
Bonica, J. (1990). *The management of pain* (Vol. 2). Philadelphia: Lea & Febiger.
Bradley, R. (1981). *Husband-coached childbirth* (3rd ed.). New York: Harper & Row.
Dick-Read, G. (1987). *Childbirth without fear.* (5th ed.). New York: Harper & Row.
Eisenberg, A., Murkhoff, H., & Hathaway, S. (1989). *What to expect when you're expecting.* New York: Workman.
Jones, C., & Jones, J. (1989). *The birth partner's handbook: How to help a woman through childbirth.* New York: Simon and Schuster.
Jones, M.E. et. al (1990). Prenatal education outcomes for pregnant adolescents and their infants using trained volunteers. *Journal of Adolescent Health Care, 11*(5), 437–444.
Karmel, M. (1983). *Thank you, Dr. Lamaze.* New York: Harper & Row.
Kieffer, J.L. (1988). *To have . . . to hold . . . .* Harrisburg, PA: Training Resource Corporation.
Kitzinger, S. (1987). *Your baby, your way, making pregnancy decisions and birth plans.* New York: Pantheon.
Kitzinger, S. (1989). *Giving birth: How it really feels.* New York: Farrar, Straus, & Giroux.
Korte, D., & Scaer, R. (1990). *A good birth, a safe birth.* New York: Bantam.

McKay, S. (1986). *The assertive approach to childbirth*. Englewood Cliffs, NJ: Prentice Hall.

NAACOG: Organization for Obstetric, Gynecologic and Neonatal Nurses. (1987). *Competencies and program guidelines for nurse providers of childbirth education*. Washington, DC: Author.

Nichols, F.H., & Humenick, S.S. (Eds.). (1988). *Childbirth education: Practice, research, and theory*. Philadelphia: Saunders.

Simkin, P. (1989). *The birth partner: Everything you need to know to help a woman through childbirth*. Boston: Harvard Common.

Cesarean Childbirth

Donovan, B. (1986). *The cesarean birth experience*. Boston: Beacon.

Norwood, C. (1984). *How to avoid a cesarean section*. New York: Simon and Schuster.

Rosen, M., & Thomas, L. (1989). *The cesarean myth: Choosing the best way to have your baby*. New York: Penguin.

Dealing With Grief and Loss in Pregnancy

Borg, S., & Lasker, J. (1981). *When pregnancy fails: Families coping with miscarriage, stillbirth and infant death:* Boston: Beacon.

Jimenez, S. (1982). *The other side of pregnancy: Coping with miscarriage and stillbirth*. New York: Prentice Hall.

Sibling Preparation

Baker, G., & Montey, V. (1981). *Special delivery: A book for kids about cesarean and vaginal birth*. Lynnwood, WA: Charles Franklin.

Malecki, M. (1982). *Mom and Dad and I are having a baby!* Seattle: Pennypress.

Breastfeeding

Ewy, D., & Ewy, R. (1985). *Preparation for breastfeeding*. New York: Doubleday.

Grams, M. (1988). *Breastfeeding source book*. Sheridan, WY: Achievement.

La Leche League International. (1987). *The womanly art of breastfeeding* (4th ed.). Chicago: La Leche.

Reukauf, D., & Trause, M.A. (1988). *Commonsense breastfeeding: Practical guide to the pleasures, problems and solutions*. New York: Macmillan.

MATERNAL-FETAL
WELL-BEING

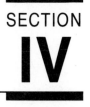

Judy E. Smith

CHAPTER

10

Age-Related Concerns

Objectives

1. Identify the risks that are related to childbearing in adolescents

2. Identify the risks that are related to advanced maternal age

3. Distinguish between the risks that can be attributed solely to biological age factors and the risks that can be attributed to sociocultural and economic factors

4. Select nursing interventions that correspond to a pregnant adolescent's developmental level

5. Design and implement health education that reflects a sensitivity to the specialized needs of younger expectant parents and older expectant parents

Introduction

Pregnancy that occurs at the two age extremes (younger than 19 years and older than 35 years) of a woman's childbearing years places the expectant mother and the fetus at risk for age-related complications. However, research has revealed that the increased risks of age extremes are related more to sociocultural and economic factors than to the biological factors of age (Mansfield, 1987). Many of these risks can be minimized through the use of current technology, education, and consistent prenatal care. Pregnancy in women 35 years and older who deliver in settings in which current technology is available may be at no higher risk for an adverse outcome than pregnancy in younger women (Kirz, Dorchester, & Freeman, 1985). With early and thorough prenatal care, adolescents older than the age of 15 years have no greater risks than those of the general pregnant population. Although the incidence of certain complications may be greater because of age extremities, the nursing diagnoses, interventions, and evaluations remain relatively unchanged from those for the general pregnant population with the same complications.

CLINICAL PRACTICE

ADOLESCENCE

A. Assessment

1. History (specifics to add related to the adolescent's age)
   a. Age at menarche
      (1) Several of the first menstrual cycles are anovulatory and irregular, making gestational dating difficult
      (2) Long bone growth is incomplete until approximately 2 years after menarche and the pelvis does not reach adult size until 1 to 3 years after menarche (Mansfield, 1987)
   b. Number of sexual partners
      (1) Having multiple sexual partners increases the risk of concurrent sexually transmitted diseases; adolescents will frequently have serial monogamous relationships (i.e., one short-term, monogamous relationship that is followed by another, and then another)
      (2) Adolescents who are 15- to 19-years old have the second highest incidence of sexually transmitted diseases in the United States
   c. Knowledge about how conception occurs
   d. Planned or unplanned pregnancy
   e. Previous pregnancies
      (1) Term or preterm
      (2) Spontaneous abortions
      (3) Therapeutic abortions
   f. Contraceptive use
      (1) Type
      (2) Frequency of use
      (3) Last time used
      (4) Non-use
   g. Dietary intake
      (1) Is frequently inadequate in adolescents
      (2) Caloric restriction can occur when the pregnant adolescent attempts to "not get fat," to control abdominal protrusion, or to deny the pregnancy to herself and others
      (3) Overeating may occur to mask the bodily changes of pregnancy
      (4) The incidence of eating disorders may be high among adolescents, as a group
   h. Prenatal care
      (1) Some adolescents have no prenatal care, may not have known they were pregnant, or continue to deny their pregnancy
      (2) Prenatal care is frequently started in middle-to-late pregnancy
      (3) Sporadic prenatal care and missed appointments
   i. Alcohol, tobacco, and illicit drug use
   j. Support system
      (1) Financial
      (2) Emotional: father of baby
      (3) Marital status
      (4) Parents' awareness of and attitude toward their teen-aged daughter's pregnancy
   k. Attendance at prenatal classes
2. Developmental assessment
   a. The overall developmental tasks of an adolescent are
      (1) Acceptance of and comfort with one's body image
      (2) Internalization of a sexual identity and role
      (3) Development of a personal value system
      (4) Development of a sense of productivity

      (5) Identification of a life's work

      (6) Achievement of a sense of independence

      (7) Development of an adult identity

    b. Early-adolescent girl (younger than 15 years)

      (1) Is a concrete thinker

      (2) Usually has some degree of discomfort with normal body changes and body image

      (3) Usually has only a minimal ability to foresee the consequences of her behavior and see herself in the future

      (4) Her locus of control is usually external

    c. Middle-adolescent girl (15 to 17 years)

      (1) Is prone to experimentation and challenges

        (a) Drugs and alcohol

        (b) Sex

        (c) Feels invulnerable

      (2) Seeks independence and frequently turns to her peer group for support, information, and advice; pregnancy at this age can force a parental dependency and interfere with her striving for independence

      (3) Is capable of formal operational thought and abstract thinking but may have difficulty anticipating the long-term implications of her actions

    c. Late-adolescent girl (17 to 19 years)

      (1) Is developing individuality

      (2) Is capable of thinking abstractly and anticipating consequences

      (3) Is capable of problem solving and decision making

      (4) Can picture herself in control

  3. Physical findings (specifics related to the adolescent girl's age)

    a. Bone growth is still incomplete in early adolescence

      (1) If pregnancy occurs before bone growth is complete, it can interfere or arrest further bone growth

        (a) The first 4 years after menarche carry the highest risk

        (b) An increase of estrogen during this time, caused by pregnancy, can lead to the early closure of the epiphysis

      (2) Pelvic bones have not reached adult female dimensions: the incidence of cephalopelvic disproportion leading to cesarean section, is increased

    b. Signs of pregnancy-induced hypertension (see Chapter 26 for a complete discussion of pregnancy-induced hypertension)

      (1) Pregnancy-induced hypertension is the most prevalent medical complication in young, pregnant adolescents

      (2) Higher incidence may be due to

        (a) Suboptimal uterine vascular development

        (b) Poor nutritional practices by adolescents

    c. Signs of intrauterine growth retardation (see Chapter 36 for a complete discussion of intrauterine growth retardation)

      (1) Adolescents have a higher incidence of low-birth-weight infants

      (2) Fundal height and gestational age discrepancy: fundal height in centimeters is normally equivalent to the number of gestational weeks

      (3) Inadequate nutritional status may be evidenced by low weight gain

      (4) Signs of infection (see Chapter 27 for a complete discussion of intrauterine infection and Chapter 39 for congenital infections of the neonate)

B. **Nursing Diagnoses**

1. Alteration in growth and development of the adolescent related to pregnancy
2. Alteration in family functioning related to the adolescent's denial of pregnancy
3. Knowledge deficit related to adequate nutrition during pregnancy
4. Noncompliance with prenatal care and instructions related to a lack of understanding of the value of prenatal care to pregnancy outcome

C. **Interventions/Evaluations**

1. Alteration in growth and development of the adolescent related to pregnancy (see Chapter 12 for a complete discussion of nutrition)
   a. Interventions
      (1) Adapt the nutritional requirements of pregnancy to the individual adolescent's likes, cultural influences, economic resources, and peer-group habits
         (a) Instruct the adolescent about how to make the most nutritious selections from fast-food menus without attracting peer attention
         (b) Instruct the adolescent about how to select and plan for healthy snacks when she is both away from home and at home
      (2) Adapt all interventions to correspond with the adolescent's developmental level
         (a) Assist her to develop and use decision-making skills that are appropriate to her developmental level
         (b) Assist her to develop and use problem-solving skills that are appropriate to her developmental level
         (c) Actively involve her in her own care
            (i) Have her listen to fetal heart tones
            (ii) Have her place her hands on palpable fetal parts in late pregnancy and help her to visualize the fetal position
   b. Evaluations
      (1) The pregnant adolescent will be able to select and consume a nutritious diet without feeling conspicuous among her peers
      (2) The pregnant adolescent will show an active involvement in her own care
      (3) The pregnant adolescent will seek information and make decisions that are appropriate for her developmental level
2. Alteration in family functioning related to the adolescent's denial of pregnancy
   a. Interventions
      (1) Develop a trusting relationship with the adolescent
         (a) Listen attentively
         (b) Maintain a nonjudgmental approach
         (c) Avoid sounding like a parent to the adolescent (i.e., avoid using the word *should,* giving unwanted advice, making decisions for her)
         (d) Recognize the unique problems of the adolescent as they relate to her individual situation
         (e) Determine her individual strengths and compliment her on these strengths
      (2) Assist her in developing and using decision-making and problem-solving skills related to her developmental level
         (a) Encourage her to include her family as a resource, if appropriate, in decision making and problem solving
         (b) If inappropriate to include her family in the decision-making process, encourage the adolescent to communicate to her family the thoughts and resources she used to arrive at her decisions
         (c) Support and encourage her well-thought-out decisions; praise her abilities and her approximations toward thoughtful decisions
      (3) Seek involvement of the adolescent's mother, older sister, or other close female relative, if appropriate
   b. Evaluations
      (1) The pregnant adolescent will develop a trusting relationship with the nurse
      (2) The pregnant adolescent will be able to include her parent(s) or another relative in the problem-solving process, if at all possible, and seek the support of her family, if appropriate

3. Knowledge deficit related to adequate nutrition during pregnancy (see Chapter 12 for a complete discussion of nutritional needs during pregnancy)
4. Noncompliance with prenatal care and instructions related to a lack of understanding of the value of prenatal care to pregnancy outcome
    a. Interventions
        (1) Give specific information about the effect or purpose of each procedure that is conducted during a prenatal visit
            (a) Explanations must be appropriate to the adolescent's developmental level
            (b) Adolescents have a tendency to be egocentric
                (i) Effects of maternal health and habits on the fetus may not be regarded as important by the adolescent
                (ii) Emphasize the effects of health maintenance and practices on herself
        (2) Adapt prenatal instructions to the adolescent's lifestyle as much as possible
    b. Evaluations
        (1) The adolescent will seek prenatal care within the first trimester of her pregnancy
        (2) The adolescent will receive consistent prenatal care throughout her pregnancy
        (3) The pregnant adolescent will demonstrate an adequate knowledge of the value of prenatal care and demonstrate compliance with instructions

ADVANCED MATERNAL AGE

A. Assessment

1. History
    a. Conception problems
        (1) Any tests, treatments, or procedures that were used to facilitate conception
        (2) Duration of the conception problem
        (3) Fertility drugs that were taken to facilitate conception
    b. Previous pregnancies
        (1) Problems conceiving
        (2) Complications during the pregnancy
    c. Planned or unplanned pregnancy
    d. Occupation or career
        (1) Women over the age of 35 years may have advanced in their careers to a level of high responsibility and high stress
            (a) Frequently are college educated
            (b) Frequently have high achievement needs
            (c) Usually have a deep psychological investment in their careers
        (2) Career women over the age of 35 years may have difficulty balancing a career with the physical and psychological demands of pregnancy (Meisenhelder & Meservey, 1987)
        (3) Women over the age of 35 years may have difficulty with or feel an increased ambivalence about changing their roles (Meisenhelder & Meservey, 1987)
            (a) During the postpartum period women must make decisions about whether to return to work and, if they plan to, when they will return
            (b) They must make decisions about obtaining adequate child care if they will return to work, and must deal with the feelings of combining motherhood and a career
    e. Chronic diseases, which are more common in women over the age of 35 years, may affect the pregnancy (e.g., arthritis, hypertension, and diabetes)

2. Physical assessment (specific to advanced maternal age)
    a. Genetic testing (see Chapter 3 for a complete discussion of genetics)
        (1) Incidence of chromosomal abnormalities increases with age
        (2) Chorionic villi sampling or amniocentesis is performed for the detection of chromosomal abnormalities
    b. Signs of diabetes (see Chapter 29 for a complete discussion of diabetes in pregnancy)
        (1) Blood glucose tolerance screening, if not done as a routine screening on all pregnant women, is usually done on pregnant women over the age of 35 years
        (2) Incidence of gestational diabetes is increased in women over 35 years old
    c. Signs of hypertension or pregnancy-induced hypertension (see Chapter 26 for a complete discussion of hypertensive disorders in pregnancy)
        (1) Incidence of pregnancy-induced hypertension is increased in women over 35 years old
        (2) Women with chronic hypertension have an increased incidence of superimposed pregnancy-induced hypertension
    d. Presence of uterine fibroids
        (1) Increased incidence in women over 35 years old
        (2) Can cause pregnancy and labor complications
    e. Fundal height and due date discrepancy
        (1) Women over 35 years old are at higher risk for term, low-birth-weight infants; however, many studies that have reached this conclusion have not controlled for the confounding factors of educational level, prenatal care, nutrition, parity, and socioeconomic level (Mansfield, 1986)
        (2) There is an increased incidence of multiple gestation in women over 35 years old
    f. Vaginal bleeding: there is an increased incidence of gestational bleeding in women over 35 years old (see Chapter 28 on hemorrhagic disorders in pregnancy for a complete discussion of bleeding during pregnancy)
        (1) Increased incidence of abruptio placentae
        (2) Increased incidence of placenta previa
        (3) Increased incidence of trophoblastic disease, particularly over the age of 40 years (Willmot, 1984)

B. **Nursing Diagnoses**

1. Anxiety and fear related to the possible complications of pregnancy
2. Anxiety and fear related to a possible chromosomal abnormality in the fetus
3. High risk for alteration in parenting related to late childbearing

C. **Interventions/Evaluations**

1. Anxiety and fear related to the possible complications of pregnancy
    a. Interventions
        (1) Treat the pregnancy as normal unless specific complications are identified
        (2) Reassure the client that good nutrition, health habits, and consistent prenatal care significantly reduce the risks associated with advanced maternal age
        (3) Stress the importance of consistent prenatal care to detect any complications early, when treatment is most effective
        (4) Review the danger signs in pregnancy and rehearse the appropriate responses to them so that the woman feels confident about what to do
    b. Evaluations
        (1) The woman with advanced maternal age will feel that her pregnancy is normal unless specific complications are identified
        (2) The pregnant woman with advanced maternal age who has identified risks and complications will feel confident in the care and treatment she receives to minimize her risks and complications

(3) The woman with advanced maternal age will seek and receive early prenatal care

2. Anxiety and fear related to a possible chromosomal abnormality in the fetus
   a. Interventions
      (1) Encourage genetic counseling to identify the risks and discuss the implications of testing to enhance decision making
      (2) Decision to have amniocentesis or a chorionic villi sampling performed may be related to beliefs and attitudes about abortion; therefore, the nurse needs to respect the woman's decision
      (3) Support the woman and encourage her to ventilate her anxiety during the days of waiting for the amniocentesis results
   b. Evaluations
      (1) The pregnant woman with advanced maternal age will make an informed choice about whether she will have genetic studies performed and will feel confident about her decision
      (2) The pregnant woman with advanced maternal age and her partner will understand what is taking place on a technical level during the waiting period after amniocentesis for a chromosomal study and will verbalize their frustration and anxiety associated with delayed results

3. High risk for alteration in parenting related to late childbearing
   a. Interventions
      (1) Encourage expectant parents' attendance at parenting classes before the baby's birth
      (2) Identify and promote individual strengths and the advantages related to late childbearing
         (a) Financial security has been achieved
         (b) Education has usually been completed
         (c) Expectant mother usually is secure in a career or occupation
         (d) Marriage or relationship has had the opportunity to stabilize (Schlesinger & Schlesinger, 1989)
         (e) Woman has had a child-free period for personal development before childbearing (Wilkie, 1981)
         (f) Personal maturity will generally result in mothers who are more accepting and feel less conflict in their parenting role (Frankel & Wise, 1982; Issod, 1987)
      (3) Anticipate the informational needs of older couples
         (a) Handling the feelings of social isolation that may occur when peers have children who are already teenagers
         (b) Coping with the energy required to care for a newborn and developing strategies to meet the added energy demands
            (i) Getting help in the house, if finances permit
            (ii) Sharing the care of the newborn with the partner
            (iii) Planning naps
            (iv) Eating simple, nutritious meals
   b. Evaluations
      (1) The pregnant woman with advanced maternal age and her partner will feel confident in their ability to parent their newborn
      (2) The expectant couple with advanced age will develop a plan to meet the high-energy demands of newborn care and tailor it to their individual lifestyle

Health Education

A. Adolescence

1. Preparation for childbirth classes focused on pregnant adolescents' special concerns
   a. Lack of knowledge about conception, pregnancy, and labor and delivery

  b. Alteration in body image issues
  c. Isolation from peer groups
  d. Alteration in education and career goals and plans
 2. Female anatomy and physiology, both before and during pregnancy
 3. Conception and contraception
 4. Information about pregnancy alternatives to assist in decision making
  a. Abortion
  b. Adoption: public and private
  c. Single parenting
 5. Parenting classes for adolescents
  a. Child development
  b. Child safety
  c. Discipline
  d. Child-care arrangements
 6. Setting realistic short-term and long-term goals
  a. Returning to school or continuing educational plans
  b. Career or life plans
  c. Adequate child care
  d. Financial considerations
  e. Social relationships

B. Advanced maternal age

 1. Preparation for childbirth and parenting skill classes developed to accommodate the special concerns and needs of older expectant parents
 2. Alteration in lifestyles and habits to adapt to a baby
 3. Combining career and quality parenting

CASE STUDIES AND STUDY QUESTIONS

Cindy is a 14½-year-old high-school student, gravida 1, para 0. Her last menstrual period was approximately 5 months ago, as best she remembers. She has had unprotected intercourse sporadically over the past year. She has had three sexual partners since she became sexually active and one steady boyfriend for the past 6 months. She states that her parents are unaware that she is sexually active and would never suspect that she might be pregnant. In fact, Cindy is surprised that her pregnancy test is positive and stated that she "doesn't do it that often." She says that her periods have always been irregular since the beginning (menarche was at 12 years of age). Skipping a few months was not unusual and Cindy did not think much about it. She states that recently it has been difficult to control her weight, that she has had to be very stringent about what she eats, and that some days she does not eat at all, just to stay at her present weight. She complains that, despite all of this effort, her clothes are uncomfortably tight and she feels fat. She denies tobacco or other drug use and states that she drinks beer only at parties. She has come to the clinic for birth control. The results of a physical examination are as follows: blood pressure, 118/60;

height, 162.6 cm (5 ft, 4 in); weight, 52.6 kg (116 lb) (prepregnant weight, 52.6 kg); urine, trace protein, no sugar; fundal height, 14 cm; ultrasound test results, intrauterine pregnancy at 16 weeks' gestation.

1. Cindy states that she cannot believe she is pregnant and that maybe a mistake has been made in the tests. This remark is not unusual because, appropriate to her age, Cindy

 a. Has the ability to foresee the consequences of her behavior but will not admit it to herself or to anybody else.

 b. Is a concrete thinker and has difficulty believing something she cannot see, such as a 16-week pregnancy.

 c. Really does know she is pregnant because she is capable of thinking abstractly but cannot deal with the thought of her parents' finding out that she is sexually active and now, pregnant.

2. From the physical findings and her history, Cindy is at greatest risk for and already showing signs of

 a. Intrauterine growth retardation.

b. Pregnancy-induced hypertension.

c. Gestational diabetes.

d. Sexually transmitted disease because of her multiple sexual partners.

3. Cindy proudly states that she has not gained any weight but complains that her clothes are fitting tighter and that she feels fat. The most appropriate intervention would be to

a. Reinforce the fact that she is pregnant and needs to eat more to support her own growth and her fetus's growth.

b. Tell Cindy not to worry about gaining weight and explain to her that after she has had the baby she will return to her normal weight.

c. Review Cindy's food intake over the past 24 hours, determine her likes and dislikes, and adapt a nutritious diet to her needs.

d. Encourage Cindy to wear looser clothing so that she will not feel so constricted.

Cindy explains that it was difficult for her to get to the clinic. She had to make an excuse to her mother and had to get an older friend to give her a ride. When given the schedule for prenatal clinic visits, Cindy states that the appointments are too frequent and, in her opinion, nothing much is done at each visit. She says she will come as often as she can, but she does not know how often that will be.

4. Cindy's anticipated missed appointments represent the largest problem in the management of adolescent pregnancy, which is

a. An adolescent seeks independence; however, the clinic represents authority and has rules.

b. The pregnant adolescent pictures herself in control and resents being told what she has to do.

c. Late and inconsistent prenatal care is the cause of most of the complications associated with adolescent pregnancy.

Mary, aged 36 years, is an accountant with a prestigious firm in a large metropolitan area. She typically works long hours and must travel, on occasion. She enjoys the responsibilities of her career as well as the authority of her position. She has been married to Brian, aged 38 years, for 10 years. They had always planned to have a family but Mary wanted time to develop her career. She is now pregnant for the first time. She has a history of uterine fibroids, one of which measures 3 cm. Physical findings are as follows: blood pressure, 130/82; height, 167.6 cm (5 ft, 6 in); weight, 64.9 kg (143 lb), prepregnant weight, 59 kg (130 lb); urine, no protein/no sugar; fundal height, 26 cm; ultrasound results, intrauterine pregnancy at 25 weeks' gestation and marginal placenta previa.

At 16½ weeks' gestation, Mary and Brian elected to have amniocentesis performed for genetic testing. They had to wait nearly 2 weeks for the results, making Mary 18½ weeks into gestation before any information was available.

5. Mary and Brian were undecided about what their actions would be if the fetus had chromosomal abnormalities. An important intervention with Mary and Brian would be

a. To assist them in clarifying and deciding what their decision is before getting the results so that their emotions will not confuse their decision.

b. To encourage them to ventilate their anxieties and concerns about the upcoming results and to delay their final decision making until the results are known.

c. To have them put their worry about the test results aside because there is nothing that they can do about it during the waiting period and they will just make themselves more anxious by worrying.

6. Because of the marginal placenta previa, Mary is instructed to report immediately any vaginal bleeding, no matter how slight. There is a possibility that the birth will have to be by cesarean section. Mary cries and wonders aloud why she just cannot be normal, like any other pregnant woman. She states she feels so out of control. The best intervention for Mary is one based on the concept that

a. This is a normal feeling for all pregnant mothers and Mary will just have to work through it psychologically.

b. Because of her age, Mary's fears are

heightened related to the fact that she may not have another chance to have a baby.

c. Mary is exaggerating her situation and creating her own anxiety.

d. Mary's career and lifestyle have elements of personal control in them to which she has become accustomed; feeling out of control is distressing for her.

7. Pregnant women over the age of 35 years have a higher incidence of all of the following except

a. Neural tube defects.

b. Gestational diabetes.

c. Multiple gestation.

d. Pregnancy-induced hypertension.

8. Women over the age of 35 years have a higher incidence of gestational bleeding related to

a. An incompetent cervix.

b. Clotting abnormalities.

c. Abruptio placentae.

d. Anemia.

Answers to Study Questions

1. b	2. a	3. c
4. c	5. b	6. d
7. a	8. c	

REFERENCES

Barkan, S., & Bracken, M. (1987). Delayed childbearing: No evidence for increased risk of low birth weight and preterm delivery. *American Journal of Epidemiology, 125*(1), 101–109.

Bobak, I., Jensen, M., & Zalar, M. (1989). *Maternity and gynecologic care* (4th ed.) (pp. 881–902). St. Louis: Mosby.

Berkowitz, G., Skovron, M., Lapinski, R., & Berkowitz, R. (1990). Delayed childbearing and the outcome of pregnancy. *New England Journal of Medicine, 322*(10), 659–663.

Degenhart-Leskosky, S. (1989). Health education needs of adolescent and nonadolescent mothers. *Journal of Obstetric, Gynecologic, and Neonatal Nursing, 18*(3), 238–243.

Dormire, S., Strauss, S., & Clarke, B. (1989). Social support and adaptation to the parent role in first-time adolescent mothers. *Journal of Obstetric, Gynecologic, and Neonatal Nursing, 18*(4), 327–337.

Frankel, S., & Wise, M. (1982). A view of delayed parenting: Some implications of a new trend. *Psychiatry, 45,* 220–225.

Issod, J. (1987, April). A comparison of "on-time" and "delayed" parenthood. *American Mental Health Counselors Association Journal,* 92–97.

Kirz, D., Dorchester, W., & Freeman, R. (1985). Advanced maternal age: The mature gravida. *American Journal of Obstetrics and Gynecology, 152,* 7–12.

Mansfield, P. (1986). Re-evaluating the medical risks of late childbearing. *Women & Health, 11*(2), 37–60.

Mansfield, P. (1987, August/September). Teenage and midlife childbearing update: Implications for health educators. *Health Education,* 18–23.

Meisenhelder, J., & Meservey, P. (1987). Childbearing over thirty. *Western Journal of Nursing Research, 9*(4), 527–541.

Olds, S., London, M., & Ladewig, P. (1988). *Maternal-newborn nursing* (3rd ed.) (pp. 398–410). Menlo Park, CA: Addison-Wesley.

Panzarine, S., & Gould, C. (1988). Knowledge about contraceptive use and conception among a group of urban, black, adolescent mothers. *Journal of Obstetric, Gynecologic, and Neonatal Nursing, 17*(4), 279–282.

Schlesinger, B., & Schlesinger, R. (1989). Postponed parenthood: Trends and issues. *Journal of Comparative Family Studies, 20*(3), 354–363.

Schlesinger, B. (1987). Postponed parenthood: A Canadian study. *Conciliation Courts Review, 25*(2), 21–26.

Sherwin, L., Scoloveno, M., & Weingarten, C. (1991). *Nursing care of the childbearing family* (pp. 1002–1022). Norwalk, CT: Appleton & Lange.

Stevens, K., & Pavlides, C. (1989). Individualized prenatal nursing care of pregnant adolescents makes a difference. *Journal of Obstetric, Gynecologic, and Neonatal Nursing, 18*(6), 521–522.

Wilkie, J. (1981, August). The trend toward delayed parenthood. *Journal of Marriage and the Family.* 583–592.

Willmot, L. (1984, February 8). Hydatidiform mole. *Nursing Times,* 40–43.

Winslow, W. (1987). First pregnancy after 35: What is the experience? *MCN: American Journal of Maternal-Child Nursing, 12,* 92–96.

Judith Noble Halle

Diagnostic Evaluation of High-Risk Pregnancies

Objectives

1. Describe the various fetal diagnostic tests performed to evaluate fetal development and well-being

2. Explain the risks and benefits of the various fetal diagnostic tests

3. Identify the high-risk pregnancy conditions that require fetal surveillance and their appropriate tests

4. List the steps in performing each test

5. Explain the sensitivities of the fetal well-being testing parameters

6. Describe the nursing diagnosis that is possible for high-risk pregnant clients undergoing a fetal diagnostic testing program and the interventions that might be helpful

Introduction

To understand how the various diagnostic tests determine fetal well-being and identify abnormal development, a basic understanding of the physiological principles of fetal life is required

A. Fetal growth and development

1. The normal length of gestation for full fetal development is 280 days (40 weeks) from the first day of the mother's last menstrual period (LMP) or 266 days (38 weeks) from actual conception. Because the conception date is usually not known, the delivery date given the mother is the estimated date of confinement (EDC), with a range of ±2 weeks to take into consideration variations in time of ovulation from LMP

2. With unknown LMP, an estimation of gestational age (EGA) can be determined by estimating fetal size; one method is to measure the distance from the upper aspect of the maternal symphysis pubis to the top of the uterus (fundal height)

   a. Given a normal uterus, normal amniotic fluid volume, and a nondiabetic singleton gestation, a 20-week fetus usually causes a fundal height of 20 cm, with a normal growth rate of 1 cm/wk until 36 weeks, after which engagement of the presenting part occurs

b. If there is more than a 2-cm discrepancy in this size-for-dates estimate between 20 and 36 weeks of gestation, an ultrasound scan can be performed
(1) The earlier the ultrasound scan is performed, the better for exact dating
(2) After 30 weeks, estimates have a 2- to 3-week range of accuracy
(3) According to Barcroft (1977), the relation of age to weight is relatively constant among fetuses up to a point of gestation, after which extremes of weight become increasingly apparent

c. Human intrauterine growth charts have been developed that are clinically useful in assessing adequate serial fetal growth; the normal fetus grows from a weight of 2 to 4 g (0.10 to 0.12 oz) and less than 2 to 3 cm (1 in) at the onset of the fetal period (the beginning of the ninth week), up to an average weight of 3000 to 3600 g (6 lb 10 oz to 7 lb 15 oz) and a length of 48 to 53 cm (19 to 21 in) at term

3. Fetal organ growth is not synchronous; fetal systems grow in staggered periods
a. Because all body organ systems are present at least in rudimentary form by the end of the embryonic stage (8 weeks), the fetal period involves tissue and organ specialization and growth, accompanied by changes in body proportions
b. Depending on their level of development, the systems have a varying degree of susceptibility to malformations caused by environmental agents and maternal conditions
c. The fetal heart is usually large enough at 18 to 20 weeks' gestation to be audible with a DeLee stethoscope; this finding is another confirmation of gestational age and, if not found, could mean the fetus is not as old as expected.

4. Viability can be defined in terms of ability or capacity of a product of conception to survive for a finite time in a defined environment
a. Most authorities believe that 23 weeks (menstrual dating) represents the time of earliest survival (Little, 1990)
b. Some systems are more immediately critical than others for survival
(1) The respiratory system is critical, since gas exchange must occur even if assisted ventilation is used
(2) The kidneys are more essential than the central nervous system (CNS)

B. Fetal physiological responses

1. Adequate tissue oxygenation in the fetus is accomplished by an umbilical vein Po_2 level of 28.9 ± 7 mm Hg (Silverman, Suidan, & Wasserman, 1985), the critical level of hypoxia that triggers an adaptive response being 17 to 18 mm Hg (Freeman & Lagrew, 1990)
2. Without adequate oxygen, the metabolism of glucose is incomplete, causing a build-up of lactic acid, a potent acid capable of rupturing brain cells; the level of lactic acid (metabolic acidosis) is measured by
a. The pH of the blood: by fetal scalp sample: reassuring, > 7.25; borderline, 7.20 to 7.25; acidosis, < 7.20; critical and potentially damaging, < 7.00 (McDuffie & Haverkamp, 1991)
b. The amount of base (HCO_3) used by the body to buffer the acid present (base deficit > 8)
3. A diminished oxygen reserve has numerous causes
a. Uteroplacental insufficiency
b. Umbilical cord compression
c. Fetal complications (e.g., sepsis, hemorrhage)
4. The fetus's attempt to adapt to a diminished oxygen supply involves a complex array of responses; these biophysical responses vary according to certain factors present in each situation
a. Severity and acuteness of onset of hypoxemia

  b. Pre-existing fetal condition
  c. Presence of compounding factors (e.g., hyperglycemia)
  d. Level of maturity of reflexes and endocrine systems
5. According to Manning and Harman (1990), asphyxia is the presence of both hypoxia and acidemia; the fetal biophysical responses to asphyxia may be divided into two categories
  a. Acute, or immediate, responses such as changes in CNS function
  b. Chronic responses, such as reduction in amniotic fluid production, impaired fetal growth, and increased probability of ischemic neonatal complications
6. Porto (1987) and others believe that there is usually a progressive response to asphyxia, following the CNS embryological developmental phases, with the area developed last being the most sensitive to hypoxia
  a. The medulla, which controls heart reactivity, is the last area to develop; thus, a loss of fetal ability to accelerate (a nonreactive nonstress test) should be the first CNS response to asphyxia
  b. Prolonged exposure is needed to lose the CNS responses of fetal movement, breathing, and then tone, which are responses regulated by neurological areas with earlier embryological development
  c. This understanding of progressive fetal biophysical response to asphyxia is useful clinically in ruling out false-positive findings; with a maternal complaint of decreased fetal movement, if testing shows presence of fetal heart accelerations (reactive nonstress test), the mother can be reassured of fetal well-being
  d. In a true case of asphyxia, the CNS would already have lost the ability to stimulate fetal heart acceleration, before the loss of the ability to stimulate movement

C. Comparison of fetal surveillance tests: sensitivity of testing parameters

1. Reflex late deceleration
  a. The most sensitive indicator of fetal hypoxia is a late deceleration of the fetal heart rate, which is triggered by chemoreceptors sensing a Po_2 of less than 20 mm Hg (Caldeyro-Barcia, Casacuberta, & Bustos, 1968; Cibils, 1981)
  b. This response occurs before changes in pH, baseline fetal heart rate (FHR), variability or reactivity (Martin, de Haan, van der Wildt, Jongsma, Dilleman, & Arts, 1979; Porto, 1987)
  c. Early work by Adamsons and Myers (1977) in monkeys showed that when late decelerations lasted for less than an hour, no neurological damage occurred; a degree of hypoxia is demonstrated without CNS depression during this clinical experience, making it an excellent time for intervention for the term or fully developed fetus to prevent neurological damage (Freeman & Lagrew, 1990)
2. Accelerations
  a. When hypoxia lasts long enough for anaerobic metabolism of glucose to cause lactic acid build-up, the pH falls below 7.22 and FHR accelerations disappear (Murata, Martin, & Ikenoue, 1982)
  b. The foundation work by Myers and colleagues (1969) demonstrated that lactic acid is a potent acid and that severe asphyxia can cause swelling in the brain and eventually rupture the cells
3. Variability
  a. After an initial period of increased FHR variability in response to mild hypoxia, variability decreases as the degree of hypoxia and acidosis increase (Boehm, 1990)
  b. When moderate FHR variability (6 to 25 beats/min) (Parer, 1989) was present 30 minutes before delivery, only 2% of newborns had Apgar scores below 7 at 5 minutes (Krebs, Petres, & Dunn, 1979)

c. This gives a 98% accuracy in predicting fetal well-being, regardless of the presence of periodic decelerations, making the presence of variability the most reassuring aspect of FHR monitoring
4. Biophysical profile
   a. Prolonged hypoxia is needed to lose the CNS response of breathing, fetal movement, and then, tone (Vintzileos, Campbell, Ingardia, & Nochimson, 1983)
   b. Chronic hypoxia can also cause a protective redistribution of cardiac output away from organ systems not vital to fetal life (lung, kidney, and gut) and toward vital organs (heart, brain, adrenals, and placenta)
   c. With decreased renal and pulmonary perfusion, urine production and lung fluid flow are decreased, which results in decreased amniotic fluid

Clinical Practice

BIOPHYSICAL ASSESSMENT

Ultrasonography

A. Introduction
1. Principles
   a. Definition: ultrasonography is a method of tissue imaging based on graphic analysis of the spectral characteristics of reflected high-frequency sound waves (Manning, 1989)
   b. Equipment
     (1) Transducer
       (a) Most scanning in obstetrics is done with 3.5- and 5-MHz transducers
       (b) The transducer contains crystals that emit ultrasound wave energy; it also receives the reflected sound energy as echoes
         (i) Linear array scanning: with a series of crystals aligned along a transducer, an electronic distributor fires the crystals in sequence to produce a broad band of ultrasound waves
         (ii) Sector scanning: scanning is done by a single transducer rotated through a prescribed arc while the ultrasound lines are being compounded
     (2) Signal display (B-scan)
       (a) Reflected sound waves are converted first into electrical signals then into a spot on the oscilloscope
       (b) The intensity (brightness) of the spot varies directly with the strength of the echo, which can be amplified by the gain controls, resulting in 64 shades of gray
2. Safety concerns: dosage levels
   a. The ratio between emitting and receiving time with diagnostic ultrasound is only 1:1000
     (1) Total exposure time during 24 hours is less than 84 seconds
     (2) Therefore, a fetus that is 8 cm from the source receives an average of 0.01 to 0.03 mW/cm^2, which is only 0.01% of the maximal safe level of 100 mW/cm^2.
   b. More than 25 years of follow-up by the American College of Radiology have shown no adverse effects of diagnostic ultrasonography

B. Assessment

1. History: according to the American College of Obstetricians and Gynecologists (ACOG) guidelines (1986), the screening (level 1) obstetric ultrasound examination includes the following parameters, which are also indications for use (American College of Radiology, 1984)
   a. Gestational dating

b. Placental evaluation and localization
c. Fetal presentation
d. Fetal number
e. Fetal viability
f. Amniotic fluid volume
g. Survey of fetal anatomy for gross anomalies
h. Detection and evaluation of maternal pelvic masses

2. Physical findings
   a. Gestational dating
      (1) Because over 45% of clients in some clinic populations have questionable menstrual histories (Gabbe, 1986), a more accurate method is needed for determining EDC than that based on LMP
      (2) This is especially true in high-risk pregnancies, in which the fetal maturity estimate weighs heavily in the risk/benefit decision in planning a delivery
      (3) In 1985 Queenan developed the scoring system given in Table 11–1 to identify a term fetus
      (4) Using measurements of various parts of fetal anatomy according to the trimester, Sabbagha (1978) and others developed equations and reference tables for serial size and age determinations (Table 11–2)
   b. Placental evaluation
      (1) Grading criteria: Grannum and colleagues (1979) reported on a method of categorizing maturation into grades 0 to III
         (a) This method was based on the identification and distribution of calcium deposits within the placenta and the increasing delineations with maturity, as in the appearance of the basal and chorionic plate of placenta and the placental substance (Fig. 11–1).
         (b) Clinical implications (Grannum, Berkowitz, & Hobbins, 1979)
            (i) Grade 0: immature placenta of less than 12 weeks' gestation
            (ii) Grade I: placenta of more than 12 weeks' gestation; associated with only 67.7% fetal lung maturity
            (iii) Grade II: placenta of more than 12 weeks' gestation associated with 87.5% fetal lung maturity
            (iv) Grade III
               • Placenta of more than 36 weeks' gestation or presence of hypertension or growth-retarded fetus; this grade was associated in one study with 100% fetal lung maturity (Grannum, Berkowitz, & Hobbins, 1979) and in another with 93% lung maturity (Harman, 1982)
               • Placenta of more than 42 weeks' gestation; this grade has a 40% incidence of villous changes, which can reduce blood

Table 11–1
FETAL MATURITY SCORING*

Parameter	Traits of Maturity
Biparietal diameter (BPD)	>9 cm
Placental grading	II–III
Amniotic fluid volume (AFV)	Normal to Crowding

* See the related findings discussions for explanation of each parameter.

Modified from Queenan, J., & Warsof, S. (1985). In J. Queenan (Ed.), *Management of high-risk prenancy* (2nd ed.). Oradell, NJ: Medical Economics.

Table 11–2
GESTATIONAL AGE DETERMINATION BY ULTRASOUND MEASUREMENTS

Parameter	Stage of Pregnancy (wk)	Accuracy (days)
Gestational sac (GS)	6–8	±0.5–3
Crown–rump length formula: cm + 6.5 = weeks	8–14	±0.5–3
Biparietal diameter (BPD) Femur length (FL) Abdominal circumference (AC)	15–26	±10
BPD, FL, AC	>30	±14–21

Modified from Queenan, J., & Warsof, S. (1985). Ultrasonography. In J. Queenan, (Ed.). *Management of high-risk pregnancy* (2nd ed.) (p. 217). Oradell, NJ: Medical Economics.

flow leading to fetal hypoxia (e.g., increased calcification, intervillous thrombosis, perivillous fibrin [Eden, 1990])

(2) Localization

    (a) Placenta previa: in the presence of vaginal bleeding episodes, diagnostic ultrasonography is used to screen for low-lying placenta or placenta previa (implantation partially or completely over the cervical os)

    (b) Placental migration: with uterine growth and the development of the lower uterine segment as the pregnancy advances, the placenta may be carried away from the os

        (i) Wexler and Gottesfeld (1977) found that, before the third trimester, 45% of pregnancies were characterized by a low-lying pla-

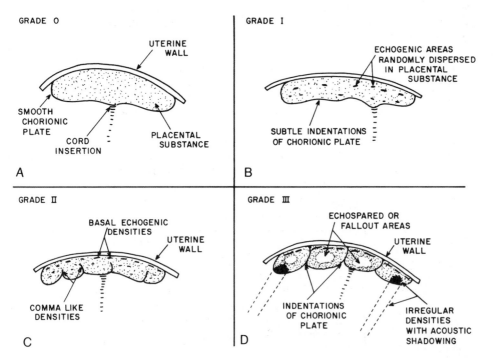

Figure 11–1
Placental grading. (From Grannum, P., Berkowitz, R., & Hobbins, J. [1979]. The ultrasonic changes in the maturing placenta and the relation to pulmonic maturity. *American Journal of Obstetrics and Gynecology, 133*(8), 916.)

centa; this contrasts with an incidence of placenta previa at birth of less than 1%

(ii) Clinical implication: Because most cases of asymptomatic placenta previa found early are cured by placental migration, restriction of activity need not be practiced unless the placenta previa persists beyond 30 weeks or becomes clinically apparent before that time

c. Fetal presentation

(1) Vertex: because malpresentations have a much higher incidence of morbidity associated with vaginal birth than do cephalic presentations, it is crucial to identify the fetal presentation in labor accurately; visualization by ultrasonography of the fetal skull outline at the maternal pelvic brim is a reassuring finding

(2) Breech: because breech presentation in the last trimester may be manipulated into a vertex presentation by an external cephalic version procedure, antepartum assessment of presentation can also be of value in enabling a timely intervention to avoid a malpresentation at delivery

d. Multiple pregnancy

(1) Risk of discordant growth: multiple pregnancies can be high risk, especially if monozygotic, in which two fetuses compete for nutrition from the same placenta and the cords can become entangled in utero

(2) Mode of delivery planning

(a) The third-trimester presentation of twin fetuses determines the mode of delivery; if vertex/vertex, a vaginal birth is considered safe by many

(b) If the first twin is vertex, some may do a version of the second transverse twin after the first has been born vaginally

(c) Cesarean birth is the preferred delivery method for all other presentations

(3) Clinical implication: antepartum surveillance of twin pregnancies, starting at 28 weeks (Manning & Harman, 1990) in multiple pregnancies, is performed for the monitoring of serial growth patterns and adequate uteroplacental function

e. Fetal viability

(1) Real-time ultrasound can be used to confirm fetal death in utero by the presence of fetal scalp edema and the overlapping of the fetal cranial bones (Gabbe, 1986)

(2) Fetal life can be confirmed by the visualization of the heart's beating and of fetal movements

f. Amniotic fluid volume

(1) Most researchers agree that less than 500 cc of amniotic fluid at term is considered oligohydramnios, or decreased fluid, and more than 2000 cc is considered polyhydramnios (Brace, 1989); the exact ultrasonographic measurement that reflects a significant decrease has varied

(2) Amniotic fluid index (AFI)

(a) The AFI is a method that was developed by Rutherford and colleagues (1987) in which the depths of amniotic fluid in all four quadrants surrounding the maternal umbilicus (in centimeters) are totaled

(b) The interpretation currently recommended is based on findings of an increased perinatal morbidity (low Apgar scores, meconium staining, fetal distress) in pregnancies with lower-than-normal measurements at term (Chervenak & Gabbe, 1991)

(i) Normal: 5 to 19 cm

(ii) Oligohydramnios: less than 5 cm

(iii) Polyhydramnios: 20 cm or greater

(3) Severe oligohydramnios: Chamberlain, Manning, and Morrison (1984)

reported severe oligohydramnios of 1 cm or less in less than 1% of more than 7500 pregnancies evaluated; this finding was associated with a 40-fold increase in perinatal mortality (187 of 1000) as compared with patients with normal fluid volumes

(4) Hydramnios was observed in approximately 2.8% of pregnancies, and major fetal malformations were found in 18% of these cases; neural tube defects, obstruction of the fetal gastrointestinal tract, multiple gestations, and fetal hydrops are associated with hydramnios (Hobbins, Grannum, & Berkowitz, 1979)

g. Congenital anomalies and follow-up directed (level 2) scans

(1) Incidence

(a) Approximately 3% of live-born infants have a major anomaly (Simpson, 1991)

(b) There are at least 500 known developmental anomalies

(c) Congenital anomalies now account for 15 to 20% of all perinatal deaths (Manning, 1989)

(d) After 36 weeks, more than 85% of all major anomalies can be detected by ultrasound test (Manning, 1989)

(e) The recognition of an anomaly may influence the location and method of delivery so that neonatal outcome may be optimized (Chervenak & Gabbe, 1991)

(2) Directed scans are performed as a thorough examination of a client suspected of carrying a physiologically or anatomically defective fetus, based on her history, clinical evaluation, or previous ultrasonography

(3) Management of anomalies depends on consideration of variables such as

(a) Expected prognosis for the lesion

(b) Demonstration of progressive pathophysiology

(c) Availability of treatment modalities, if any

(d) Fetal age at the time of diagnosis (Manning, 1989)

Biophysical Profile

A. Assessment

1. History: in 1980, Manning, Platt, & Sipos introduced the biophysical profile (BPP) test as a form of an intrauterine Apgar score
2. Physical findings
   a. Of the five biophysical parameters, each has been studied alone to correlate with fetal well-being (Table 11–3) (Gabbe, 1991)

Table 11–3
BIOPHYSICAL PROFILE

Criteria	Points	
	None	*Present*
Reactive nonstress test	0	2
Fetal breathing movements (one or more episodes of 30 seconds or more in 30 minutes)	0	2
Fetal movements (three or more discrete body or limb movements in 30 minutes)	0	2
Fetal tone (one or more episodes of extension with return to flexion)	0	2
Quantitation of amniotic fluid volume (one or more pockets of 2 cm or more in two perpendicular planes)	0	2
Interpretation		
Normal	8–10 (in a the absence of oligohydramnios)	
Equivocal	6	
Abnormal	≤4	

  b. Interpretation
     (1) Normal: 8 to 10 (in the absence of oligohydramnios)
     (2) Equivocal: 6
     (3) Abnormal: 4 or less

Doppler Ultrasound Blood Flow Assessment

A. Introduction: one of the major new advances in perinatal medicine is the ability to study blood flow noninvasively in the fetus and placenta. In pregnancies suspected of uteroplacental insufficiency, analysis of Doppler wave forms can allow identification of jeopardized fetuses before asphyxial compromise has occured (Sonek, Reiss, & Gabbe, 1990)

B. Assessment

1. History: the Doppler principle
   a. When an ultrasound wave is directed at an acute angle to a moving target, as with blood flowing through a vessel, the frequency of the echoes is altered in response to the systolic and diastolic components of the cardiac cycle
   b. This change, referred to as the Doppler shift, indicates forward movement of blood within the vessel; Doppler shifts can be analyzed and displayed as velocity wave forms (Fig. 11–2)
2. Physical findings
   a. According to Cundiff and associates (1990), visual representation of the blood flow can be calculated at the time of the procedure by dividing the systolic (S) peak by the end diastolic (D) component
   b. The normal S/D ratio declines from 2.8 to 2.2 between midpregnancy and term
      (1) When uteroplacental perfusion is reduced, diastolic flow decreases, resulting in an elevated S/D ratio
      (2) Elevations above 3 are abnormal

Fetal Movement Assessment by Client

A. Assessment

1. History: physiological basis
   a. Fetal activity expresses fetal condition in utero, and daily evaluation of fetal movements provides an inexpensive, noninvasive way of assessing fetal well-being
   b. Decreased activity in a previously active fetus may reflect disturbance of placental function and may be a clue to impending demise (Sadovsky, 1985a)
   c. Many variables (e.g., fetal resting state, maternal glucose load, medications, exercise), however, make the interpretation of fetal movement (FM) patterns confusing (Queenan, 1985)
2. Physical findings
   a. According to Sadovsky (1990), the mean daily fetal movement recording (DFMR) rises from about 200 in the 20th week to a maximum of 575 in the 32nd week of gestation, and then decreases gradually thereafter until delivery, with a mean of 282 daily FMs
   b. The periods of decreased activity at term may be related to fetal sleep states, which increase with maturity (Timor-Tritech, Dierker, & Hertz, 1979)
   c. Except for very low DFMRs, and especially where there is a definite trend toward decreasing motion, the clinical value of the absolute number of FMs has not been established; the only exception is when FMs cease entirely for 12 hours
   d. Interpretation is complicated because every pregnancy has its own rhythm

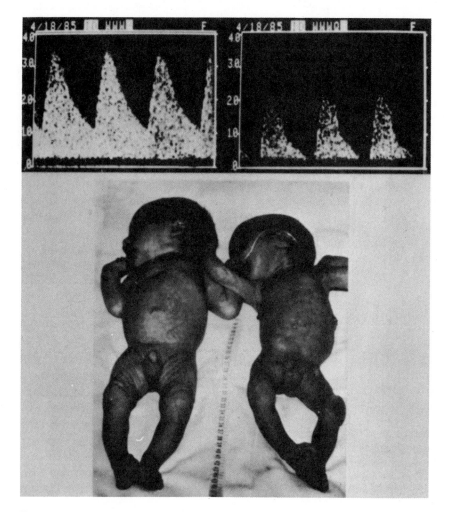

Figure 11–2
Doppler ultrasound comparison of N1 twin to twin with intrauterine growth retardation (IUGR). (From Schulman, H. [1990]. Doppler ultrasound. In R. Eden & F. Boehm [Eds.], *Assessment and care of the fetus: Physiological, clinical and medicolegal principles* [p. 402]. Norwalk, CT: Appleton & Lange.)

     and a woman's perception is subjective; when compared with an FM-sensing device, however, there was an 80 to 90% correlation with maternal perception of FM (Sadovsky, 1990)

    e. Many women report that fetal activity during the day is not constant. Therefore, it would be incorrect to evaluate FM only once a day for a short period

3. Interpretation: various protocols are used by practitioners to identify clinically significant decreased FM; based on his research, Sadovsky (1985b) developed the following protocol

    a. Normal

      (1) Assess FM for 30 minutes three times a day

      (2) The perception of four or more FMs in a 30-minute period is normal; assess FM during the next counting period

    b. Requiring follow-up

      (1) If fewer than four FMs are noted, the patient should continue counting for up to 6 hours

      (2) If there are fewer than 10 FMs or all movements are weak, the client should undergo a nonstress test (NST), a contraction stress test (CST), and an ultrasound

BIOCHEMICAL ASSESSMENT

Amniocentesis

A. Assessment

1. History
    a. Definition: amniocentesis involves removal of a small amount of amniotic fluid by a needle inserted with ultrasound guidance through the abdominal wall, the uterine wall, and the amniotic sac (Gilbert & Harman, 1986) (Fig. 11–3)
    b. Safety concerns: risks—amniocentesis is a relatively safe procedure with almost no severe maternal complications. The following list shows various risks involved and incidence in experienced hands
        (1) Infection (amnionitis): 0.01% (Elias & Simpson, 1986)
        (2) Pregnancy loss 0.2 to 0.5% higher than spontaneous loss of 3% at 16 weeks (Evans & Schulman, 1986)
        (3) Needle injuries with ultrasound guidance: rare (Drugan, Johnson, & Evans, 1990)
    c. Accuracy: according to the National Institute of Child Health and Human Development (1976), the overall accuracy of prenatal diagnosis was 99.4%
    d. Indications
        (1) Detection of chromosomal abnormalities
        (2) Assessment of fetal lung maturity
        (3) Confirmation of amnionitis
        (4) Evaluation of Rh-sensitized pregnancies
2. Physical findings
    a. Detection of chromosomal abnormalities
        (1) Most common indication
        (2) Usually done between 15 and 17 weeks to allow
            (a) Uterus to be above the symphysis

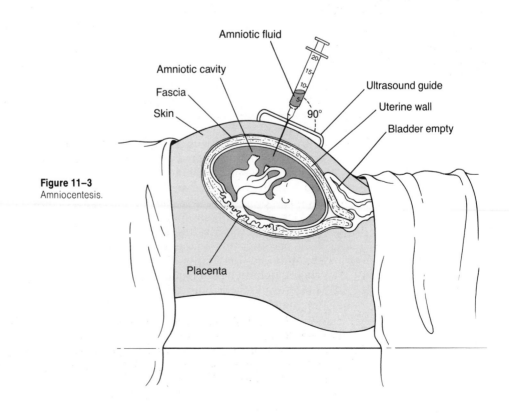

Figure 11–3
Amniocentesis.

(b) Adequate amniotic fluid volume (200 cc)

(c) Time for cell cultures and laboratory completion before it is too late for pregnancy termination at 20 weeks, if indicated

(3) Early amniocentesis at 10 to 15 weeks

(a) To minimize uterine irritability resulting from changes in fluid pressure after fluid withdrawal, total amount withdrawn is limited to 1 cc of fluid for each week of pregnancy (i.e., if the patient is at 12 weeks, only 12 cc would be removed) (Rodriguez, 1991)

(b) Earlier results make earlier termination possible, if so elected

(c) Advantages over chorionic villi sampling (CVS) includes the ability to also measure fetal alpha-fetoprotein (AFP)

b. Determination of fetal lung maturity

(1) There is a 98% chance of lung maturity if the concentration of lecithin is twice that of sphingomyelin in lung surfactant secreted by the fetus into the amniotic fluid (L/S ratio over 2:1) in the nondiabetic client

(2) For diabetic clients, or in specimens contaminated with blood or vaginal fluids, the additional presence of phosphatidylglycerol (PG), which appears after 35 weeks' gestation, is required for definitive maturity assessment

(3) Foam stability index (FSI)

(a) Exact amounts of 95% ethanol, isotonic saline, and amniotic fluid are combined and the test tube is shaken

(b) The persistence of a complete ring of bubbles on the surface of the liquid after 15 minutes indicates a positive shake test, signifying lung maturity

(4) Fluorescence polarization test (microviscosimetry)

(a) The microviscosity of lipid aggregates in the amniotic fluid may be assayed by mixing the fluid with a specific fluorescent dye that incorporates into the hydrocarbon region of the lipids in the surfactant (Barkai, Reichman, Modan, Goldman, Serr, & Mashiach, 1988)

(b) The intensity of the fluorescence induced by polarized light is measured

(c) Polarization value of 0.320 is associated with fetal lung maturity (Garite & Freeman, 1986)

(d) The technique is rapid and simple to perform, but the instrumentation is expensive

c. Confirmation of amnionitis: Gram's stain of fluid for bacteria can confirm the presence of amnionitis in a pregnancy suspected of infection

d. Evaluation of Rh-sensitized pregnancies

(1) Rationale

(a) If an Rh-negative woman is exposed to Rh-positive blood, either through transfusion or a prior pregnancy, she produces immunoglobulin (Ig)G antibody (anti-Rh[D])

(b) She is then considered sensitized, and the amount of maternal Rh antibody produced (titer) can be measured. Antibody titers measured by albumin agglutination techniques that are 16 or more indicate the fetus is at risk (Morrison & Pryor, 1990)

(c) If she becomes pregnant with an incompatible Rh-positive fetus, her Rh antibodies may cross the placenta and destroy fetal blood cells, causing hemolytic anemia in the fetus

(d) Concentrations of bilirubin and other breakdown products from destroyed RBCs can be detected in amniotic fluid by spectrophotometry. (Optical density [OD] reading at delta 450 mμ setting)

(e) This measurement is then plotted on a Liley graph, which takes gestational age into consideration for the interpretation, since there is a normal small amount of red blood cell (RBC) breakdown that decreases with fetal age; zone I is normal (Liley, 1961)

(2) Interpretation and management regimen
  (a) Zone I: the fetus is either unaffected or only mildly involved; no intervention is required and another amniocentesis is needed in 2 to 3 weeks
  (b) Zone II: there is moderate involvement and the need for closer observation by more frequent testing so the trend can be determined; the age of the fetus and trend in optical density determine the mode of therapy
  (c) Zone III: there is severe fetal involvement necessitating either intra-uterine transfusion or delivery if fetal maturity allows
(3) Test reliability
  (a) Although frequent, serial amniotic fluid OD 450 readings have been reported by Bowman (1990) to be 95% predictive of fetal anemia, a single reading may not be accurate
  (b) Direct fetal blood sampling has been advocated as an alternative, especially in clients with poor immunization histories or high zone II readings

Cordocentesis and Percutaneous Umbilical Blood Sampling

A. Assessment

1. History
  a. Definition: cordocentesis involves obtaining fetal blood through ul-trasound-guided puncture of the umbilical cord vessel (Daffos, Capella-Pavlovsky, & Forestier, 1983)
  b. Indications
    (1) Detection of inherited blood disorders
    (2) Detection of fetal infection
    (3) Karyotyping of fetuses
    (4) Assessment and treatment of RBC-isoimmunized and thrombocytope-nic pregnancies
    (5) Determination of acid–base balance of small-for-gestational age fetuses (Nicolaides et al, 1990)
  c. Safety concerns: risks
    (1) The risk of fetal death after cordocentesis depends on the indication for blood sampling and the experience of the operator
    (2) The combined experience from 14 U.S. centers with 1600 clients shows a 1.6% mean fetal loss rate (Ludomirski & Weiner, 1988)
  d. Technique (Fig. 11–4)
    (1) Sampling
      (a) With ultrasound-guided needle insertion, the cord is punctured close to its placental insertion
        (i) Between 1 and 4 ml of blood is removed for testing
        (ii) If the hemoglobin is normal, the needle is withdrawn
      (b) After needle withdrawal,the duration of bleeding from the umbilical cord usually is short and can be monitored ultrasonically (Cun-ningham, MacDonald, & Gant, 1989)
      (c) Daffos and colleagues (1985) recommend continuous FHR monitor-ing for a few minutes and then a second ultrasound examination 1 hour later to ensure that no further bleeding or hematoma occurred
    (2) Intrauterine transfusion
      (a) If the hemoglobin concentration is below the normal range, the tip of the needle is kept in the lumen of the umbilical cord vessel and fresh, packed Rh-negative blood compatible with that of the mother is infused into fetal circulation through a 10-ml syringe
      (b) The FHR and flow of the infused blood are monitored continually by ultrasonography; at the end of the transfusion, a fetal blood sample is aspirated for determination of the hemoglobin concentration

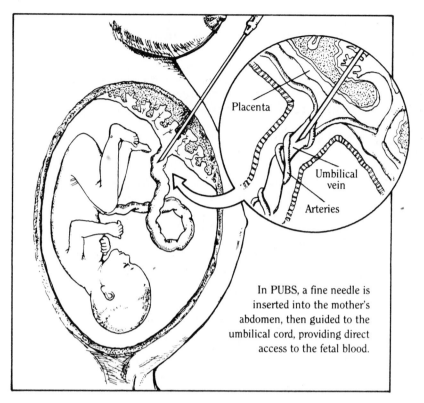

Placenta

Umbilical vein

Arteries

In PUBS, a fine needle is inserted into the mother's abdomen, then guided to the umbilical cord, providing direct access to the fetal blood.

Figure 11–4
Percutaneous umbilical blood sampling (PUBS). (Drawing by Jonel Sofian for Pennsylvania Hospital, Philadelphia, PA.)

2. Physical findings
   a. Fetal infection
      (1) Viral particles may be identified directly by electron microscopy of fetal blood, ascites, or urine specimens
      (2) Fetal blood and amniotic fluid may be cultured for further diagnosis (Weiner, 1988)
   b. Genetic disorders
      (1) An ultrasound-detected structural anomaly may be caused by fetal chromosome abnormalities
      (2) Benefits of documenting an abnormal karyotype
         (a) Cesarean section for fetal distress may be avoided
         (b) Recurrence risks are identified for counseling
      (3) Advantages
         (a) A preparation not requiring confirmation is available within 48 hours
         (b) Other causes of certain structural anomalies (e.g., congenital infections) may be sought
         (c) The fetal metabolic condition can also be assessed (Weiner, 1988)
   c. RBC isoimmunization
      (1) Normal mean fetal hemoglobin values range from 11 g/dl at 16 weeks to 15.5 g/dl at 40 weeks (Nicolaides, Soothill, Clewell, Rodeck, & Campbell, 1988)
         (a) Fetuses with hemoglobin deficits greater than 2 g/dl require transfusion
         (b) Severe isoimmunized fetuses may have deficits of greater than 7 g/dl (Nicolaides et al., 1988)

(2) Advantages
   (a) Permits definition of fetal blood type and count precisely, including degree of fetal anemia
   (b) Avoid unnecessary further intervention if the fetus is antigen-negative
   (c) If fetus is antigen-positive, a direct Coombs' test confirms the risk of hemolysis and need for further study (Ludomirski & Weiner, 1988)

Chorionic Villus Sampling

A. Assessment

1. History
   a. Rationale
      (1) At the time that the CVS is performed (usually between 9 and 12 menstrual weeks), the placenta is a heterogenous organ in which active and vigorous villus proliferation is noted in the central parts of the cotyledon (Golbus & Appelman, 1990)
      (2) Proliferative villi at the embryonic pole that faces the decidua basalis constitute the chorion frondosum (Fig. 11–5)
      (3) Villi in the chorion frondosum are believed to reflect fetal chromosome, enzyme, and DNA content, thereby permitting earlier diagnosis than can be obtained by amniocentesis (Brambati & Oldrini, 1985)
   b. Indications
      (1) In 90% of clients, the indication is advanced maternal age (Hogge, Schonberg, & Golbus, 1986)
      (2) The other major indication for CVS involves biochemical or molecular assays
   c. Safety concerns: risks

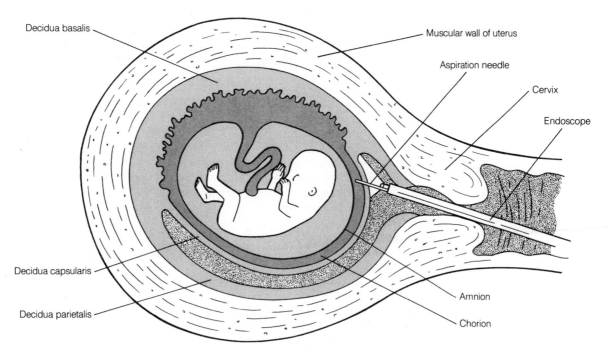

Figure 11–5
Diagram of an 8-week pregnancy showing endoscopic needle aspiration of extraplacental villi. (From Rodeck, C.H., & Morsman, J.M. [1983]. First trimester biopsy. In M.A. Ferguson-Smith [Ed.], *Early prenatal diagnosis* [p. 338]. Edinburgh: Churchill Livingstone.)

(1) CVS is a relatively new procedure, and data are still being accumulated about both short- and long-term complication rates

(2) Immediate complications of CVS are uncommon, except for some spotting or bleeding that usually subsides without consequences

(3) The short-term complication of CVS is pregnancy loss

    (a) The overall spontaneous abortion rate for all pregnancies to 28 menstrual weeks is 4.67%

    (b) The incidence of spontaneous abortion in those sampled from 9 to 12 weeks is only 3.8%

    (c) According to the recently published NIH, CVS Study Group (1989) results based on 2292 patients having CVS and 669 clients selecting amniocentesis, the CVS procedure-related pregnancy loss rate is 0.6% higher than that for clients undergoing amniocentesis for prenatal diagnosis

(4) Other short-term complications are chorioamnionitis, oligohydramnios (0.5%), and fetal-maternal hemorrhage

d. Techniques

(1) Technique for transcervical sampling

    (a) The morning of the procedure, the client is asked to fill her bladder, since displacement of an anteverted uterus may aid in positioning the uterus for catheter insertion

    (b) A high-resolution linear-array or sector ultrasound is used to determine uterine position, cervical position, size of the gestational sac, and crown–rump length measurement, and to identify the area of placental formation and cord insertion

    (c) The client is placed in the lithotomy position; the vulva, vaginal vault, and cervix are cleansed with povidone-iodine (Betadine); and a sterile speculum is inserted into the vagina

    (d) The catheter with its encircled metal obturator is introduced transcervically under simultaneous ultrasonographic visualization

    (e) The device is directed into the placenta, parallel to the long axis and away from either gestational sac or decidua

    (f) The obturator is then removed and the catheter connected to a 20- to 30-cc syringe containing 5 cc of tissue culture medium; by negative pressure, 10 to 25 cc of chorionic villi is aspirated (Elias, Simpson, & Martin, 1986)

(2) Transabdominal technique

    (a) Using concurrent ultrasound, a spinal needle with stylet is passed into the placenta, with the device inserted lengthwise to the long axis of the placenta

    (b) After removal of the stylet, the spinal needle is connected to a 20- to 30-cc syringe containing 5 cc of medium and heparin

    (c) The syringe is connected to a breast biopsy aspiration device that facilitates the application of negative pressure in aspirating villi (Simpson & Elias, 1989)

(3) Precautions

    (a) To protect against infection, if more than one attempt is necessary, a new catheter should be used before each attempt at passage through the cervix

    (b) Rh-negative women should be given RhoGAM to avoid possible isoimmunization

2. Physical findings

a. Analysis of fetal cells

(1) Chorionic villi cells divide so rapidly that metaphases can accumulate within hours, and, therefore take fewer days for growth than do amniotic fluid cells

(2) Therefore, results are obtained in 3 hours to 7 days as compared with 2 to 4 weeks for amniocentesis

BIOCHEMICAL ASSESSMENT

Maternal Serum Alpha-Fetoprotein Screening

A. Assessment

1. History
   a. Background physiology
      (1) Alpha-fetoprotein (AFP) is the major protein in the serum of the embryo and early fetus; initially produced by the yolk sac, it is primarily of hepatic origin by the end of the first trimester
      (2) The concentration in fetal serum is about 150 times that found in amniotic fluid, where it is secreted by the fetal kidney
      (3) The normal level of the protein that crosses the fetal membranes into maternal circulation is only 1/100th to 1/1000th of that in fetal serum
      (4) After 13 weeks, levels in fetal serum and amniotic fluid decrease rapidly, whereas those in maternal serum (msAFP) continue to rise until late in pregnancy (Cunningham, MacDonald, & Gant, 1989)
   b. Rationale
      (1) Some of the most common reasons for an elevated AFP level in either amniotic fluid or maternal serum are in fetuses in whom the following circumstances occur
         (a) A failure of neural tube closure during embryogenesis, as the result of multifactorial or polygenetic causes, that allows the protein to leak from capillaries into the amniotic fluid (anencephaly, spina bifida)
         (b) Increased amount leaked by the fetal kidney (hydronephosis and other renal anomalies)
         (c) Abdominal wall (oomphalocele and gastroschisis) and gastrointestinal defects (intestinal atresias)
         (d) Undetected fetal demise
         (e) Normal fetuses in conjunction with one or more of the following
            (i) Amniotic fluid contaminated with fetal blood. Most laboratories routinely perform a Kleihauer-Betke stain or hemoglobin phoresis on bloody amniotic fluid
            (ii) Underestimated gestational age
            (iii) Multiple gestation
            (iv) Placenta that contains an increased number of thin-walled blood vessels that leak into the amniotic fluid
            (v) Decreased maternal weight
            (vi) Mother who is an insulin-dependent diabetic
      (2) Conditions associated with abnormally low levels include
         (a) Chromosomal trisomies
         (b) Normal fetuses with
            (i) Overestimated gestational age
            (ii) Increased maternal weight
         (c) Gestational trophoblastic disease
   c. Screening program recommendation: in 1986, ACOG recommended that screening programs be established within a coordinated system and have quality control, counseling, follow-up, and directed sonographic facilities; msAFP screening at 15 to 18 weeks is now mandatory in some states
2. Physical findings
   a. Interpretation and diagnostic work-up
      (1) Incidence of elevated AFP and follow-up
         (a) About 5% of all women have abnormally high levels, defined as more than 2.5 multiples of the median (MOM) for the population being studied (MOM is defined by each laboratory)
         (b) For initial high, abnormal results, some centers repeat the msAFP screen before follow-up testing is done. According to Cunningham and colleagues (1989), 2% of the original 5% are eliminated by re-

peated testing and the remaining 3% are referred for directed ultra-sound

(c) In 1% of the total, multiple gestation, inaccurate gestational age, or missed abortion are identified, leaving only 2% of all women screened who undergo amniocentesis for acetylcholinesterase, which is present only if there is an open neural tube defect (NTD)

(2) Incidence of NTD and routine screening controversy

  (a) Because the incidence of newborns with NTDs is 1 in 1000 in the general population in the United States (Queenan, 1985), the cost/benefit ratio of routine screening for all prenatal clients as a public health screening policy is controversial

  (b) Some believe that only at-risk clients should be screened

    (i) Previous child with NTD

      ● With one affected child, the risk of recurrence is 2 to 3% (10 to 15 times that of the general population)

      ● After two affected children, the risk increases to 6 to 8%

    (ii) Close relatives (siblings, aunts, uncles) of a client with an NTD are at increased risk (Burton, 1988)

(3) Incidence of low-msAFP results

  (a) Simpson and colleagues (1986) reported screening results for more than 1400 women, of which 9% had abnormally low levels, defined as less than 0.4 MOM

  (b) Half were eliminated by repeating the test

  (c) Of those who still had low values and underwent amniocentesis, three had chromosomally triploid fetuses

b. Anencephaly

(1) Anencephaly is a malformation characterized by an absence of the skull and cerebral hemispheres that are either rudimentary or absent

(2) It is also the most common cause of gross hydramnios and may require therapeutic amniocentesis of as much as 2 to 3 l to reduce the risk of abruptio placentae after spontaneous rupture of the membranes with sudden loss of amniotic fluid and marked uterine decompression

(3) It is a lethal anomaly with a 100% neonatal death rate

c. Spina bifida and meningomyelocele

(1) Spina bifida consists of an opening in the lumbosacral vertebrae through which a meningeal sac may protrude, forming a meningocele

(2) If the sac contains the spinal cord, the anomaly is called a meningomyelocele

(3) The neonatal outcome depends on whether it is an open or closed tube defect (ACOG, 1986)

  (a) Open defects: 33% death rate and 65% long-term disability

  (b) Closed defects: 7% death rate and 10% long-term disability

Estriol Assays

A. Assessment

1. History: this assay appears to have no clinical use in the management of complicated pregnancies; it is mentioned only for historical purposes because its usefulness as a test of fetal well-being has been superseded by more sensitive and specific tests using electronic FHR monitoring, sonography, or combinations of these two techniques

ELECTRONIC ASSESSMENT

A. Introduction

1. Whereas first and second trimester antenatal assessment is directed primarily at the diagnosis of fetal congenital anomalies, the goal of third-trimester test-

ing is to determine whether the intrauterine environment continues to be supportive to the fetus

2. The testing is often used to determine the timing of the delivery of patients at risk for uteroplacental insufficiency
3. The goals of antepartum heart rate monitoring are to "prevent in utero demise and perinatal morbidity while avoiding unnecessary iatrogenic prematurity" (Sonek, Reiss, & Gabbe, 1990)
4. Both the regimen and intepretation of tests must always be done with consideration of the client's risk factors and the gestational age of the fetus

Nonstress Test

B. Assessment

1. History
   a. Definition: the nonstress test (NST) involves observation of accelerations of the fetal heart by the electronic fetal monitor, as they occur either spontaneously or in association with fetal movements, to determine adequacy of fetal oxygenation and autonomic function
   b. Rationale
      (1) In the healthy fetus with an intact CNS, 90% of gross fetal body movements are associated with fetal heart accelerations (Devoe, 1990)
      (2) This response can be blunted by hypoxia or acidosis, drugs (analgesics, barbiturates, and beta-blockers), fetal sleep, and some congenital anomalies (Sonek, Reiss, & Gabbe, 1990)
      (3) Loss of reactivity may reflect the metabolic consequences of profound or protracted hypoxemia (ACOG, 1987)
   c. Advantages
      (1) The NST is easy to perform in an outpatient setting
      (2) The test has no known contraindications
      (3) The NST is relatively inexpensive, rapid, noninvasive, and, therefore, is a good screening test
   d. Disadvantages
      (1) The NST has a high false-positive rate for nonreactive findings, reportedly as high as 75 to 90% (Sonek, Reiss, & Gabbe, 1990), secondary to sleep cycles, medications, and fetal immaturity
      (2) The NST has slightly lower sensitivity to fetal compromise than the contraction stress test (CST) or biophysical profile
   e. Technique
      (1) The client rests in a semi-Fowler's or left-lateral position
      (2) An external fetal heart ultrasound transducer and tocodynamometer are applied
      (3) On sensing fetal movement, the mother presses the marker, which records the time of movement on the same strip on which the FHR is recorded; some fetal hearts accelerate without perceived movement by the mother, and that acceleration is also a valid finding
      (4) Monitoring is continued for at least 40 minutes or until criteria for reactivity is met
      (5) Acoustic stimulation test (Freeman, Garite, & Nageotte, 1991)
         (a) Rather than wait 40 minutes for a spontaneous fetal response, this technique uses sound stimulation to elicit accelerations
         (b) Procedure
            (i) Establish the baseline measurement for at least 10 minutes without spontaneous accelerations
            (ii) Apply an artificial larynx over the fetal head and stimulate for 1 second

(iii) Restimulate if no acceleration occurs within 10 seconds (may be repeated up to four times)

(iv) Continue to monitor for 15 minutes after accelerations

2. Physical findings
   a. Interpretation: ACOG (1987) and Devoe (1990) recommend the following threshold for grading reactivity
      (1) Criteria for a reactive tracing
         Two or more fetal heart rate accelerations of at least 15 beats/min (each with a duration of at least 15 seconds) within a 20-minute period
      (2) Nonreactive: if the test does not meet the criteria in a minimum of 40 minutes, it is nonreactive and requires further evaluation
   b. Suggested testing regimen
      (1) According to Porto (1987), the recommended NST regimen is as follows
         (a) Twice weekly in some of the higher risk conditions
             (i) Prolonged pregnancy (more than 41 weeks)
             (ii) Intrauterine growth retardation (IUGR)
             (iii) Insulin-dependent diabetes
         (b) Weekly testing in high-risk pregnancies not included in the above list
         (c) Same-day testing for complaint of decreased fetal movement (Freeman, Garite, & Nageotte, 1991)
      (2) This testing regimen is based partly on findings reported by Boehm in 1986, which showed that by increasing the frequency of NSTs to twice weekly, the corrected stillbirth rate dropped from 6.1 to 1.9 per 1000 after a reactive test

Contraction Stress Test

A. Assessment

1. History
   a. Definition: "A contraction stress test (CST) provides a method for observing the response of the fetal heart rate to the stress of uterine contractions: the desired result is a negative test" (Olds, London, & Ladewig, 1988)
   b. Rationale
      (1) The CST is based on the premise that fetal oxygenation that is only marginally adequate with the uterus at rest is transiently worsened by uterine contractions
      (2) The resultant intermittent fetal hypoxemia, in turn, leads to the fetal heart rate pattern of late decelerations (ACOG, 1987)
   c. Technique
      (1) With the mother sitting in a semi-Fowler's position, the electronic fetal monitor's ultrasonic transducer and tocotransducer are applied to the maternal abdomen, and a baseline tracing is obtained for at least 15 minutes
      (2) If three spontaneous, 40- to 60-second contractions of good quality occur in a 10-minute period, the results are evaluated and the test is concluded
      (3) If inadequate contractions occur, nipple stimulation or IV oxytocin is used
         (a) Nipple stimulation
             (i) The client brushes her palm across one nipple through her shirt for 2 to 3 minutes, stopping if a contraction begins
             (ii) The nipple stimulation continues after a 5-minute rest period, with the same process repeated if no contractions occur
             (iii) To avoid hyperstimulation (uterine contractions lasting more than 90 seconds or occurring more frequently than every 2 minutes), bilateral stimulation should not be instituted unless unilateral stimulation fails to induce contractions
         (b) Oxytocin challenge test (OCT)

       (i) If the nipple stimulation test is either unsatisfactory or contraindicated, a titrated IV pitocin infusion can be initiated according to the institution's protocol

      (ii) Oxytocin is administered until three contractions, each lasting 40 to 50 seconds, occur in a 10-minute period

      (iii) Oxytocin is discontinued
- If no response occurs when levels reach 10 μ/min or
- If repetitive late decelerations occur

2. Physical findings
  a. Interpretation of CST (ACOG, 1987; Freeman & Lagrew, 1990)
    (1) Positive results
      (a) Late decelerations after 50% or more of contractions
      (b) When the fetal pO_2 consistently falls below the critical level, late decelerations become persistent, and the CST becomes positive
    (2) Suspicious or equivocal results
      (a) Nonrepetitive late decelerations occurring with fewer than half of contractions are inconclusive
      (b) When the oxygen level fluctuates between low and normal, late decelerations are intermittent, and the test is equivocal
    (3) Hyperstimulation
      (a) Contractions closer than every 2 minutes apart or that last more than 90 seconds with a late deceleration indicate hyperstimulation
      (b) If a late deceleration occurs after a contraction lasting more than 90 seconds, it may not indicate a diminished reserve, because fetuses with normal reserves also decelerate with uteroplacental flow that has been interrupted for too long
    (4) Negative results
      (a) Three contractions of good quality lasting more than 40 seconds without late decelerations is a normal result
      (b) If the fetus never demonstrates a late deceleration when contractions are 3 minutes apart (three contractions in 10 minutes), last at least 40 to 60 seconds, and are of palpable strength, the test is considered negative
  b. Consideration in interpretation
    (1) Even if there is a 10-minute window of three contractions in which no decelerations occur, if a contraction is associated with a late deceleration elsewhere in the tracing, Freeman and Lagrew (1990) believe this should be considered a suspicious test
    (2) The perinatal mortality rate with this criteria for negative was 0.0 to 2.2 per 1000 compared with 10 per 1000 when the window interpretation was used

B. Nursing Diagnoses

1. High risk for maternal-fetal injury related to test complications
2. Knowledge deficit related to
  a. Specific high-risk pregnancy condition and treatment options
  b. Fetal diagnostic tests and surveillance regimen
3. Anxiety related to
  a. Poor outcome from disease process
  b. Fear of pain and unknown outcome
  c. Lack of support in stressful circumstances
4. High risk for ineffective coping
  a. Individual, related to
    (1) Financial and time demands of serial testing regimen
    (2) Denial of the severity of the health risk involved
  b. Family, related to
    (1) Significant other excluded from testing sessions
    (2) Fear of loss of fetus

C. Interventions/Evaluations

1. High risk for maternal-fetal injury related to test complications
   a. Interventions
      (1) Use sterile technique to prevent chorioamnionitis
      (2) Position patient properly (in lateral or wedged position) to avoid supine hypotension during fetal monitoring tests
      (3) Have terbutaline, 0.25 mg, available for subcutaneous (or IV) injection for hyperstimulation response to contraction stress test
   b. Evaluation: no complications were caused by the diagnostic procedures
2. Knowledge deficit related to high-risk pregnancy condition and fetal testing and surveillance regimen
   a. Interventions
      (1) Provide simple, clear explanations of the condition's pathophysiology and the maternal-fetal implications
      (2) Clarify the treatment options
      (3) Explain what the fetal test measures
      (4) Describe the purpose and frequency of the tests, what the results mean, and the estimated length of the sessions
   b. Evaluations
      (1) Client verbalized awareness of the condition placing her at risk and of possible preventive measures, and she becomes a participant in achieving the best possible pregnancy outcome (Doenges, 1988)
      (2) Client understands what treatments are available to improve her pregnancy outcome
      (3) Client understands how, why, and when she is to be tested (Olds, London, & Ladewig, 1988)
3. Anxiety related to (1) poor pregnancy outcome, (2) fear of pain and unknown outcome, and (3) being alone during a stressful situation
   a. Interventions
      (1) Allow the client to vent her frustrations with the discomfort, time-consuming demands, and limitations imposed by this high-risk pregnancy and fetal surveillance program
      (2) Assist the client in setting realistic goals for progress in her pregnancy so that she experiences a sense of accomplishment
         (a) Each day in utero is beneficial to the normal development of her fetus
         (b) The fetus has improved chances for survival as long as the testing remains reassuring
         (c) Compliance with treatment and testing regimens is beneficial to the fetus
      (3) Encourage interaction (if appropriate) with other high-risk mothers in informal or structured groups
      (4) Administer local anesthesia when starting an IV, as permitted by institution's protocol
      (5) Use comforting measures, such as touch, during difficult procedures
      (6) Explain procedures step by step
      (7) Encourage the client's significant others to be with her if she requests it during procedures
      (8) Remain with the client if significant others are not available
   b. Evaluations
      (1) Client verbalizes her fears and concerns related to the high-risk pregnancy, and she feels cared for (Doenges, 1988)
      (2) Client experiences minimal pain and fear during testing
      (3) Client is comforted by the presence of her significant others
      (4) Client agrees to continue treatment and testing regimens
4. High risk for ineffective coping, related to the stress of antepartum surveillance regimen
   a. Interventions

(1) Review sources of conflict for the client, such as financial limitations and family commitments
(2) Arrange for social service counseling to assist with problem solving
(3) Schedule testing appointments at the client's convenience when possible
(4) Follow up when the client does not keep an appointment
  (a) Reinforce the value of testing
  (b) Identify the cause of noncompliance
(5) Include significant others during testing and teaching sessions
  b. Evaluations
(1) Client attends all scheduled testing sessions and gains reassurance of fetal well-being from the good results
(2) Significant others are coping well and being supportive

Health Education

A. Several client education issues have already been addressed under the nursing diagnosis of knowledge deficit and during the description of the various tests; therefore, refer to those sections for a complete review of this topic

B. Because certain high-risk pregnancy conditions are preventable and relate to lifestyle choices that are hazardous to the fetus, counseling during some testing sessions can be done to assist clients in making better choices

1. Obtain prenatal care within the first trimester
  a. Prenatal care increases the accuracy of gestational age assessment
  b. It allows more timely intervention in true cases of post-term pregnancies
  c. It improves determination of inadequate fetal growth for a given fetal age
2. Avoid alcohol, illegal drugs, caffeine, and over-the-counter drugs during pregnancy, especially during the first trimester, to prevent teratogenic effects
3. Normal fetal growth can result if smoking is stopped during pregnancy

CASE STUDIES AND STUDY QUESTIONS

Ms. Jones is a 37-year-old gravida 1, para 0 (G1,P0) whose last menstrual period was March 17. Her first prenatal visit was on July 3, at which time her fundal height was 22 cm. Fetal heart tones were audible by Doppler ultrasonography but not by DeLee stethoscope, and she has not yet felt fetal movement. Select from among the following items those that apply to Ms. Jones or the issue addressed.

1. High-risk factors
  a. Fetal cardiac anomaly.
  b. Advanced maternal age.
  c. Size greater than dates.
  d. IUGR.
  e. Decreased fetal movement.

2. Differential diagnosis for size greater than dates
  a. Oligohydramnios.

  b. Polyhydramnios.
  c. Twins.
  d. Uterine fibroids.
  e. Inaccurate date of LMP.
  f. Pregnancy-induced hypertension (PIH).

3. Diagnostic testing options
  a. CST.
  b. Amniocentesis for genetics.
  c. NST.
  d. Ultrasonography for dating.

4. Risk of miscarriage because of amniocentesis
  a. Less than 1%.
  b. 10%.
  c. 5%.
  d. 8%.

Ms. Smith is a 30-year-old gravida 3 (G3) at 43 weeks' gestation (by poor dates) with late prenatal care. Her obstetric ultrasonography at 42½ weeks showed a grade III placenta and biparietal diameter of 9.2. She has complained of decreased fetal movement since the previous night. Her next scheduled office visit is in 3 days. Select from among the following items those that apply to Ms. Smith or the issue addressed.

5. High-risk factors

   a. Preterm labor.

   b. Postdate pregnancy.

   c. Abruptio placentae.

   d. Decreased fetal movement.

   e. Grand multipara.

6. Possible diagnosis

   a. Post-term pregnancy.

   b. Term pregnancy.

   c. Placenta previa.

   d. Inaccurate maternal perception of fetal movement.

   e. Uterine dystocia.

   f. Fetal distress.

   g. Preterm pregnancy.

7. Diagnostic testing options

   a. Chorionic villi sampling.

   b. Percutaneous umbilical blood sampling. (PUBS)

   c. Amniocentesis for lecithin/sphingomyelin ratio (L/S).

   d. NST.

   e. CST.

   f. Amnionic fluid index (AFI).

   g. OD delta 450.

   h. Biophysical profile.

8. Is it true or false that Ms. Smith is at no additional risk if she waits until her next scheduled office visit to be evaluated?

9. Is it true or false that all patients should be induced for post-term pregnancy at 42 weeks by dates, regardless of the accuracy of their EGA dating method, fetal surveillance results, or evidence of fetal maturity?

Ms. Garcia is a 25-year-old gravida 2, para 1 (G2,P1) at 32 weeks' EGA. She is Rh-negative and was delivered of an Rh-positive infant 2 years previously without receiving postpartum RhoGAM. Her current Rh titer is 1:30. Select from among the following items those that apply to Ms. Garcia or the issue addressed.

10. High-risk factor

    a. Pre-eclampsia.

    b. Rh sensitization.

    c. Maternal anemia.

    d. IUGR.

11. Diagnostic testing options for Rh-sensitized pregnancy

    a. Aminocentesis for OD delta 450.

    b. Early amniocentesis for genetics.

    c. PUBS.

    d. Alpha-fetoprotein (AFP) screen.

    e. NST.

12. Is it true or false that if the results were zone III on the Liley graph, intrauterine transfusion would be an option for therapy in the absence of hydrops?

Ms. Lopez is a 25-year-old gravida 4, para 3 (G4,P3) at 34 weeks' gestation (by good dates) who has a history of drug abuse and smoking. Fetal serial ultrasound tests show poor interval growth, with a current biparietal diameter (BPD) of 7.8 cm and femur length of 6 cm, both consistent with 30 weeks' gestation. Select from among the following items those that apply to Ms. Lopez or the issue addressed.

13. High-risk factor

    a. Pre-eclampsia.

    b. Diabetes.

    c. IUGR.

    d. Multiple pregnancy.

    e. Substance abuse.

14. Diagnostic testing for IUGR pregnancy and treatment planning

   a. Cervical culture.

   b. Biophysical profile.

   c. Amniocentesis for lung profile.

   d. Maternal urine toxicology screen.

   e. Maternal glucose testing.

   f. NST and AFI.

15. Is it true or false that if Ms. Lopez were to stop smoking now, her fetus would have an improved blood supply and would gain weight more rapidly?

Answers to Study Questions

1. b,c	2. b,c,d,e	3. b,d
4. a	5. b,d	6. a,b,d,f
7. c,d,e,f,h	8. False	9. False
10. b	11. a,c,e	12. True
13. c,e	14. b,c,d,f	15. True

REFERENCES

Adamsons, K., & Myers, R. (1977). Late decelerations and brain tolerance of the fetal monkey to intrapartum asphyxia. *American Journal of Obstetrics and Gynecology, 128,* (8), 893–900.

American College of Obstetricians and Gynecologists. (1987). Antepartum fetal surveillance. *Technical Bulletin,* No. 107.

American College of Obstetricians and Gynecologists. (1986). Prenatal detection of neural tube defects. *Technical Bulletin,* No. 99.

American College of Radiology. (1984). Policy statement: Antepartum obstetric ultrasound examination guidelines. Adopted by ACOG (1986) as reported in F. Zuspan & T. Quilligan (Eds.), (1990). *Manual of obstetrics and gynecology* (2nd ed.). St. Louis: Mosby.

Ballard, P., & Ballard, R. (1972). Glucocorticoid receptors and the role of glucocorticoids in fetal lung development. *Proceedings of the National Academy of Science USA, 69,* 2668–2672.

Barkai, G., Reichman, B., Modan, M., Goldman, B., Serr, D., & Mashiach, S. (1988). The influence of abnormal pregnancies on fluorescence polarization of amniotic fluid lipids. *Obstetrics and Gynecology, 72*(1), 39–43.

Barcroft, J. (1977). *Researchers on pre-natal life* (Vol. 1). Columbus, OH: Ross Laboratories.

Boehm, F. (1990). Fetal distress. In R. Eden & F. Boehm (Eds.), *Assessment and care of the fetus: Physiological, clinical, and medicolegal principles* (pp. 809–822). Norwalk, CT: Appleton & Lange.

Boehm, F., Salyer, S., Shah, D., & Waughn, W. (1986) Improved outcome of twice weekly nonstress testing. *Obstetrics and Gynecology, 67*(4), 566–568.

Bowman, J. (1990). Maternal blood group immunization. In R. Eden & F. Boehm (Eds.), *Assessment and care of the fetus: Physiological, clinical, and medicolegal principles* (pp. 749–766). Norwalk, CT: Appleton & Lange.

Brace, R. (1989). Amniotic fluid dynamics. In R. Creasy & F. Boehm (Eds.), *Maternal-fetal medicine: Principles and practice* (pp. 128–140). Philadelphia: Saunders.

Brambati, B., & Oldrini, A. (1985, May). CVS for first-trimester fetal diagnosis. *Contemporary Obstetrics and Gynecology, 25,* 94–97.

Burton, B. (1988). Elevated serum alpha-fetoprotein (MSAFP): Interpretation and follow-up. *Clinical Obstetrics and Gynecology, 31*(2), 283–305.

Caldeyro-Barcia, R., Casacuberta, C., & Bustos, R. (1968). Correlation of intrapartum changes in fetal heart rate with fetal blood oxygen and acid-base state. In K. Adamsons (Ed.), *Diagnosis and treatment of fetal disorders* (pp. 25–37). New York: Springer-Verlag.

Cassmer, O. (1959). Hormone production of the isolated human placenta (supplement). *Acta Endocrinol, 32,* 45–40.

Chamberlain, P., Manning, F., & Morrison, I. (1984). Ultrasound evaluation of amniotic fluid volume. Part I: The relationship of marginal & decreased amniotic fluid volumes to perinatal outcome. *American Journal of Obstetrics Gynecology, 150*(3), 245–249.

Chamberlain, P., Manning F., & Morrison I. (1984). Ultrasound evaluation of amniotic fluid volume. Part II: The relationship of increased amniotic fluid volume to perinatal outcome. *American Journal of Obstetrics and Gynecology, 150*(3), 250–254.

Chervenak, F., & Gabbe, S. (1991). Obstetric ultrasound: Assessment of fetal growth and anatomy. In S. Gabbe, J. Neibyl, & J. Simpson (Eds.), *Obstetrics: Normal and problem pregnancies.* (2nd ed.) (pp. 329–376). New York: Churchill Livingstone.

Chudleigh, P., & Pearce, M. (1986). *Obstetric ultrasound: How, why and when.* New York: Churchill Livingstone.

Cibils, L.A. (1981). *Electronic fetal-maternal monitoring: Antepartum and intrapartum.* Boston: PSG.

Clark, S., Gimovsky, M., & Miller, F. (1982). Fetal heart rate response to scalp blood sampling. *American Journal of Obstetrics and Gynecology, 144*(6), 706–708.

Clark, S., Gimovsky, M., & Miller, F. (1984). The scalp stimulation test: A clinical alternative to fetal scalp blood sampling. *American Journal of Obstetrics and Gynecology, 148*(3), 274–284.

Clements, J., Platzker, A., Tierney, D., Hobel, C., Creasy, R., Margolis, A., Thibeault, D., Tooley, W., & Oh, W. (1972). Assessment of the risk of respiratory distress syndrome by a rapid test for surfactant in amniotic fluid. *New England Journal of Medicine, 286*(20), 1077–1081.

Cohn, H.E., Sacks, E.T., & Heymor, M.A. (1974). Cardiovascular responses to hypoxemia and acidemia in fetal lambs. *American Journal of Obstetrics and Gynecology, 120*(7), 817–824.

Cundiff, J., Haubrich, K., & Hinzman, N. (1990). Umbilical artery doppler flow studies during pregnancy. *Journal of Obstetric, Gynecologic, and Neonatal Nursing, 19*(6), 475–481.

Cunningham, F.G., MacDonald, P.C., & Gant, N.F. (1989). *Williams obstetrics* (14th ed.). Norwalk, CT: Appleton & Lange.

Daffos, F., Capella-Pavlovsky, M., & Forestier, F. (1985). Fetal blood sampling during pregnancy with the use of a needle guided by ultrasound: A study of 606 consecutive cases. *American Journal of Obstetrics and Gynecology, 153*(6), 655–660.

Daffos, F., Capella-Pavlovsky, M., & Forestier, F. (1983). A new procedure for fetal blood sampling in utero: Preliminary results of 53 cases. *American Journal of Obstetrics and Gynecology, 146*(8), 985–987.

Devoe, L. (1990). The nonstress test. In R. Eden & F. Boehm (Eds.), *Assessment and care of the fetus: Physiological, clinical, and medicolegal principles.* (pp. 365–383). Norwalk, CT: Appleton & Lange.

Doenges, M., Kenty, J., & Moorhouse, M.F. (1988). *Maternal-newborn care plans: Guidelines for client care.* Philadelphia: Saunders.

Drugan, A., Johnson, J., & Evans, M. (1990). Amniocentesis. In R. Eden & F. Boehm (Eds.), *Assessment and care of the fetus: Physiological, clinical, and medicolegal principles* (pp. 283–290). Norwalk, CT: Appleton & Lange.

Dunn, A., Weiner, S., & Ludomirski, A. (1988). Percutaneous umbilical blood sampling. *Journal of Obstetrics, Gynecologic, and Neonatal Nursing, 17*(5), 308–313.

Eden, R. (1990). Postdate pregnancy. In R. Eden & F. Boehm (Eds), *Assessment and care of the fetus: Physiological, clinical and medicolegal principles* (pp. 767–778). Norwalk, CT: Appleton & Lange.

Elias, S., & Simpson, J.L. (1986). Amniocentesis. In A. Milunski (Ed.), *Genetic disorders and the fetus* (2nd ed.) (pp. 31–52). New York: Plenum.

Elias, S., Simpson, J., & Martin, A. (1986). Chorionic villus sampling in continuing pregnancies. I. Low fetal loss rates in initial 109 cases. *American Journal of Obstetrics and Gynecology, 154*(6), 1349–1352.

Evans, M., & Schulman, J. (1986). Prenatal diagnosis: Invasive techniques and alpha-fetoprotein screening. In G. Avery (Ed.), *Neonatology: Pathophysiology and management of the newborn* (pp. 574–594). Philadelphia: Lippincott.

Freeman, R., Garite, T., & Nageotte, M. (1991). *Fetal heart rate monitoring* (2nd ed.). Baltimore: Williams & Wilkins.

Freeman, R., & Lagrew, D. (1990). The contraction stress test. In R. Eden & F. Boehm (Eds.), *Assessment & care of the fetus: Physiological, clinical, and medicolegal principles* (pp. 351–363). Norwalk, CT: Appleton & Lange.

Gabbe, S. (1991). Antepartum fetal evaluation. In S. Gabbe, J. Niebyl, & J. Simpson (Eds.), *Obstetrics: Normal and problem pregnancies* (2nd ed.) (pp. 377–424). New York: Churchill Livingstone.

Gabbe, S. (1986). Antepartum fetal evaluation. In S. Gabbe, J. Niebyl, & J. Simpson (Eds.), *Obstetrics: Normal and problem pregnancies* (pp. 269–322). New York: Churchill Livingstone.

Garite, T., & Freeman, R. (1986). Fetal maturity cascade: A rapid and cost effective method for fetal lung maturity testing. *Obstetrics and Gynecology, 67*(4), 619–622.

Garite, T. (1990). Theory of antepartum testing. Presentation at Advanced Fetal Monitoring Conference. Co-sponsored by Memorial Medical Center of Long Beach, University of California, Irvine; and Saddleback Memorial Hospital, Newport Beach, CA.

Gilbert, E., & Harmon, J. (1986). *High-risk pregnancy and delivery.* St. Louis: Mosby.

Gluck, L., Kulovich, M., Borer, R., Brenner, P., Anderson, G., & Spellacy, W. (1971). Diagnosis of the respiratory distress syndrome by amniocentesis. *American Journal of Obstetrics and Gynecology, 109*(3), 440–445.

Golbus, M., & Appelman, Z. (1990). Chorionic villus sampling. In R. Eden & F. Boehm (Eds.), *Assessment and care of the fetus: Physiological, clinical, and medicolegal principles* (pp. 259–265). Norwalk, CT: Appleton & Lange.

Grannum, P., Berkowitz, R., & Hobbins, J. (1979). The ultrasonic changes in the maturing placenta and their relation to fetal pulmonic maturity. *American Journal of Obstetrics and Gynecology, 133*(8), 915–922.

Harding, R., Sigger, N., & Wickham, P. (1987). Fetal and maternal influences on arterial oxygen levels in the sheep fetus. *Journal of Developmental Physiology, 5,* 267–269.

Harman, C., Manning, F., Stearns, E., & Morrison, I. (1982). The correlation of ultrasonic placental grading and fetal pulmonary maturation in five hundred sixty-three pregnancies. *American Journal of Obstetrics and Gynecology, 143*(8), 941–943.

Herbert, W., Chapman, J. & Cefalo, R. (1984, February). Reliability of the foam stability index text in assessing fetal lung maturation. Paper presented at the annual meeting of the Society for Perinatal Obstetricians, San Antonio, TX.

Higgins, L. (1954). Prolonged pregnancy. *Lancet, 2,* 1154–1160.

Hobbins, J., Grannum, P., & Berkowitz, R. (1979). Ultrasound in the diagnosis of congenital anomalies. *American Journal of Obstetrics and Gynecology, 134*(3), 331–345.

Hogge W., Schonberg S., & Golbus M. (1986). Chorionic villi sampling: Experience of the first 1,000 cases. *American Journal of Obstetrics and Gynecology. 154*(6), 1249–1252.

Hook, E., Cross, P., & Schreinemachers, D. (1983). Chromosomal abnormality rates at amniocentesis and in liveborn infants. *Journal of the American Medical Association, 249*(15), 2034–2038.

Hook, E. (1981). Rates of chromosome abnormalities at different maternal ages. *Obstetrics and Gynecology. 58*(3), 282–285.

Kochenour, N. (1982). Estrogen assay during pregnancy. *Clinical Obstetrics and Gynecology, 25*(4), 659–672.

Krebs, H., Petres, R., & Dunn, L. (1979). Intrapartum fetal heart rate monitoring. I. Classification and prognosis of fetal heart rate patterns. *American Journal of Obstetrics and Gynecology, 133*(7), 762–772.

Liggins, G., & Howie, M. (1972). A controlled trial of antepartum glucocorticoid treatment of prevention of the respiratory distress syndrome in premature infants. *Pediatrics, 50*(4), 515–525.

Liley, A. (1961). Liquor amnii analysis in the management of the pregnancy complicated by rhesus sensitization. *American Journal of Obstetrics and Gynecology, 82*(6), 1359–1370.

Little, G. (1990). Fetal growth and development. In R. Eden & F. Boehm (Eds.), *Assessment and care of the fetus: Physiological, clinical, and medicolegal principles* (pp. 3–15). Norwalk, CT: Appleton & Lange.

Ludomirski, A., & Weiner, S. (1988). Percutaneous fetal umbilical blood sampling. *Clinical Obstetrics and Gynecology, 31*(1), 19–26.

Manning, F., & Harman, C. (1990). The fetal biophysical profile. In R. Eden & F. Boehm (Eds.), *Assessment and care of the fetus: Physiological, clinical, and medicolegal principles* (pp. 385–396). Norwalk, CT: Appleton & Lange.

Manning, F. (1989). General principles and application of ultrasound. In R. Creasy & R. Resnick (Eds.), *Maternal-fetal medicine* (2nd ed.) (pp. 195–253). Philadelphia: Saunders.

Manning, F., Platt, L., & Sipos, L. (1980). Antepartum fetal evaluation: Development of a fetal biophysical profile. *American Journal of Obstetrics and Gynecology. 136*(6), 787–795.

Martin, C., de Haan, J., van der Wildt, B., Jongsma, H., Dilleman, A., & Arts, T. (1979). Mechanisms of late deceleration in the fetal heart rate. A study with autonomic blocking agents in fetal lambs. *European Journal of Obstetrics, Gynaecology, and Reproductive Biology. 9*(6), 361–365.

Martin, C., Murata, Y., & Petrie, P. (1974). Respiratory movements in fetal rhesus monkeys. *American Journal of Obstetrics and Gynecology. 119*(7), 939–948.

McDuffie, R. & Haverkamp, A. (1991). Intrapartum fetal surveillance. In J. Frederickson & L. Wilkins-Haug (Eds.) *Ob-gyn secrets* (pp. 253–256). St. Louis: Mosby.

Morrison, J., & Pryor, J. (1990). Hemolytic disorders. In R. Eden & F. Boehm (Eds.), *Assessment and care of the fetus: Physiological, clinical, and medicolegal principles* (pp. 737–748). Norwalk, CT: Appleton & Lange.

Murata, Y., Martin, C., & Ikenoue, T. (1982). Fetal heart rate accelerations and late decelerations during the course of intrauterine death in chronically catheterized rhesus monkeys. *American Journal of Obstetrics and Gynecology, 144*(2), 218–223.

Murray, M. (1988). *Antepartal and intrapartal fetal monitoring.* Washington, DC: Nurses Association of American College of Obstetrics and Gynecology.

Myers, R., Beard, R., & Adamson, K. (1969). Brain swelling in the newborn rhesus monkey following prolonged partial asphyxia. *Neurology, 19*(10), 1012–1018.

Natale, R., Clewlow, F., & Dawes, G. (1981). Measurement of fetal forelimb movements in lambs in utero. *American Journal Obstetrics and Gynecology, 140*(5), 545–551.

National Institute of Child Health and Human Development, National Registry for Amniocentesis Study Group. (1976). Midtrimester amniocentesis for prenatal diagnosis: Safety and accuracy. *Journal of the American Medical Association. 236*, 1471–1476.

National Institute of Health CVS Study Group (1989). The safety and efficacy of chorionic villus sampling compared to amniocentesis for prenatal diagnosis. *New England Journal of Medicine, 320*(10), 609–617.

Nicolaides K., Thorpe-Beeston, J., & Noble P. (1990). Cordocentesis. In R. Eden & F. Boehn (Eds.), *Assessment and care of the fetus: Physiological, clinical, and medicolegal principles* (pp. 291–306). Norwalk, CT: Appleton & Lange.

Nicolaides, K., Soothill, P., Clewell, W., Rodeck, C., Campbell, S. (1988). Fetal hemoglobin measurement in the assessment of red cell isoimmunization. *Lancet, 1*, 1073–1075.

Nicolaides, K., Soothill, P., Rodeck, C., & Campbell, S. (1986). Ultrasound-guided sampling of umbilical cord and placental blood to assess fetal wellbeing. *Lancet, 1*, 1065–1067.

Niswander, K., & Gordon, M. (1970). *Women and their pregnancies.* Philadelphia: Saunders.

Olds, S., London, M., & Ladewig, P. (1988). *Maternal-newborn nursing* (3rd ed.). Menlo Park, CA: Addison-Wesley.

Parer, J. (1989). Fetal heart rate. In R. Creasy & R. Resnick (Eds.). *Maternal-fetal medicine: Principles and practice* (2nd ed.) (pp. 314–343). Philadelphia: Saunders.

Porto, M. (1987). Comparing and contrasting methods of fetal surveillance. *Clinical Obstetrics and Gynecology, 30*(4), 956–967.

Poseiro, J., Mendez-Bauer, C., Pose, S., & Caldeyro-Barcia R. (1969). *Effect of uterine contractions on maternal blood flow through the placenta.* Pub. No. 18, 161–171. Washington, DC: Pan American World Health Organization.

Queenan, J. (1985). *Management of high-risk pregnancy* (2nd ed.). Oradell, NJ: Medical Economics.

Queenan, J., & Hobbins, J. (1982). *Protocols for high-risk pregnancies.* Oradell, NJ: Medical Economics.

Queenan, J. (1970). Recurrent acute polyhydramnios. *American Journal of Obstetrics and Gynecology. 106*(4), 625–626.

Robinson, H. (1975). Gestational sac volume as determined by sonar in first trimester of pregnancy. *British Journal of Obstetrics and Gynecology, 82*(2), 100–107.

Robison, H., & Flemming, J. (1975). A critical evaluation of sonar crown rump length measurement. *British Journal of Obstetrics and Gynecology, 82*(9), 702–710.

Rodriquez, H. (1991). Early amniocentesis. Paper presented at the PAC/LAC subregion VI monthly meeting, Pomona Valley Medical Center, Pomona, CA.

Rutherford, S., Phelan, J., Smith, C., & Jacobs, N. (1987). The four-quadrant assessment of amniotic fluid volume: An adjunct to antepartum fetal heart rate testing. *Obstetrics and Gynecology, 70*(3), 353–356.

Sabbagha, R. (1978). Standardization of sonar cephalometry and gestational age. *Obstetrics and Gynecology, 52*(4), 402–409.

Sadovsky, E. (1990). Fetal movements. In R. Eden & F. Boehm (Eds.), *Assessment and care of the fetus: Physiological, clinical, and medicolegal principles* (pp. 341–349). Norwalk, CT: Appleton & Lange.

Sadovsky, E. (1985). Fetal movements. In J. Queenan (Ed.), *Management of high-risk pregnancy* (2nd ed.) (pp. 183–193). Oradell, NJ: Medical Economics.

Sadovsky, E., (1985). Monitoring fetal movements: A useful screening test. *Contemporary Obstetrics and Gynecology, 25,* 123–127.

Sadovsky, E. (1981). Fetal movements and fetal health. *Seminars in Perinatalogy, 5*(2), 131–143.

Schulman, H. (1990). Doppler ultrasound. In R. Eden & F. Boehm (Eds.), *Assessment and care of the fetus: Physiological, clinical and medicolegal principles* (pp. 397–407). Norwalk, CT: Appleton & Lange.

Shepard, M., Richards, V., & Berkowitz, R. (1982). An evaluation of two equations for predicting fetal weight by ultrasound. *American Journal of Obstetrics and Gynecology, 142*(1), 47–54.

Silverman, F., Suidan, J., & Wasserman, J. (1985). The Apgar score: Is it enough? *Obstetrics and Gynecology, 66*(3), 331–336.

Simpson, J., (1991). Genetic counseling and prenatal diagnosis. In S. Gabbe, J. Niebyl, & J. Simpson (Eds.), *Obstetrics: Normal and problem pregnancies* (2nd ed.) (pp. 269–298). New York: Churchill Livingstone.

Simpson, J., & Elias, S. (1989). Prenatal diagnosis of genetic disorders. In R. Creasy & R. Resnick (Eds.), *Maternal-fetal medicine* (2nd ed.) (pp. 78–107). Philadelphia: Saunders.

Simpson, J. (1985). Antenatal diagnosis of chromosomal abnormalities. In J. Queenan (Ed.), *Management of high-risk pregnancy* (2nd ed.) (pp. 29–39). Oradell, NJ: Medical Economics.

Smith, D. (1990). Fetal rights. In R. Eden & F. Boehm (Eds.), *Assessment and care of the fetus: Physiological, clinical, and medicolegal principles* (pp. 931–938). Norwalk, CT: Appleton & Lange.

Sonek, J., Reiss, R., & Gabbe, S. (1990). Antenatal fetal assessment. In F. Zuspan & E. Quilligan (Eds.), *Manual of obstetrics and gynecology* (2nd ed.) (pp. 57–95). St. Louis: Mosby.

Timor-Tritech, I., Dierker, L., & Hertz R. (1979). Fetal movements: A brief review. *Clinical Obstetrics and Gynecology, 22*(3), 583–592.

Trudinger, B. (1989). Doppler ultrasound assessment of blood flow. In R. Creasy & R. Resnick (Eds.), *Maternal-fetal medicine.* (2nd ed.) (pp. 254–267). Philadelphia: Saunders.

Vintzileos, A., Campbell, W., Ingardia, C., & Nochimson, D. (1983). The fetal biophysical profile and its predictive value. *Obstetrics and Gynecology. 62*(3), 271–278.

Weiner, C., (1988) The role of cordocentesis in fetal diagnosis. *Clinical Obstetrics and Gynecology. 31*(2), 285–292.

Wexler, P., & Gottesfeld, K.R. (1977). Second-trimester placenta previa: An apparently normal placentation. *Obstetrics and Gynecology, 50*(6), 706–709.

White, E., Sky, K., & Benedetti T. (1986). Chronic fetal stress and the risk of infant respiratory distress syndrome. *Obstetrics and Gynecology, 67*(1), 57–62.

Other

NAACOG (1991). Antepartum fetal surveillance and intrapartum fetal heart monitoring. In *Nursing practice competencies and educational guidelines* (2nd ed.). Washington, DC: Author.

Lillian Lew

Nutrition

Objectives

1. Recognize the maternal kilocalorie and nutrient needs during the different stages of a normal pregnancy

2. Determine those expectant mothers who are at nutritional risk from an initial health history

3. Identify the appropriate weight gain during pregnancy

4. Determine the nutrient needs of the fetus during the various stages of growth

5. Recognize the influence of nutrition on pregnancy outcomes

6. Identify substances that are ingested orally but that either may have no nutritional value or may be detrimental

7. Understand the circumstances in which ethnocultural consideration is important

8. Correlate nutritional needs with food recommendations

9. Examine pregnancy complications for which diet is a factor

10. Formulate a nutritional educational plan to meet the needs of each pregnancy

11. Distinguish ethnocultural considerations in the maternal diet to enhance nutritional compliance

Introduction

A. Background

1. The ethics of human research state that most of our current nutritional knowledge must be drawn from animal studies and observations of humans within an historical "laboratory"
2. Animal studies have determined the maternal needs for fetal well-being
3. Observations during historical events, such as famines or food deprivation during times of war, have led to the conclusion that maternal nutritional status has a major influence on the pregnancy outcome
4. There is evidence to indicate that the nutrition of the mother is one of the major determinants of fetal growth and, therefore, of the weight and health of the infant at birth

5. The nurse is often the sole observer of maternal dietary intake and is in a position to regularly provide nutritional education and encourage client compliance
6. It is important for the nurse to understand the basics of maternal–fetal nutrition

B. Nutritional consideration during pregnancy: a good maternal diet has long been considered important to the developing fetus; although attitudes have varied over the years and within cultures about a desirable weight gain and the adverse consequences of an inadequate or excessive weight gain, much of the recent scientific body of knowledge allows some general observations

1. Prepregnancy weight and weight gain: weight gain and loss before and during pregnancy are directly related to the birth weight of the infant
   a. A weight gain of between 11.4 and 15.9 kg (25 and 35 lb) is recommended for pregnant women in developed countries
      (1) Weight gain should be steady throughout the pregnancy and not sudden and excessive
      (2) Approximately 200 to 450 g/wk (½ to 1 lb/wk) should be adequate during the second and third trimesters
   b. If prepregnancy weight is estimated at 20% or more above ideal body weight, the mother is considered overweight or obese; weight gain for overweight women is recommended at between 6.8 and 11.4 kg (15 and 25 lb), depending upon nutritional status and degree of obesity
   c. If prepregnancy weight is estimated at 10 to 20% below ideal body weight, the mother is considered to have poor nutritional status
      (1) This may also indicate an inability to attain proper weight or the presence of poor or unusual dietary habits
      (2) It is usually recommended that underweight women during pregnancy gain the amount of weight to reach their ideal weight plus 11.4 to 15.9 kg (25 to 35 lb)
2. Energy and calorie requirements are increased during pregnancy for deposition of new tissue, increased metabolic expenditure, and increased energy needed to move the pregnant body around
   a. The recommended daily allowance (RDA) states that pregnant women need an additional 300 kilocalories/day
   b. These additional kilocalories can be adequately met by doing the following
      (1) Increasing recommended milk (calcium) intake from 480 ml (2 c) prepregnancy to the recommended 960 ml (4 c) during pregnancy
      (2) Meeting increased protein needs
      (3) Ensuring intake of fruits and vegetables
3. Protein requirements are increased for the development of new tissue; currently, the RDA for pregnant women includes an additional 10 g of protein per day or a total of 60 g of protein per day
4. Vitamins and mineral requirements are usually increased during pregnancy
   a. Folic acid
      (1) Needs to be increased from 180 to 400 mg/day because of the demand for maternal erythropoiesis and fetal-placental growth
      (2) This need may be met by an increased intake of leafy green vegetables and citrus fruits
   b. B vitamin requirements are increased because of increased energy needs
      (1) Adequate intake of protein foods and grains should meet this requirement
      (2) The RDA for the B vitamins is as follows
         (a) Riboflavin (B_2): 1.6 mg
         (b) Thiamine (B_1): 1.1 mg
         (c) Pyridoxine (B_6): 2.2 mg
         (d) B_{12}: 2.2 mg
   c. Ascorbic acid (vitamin C)

(1) Currently, the RDA during pregnancy is 70 mg/day of vitamin C, or 10 mg/day more than the prepregnancy intake

(2) This need is easily met by a minimal increase of rich in vitamin C foods (e.g., citrus fruits, certain melons, peppers, and leafy green vegetables)

d. Vitamin A

(1) The RDA does not currently indicate an increase for vitamin A during pregnancy

(2) Adequate vitamin A can be obtained from consuming, at least every other day, a yellow, orange, or red vegetable or fruit or a leafy green vegetable

e. Vitamin K

(1) Parenteral vitamin K is often administered to the newborn because the newborn has a sterile gut and bacterial synthesis of vitamin K is unreliable during the neonatal period

(2) This parenteral administration is controversial because of the infant's increased tendency to develop hyperbilirubinemia, which may result from excess dosage

(3) Alternative recommendations have included treatment of the newborn with natural vitamin K and oral administration of vitamin K to the mother during the last week of pregnancy

f. Calcium

(1) Requirement remains at 1200 mg/day to ensure adequate calcium for changes in bone metabolism during pregnancy

(2) Phosphorus and vitamin D are also involved in bone and calcium metabolism and imbalances of either may affect calcium requirements

(3) Phosphorus requirement is increased during pregnancy by 400 mg to 1200 mg/day

(4) Daily intake of 10 mg of vitamin D is recommended

g. Iron requirements are greatly increased during pregnancy because of increased maternal blood volume

(1) Inadequate iron intake, which may lead to moderate or severe anemia, has been associated with the increased incidence of spontaneous abortion, premature delivery, low birth weight, stillbirth, and perinatal death

(2) The current RDA for iron is 30 mg/day

(a) It is difficult to get adequate iron intake from food sources during pregnancy; generally, iron supplements are given prenatally to increase daily intake

(b) Good food sources of iron include liver and all animal proteins

(c) Although vegetable proteins and most leafy green vegetables have iron, its bioavailability is often inhibited by the presence of phytate

h. Sodium

(1) Is currently not restricted unless a medical condition so warrants

(2) Not less than 2 to 3 g of sodium should be consumed daily during pregnancy

i. Other requirements include

(1) Vitamin E (10 mg/day)

(2) Zinc (15 mg/day)

(3) Iodine (175 mg/day)

(4) Selenium

(5) These requirements can be met by a good varied diet

C. Nutrition for optimal fetal health

1. The fetus is dependent on the maternal host for nutrients
2. Because the fetus is in a state of growth and development, deprivation of essential nutrients can lead to stunted growth, various birth abnormalities, or spontaneous abortions
3. Nutritional knowledge in this area is not yet complete

4. The following evidence is based on animal studies and is not all-conclusive or all-inclusive
   a. Riboflavin (vitamin B_2) deficiency has been associated with poor skeletal formation
   b. Pyridoxine (vitamin B_6) deficiency has been associated with neuromotor problems
   c. Vitamin B_{12} deficiency has been associated with hydrocephalus
   d. Niacin and folic acid deficiencies have been associated with cleft palate
   e. The fetal growth stage known as hyperplasia, the time during the first trimester when the cells are rapidly dividing and multiplying, requires folic acid and vitamin B_{12}, which play a role in the synthesis of nucleic acids
   f. The next fetal growth stage, known as hypertrophy, occurs during the second and third trimesters of pregnancy when the cells increase in size, and requires amino acids and vitamin B_{12} for protein synthesis
   g. Iron is essential to maintain the maternal hemoglobin levels which, in turn, supply oxygen to the developing fetus
   h. Deprivation of kilocalories can lead to a low birth weight in infants

Clinical Practice

A. Assessment

1. History
   a. A 24-hour recall: a verbal or written recollection of all foods, meals, and snacks eaten within the last 24-hour period
   b. Food frequency analysis: the number of times each week a basic food is eaten
   c. Additional factors to be considered
      (1) Where food is eaten
      (2) How much is eaten
      (3) How food is prepared (e.g., fried with a bread coating)
      (4) Which foods or odors seem to precipitate discomfort
      (5) Which foods are limited and for what reasons
   d. Compare data with the basic four food groups and daily food guide recommendations for pregnancy and lactation [Table 12–1] (it is not necessary for the nurse to compute the RDA because it has been calculated into the food groups and daily guide)

Table 12–1
DAILY FOOD GUIDE FOR NONRISK PREGNANCY

Food	Amount
Meat	Minimum of 2 servings per day
Milk/milk products	Minimum of 3 or 4 servings per day (1 serving is 240 ml (8 oz)
Eggs	1
Bread/cereals	4 or 5 servings per day
Citrus fruits	2 servings per day (e.g., ½ grapefruit and ½ cup of orange juice)
Yellow or dark-green vegetables and fruits	1 or 2 servings per day
Other fruits and vegetables	1 or 2 servings per day
Fats	15 ml (1 tablespoon)
Fluids	Minimum 1440 ml (48 oz) daily (including milk)

  e. Age (e.g., adolescents may have poor eating habits)
  f. Number of previous pregnancies (especially including a history of miscar-
     riages) may indicate poor nutritional status
  g. Economic and social background: may indicate inability to obtain adequate
     nutrition
  h. Ethnic and cultural and religious background: may determine which foods
     are customarily desirable and those that are not consumed
  i. History of obstetrical care and fetal condition
  j. Medical history: mothers with chronic diseases, such as hypertension,
     diabetes, and cardiovascular disease, may need special dietary consider-
     ation (see section in this chapter that discusses alteration in nutrition
     related to pregnancy complications)
  k. Mental status: increased psychological stress during pregnancy may in-
     crease the need for kilocalories and additional nutrients
  l. Medications: may have to be adjusted (e.g., insulin) or discontinued dur-
     ing pregnancy
  m. Allergies: may determine the need for dietary substitutions or supplements
  n. Use of tobacco, alcohol, or both
2. Physical findings
  a. Blood pressure: readings above 140/90 mm Hg or an increase of 30 mm Hg
     systolic or 15 mm Hg diastolic over baseline blood pressure may indicate
     pregnancy-induced hypertension (PIH), if combined with other signs
  b. Temperature: readings above 37.0°C (98.6°F) may indicate infection, which
     may increase basal metabolic rate and protein requirements
  c. Weight and height
     (1) Ideal body weight (IBW): compare maternal height and weight with
         recommended standard height-and-weight charts
3. Diagnostic procedures
  a. Blood analysis
     (1) Anemia can be the result of nutritional deficiencies, including an iron
         deficiency; during pregnancy, anemia is most commonly caused by an
         iron or folic acid deficiency
         (a) Hemoglobin value of less than 11 g/dl may indicate iron-deficiency
             anemia
         (b) Hematocrit of less than 35% may indicate iron-deficiency anemia
         (c) Mean corpuscular volume (MCV)
             (i) Of less than 80 μm^3 may indicate iron-deficiency anemia
             (ii) Of greater than 94 μm^3 may indicate vitamin B_{12} deficiency, folic
                  acid deficiency, or both
     (2) Serum albumin level may indicate poor nutritional status
         (a) During pregnancy, albumin should remain at the prepregnancy
             level of 4 to 5 g/dl
         (b) Failure to improve albumin levels may induce early delivery or the
             birth of a low-birth-weight infant
     (3) Glucose: abnormal findings may indicate diabetes (see Chapter 29 on
         endocrine disorders)
  b. Urinary analysis
     (1) Ketone and glucose: levels elevated above normal may indicate gesta-
         tional or overt diabetes mellitus; low intake or absorption of ketones
         may indicate starvation ketosis
     (2) Protein (albumin): increased levels after 20 weeks may indicate pre-
         eclampsia (PIH)

B. Special consideration/problems

1. Diet and food restrictions
  a. During pregnancy, food intake should not be restricted for the purpose of
     losing weight; adequate education about health and nutrition is required to
     prevent this from occurring

   b. Food fads (e.g., the excessive intake of one kind of food or the total avoidance of a food group) should be discouraged
   c. A vegetarian diet needs special consideration because it is a growing practice
      (1) Generally, a vegetarian diet is practiced because of physiological, philosophical, or religious commitments
      (2) Ensuring adequate protein and vitamin intake is an important consideration
      (3) Food combinations are usually practiced to ensure enough protein in the diet (examples: legumes and grains; legumes and seeds; and seeds and grains)
      (4) The vegetarian classifications are
         (a) Lacto-ovo: excludes all animal protein but includes eggs and dairy products and all plant foods
         (b) Lacto: excludes all animal protein and eggs but includes dairy products and all plant foods
         (c) Vegan: excludes all animal products, including eggs and dairy products; diet consists of plant foods only
2. Obesity: recent research has confirmed that obese pregnant women have a higher incidence of obstetrical complications
   a. These women are at an increased risk of developing PIH, diabetes, wound complications, and thromboembolism
   b. However, weight loss is not recommended during pregnancy
3. Eating disorders, such as anorexia nervosa or bulimia, can lead to poor maternal and fetal nutrition, fetal growth retardation, and fetal organ damage
   a. Anorexia nervosa is a life-threatening condition: individuals fear food and perceive their bodies as obese when in fact they are dangerously thin from self-induced starvation
      (1) Laxatives, diuretics, induced vomiting, and excessive exercise are some of the methods used to prevent weight gain
      (2) Many women with this condition are infertile, but those who have a body fat composition of at least 22% can become pregnant
   b. Bulimia is a patterned behavior of binge eating followed by self-induced vomiting; this behavior may be combined with other methods to prevent weight gain (e.g., laxatives, diuretics, fasting, and enemas)
   c. Indications of a current or past eating disorder are an underweight condition or a history of weight fluctuations
      (1) These conditions alone do not denote an eating disorder because the pregnant woman may be neither underweight nor willing to admit to a past eating disorder
      (2) For women with either anorexia or bulimia, psychological and nutritional counseling is recommended at the earliest stage of prenatal care
4. Hyperemesis is excessive vomiting, nausea, or both, which may begin in the first trimester of pregnancy but persists, causing an altered nutritional status, and possibly, dehydration and starvation
   a. Women at risk for hyperemesis include
      (1) Women younger than 20 years old
      (2) Primigravidas
      (3) Overweight women
      (4) The condition may repeat in the following instances
         (a) Subsequent pregnancies
         (b) Women who have had a spontaneous abortion
         (c) Women who have had multifetal pregnancies
   b. The cause of hyperemesis is believed to be a combination of physical and psychological factors, for example
      (1) The increased levels of estrogen and human chorionic gonadotropin (HCG) secreted by the placenta are a possible physiological cause

(2) Stress and an unconscious fear or rejection of the pregnancy are among the possible psychological conditions precipitating the onset of hyperemesis

c. The pregnant woman may need to be hospitalized to treat dehydration and starvation; if hospitalization is required, a psychological evaluation should be conducted

5. Alcohol intake should be restricted
   a. The reason is that alcohol can pass through the placenta and induce fetal alcohol syndrome (FAS) in the fetus or in the infant
   b. Some signs of fetal alcohol syndrome include prenatal and postnatal growth failure, developmental delay, microcephaly, slanted eyes (including the epicanthal fold), facial abnormalities, skeletal joint abnormalities, and mental retardation (see Chapter 32 on substance abuse)
6. Tobacco use should be restricted or stopped; smoking of tobacco has been found to restrict the oxygen flow to the fetus (see Chapter 32 on substance abuse)
7. Caffeine intake should be limited to approximately the equivalent of 480 ml (16 oz) of coffee per day because caffeine
   a. Curbs appetite
   b. Increases gastrointestinal motility, which decreases maternal absorption of essential nutrients
   c. Increases hydrochloric acid production, which may induce vomiting and nausea
8. Artificial sweeteners, such as saccharin and aspartame, are not recommended during pregnancy
   a. Based on animal studies, saccharin is believed to be a carcinogen
      (1) Saccharin has also been found in the placenta after maternal concentrations have been absorbed
      (2) Warning labels are required on all food products containing saccharin, and pregnant women should be advised to avoid these products until conclusive studies illustrate that ingestion of saccharin does not harm the mother or the fetus
   b. Aspartame is manufactured under the product names of Nutrasweet and Equal
      (1) Research has been inconclusive about whether aspartame once ingested passes through the placenta
      (2) Current label warnings suggest that those with the genetic disorder phenylketonuria (PKU) should not use food products containing aspartame
9. Food contaminants: a number of heavy metals that are embryotoxic have found their way into the food chain through natural and artificial contamination of the water, air, and soil
   a. Metals are mercury, lead, cadmium, and possibly, nickel and selenium
   b. As an example, high levels of mercury have been found in some deep-sea fish (see Chapter 13 on environmental hazards)
10. Pica is the compulsive ingestion of nonfood substances with little or no nutritive value; one suggested reason for pica is that the body is lacking in some essential nutrient
    a. The most commonly ingested substances are
       (1) Dirt
       (2) Clay
       (3) Starch
       (4) However, a variety of other substances have also been known to be eaten, such as
          (a) Ice
          (b) Hair
          (c) Gravel

          (d) Charcoal

          (e) Antacid tablets

          (f) Baking soda

          (g) Coffee grounds

          (h) Inner tubes

     b. Pica is neither a new phenomenon nor one that is correlated to a geographical area, race, creed, culture, gender, or socioeconomic status

     c. Etiology and medical implications are not well understood, but the practice may lead to

        (1) Inadequate intake of essential nutrients

        (2) Intake of substances that may contain toxic compounds

        (3) Interference with the absorption of certain minerals (e.g., iron)

11. Megavitamins are not recommended because most of the nutritional requirements can be met in food and vitamin supplements prescribed during prenatal care

     a. Ingestion of megavitamins can have a reverse effect and actually harm the mother and fetus; for example, megadoses of vitamin C, a water-soluble vitamin, may cause rebound scurvy

     b. Body may also become dependent on megadoses and experience withdrawal once dosage is curtailed

     c. Fat-soluble vitamins, such as vitamins A, D, E, and K, are toxic in megadoses; the body does not excrete the excess, but stores the unused vitamin in the fat cells

12. Lactose intolerance should not hinder the pregnant woman's ingestion of calcium-fortified foods during pregnancy

     a. Suggested substitutions for milk or dairy products are calcium-fortified tofu, soy milk, and canned salmon with bones

     b. Although leafy green vegetables are high in calcium, the bioavailability of calcium may be inhibited by phytates

13. Food beliefs, avoidances, cravings, and aversions (prenatal and postpartum periods)

     a. An important group of beliefs surround dietary restriction for avoidance of excessive weight gain to ensure a smaller baby and easier delivery; although at one time this belief prevailed, it is now considered a folk belief that is still practiced by some groups (e.g., rural Southeast Asians)

     b. Food avoidances are conscious choices not to consume certain foods, generally for reasons associated with personal taste, cultural practices, religious beliefs, or family preferences

     c. Cravings and aversions are powerful urges for or avoidance of certain foods; the most commonly reported cravings are those for sweets and dairy products, but these are not all-inclusive

     d. Nutritional significance of these food-related behaviors is difficult to evaluate because most of the information available is anecdotal; currently, most behavior must be analyzed on an individual basis

B. Nursing Diagnoses

1. Altered nutrition: less than body requirements
2. Altered nutrition: more than body requirements
3. Altered nutrition requirements related to pregnancy

C. Interventions/Evaluations

1. Altered nutrition: less than body requirements

     a. Interventions

        (1) Eat small meals frequently to obtain adequate kilocalories for weight gain and protein conservation

        (2) Excessive exercise may have to be eliminated if maternal weight is too low

   (3) Women who are malnourished or underweight before pregnancy have a higher risk of adverse birth outcomes; these women should gain at least 11.4 to 15.9 kg (25 to 35 lb) plus the amount of weight under their ideal weight; dietary recommendations follow
      (a) Encourage a well-balanced diet that includes concentrated sources of calories
      (b) Recommend an increased intake of nutrient-dense foods that have nutritional value and are high in kilocalories (e.g., sauces, gravies, juices, and milkshakes)
      (c) Limit foods that have empty calories
      (d) Recommend eating between meals
      (e) Follow all other recommendations for a nonrisk pregnancy (see earlier)
   (4) Daily dietary considerations for the lacto-ovo vegetarian include
      (a) A minimum of 960 ml (32 oz) of milk per day
      (b) A minimum of four servings of eggs, dried beans, peas, or soybean curd (tofu), and nuts per day
      (c) At least five servings of fruit and vegetables, including those that are high in vitamins C and A
      (d) At least six servings of whole-grain or enriched cereal products
      (e) Three servings of fats or oils (serving size = 5 ml (1 tsp)
   (5) Daily dietary consideration for the lacto vegetarian is the same as that for the lacto-ovo vegetarian, except that a minimum of 960 ml (32 oz) fortified soy milk replaces eggs
  b. Evaluations
   (1) Adequate kilocalorie, vitamin, and mineral intake is evidenced by an appropriate amount of weight gain by the woman and fetus
   (2) Vegetarian demonstrates an understanding of combining proteins to ensure adequate intake
2. Altered nutrition: more than body requirements
  a. Interventions
   (1) Recommend a well-balanced diet that is high in nutrient-dense foods and low in fats and complex carbohydrates
   (2) Avoid foods that provide empty calories
   (3) Limit snacking if it increases kilocaloric intake
  b. Evaluations
   (1) There is a weight gain of 6.8 to 11.4 kg (15 to 25 lb)
   (2) There is no evidence of ketoacidosis (from dieting so that fat is being used for energy), intrauterine growth retardation (IUGR), low-birth-weight baby or other signs of fetal compromise
3. Altered nutritional requirements related to pregnancy complications
  a. Interventions
   (1) Nausea and vomiting
      (a) Morning sickness or nausea is common during the early months of pregnancy; it usually disappears as the pregnancy advances
      (b) When there is excessive vomiting, an acute protein and energy deficiency and loss of minerals, vitamins, and electrolytes may result
      (c) In cases of pernicious vomiting, a dietary regimen that includes the following is recommended
         (i) Frequent small meals, consisting of dry foods such as thickly cooked cereal (including rice), Melba toast, saltines, and baked potatoes
         (ii) Withholding of fluids from 1 to 2 hours before and after meals
         (iii) If food and fluids are retained, a soft, dry diet may be given; a soft, dry diet is expanded to include breads, eggs, pasta, and lean meats
         (iv) A low-fat diet should also be followed until fats can be tolerated

(v) Other foods are slowly added as they become tolerated
(vi) The pregnant woman should be advised to eat as much as possible when she is not nauseated, and to include concentrated sources of kilocalories such as butter or margarine, jelly and jams, dried fruits, nuts, gravies, sauces, and dressings
(2) Heartburn
  (a) Is a common complaint during the latter months of pregnancy, when the pressure of the enlarging uterus pushes on the stomach
  (b) This complaint can usually be relieved by limiting the amount of food consumed at one time
(3) Constipation
  (a) Is a common problem in the latter stages of pregnancy
  (b) Causes include reduced gut motility, physical inactivity, and pressure exerted on the bowel by the enlarged uterus; it is also a side effect of ingesting iron supplements
  (c) Dietary recommendations include increased intake of fluids and fiber-rich foods, such as whole-grain cereals and fruit with an edible peel, and vegetables
(4) Hypertension
  (a) Chronic hypertension is often confused with preeclampsia (PIH) if it is diagnosed during pregnancy
    (i) Dietary recommendations include a varied and balanced diet to ensure a mixture of essential nutrients and a sodium restriction of about 2000 mg/day
    (ii) The client should be counseled to eat high-potassium foods, such as potatoes, avocados, dairy products, bananas, and leafy green vegetables
  (b) Preeclampsia (PIH)
    (i) Hypertension with proteinuria or edema usually appear after the 20th week of pregnancy
    (ii) Symptoms include rapid weight gain (edema), dizziness, headaches, visual disturbances, anorexia, nausea, vomiting, upper abdominal pain, and eventually, convulsions (eclampsia) if PIH is not treated
      • Increase kilocaloric, protein, and calcium intake and decrease sodium and water intake if pulmonary edema is present
      • In severe PIH, parenteral solutions may be required (see Chapter 26 on hypertensive disorders during pregnancy)
(5) Cardiovascular disease from a dietary perspective is treated similarly in the pregnant state and the nonpregnant state
  (a) The client should be under the care of a physician and a dietition to determine the stage of the disease and the diet therapy that is necessary
  (b) Dietary regulation in pregnant cardiac clients is primarily concerned with limiting kilocalories to control obesity and vascular congestion (retention of water, enlarged heart), which can lead to congestive heart failure
  (c) Adequate iron intake is important
(6) Diabetes: dietary intervention is essential
  (a) Usual intake recommendations (based on a 2200 calorie/day diet) are
    (i) Protein: 12 to 24% of daily intake or 264 to 528 calories/66 to 132 g/day
    (ii) Carbohydrates: 45 to 55% of daily intake or 990 to 1210 calories/ 247.5 to 302.5 g/day
    (iii) Fat: 25 to 35% of daily intake or 550 to 770 calories/61 to 85.5 g/day
  (b) Saturated fats are limited to 12 to 18% of total fats
  (c) Limit all foods that induce nausea and vomiting, or ketosis may result

    (d) Meals are usually divided into three meals and three snacks; carbo-hydrates are usually divided as follows (see Chapter 29 on metabolic and endocrine disorders for further discussion)

      (i) Breakfast: 25% (save some for a midmorning snack)

      (ii) Lunch: 30% (save some for a midafternoon snack)

      (iii) Dinner: 30%

      (iv) Bedtime: 15%

(7) Multiple pregnancy

    (a) Theoretically, the nutritional needs of a woman carrying more than one fetus should be greater to support extra blood volume and placental/fetal tissue

    (b) However, there has been no formal evaluation of needs and specific guidelines have not been developed; nutritional needs are unlikely to be doubled

    (c) General dietary recommendations include the following

      (i) Follow all dietary recommendations of nonrisk pregnancy (see earlier)

      (ii) Eat nutrient-dense foods

      (iii) Possibly increase protein and calcium intake

(8) Teen-age pregnancy

    (a) The incidence of teen-age pregnancy has increased over the last few decades

    (b) Low-birth-weight infants are more common among these preg-nancies (see Chapter 10 on risks associated with age for further discussion)

    (c) Dietary recommendations include

      (i) Follow all recommendations for nonrisk pregnancy (see preceding section)

      (ii) Eat nutrient-dense foods

      (iii) Increase protein and calcium intake

      (iv) Substitute complex carbohydrates for refined carbohydrates

      (v) Limit highly processed and fried foods

      (vi) Limit empty-calorie foods (e.g., carbonated sodas, potato chips)

      (vii) Limit snacking if it interferes with meals

      (viii) Need to build rapport with the adolescent to determine the type of nutritional counseling that may be necessary; know the teen-ager's

- Family history
- Marital status
- Support system
- Amount of control she has over food purchasing and prepa-ration
- Eating and food habits
- Fears and myths related to pregnancy

      (ix) Nutritional counseling: focus on the following

- Establish teenager's priorities and work with her priorities (e.g., encourage the addition of nutrient-dense foods to en-courage weekly weight gain, which may seem less threaten-ing than a total weight-gain goal)
- Prepare a dietary care plan that is simple and realistic
- Work with individual food preferences; empty-calorie foods may be used as a bargaining tool to encourage the teen-ager to eat nutrient-dense foods (e.g., for every soda she drinks, she must also consume two glassfuls of juice and/or milk)
- Direct emphasis toward the dietary benefits for herself (e.g., hair and skin, rather than solely on the welfare of the baby)

(9) Food intake during labor: recommendations vary and no universal practice exists

    (a) Some birth centers encourage women to eat lightly and maintain fluid intake in latent and early labor; others advise women to continue intake of solids and fluids throughout labor, depending on the woman's preference

    (b) Another recommendation may be the avoidance of solid foods and liquids once labor begins, so the client will not vomit food that she ingested during the past 24 to 48 hours, or in case a general anesthetic is required

    (c) In the event of a prolonged labor, parenteral feedings are advised

b. Evaluations

  (1) Nausea and vomiting are avoided or prevented

  (2) Heartburn and constipation are decreased or diminished

  (3) Blood pressure, edema, and weight gain remain within limits

  (4) No ketoacidosis is reported

  (5) Teen-aged mother gains the appropriate amount of weight

Health Education

A. Food allowances for a normal pregnancy (see Table 12–1 for a nonrisk pregnancy)

1. The guide in Table 12–1 is designed to provide the basic minimal requirements for optimal nutrition during pregnancy
2. For most normal nonrisk pregnancies, the pregnant woman needs only 300 kilocalories/day more than a nonpregnant woman; these kilocalories should be consumed to meet the increased requirements for calcium and protein
3. The other requirements can be easily met by eating more nutrient-dense foods, such as dark-green leafy and deep-yellow vegetables, citrus fruits, lean meats, fish, and legumes

B. Ethnocultural considerations: the United States is a multicultural society

1. Health care must be adapted to gain client compliance and to attain the goal of optimal health for the client
2. As was stated in an earlier section, a number of factors govern food intake, from folk beliefs and culture to individual preference
3. When doing nutritional assessment, counseling, and education, the nurse must work with the individual client's preferences to ensure her compliance: food habits are often the last of all cultural habits to change
4. The following is an amalgam of suggestions for working with culturally diverse clients

  a. Use bilingual, bicultural members of the community; work with your local university and hospital medical anthropologist

  b. Contact your dietary department, local university nutrition program, or local public health department for resource information on the food habits of the ethnic group(s) that you work among

  c. If you have access to a medical library, run a MEDLINE search

  d. If possible, when doing nutritional assessment, counseling, and education, use visual aids (e.g., photographs) of ethnic foods and food models

  e. Simply asking a client if she eats a certain type of food before recommending it will go a long way to ensure cultural sensitivity; in many cases, if a food is not a cultural preference, the client will respond that she does not know how to eat it

  f. Work with the client's cultural preferences; for example, many Asian clients do not like to drink milk

    (1) Fresh milk is not available throughout most of Asia and many Asian women are lactose intolerant

(2) Therefore, to ensure that Asian women fulfill the calcium requirements, the nurse might recommend eating more servings of sardines, canned salmon with bones (similar to some ethnic fish products with edible bones), and soybean curd (tofu), all of which are high in calcium and protein

g. Another example is the Asian and Hispanic medical folk beliefs in the polar opposites of energy

   (1) The body state, medicines, herbal remedies, the mental state (emotions), and food substances are either hot or cold (this is a metaphysical concept of hot and cold and is not necessarily related to temperature)

   (2) For the body to be healthy, there must be a balance of the hot and cold forces

   (3) Asian and Hispanic women believe that the body state becomes cold after birth and delivery; therefore, if the food that is recommended and/or is on the hospital tray is considered to be cold, the client will not eat it at this time

CASE STUDIES AND STUDY QUESTIONS

An 18-year-old woman is 12 weeks' pregnant. She is 162.6 cm (5 ft, 4 in) tall and weighs 44.5 kg (98 lb). Her blood analysis indicates that her hemoglobin count was 10 g/dl and her hematocrit was 31%. She is suffering from severe nausea and vomiting. Her dietary history shows that she generally eats two meals a day with frequent snacking on carbonated beverages, chips, cookies, and occasionally, some fruit. Lately, however, she is unable to hold any food in her system.

1. The young pregnant woman in the case study needs to control the nausea and vomiting. She should do which of the following except

   a. Eat frequent small meals consisting of dry foods.

   b. Eat concentrated sources of kilocalories.

   c. Eat a high-fat diet.

   d. Withhold liquids 1 or 2 hours before and after meals.

2. What diet adjustments or recommendations need to be made once the nausea and vomiting are under control?

   a. Limit empty-calorie foods and snacking.

   b. Eat three balanced meals per day.

   c. Increase protein and calcium intake.

   d. All of the above.

3. In the case study, the pregnant woman has a hemocrit reading of 31%. She is at risk for

   a. PIH.

   b. Iron-deficiency anemia.

   c. Vitamin B_{12} deficiency.

   d. Malnutrition.

4. How much weight should this pregnant teen-ager gain to ensure healthy fetal growth?

   a. 16 to 25 kg (35 to 55 lb)

   b. 7.25 kg (16 lb)

   c. 11 to 16 kg (25 to 35 lb)

   d. more than 25 kg (more than 55 lb)

A 35-year-old Vietnamese woman is found to have gestational diabetes after a 3-hour oral glucose tolerance test. She is 24 weeks pregnant. The physician has indicated that insulin is not necessary: her blood sugar level may be regulated by diet only. The client's history taken at the beginning of prenatal care indicates that she has been in the United States for 3 years and cannot speak or understand English very well. Further questioning and observation disclose that she cannot read or write Vietnamese; however, the client's husband appears to speak more English than his wife.

5. To communicate the necessary medical and nutritional information to this Viet-

namese woman, it would be best to do which of the following?

a. Utilize the woman's husband as a translator and give him the needed information in English.

b. Give the patient some pamphlets translated into Vietnamese on nutrition and diabetes.

c. Use the services of a Vietnamese-speaking medical translator.

d. Both a and b.

6. If you, as the nurse, are unfamiliar with the food preferences and avoidances of the Vietnamese culture, how could you find out the needed information on nutrition?

a. Ask the patient through the interpreter about particular foods.

b. Contact the hospital's dietary department, the local university nutrition program, or the local public health department or medical anthropologist.

c. Run a MEDLINE search in the hospital library, if available.

d. All of the above.

7. Inadequate iron intake has been associated with which of the following?

a. Premature delivery and low birth weights.

b. Fetal retardation.

c. Spontaneous abortion.

d. Both a and c.

8. Obese pregnant women are at a greater risk for developing which of the following?

a. Iron deficiency.

b. Anemia.

c. Constipation.

d. Diabetes.

9. When assessing the nutritional status of a pregnant woman during intake, which strategy would provide the best possible information?

a. Ask her husband or family what she eats.

b. Give the pregnant woman written information on nutrition to take home.

c. Obtain a verbal or written recall of all foods eaten in the last 24 hours.

d. Ask the pregnant woman where she usually eats meals.

10. If a pregnant woman in approximately her 20th week of pregnancy displays the symptoms of dizziness, headaches, nausea, vomiting, and edema, she may be suffering from which of the following?

a. Preeclampsia (PIH).

b. Vitamin A deficiency.

c. Cardiovascular disease.

d. Food contamination.

Answers to Study Questions

1. c	2. d	3. b
4. a	5. c	6. d
7. d	8. d	9. c
10. a		

REFERENCES

Dimperio, D. (1988). *Prenatal nutrition: Clinical guidelines for nurses.* White Plains, NY: March of Dimes Birth Defects Foundation.

Escott-Stump, S. (1988). *Nutrition and diagnosis-related care.* Philadelphia: Lea & Febiger.

Guthrie, H. (1983). *Introductory nutrition.* St. Louis: Mosby.

Krause, M., & Mahan, L. (1984). *Food, nutrition and diet therapy.* Philadelphia: Saunders.

Kreutler, P. (1980). *Nutrition in perspective.* Englewood Cliffs, NJ: Prentice-Hall.

Morrissey, B. (1984). *Quick reference to therapeutic nutrition.* Philadelphia: Lippincott.

National Research Council. (1989). *Recommended dietary allowances.* Washington, DC: National Academy Press.

Sherwen, L., Scoloveno, M., & Weingarten, C. (1991). *Nursing care of the childbearing family.* Norwalk, CT: Appleton & Lange.

Arlene Gray Blix

Environmental Hazards

Objectives

1. Recognize potential environmental hazards and the possible risks to the fetus

2. Identify people who have had exposure to potential environmental hazards and refer them for appropriate follow-up

3. Recognize the need to take a complete occupational history on all prenatal clients

4. Assist prenatal clients in handling their fears about environmental risks

5. Use community resources for health education and referral relevant to environmental hazards

6. Educate women of childbearing age about potential environmental hazards and how to protect against or minimize exposure

Introduction

A. Scope of the problem: as many as 85% of health problems may be attributed to environmental factors; pregnancy is greatly affected by the environment; refer to health history guide (Table 13–1)

1. Exposure has reproductive implications for both parents
2. Embryo is most vulnerable during the first trimester
3. Negative outcomes
   a. Altered fertility
   b. Genetic defects
   c. Reproductive wastage (spontaneous abortions, stillbirths, and neonatal deaths)
   d. Altered gestational lengths
   e. Growth retardation
   f. Congenital malformations
   g. Conditions that develop later in life (developmental disabilities, behavioral disorders, chronic diseases, and malignancies)

B. Consider the following when evaluating potential risks

1. Susceptibility varies with the developmental stage at the time of exposure
2. Susceptibility depends on the genetic makeup of the mother and embryo/fetus and the manner in which it responds to environmental factors

Table 13–1
ENVIRONMENTAL HEALTH HISTORY

Occupational
1. What do you and your partner do for a living?
2. How long has each of you worked at your job?
3. What are the specific tasks each job involves?
4. What product or service is produced?
5. Are either of you exposed to any of the following at work?
   Chemicals
   Loud noise
   Radiation
   Heavy metals
   Vibration
   Prolonged standing
   Extreme heat or cold
6. Do you or your partner use protective clothing or equipment at work? If yes, describe.

Other exposures
1. Does either of you have hobbies that involve exposure to any of the above?
2. Are you exposed to secondhand cigarette smoke? If yes, how frequently and for how long?
3. What medications do you take or use? How long have you been taking them? Is your health care provider aware of your use?

3. Outcome depends on the nature of the agent, amount and duration of the exposure, and mode of transmission
4. Benefits must be weighed against the potential risks
5. Causal relations between exposure and negative outcomes are difficult to confirm, because there may be exposure to more than one agent at a time and it is difficult to determine and quantify exposures

C. **Stages of susceptibility to exposure**

1. First stage is during the first 2 weeks before implantation; the fetus is likely to experience little structural damage, but lethality risk may be great
2. Second stage is from 3 to 8 weeks' gestation during organogenesis; the fetus is susceptible to structural damage; major malformations usually occur between 14 and 56 days' gestation
3. Third stage is when organogenesis is complete; growth retardation and functional problems are the most common anomalies.

D. **Categories of environmental risks in this chapter**

1. Occupational hazards
2. Temperature extremes
3. Pharmaceuticals
4. Passive smoking

E. **Definition of terms used in this chapter**

1. Mutagen: chemical or physical agent that causes alterations in deoxyribonucleic acid (DNA), changing the genetic material of the fetal cells
2. Teratogen: agents that act directly on the developing fetus, causing abnormal embryonic or fetal development: with low doses, there may be no effect; with intermediate doses, malformation may result; and with high doses, death of the embryo may occur
3. Carcinogen: an agent that results in cancer in children and that is attributable to parental exposure

Clinical Practice

Occupational Hazards

A. **Introduction**

1. Labor force profile: over 60% of all women 18 to 64 years of age are in the civilian labor force

2. The workplace has been designed predominantly for men
3. Work exposures affect the reproductive health of both men and women

B. Assessment

1. History of occupational exposure
   a. Time: when during the pregnancy did exposure occur?
   b. Duration: for how long was the woman exposed?
   c. Mode: what was the mode of exposure (respiratory, gastrointestinal, skin)?
   d. Precautions: were precautions taken to control exposure (e.g., was protective clothing or equipment used)?
   e. Exposure level: what were the exposure levels in the workplace?
2. Exposure agent
   a. Ethylene oxide (ETO): may produce mutagenic effects and cause spontaneous abortion
      (1) Use: used in the production of ethylene glycol for antifreeze, polyester fibers and films, and detergents; in sterilizing equipment and supplies in health care facilities; as a fumigant in the manufacture of medical products and foodstuffs; in libraries and museums
      (2) Establish a history of exposure: exposure during all stages of cell division is important
   b. Halogenated hydrocarbons: several have been implicated as mutagenic, teratogenic, and carcinogenic; paternal exposure may lead to early fetal death and birth defects; women may be more susceptible to the effects, because of their increased metabolic rate
      (1) Use: used in the laundry and dry cleaning industries and in the rubber industry
      (2) Establish a history of exposure of either the mother or the father to tetrachloroethylene, vinyl chloride, and chloroprene
         (a) Timing of exposure
            (i) Mutagen: exposure is important during all stages of cell division
            (ii) Teratogen: exposure is most important during early differentiation
            (iii) Carcinogen: exposure is important any time during pregnancy
            (iv) Paternal exposure before pregnancy may have a negative impact in some cases
   c. Heavy metals: cadmium, lead, and mercury may be teratogenic; cadmium may affect male fertility; lead may lead to spontaneous abortions, premature birth, and early fetal death; mercury may result in spontaneous abortions, developmental disabilities, and cerebral palsy
      (1) Use
         (a) Cadmium: used in batteries, pigments, paints, soldering liquids, semiconductors, photo cells, insecticides, and fungicides
         (b) Lead: used in gasoline, batteries, paints, ink, ceramics, pottery, ammunition, and textiles
         (c) Mercury: used in mercury vapor lamps, paint, and thermometers
      (2) Establish a history of exposure: exposure at any time may be dangerous, especially during the first trimester
   d. Ionizing radiation: exposure to x-rays and gamma rays is usually well controlled and with proper protection do not pose a major threat; evidence about the dangers of video display terminals (VDTs) is inconclusive; further research is necessary
      (1) Use: used diagnostically and therapeutically in the health care industry
      (2) Establish a history of exposure: a dose to a pregnant woman should not exceed 1.5 rad during pregnancy
         (a) Timing of exposure
            (i) Mutagen: exposure is important during any stage of cell division
            (ii) Teratogen: exposure is most important during early differentiation

(b) Establish workplace levels
   (i) High doses may lead to spontaneous abortion, late fetal death, neonatal death, low birth weight, microcephaly or mental retardation, and childhood mortality
   (ii) Low doses may lead to altered sex ratio, childhood malignancies, and childhood mortality
e. Noise: sound transmits to the fetus, but the effects on the fetus are inconclusive; exposure is linked to growth retardation in the fetus, low birth weight of infant, prematurity, and an increase in the child's risk of having high-frequency hearing losses
   (1) Use: used in many manufacturing processes and heavy-equipment operation, for example
   (2) Establish a history of exposure: exposure above 85 decibels (dB) may be dangerous (Table 13–2); cumulative noise exposure must include exposure to recreational noise, such as to loud music; noise levels above 85 dB usually interfere with communication
      (a) Timing of exposure: it is uncertain which time is most critical—possibly is dangerous at all stages
f. Organic solvents: benzene may act as a teratogen and carcinogen
   (1) Use: used in chemical laboratories
   (2) Establish a history of exposure
      (a) Teratogen: exposure is most important during stage of early undifferentiation
      (b) Carcinogen: exposure is important during any stage
g. Pesticides: there is no conclusive evidence about the potential harmful effects of pesticides; exposure to chlorinated hydrocarbons, such as chlordane, may be mutagenic and carcinogenic
   (1) Use: used to control unwanted pests in crops; commonly used by farm workers
   (2) Establish a history of exposure: exposure at any stage may be important
h. Herbicides: exposure to 2,4,5,-T in the United States has been associated with an increased spontaneous miscarriage rate
   (1) Use: used to control unwanted vegetation
   (2) Establish a history of exposure: exposure during the first trimester is most important
i. Physical energy demands: exertion may increase the risk of early fetal death, prematurity, and low birth weight; exposure to vibration may be related to stillbirths; no conclusive evidence links heavy work and pregnancy outcome
   (1) Use: physical effort occurs at work or during prolonged standing
   (2) Establish a history of exposure: tolerance of strenuous exertion, such as lifting, pulling, pushing, or climbing, varies greatly among women on

Table 13–2
TYPICAL NOISE LEVELS

Level	Example
30 dB	Quiet library, soft whisper
40 dB	Quiet office, living room, bedroom away from traffic
50 dB	Light traffic at a distance, refrigerator
60 dB	Air conditioner at 6.1 m (20 ft), conversation, sewing machine
70 dB	Busy traffic, noisy restaurant (constant)
80 dB	Subway, heavy city traffic, alarm clock at 0.6 m (2 ft), factory noise; dangerous if more than an 8-hour exposure
90 dB	Truck traffic, noisy home appliances, shop tools, lawnmower; dangerous if more than an 8-hour exposure
100 dB	Chainsaw, boiler shop, pneumatic drill; dangerous if more than a 2-hour exposure

the basis of physical fitness and strength, the load handled, and the environment

  (a) Time of exposure: exposure is important at any stage, especially late in a pregnancy

j. Waste anesthetic gases: gases can cross the placental barrier; exposure may cause early fetal death, altered sex ratio, late fetal death, low birth weight, and birth defects; exposure to halogenated gases may be carcinogenic, teratogenic, or mutagenic, and may also reduce fertility in men

  (1) Use: commonly used by health care workers, dentists, laboratory personnel, and veterinarians

  (2) Establish a history of exposure

    (a) Timing of exposure: exposure may be important at any stage, including before pregnancy

3. Diagnostic procedures

  a. Establish client's level of exposure through review of records when possible; review biological samples when appropriate (e.g., urine, to determine levels of organic solvents and pesticides; blood, to determine lead levels)

  b. Establish level of exposure through environmental monitoring of workplace (e.g., use of dosimeter for noise level)

C. Nursing Diagnoses

1. Injury, high risk for fetus
2. Knowledge deficit and learning need
3. Anxiety

D. Interventions/Evaluations

1. Injury, high risk for fetus

  a. Interventions

    (1) Assess for exposure to potential hazards

    (2) Evaluate risk, taking into account the specificity of the agent, the developmental stage, the dose and length of exposure, the health of the mother, and the type of protection that was used to control exposure

    (3) Use occupational health nurse and physician in the workplace to assess and plan for exposure control

    (4) Refer client to health care provider for further evaluation

    (5) Refer client to appropriate agencies for further information about the potential hazard or to report exposure

    (6) Refer client for genetic counseling, as needed

    (7) Reassure client that not every exposure results in a negative outcome—many uncertainties exist

  b. Evaluations

    (1) Client follows through on referrals made

    (2) Client obtains information to more clearly understand exposure to potential hazards

    (3) Client avoids exposure to potential hazards and controls exposure to minimize negative effects

2. Knowledge deficit

  a. Interventions

    (1) Provide client with information about the possible effects of exposure to environmental hazards, putting the information in proper perspective

    (2) Refer client to material safety data sheets, available at the workplace, which describe possible hazards

    (3) Advise client to use appropriate safety precautions to control exposure

    (4) Advise client to inform the health care provider of possible or real exposure

    (5) Advise client to inform the occupational health office of pregnancy as

soon as possible, and discuss possible options to prevent or minimize exposures

(6) Advise expectant father to also control exposure to potential reproductive hazards

(7) Advise client to cooperate in biological monitoring while at the workplace

(8) Refer client to appropriate agencies for further information

(9) Educate client about the importance of avoiding potential environmental hazards at all times, not just while pregnant

(10) Advise client to plan pregnancies to avoid potentially harmful exposures before she becomes pregnant because the first trimester is so important in determining outcome of exposure

(11) Advise client to avoid prolonged standing and exertion

(12) Encourage client to share information with others to serve as an advocate for healthy pregnancies

b. Evaluations

(1) Client is able to describe potential harmful effects of exposures

(2) Client uses protective equipment when advised to control exposure

(3) Client follows through on referrals and advice

(4) Client establishes healthy behaviors to maximize pregnancy outcome

3. Anxiety

a. Interventions

(1) Listen to client's fears

(2) Reassure client that not all exposures result in negative consequences to the fetus

(3) Provide information honestly

(4) Refer client for counseling, as needed

(5) Assist client in finding support system

b. Evaluations

(1) Client is more calm and has realistic perspective

(2) Client avoids further risks

(3) Client is able to communicate concerns with appropriate health professionals and significant others

Temperature Extremes

A. Introduction

1. Extreme heat and humidity may lead to impairment of alertness, mental function, and physical capacity

2. Pregnant women may be more sensitive to heat and humidity

3. Controversy exists about the possible risk

B. Assessment

1. History

a. Hyperthermia: hyperthermia increases the body's core temperature, and prolonged high temperature may affect the central nervous system (CNS) of the fetus; hyperthermia is considered a suspected teratogen by some authorities; others have concluded there is no reproductive hazard

(1) Use: hyperthermia may result from exposure to high temperatures in hot tubs, jacuzzis, or saunas, or from febrile illness

(2) Establish history of exposure

(a) Timing of exposure: as a suspected teratogen, the greatest harm is produced during early differentiation; exposure during all stages of pregnancy may be dangerous

(b) Establish temperature level of client and environment

2. Physical findings

a. Symptoms of heat exhaustion

      (1) Syncope, dizziness, weakness
      (2) Nausea and vomiting
      (3) Increased pulse rate
      (4) Shortness of breath
      (5) Skin is moist and clammy
   b. Symptoms of heat stroke
      (1) Hot, dry skin
      (2) Confusion
      (3) Convulsions
      (4) Loss of consciousness
3. Psychosocial findings
   a. Disorientation
   b. Diminished mental alertness and functioning

C. **Nursing Diagnoses**

1. Injury, high risk for fetus
2. Knowledge deficit, learning need

D. **Interventions/Evaluations**

1. Injury, high risk for fetus
   a. Interventions
      (1) Assess for exposure to extreme heat
      (2) Provide cooling measures immediately
      (3) Provide extra liquids
      (4) Refer client to her health care provider for further evaluation
   b. Evaluation: client avoids exposure to extreme heat conditions
2. Knowledge deficit
   a. Interventions
      (1) Provide information about the possible dangers of prolonged exposure to heat
      (2) Advise against the use of spas, jacuzzis, saunas, and other activities that expose the client to extreme heat
      (3) Discourage strenuous physical activities, which might increase body temperature
   b. Evaluations
      (1) Client is able to describe potential dangers of hyperthermia to pregnancy
      (2) Client avoids exposure to extreme heat conditions

Pharmaceuticals

A. **Introduction**

1. Pharmaceuticals may be prescribed as part of a treatment regimen or over-the-counter drugs may be taken to relieve symptoms
2. No safe dose has been determined in most cases
3. The most critical time for exposure to pharmaceuticals is during early differentiation
4. Drugs may have a variety of effects on the fetus; the dose of the agent, timing of exposure, agent synergism, rate of metabolism, and host susceptibility of both mother and fetus play a role in fetal outcome; polydrug use further complicates the problem
5. Dose and method of administration must be considered in evaluating risk
6. Each drug taken must be evaluated based on its potential effect as a carcinogen, mutagen, or teratogen
7. Drugs that are either absorbed systemically or known to be potentially harmful to the fetus are required by the U.S. Food and Drug Administration (FDA) to be categorized according to one of five pregnancy categories as follows (the letter signifies the level of risk to the fetus)

a. Category A drugs are those that have failed to demonstrate risk to the fetus based on controlled studies in women

b. Category B refers to drugs that have not demonstrated fetal risk but for which there are no controlled studies in pregnant women

c. Category C drugs are those that have had adverse effects on the fetus in animal studies but for which there are no controlled studies in women; category C also includes drugs for which no studies are available; most drugs are in this category because of the lack of available studies

d. Category D refers to those drugs for which there is evidence of human fetal risk but for which the benefits might outweigh the risk if no safer, effective drugs are available

e. Drugs in category X have been deemed contraindicated in women who are or may become pregnant; the risk of use clearly outweighs any possible benefit

8. Because of space constraints, priority has been given to drugs found in categories D and X

B. Assessment

1. History
   a. Amphetamines
      (1) Action: CNS stimulant
      (2) Effects
         (a) Dextroamphetamine (Dexedrine): effects may include congenital heart defects (no conclusive evidence is available to support this)
         (b) Methamphetamine: effects are prematurity, abruptio placentae, fetal distress, and postpartum hemorrhage; developmental delays; tremulousness, startle reflex, and alterations in visual processing and quality of alterness in infants; and frontal lobe dysfunction that becomes manifest at school age; methamphetamine is also a teratogen
         (c) Benzphetamine hydrochloride (Didrex): effects in pregnant women have not been established
      (3) Timing of exposure: exposure is important at any stage, with greatest damage occurring during the stage of early differentiation
   b. Analgesics
      (1) Action: nonnarcotic pain relievers
      (2) Aspirin and phenylbutazone (butagesic, butazolidin) have been classified as category D drugs; safe use during pregnancy has not been demonstrated, particularly during the third trimester; both should be avoided during pregnancy when possible
      (3) Effects of aspirin include a potential decrease in blood clotting time near delivery; prolonged gestation has also been reported
   c. Antialcohol agents
      (1) Action: deterrence of alcohol ingestion
      (2) Disulfiram (Antabuse) is classified as a category X drug and is contraindicated during pregnancy; specific risks are not well documented
   d. Antibiotics
      (1) Action: infection control
      (2) Effects
         (a) Streptomycin: effects may include damage to the auditory nerve that leads to fetal deafness
         (b) Ribavirin (Tribavirin, Viramid): an antiviral, ribavirin is associated with fetal abnormalities
         (c) Quinine sulfate: an antimalarial drug, quinine sulfate is contraindicated as a category X drug
         (d) Tetracycline: when administered in last half of pregnancy, effects may include tooth discoloration in infant

(e) The following anti-infective agents are included in category D: ethionamide (Trecator S.C.), kanamycin (Anamid, Kantrex, Klebcil), povidone-iodine (Betadine), tobramycin sulfate (Nebcin, Tobradex), netilmicin sulfate (Netromycin), and emetine hydrochloride; specific effects on the fetus have not been described

e. Anticoagulants
  (1) Action: decrease in clotting time
  (2) Effects
     (a) Coumarin derivatives (Warfarin, Dicumarol, Phenindione): effects include decreased synthesis of the vitamin K–dependent clotting factors II, VII, IX, and X, as well as interference with protein binding of calcium; coumarin is also considered to be teratogenic
     (b) Warfarin
        (i) Exposure during the first trimester increases the risk for warfarin embryopathy (nasal hypoplasia because of the lack of development of the nasal septum and stippling of the epiphyses); effects may include growth and developmental retardation, scoliosis, deafness, and congenital heart disease
        (ii) Exposure during the second and third trimesters is associated with eye anomalies, hydrocephaly, and other CNS defects; spontaneous abortions; stillbirth; and neonatal hemorrhage
     (c) Phenindione in breast milk has been associated with neonatal hemorrhage

f. Anticonvulsants
  (1) Action: treatment of tonic-clonic and psychomotor seizures; it is difficult to assign teratogenic potential because epilepsy and anomalies may be interrelated
  (2) Effects
     (a) Effects of exposure to anticonvulsants include seizure-related hypoxia and acidosis in the developing embryo/fetus
     (b) Dilantin, diazepam (Valium), and trimethadione have been implicated as teratogens
     (c) Dilantin: effects include intrauterine and extrauterine growth retardation, mental impairment, congenital heart lesions, facial dysmorphisms (cleft lip or palate, low-set ears, depressed nasal bridge, and short nose), hernias, distal digital and nail hypoplasias, and limb anomalies; Dilantin is also associated with increased risk for childhood neuroectodermal tumors and neonatal coagulopathy
     (d) Trimethadione may cause developmental delay, mental impairment, and craniofacial abnormalities; spontaneous abortion has also been associated
     (e) Diazepam (Valium) has been associated with an increase in congenital malformations when taken during the first trimester
     (f) The following drugs are classified as category D drugs and should be used with caution: paramethadione (Paradione), phenacemide (Phenurone), phensuximide (Milontin), primidone (Myiodone), and valproic acid (Depakene)
  (3) Timing of exposure: first trimester poses the greatest risk; use of anticonvulsants is contraindicated during any stage of pregnancy

g. Antidepressants and psychotropics
  (1) Action: treatment of depression
  (2) Effects
     (a) Lithium has been linked to cardiac abnormalities
     (b) Meprobamate (Equanil, Miltown) has been implicated in cardiac abnormalities
     (c) Chlordiazepoxide hydrochloride (Librium) may cause mental retardation, spastic diplegia, deafness, microcephaly, and duodenal atresia

    (d) Haloperidol (Haldol, Peridol) has been implicated in limb deformity
    (e) Other category D drugs are nortriptyline hydrochloride (Aventyl), alprazolam (Xanax), lorazepam (Ativan, Alzapam); specific risks have not been documented

  h. Antiemetics
   (1) Action: control of nausea and vomiting
   (2) Effects: thiethylperazine maleate (Torecan) is contraindicated during pregnancy as a category X drug; specific effects are not well documented

  i. Antihypertensives
   (1) Action: treatment of hypertension
   (2) Effects
    (a) Reserpine may cause nasal congestion, lethargy, depressed Moro reflex, and bradycardia in infants
    (b) Metolazone (Diulo, Zaroxolyn), benzthiazide (Hydrex, Aquatag, Marazide), and polythiazide (Renese) may result in neonatal jaundice, thrombocytopenia, and other adverse reactions

  j. Antimigraine agents
   (1) Action: prevention or abortion of migraine, cluster headache, and other vascular headaches
   (2) Effects: exposure to ergotamine tartrate (Ergostat, Ergomar) is clearly contraindicated during pregnancy as a category X drug because of the potential uterotonic effects of the ergot alkaloids

  k. Antineoplastics
   (1) Action: alkylating agents commonly used in the treatment of cancers
   (2) Effects
    (a) Aminopterin is associated with a number of birth defects—hydrocephaly, cleft palate, meningomyelocele, and cranial abnormalities
    (b) Methotrexate may cause fetal death and congenital anomalies that have not been well described
    (c) Most antineoplastics are classified as category X drugs and are clearly contraindicated during pregnancy; fetal death and unspecified congenital anomalies are the common risks of exposure
   (3) Timing of exposure: exposure is most critical during the first trimester; exposures during the second and third trimesters do not seem to be associated with congenital malformations

  l. Antithyroid drugs
   (1) Action: inhibits the excess production of thyroid hormone
   (2) Effects
    (a) Propylthiouracil (PTU) is capable of inducing mild fetal hypothyroidism, which usually resolves within several days; enlargement of the thyroid gland in the fetus may also result
    (b) Methimazole (Tapazole) and propylthiouracil can induce goiter and even cretinism in the developing fetus; therefore, caution is recommended in determining a small but effective dose; it may be withdrawn 2 or 3 weeks before delivery
    (c) Potassium iodide may cause fetal goiter development
    (d) Radioactive iodine may result in congenital hypothyroidism in neonates; its use is contraindicated
   (3) Timing of exposure: exposure is most critical during the first and second trimesters; minimal doses are recommended, especially in the third trimester

  m. Diethylstilbestrol (DES)
   (1) Action: a potent, synthetic nonsteroidal estrogen widely used between 1940 and 1971 for the treatment of various complications of pregnancy
   (2) Effects

      (a) Increased risk for female reproductive tract abnormalities

      (b) Increased risk for male reproductive tract defects, including epididymal cysts, hypotrophic testes, varicocele, and altered semen

      (c) Early fetal death and childhood malignancies

      (d) All forms of estrogen are contraindicated during pregnancy

    (3) Timing of exposure: exposure is most critical during the first trimester, when it is most commonly associated with abnormalities

  n. Retinoids

    (1) Action: vitamin A analogues used for the treatment of chronic cystic acne.

    (2) Effects

      (a) Isotretinoin (Accutane) may cause birth defects and early or late fetal death; hydrocephalus, craniofacial anomalies, cardiovascular anomalies, and thymus abnormalities are common results

      (b) Childhood mortality is high among those exposed in utero

        (i) Exposed infants are approximately 27 times more likely to die during the first year of life than unexposed infants

        (ii) Specific causes of death have not been well documented

      (c) Retinoids are considered some of the most potent human teratogens; the risks of retinoic acid are similar to those posed by prenatal Thalidomide exposure in the 1960s

    (3) Timing of exposure: exposure is most critical during the first trimester of pregnancy, resulting in a risk of giving birth to a baby who has a CNS, cardiovascular, or craniofacial abnormality that is 25 times that in those not exposed

  o. Sedative-hypnotics

    (1) Action: control of agitation

    (2) Effects: exposure to barbiturates can cause fetal damage and are associated with a higher incidence of fetal abnormalities; the highest concentration of barbiturates have been found in the placenta, fetal liver, and brain; withdrawal symptoms occur in infants born exposed

    (3) Examples of barbiturates include pentobarbital (Nembutal), phenobarbital, triazolam (Halcion), butabarbital (Barbased, Butatran), and amobarbital (Amytal)

    (4) Timing of exposure: exposure is most critical during the first 6 weeks in influencing fetal development; exposure during the third trimester is of concern for withdrawal symptoms in the infant at time of birth

  p. Thalidomide

    (1) Action: widely used in the 1960s as a sedative in other countries but banned in the United States

    (2) Effects: exposure leads to birth defects

2. Diagnostic procedures

  a. Take a urine sample from newborn to detect level of drug

  b. Perform a fetal ultrasound evaluation as necessary

C. Nursing Diagnoses

1. Injury, high risk for fetus
2. Knowledge deficit and learning need
3. Anxiety

D. Interventions/Evaluations

1. Injury, high risk for fetus

  a. Interventions

    (1) Advise of potential reproductive dangers of pharmaceuticals, whether prescribed or over-the-counter

    (2) Advise patient to consult health care provider before taking any drugs

    (3) Refer pregnant women exposed to potentially hazardous pharmaceuti-

cals before and early in the pregnancy to teratogen registries, March of Dimes, and other agencies who are interested in collecting data to generate or support hypotheses about the link between the use of pharmaceuticals and pregnancy outcome
  b. Evaluations
    (1) Client obtains information about potentially hazardous pharmaceuticals
    (2) Client informs health care provider of medications used
    (3) Client discontinues all drugs not approved by health care provider
    (4) Client follows through on all referrals
  2. Knowledge deficit and learning need
    a. Interventions
      (1) Advise client of potential dangers during pregnancy of any drug use, including over-the-counter drugs and drugs prescribed by other health care providers
      (2) Advise client to read all labels and adhere to their precautions
      (3) Advise client to inform health care provider of plans for pregnancy so implications of prescribed drugs can be discussed
    b. Evaluations
      (1) Client avoids using drugs except those approved by health care provider
      (2) Client informs all health care providers of pregnancy
      (3) Client reads drug labels
      (4) Client uses drugs as directed
      (5) Client disposes of drugs appropriately
  3. Anxiety
    a. Interventions
      (1) Provide emotional support and factual information to give a realistic perspective to pregnant women concerned about potentially hazardous exposures to pharmaceuticals
      (2) Participate in or support research on the correlation between pharmaceutical use and pregnancy outcome
    b. Evaluations
      (1) Client is calmer and has a realistic perspective of dangers
      (2) Client avoids further exposure
      (3) Client communicates concerns to appropriate health professionals and significant others

Passive Smoking

A. Introduction

1. Passive smoking refers to exposure to approximately 15% of mainstream smoke (from the smoker) and approximately 85% of sidestream smoke (from the cigarette)
2. There are approximately 3800 chemicals in cigarette smoke
3. Because active smoking is linked to low birth weight in infants, early fetal death, and prematurity, it is likely that passive smoking may have similar effects with sufficient exposure
4. Passive smoking has been implicated in an increase of respiratory infections and may be a risk factor for sudden infant death syndrome (SIDS) in children exposed to passive smoking

B. Assessment

1. History
   a. Effects on pregnancy of exposure to environmental tobacco smoke at work or at home have not been clearly documented; one must consider the length and frequency of exposure
   b. Timing of exposure: exposure is important during any stage of pregnancy
2. Diagnostic procedures: none known

C. Nursing Diagnoses

1. Injury, high risk for fetus
2. Knowledge deficit, learning need

D. Interventions/Evaluations

1. Injury, high risk for fetus
   a. Interventions
      (1) Specific effects from passive smoking on the fetus have not been documented (research is needed in this area); it is safe to assume that the dangers may be similar, on a lesser scale, to active smoking (i.e., prematurity, low birth weight) given adequate exposure; see Chapter 32 for further discussion
      (2) Advise client to insist on a healthy work environment that is free of smoke
      (3) Encourage client to avoid settings where exposure to environmental tobacco smoke is great
      (4) Inform client of laws and legislation that provide smoke-free environments
      (5) Encourage client to be assertive in not allowing smoking in environments she can control
   b. Evaluations
      (1) Client protects fetus from exposure to passive smoking when possible
      (2) Client informs employer of potential dangers of exposure to passive smoking, if necessary
2. Knowledge deficit, learning need
   a. Interventions
      (1) Advise client of potential dangers from both active and passive smoking
      (2) Advise client to evaluate environments she is frequently exposed to for potential hazards and to avoid them if possible
      (3) Advise client of increased risk of respiratory problems and possibly SIDS in infants and children resulting from exposure to passive smoking
   b. Evaluations
      (1) Client avoids smoke-polluted environments when possible
      (2) Client selects nonsmoking areas in public places
      (3) Client restricts smoking in personal environments at home and work during and after pregnancy

Health Education

The following health educational needs for the patient and family have been identified. Refer to previous nursing interventions for additional detail. Community resources are listed in Table 13–3.

Table 13–3
COMMUNITY RESOURCES THAT MAY PROVIDE USEFUL INFORMATION ABOUT ENVIRONMENTAL HAZARDS

American Lung Association
Genetic Counseling Services
March of Dimes
National Institute of Occupational Safety and Health
Occupational Safety and Health Administration (federal and state)
Teratogen registries
Pesticide Clearing House (800-858-7378)

A. Occupational hazards

1. Accurate, current information on potential reproductive risks in the workplace and possible negative outcomes
2. Importance of informing health care provider of potential occupational exposures
3. Importance of informing occupational health office at work of pregnancy or plans for pregnancy
4. Safety precautions to take at work to minimize exposure
5. Importance of biological monitoring for exposure levels in the workplace
6. Information about potential reproductive risks at work for spouse
7. Precautions to control exposures to environmental hazards at home (e.g., with chemicals and noise)

B. Pharmaceuticals

1. Dangers of taking any medication, over-the-counter or prescribed, unless discussed with the health care provider
2. Importance of informing all health care providers of pregnancy before treatment is prescribed
3. Importance of taking drugs as directed
4. Dangers of drug interactions
5. Importance of planning pregnancies and avoiding use of potentially harmful drugs before becoming pregnant

C. Temperature extremes

1. Dangers of exposure to extreme hot or cold temperatures
2. Importance of avoiding hot tubs, jacuzzis, spas, tanning booths, and saunas
3. Importance of avoiding strenuous physical activity that may increase the body's core temperature

D. Passive smoking

1. Dangers of passive smoking to mother, fetus, and others exposed
2. Importance of selecting nonsmoking areas in public places
3. Importance of being assertive in maintaining a smoke-free environment
4. Importance of supporting legislation limiting smoking
5. Importance of attaining or maintaining nonsmoker status
6. Importance of informing friends and relatives of the dangers of smoking to fetus and children

CASE STUDIES AND STUDY QUESTIONS

Occupational Hazards

Michelle is a 25-year-old woman who has been employed by the research and development office of a major oil company for the past 2 years. Her work involves standing about half of the time. She has just learned that she is 6 weeks pregnant. Her husband, Steve, is a chemist for the same company. Both Michelle and Steve have graduate degrees and have planned this pregnancy. Michelle plans to resume working after the baby is born. Michelle attends aerobic classes for exercise three times each week.

1. Which of the following would you include in an occupational history of Michelle?

   (1) Chemicals that Michelle works with.

   (2) Precautions taken to control exposure.

   (3) Chemicals that Steve works with.

   (4) Amount of time Michelle spends standing and sitting at work.

   a. 1, 2.

   b. 1, 3.

   c. 1, 2, 3.

   d. All of the above.

2. Which of the following would you include in health education for Michelle?

   (1) Importance of reviewing material safety data sheets on each chemical that she and Steve are exposed to.

(2) Importance of using recommended protective equipment.

(3) Importance of informing the company's health office of pregnancy.

(4) Importance of taking 5- to 10-minute activity breaks every hour to avoid prolonged standing and sitting.

a. 1, 2.

b. 1, 2, 4.

c. 1, 3.

d. All of the above.

3. Which of the following would you advise regarding Michelle's recreational activities?

a. Aerobic class activities should be evaluated to determine level of safety.

b. Advise discontinuation of aerobic classes because they are too strenuous.

c. Advise Michelle to continue aerobic classes because they do not pose a potential health threat.

d. Recommend that Michelle discuss her pregnancy with her aerobics instructor.

Pharmaceuticals

Janet is a 33-year-old woman who is 8 weeks pregnant. This pregnancy is not wanted, and she is extremely depressed. Her obstetrician has referred her to a psychiatrist for evaluation. She has three other children and is unemployed. Her family physician prescribed lithium 2 years earlier for "her nerves." She uses it when needed. Since she became pregnant, she has taken aspirin for headaches and antihistamines for allergy symptoms. She also uses antacids occasionally. Janet's husband, Leonard, is an executive for a savings and loan company.

4. Which of the following drugs that Janet may be using would concern you?

a. Lithium

b. Aspirin

c. Both

d. Neither

5. Which of the following would you recommend for Janet to ease her depression and manage stress?

a. Become involved with a social support group.

b. Follow through on referral for psychiatric evaluation and counseling.

c. Learn and practice stress management techniques such as relaxation, meditation, and biofeedback.

d. All of the above.

Temperature Extremes

Julie is a pregnant, 31-year-old mother of three children. She and her husband live in a large home in an affluent neighborhood. They have a swimming pool and Jacuzzi. They enjoy relaxing in the Jacuzzi nightly before retiring.

6. Which of the following would you advise Julie to do to control her exposure to high temperatures?

(1) Stop using the Jacuzzi.

(2) Use the Jacuzzi only if the temperature is 100°F or lower.

(3) Sit with only her legs or feet dangling in the hot water.

(4) Suggest she take an evening walk with her husband instead of using the Jacuzzi.

a. 1.

b. 2.

c. 2, 3, 4.

d. 4.

7. Julie inquires about the use of hot showers. Which of the following would you recommend?

a. Hot showers should be avoided altogether.

b. Hot showers are relatively safe if they last only for 5 minutes.

c. Hot showers are safe.

d. Refer Julie to her health care provider.

Passive Smoking

Brenda is a 22-year-old pregnant single mother who works for a metropolitan newspaper in the newsroom. She quit smoking when she first discovered she was pregnant with her second child. Smoking is permitted in the newsroom because most of the people in that department smoke: they claim that smoking relieves the tension of having deadlines to meet. Brenda usually dates every Friday and Saturday evenings. She especially enjoys dancing. Brenda does not permit smoking in her home or car.

8. Which of the following responses to Brenda's work situation would you support?

   a. Quit her job and find one in a smoke-free workplace.

   b. Discuss with her employer the potential dangers of passive smoking to the fetus and request a separate office that would be smoke-free.

   c. Use a fan to vent the smoke away from her.

   d. Request a transfer to a different department immediately.

9. What health teaching would you include about her social life?

   a. Suggest she stop dating because of potential dangers to the fetus.

   b. Advise her to avoid dancing because it is impossible to find a dance floor free of smoke.

   c. Encourage her to discuss her concern about the effects of passive smoking with her date and consider alternatives that would be safe.

   d. Do nothing because the dangers of passive smoking to the fetus have not been well documented.

Answers to Study Questions

1. d	2. d	3. a
4. c	5. d	6. c
7. b	8. b	9. c

REFERENCES

Occupational Hazards

American Medical Association, Council on Scientific Affairs. (1984). Effects of pregnancy on work performance. *Journal of the American Medical Association, 251*(15), 1997.

American Medical Association, Council on Scientific Affairs. (1985). Effects of toxic chemicals on the reproductive system. *Journal of the American Medical Association, 253*(23), 3431–3437.

Bernhardt, J.H. (1990). Potential workplace hazards to reproductive health: Information for primary prevention. *Journal of Obstetrics, Gynecologic, and Neonatal Nursing, 19*(1), 53–62.

Buffler, P.A., & Aase, J.M. (1982). Genetic risks and environmental surveillance: Epidemiological aspects of monitoring industrial populations for environmental mutagens. *Journal of Occupational Medicine, 24*(4), 305–314.

Chamberlain, G., & Garcia, J. (1983). Pregnant women at work. *Lancet 1*(8318), 228–230.

Clarkson, W. (1987, October). Developmental problems: Effect of environmental problems on the newborn. *Environmental Health Perspectives, 74*, 103–107.

Drinville-Shank, G. (1987). The pregnant OR employee. Part I: Ensuring maternal health. *Association of Operating Room Nurses Journal, 45*(2), 404–410.

Frank, A. (1983). Occupational history and examination. In W. Rom (Ed.), *Environmental and occupational medicine* (pp. 21–26). Boston: Little, Brown.

Kochenour, N. (1984). Adverse pregnancy outcome: Sensitive periods, types of adverse outcomes, and relationships with critical exposure periods. In J. Lockey, G. Lemaster, & W. Keye (Eds.), *The new frontier in occupational and environmental health research.* New York: Liss.

Lalande, N., Hetu, R., & Lambert, J. (1986). Is occupational noise exposure during pregnancy a risk factor of damage to the auditory system of the fetus? *American Journal of Industrial Medicine, 10*(4), 427–435.

Lindbohm, M.L., Taskinen, H., & Hemminki, K. (1985). Reproductive health of working women: Spontaneous abortions and congenital malformations. *Public Health Review, 13*, 55–87.

McCloy, E.C. (1989). Work, environment, and the fetus. *Midwifery, 5*(2), 53–62.

McCloy, E.C. (1987). Reproduction and work. In P.A.B. Raffle, W.R. Lee, R.I. McCallum, & R. Murray (Eds.), *Diseases of occupations.* London: Hodder & Stoughton.

McDonald, A., McDonald, J.C., & Armstrong, B. (1988). Fetal death and work in pregnancy. *British Journal of Industrial Medicine, 45*(3), 148–157.

Messite, J., & Bond, M. (1980). Reproductive toxicology and occupational exposure. In C. Zienz (Ed.), *Developments in occupational medicine.* Chicago: Year Book.

Nurminen, T., & Kurppa, K. (1989). Occupational noise exposure and course of pregnancy. *Scandinavian Journal of Work, Environment, and Health, 15*(2), 117–124.

Savitz, D.A., Whelan, E.A., & Kleckner, R.C. (1989). Effect of parents' occupational exposures on risk of stillbirth, preterm delivery, and small-for-gestational-age infants. *American Journal of Epidemiology, 129*(6), 1201–1218.

Sever, L.E. (1981). Reproductive hazards of the workplace. *Journal of Occupational Medicine, 23*(10), 161–165.

Slone, D., Shapiro, D., & Mitchell, A.A. (1980). Strategies for studying the effects of the antenatal chemical environment on the fetus. In R.H. Schwarz & J.Y. Sumner (Eds.), *Drug and chemical risks to the fetus and newborn.* New York: Liss.

Stasiewicz, J.H. (1980, May). Pregnancy in the workplace. *Occupational Health Nursing, 28*(5), 13–17.

Stellman, J. (1983). The occupational environment and reproductive health. In W. Rom (Ed.), *Environmental and occupational medicine.* Boston: Little, Brown.

Tannenbaum, T., & Goldberg, R. (1985). Exposure to anesthetic gases and reproductive outcomes. *Journal of Occupational Medicine, 27*(9), 659–668.

U.S. Congress, Office of Technology Assessment. (1985). *Reproductive hazards in the work-place* (OTA-BA-266). Washington, DC: U.S. Government Printing Office.

Pharmaceuticals

Chasnoff, I.J. (1988). Drug use in pregnancy: Parameters of risk. *Pediatric Clinics of North America, 35*(6), 1403–1412.

Dicke, J.M. (1989). Teratology: Principles and practice. *Medical Clinics of North America, 73*(3), 567–582.

Edelman, D.A. (1989). Diethylstilbestrol exposure and the risk of clear cell cervical and vaginal adenocarcinoma. *International Journal of Fertility, 34*(4), 251–255.

Hall, J.E., Pauli, R.M., & Wilson, K.M. (1980). Maternal and fetal sequelae of anticoagulation during pregnancy. *American Journal of Medicine, 68*(1), 122.

Hanson, J.W., Myrianthopoulos, N.C., & Sedgwick, M.A. (1976). Risks to the offspring of women treated with hydantoin anticonvulsants, with emphasis on the fetal hydantoin syndrome. *Journal of Pediatrics, 89*(4), 662.

Jahn, A.F., & Ganti, K. (1987). Major auricular malformations due to Accutane (isotretinoin). *Laryngoscope, 97*(7), 832–835.

Kasilo, O., Romero, M., Bonati, M., & Tognoni, G. (1988). Information on drug use in pregnancy from the Viewpoint Regional Drug Information Centre. *European Journal of Clinical Pharmacology, 35*(5), 447–453.

Kooker, B.M. (1987, April). Four million female hospital workers face reproductive health hazards. *Occupational Health and Safety, 56*(4), 61–64.

McDonald, A.D., McDonald, J.C., Armstrong, B., Cherry, N.M., Cote, R., LaVoie, J., Nolin, A.D., & Robert, D. (1988). Fetal death and work in pregnancy. *British Journal of Industrial Medicine, 45*(3), 148–157.

Milunsky, A., Graef, J.W., & Gaynor, M.F. (1968). Methotrexate-induced congenital malformations. *Journal of Pediatrics, 72*(6), 790.

Nurminen, T., & Kurppa, K. (1989). Occupational exposure and course of pregnancy. *Scandinavian Journal of Work and Environmental Health, 15,* 117–124.

Rane, A., Tomson, G., & Bjarke, B. (1978). Effects of maternal lithium therapy in newborn infant. *Journal of Pediatrics, 93*(2), 296.

Rayburn, W.F., McNulty, R.M., & O'Shaughnessy, R.W. (1986). *Drug therapy in obstetrics and gynecology.* Norwalk, CT: Appleton-Century-Crofts.

Ruthnum, P., & Tolmie, J.L. (1987). Atypical malformations in an infant exposed to warfarin during the first trimester of pregnancy. *Teratology, 36*(3), 299–301.

Shepard, T.H. (1986). *Catalog of teratogenic agents.* Baltimore: Johns Hopkins University Press.

Sonawane, B.R., & Yaffee, S.J. (1986). *Drug and chemical action in pregnancy: Pharmacologic and toxicologic principles.* New York: Dekker.

Stevens, D., Burman, D., & Midwinter, A. (1974). Transplacental lithium poisoning. *Lancet, 2*(7880), 595.

Thomson, E.J., & Cordero, J.F. (1989). The new teratogens: Accutane and other vitamin-A analogs. *Maternal-Child Nursing, 14*(4), 244–248.

Warkany, J. (1981). Teratogenicity of folic acid antagonists. *Cancer Bulletin, 33*(2), 76.

Temperature Extremes

Bernhardt, J.H. (1990). Potential workplace hazards to reproductive health: Information for primary prevention. *Journal of Obstetrics, Gynecologic, and Neonatal Nursing, 19*(1), 53–62.

McDonald, A.D., McDonald, J.C., Armstrong, B., Cherry, N.M., Cote, R., LaVoie, J., Nolin, A.D., & Robert, D. (1988). Fetal death and work in pregnancy. *British Journal of Industrial Medicine, 45*(3), 148–157.

Passive Smoking

Byrd, J.C., Shapiro, R.S., & Schiedermayer, D.L. (1989). Passive smoking: A review of medical and legal issues. *American Journal of Public Health, 79*(2), 209–215.

Miller, G.H. (1984). Cancer, passive smoking and nonemployed and employed wives. *Western Journal of Medicine, 140*(4), 632–635.

U.S. Department of Health and Human Services, Report of the Surgeon General. (1987). *Health consequences of involuntary smoking* (DHHS Publication No. 87-8309). Washington, DC: U.S. Government Printing Office.

Weiss, S.T., Tager, I.B., Schenker, M., Speizer, F.E. (1983). The health effects of involuntary smoking. *American Review of Respiratory Diseases, 128*(5), 933–942.

THE INTRAPARTUM PERIOD

Gail M. Turley

CHAPTER

14

Essential Forces and Factors in Labor

Objectives

1. List the forces affecting labor

2. Identify the possible causes of the onset of labor

3. Discuss the oxytocin release theory of labor onset

4. Discuss the fetal prostaglandin theory of labor onset

5. Describe the amount of uterine activity required to effect cervical changes

6. Differentiate between muscle contraction and muscle retraction, and discuss the significance of both to the progress of labor

7. List the techniques used for assessing uterine activity and uterine efficiency

8. Differentiate between true labor and false labor, using information gathered by history and physical examination

9. Identify the basic pelvic shapes

10. Recognize adequate pelvic dimensions

11. Describe methods for assessing pelvic capacity

12. Compare and contrast the anticipated progress of labor for each of the four pelvic shapes

13. Identify and discuss maternal conditions that may alter or influence pelvic capacity

14. Analyze the relation between maternal posture and the pelvic passage

15. Define fetal lie, attitude, presentation, presenting part, position, and station

16. List the mechanisms of spontaneous vaginal delivery

17. Discuss the significance of breech presentation or transverse lie to the progress of labor

18. Recognize fetal variables that may interfere with the progress of labor

19. Discuss the significance of fetal malpositioning to the course and outcome of labor

20. Describe the characteristic emotions associated with labor

21. Identify variables that determine a couple's expectations for the labor and birth experience

22. Distinguish between adaptive coping and maladaptive coping during labor

23. Identify the nursing diagnoses associated with the forces of labor

24. Describe the nursing actions that maximize the forces of labor

25. Predict when a woman is at risk for a difficult labor as the result of an alteration in one of the forces of labor

---

Introduction

A. Four essential forces

1. Power: the power of labor is provided by the uterine muscle, and the onset and establishment of a satisfactory contraction pattern is a readily recognized force of labor
2. Passage: the labor passage is defined by the bony boundaries of the pelvis, and its shape and configuration determine the ease with which the baby is expelled from the uterus
3. Passenger: the baby, or passenger, is an active participant in the labor process as it moves and turns to accommodate the maternal pelvis
4. Psyche: finally, a woman's psyche, or emotional system, determines her total response to labor and influences both physiological and psychological functioning

Clinical Practice

POWER OF LABOR

A. Assessment

1. History
   a. Onset of contractions
      (1) Maternal factor theories
         (a) The uterus is stretched to threshold point, leading to synthesis and release of prostaglandin
         (b) The pressure on the cervix and its nerve plexus reaches threshold point
         (c) Oxytocin stimulation theory
            (i) Exogenous oxytocin is known to stimulate myometrial contractions, but no evidence clearly documents its role in the onset of labor
            (ii) Progesterone inhibits myometrial response throughout pregnancy
            (iii) Estrogen at term enhances myometrial sensitivity to oxytocin
            (iv) A surge of oxytocin may be released by stretching of the cervix at term (Ferguson's reflex), but studies do not agree about this
         (d) Progesterone withdrawal theory
            (i) In animals, a decrease in progesterone is followed by evacuation of the uterus
            (ii) In humans, no firm evidence documents that progesterone is decreased at term
            (iii) However, many researchers support the view that an altered progesterone/estrogen ratio leads to increased myometrial contractility

(2) Fetal factor theories
  (a) Placental aging and deterioration trigger initiation of contractions
  (b) Fetal cortisol theory
      (i) It is reasoned that normal fetal adrenal glands produce a steroid, cortisol, that stimulates the onset of labor
      (ii) It is recognized that anencephaly causes adrenal dysfunction secondary to pituitary dysfunction
      (iii) Empirically, anencephalic fetuses tend to have prolonged gestations
  (c) Prostaglandin synthesis theory
      (i) Prostaglandins are known to stimulate uterine contractions at any gestational age
      (ii) Prostaglandin is present in increased quantities in blood and amniotic fluid during labor
      (iii) Prostaglandin production requires the precursor arachidonic acid
      (iv) Esterified arachidonic acid is stored in fetal membranes
      (v) It is postulated that free arachidonic acid is released at term and is then converted by agents in the uterine decidua to prostaglandin
b. Physiology of contractions
  (1) Myometrium
      (a) Uterine muscle is controlled by involuntary innervation
      (b) Alpha-receptors stimulate uterine contractions
      (c) Beta-receptors stimulate uterine relaxation
      (d) Norepinephrine and epinephrine stimulate both alpha- and beta-receptors
          (i) When progesterone is present, beta-receptors are stimulated
          (ii) When estrogen is present, alpha-receptors are stimulated
  (2) Contraction: the shortening of a muscle in response to a stimulus, with return to its original length (Fig. 14–1)
      (a) Increment: building up; the longest phase of a contraction
      (b) Acme: peak
      (c) Decrement: letting up
  (3) Retraction: the shortening of a muscle in response to a stimulus, without return to its original length; the muscle becomes fixed at a relatively shorter length, but there is no increase in baseline tension after the contraction (also known as brachystasis)
      (a) With each uterine contraction, the upper segment of the uterus becomes shorter and thicker, while the lower segment of the uterus becomes longer, thinner, and more distended
      (b) The division between the contractile upper segment of the uterus and the passive lower uterine segment is the physiological retraction ring
      (c) Longitudinal traction on the cervix by the upper portion of the uterus as it contracts and retracts leads to cervical effacement and dilatation
      (d) The shortening and thickening of the upper uterine segment leads to fetal descent
  (4) Tonus: the degree of pressure exerted by the uterine musculature as measured by intrauterine pressure
      (a) Tonus is measured in millimeters of mercury (mm Hg), which is also referred to as torr
      (b) Normal baseline tonus between contractions is 8 to 12 mm Hg
      (c) Pressure at peak of a contraction ranges from 35 to 75 mm Hg
  (5) Intensity: the rise in intrauterine pressure above baseline brought about by a contraction

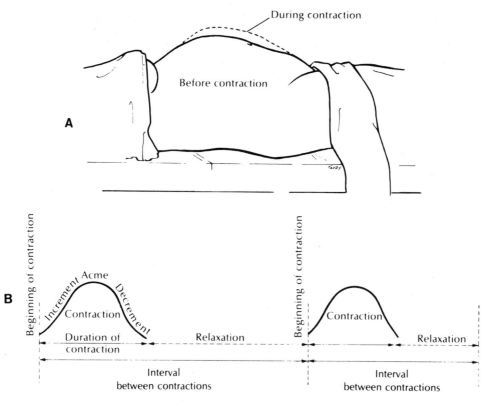

Figure 14–1
Wavelike pattern of contractile activity. (From Bobak, I., Jensen, M.D., & Zalar, M.K. [1989]. *Maternity and gynecologic care* [4th ed., p. 391]. St. Louis: Mosby.)

(a) Intensity is measured as the difference between peak pressure and baseline pressure
(b) Normally, 30 to 50 mm Hg intensity is necessary for effective labor
(6) Pacemaker: the site of electrical activity that is responsible for triggering a uterine contraction
  (a) Pacemakers are generally located in the fundus of the uterus (fundal dominance)
    (i) It was previously theorized that specialized cells existed that acted as pacemakers
    (ii) Current research indicates that the cells responsible for initiating electrical stimuli are not different from surrounding myometrial cells
    (iii) Because the fundus contains a greater number of myometrial cells, it is reasonable that the cells primarily responsible for triggering electrical activity would be located there
  (b) The wave of the contraction begins in the fundus, then proceeds downward to the rest of the uterus (descending gradient)
    (i) The duration of the contraction diminishes progressively as the wave moves away from the fundus; therefore, during any contraction, the upper portion of the uterus is contracted for a longer time
    (ii) The intensity of the contraction diminishes from top to bottom, so that the upper segment contracts more strongly than the lower segment

(iii) If the duration and intensity of the contraction were constant throughout, effacement and dilatation could not occur

(c) Asymmetry results when the uterine halves function independently, leading to ineffective contractions with minimal dilatation

(d) Ectopic pacemakers (i.e., pacemakers located outside of the uterine fundus) result in spasmodic myometrial contractions, which are disorganized and colicky, and rarely effective in producing dilatation

c. False labor

(1) Discomfort is perceived, but cervical changes do not occur

(2) Discomfort is usually perceived more in lower abdomen than in back

(3) Discomfort may be caused by uterine contractions, intestinal or bladder spasm, or abdominal wall muscle tension

(4) Despite perceived discomfort, the uterus is often relaxed, although mild contractions may be palpated

(5) Contractions are irregular and of short duration

(6) The interval between contractions is long and irregular, and it does not decrease as discomfort continues

(7) The intensity does not increase with time

(8) Contractions are easily interrupted by medication and activity, such as walking

(9) There is an absence of cervical bloody show

(10) Is mentally and physically tiring for the client

d. True labor

(1) By definition, true labor is the onset of contractions that leads to progressive cervical effacement and dilatation

(2) Discomfort is perceived in both front and back

(3) Hardening of the uterus is palpable

(4) Contractions occur at regular intervals, usually begin 20 to 30 minutes apart, last 10 to 20 seconds, and are of mild intensity

(5) As contractions continue, frequency, duration, and intensity increase

(6) True labor is not easily disrupted by medication

(7) Intensity is increased by walking

(8) Presenting part descends

(9) Bulging of the membranes may occur

(10) Bloody show is present

2. Physical examination

a. Contraction strength

(1) Myometrial activity

(a) Myometrial activity is solely responsible for effacement and dilatation of the first stage of labor

(b) Uterine contractions create increased intrauterine pressure, which exerts tension on cervix and pressure on the descending fetus

(c) Myometrial effectiveness is improved by good uterine blood flow

(i) Lateral positions avoid the vena caval syndrome

(ii) Walking and activity increase circulating blood to the uterus

(2) Expulsive activity

(a) During the second stage of labor, both involuntary and voluntary forces are present

(b) Involuntary myometrial activity continues to create increased intrauterine pressure, which exerts pressure against the fetus

(c) Full dilatation causes involuntary reflex desire to bear down, which increases intra-abdominal pressure, thereby increasing intrauterine pressure

(d) Voluntary efforts to bear down increase intra-abdominal pressure, thereby increasing intrauterine pressure

(e) Positions that flex the legs on the abdomen increase intra-abdominal pressure, thereby increasing intrauterine pressure

   b. Contraction frequency

     (1) Contraction frequency is measured from the beginning of one contraction to the beginning of the next contraction

     (2) Typical frequency of contractions during active labor is two to five contractions per 10 minutes

   c. Contraction duration

     (1) Contraction duration is measured from the beginning of the increment to the end of the decrement

     (2) Typical duration of contractions during active labor is 30 to 90 seconds

3. Diagnostic studies and techniques

   a. Manual palpation of contractions

     (1) Judge indentability of the uterine wall and assign a rating of mild, moderate, or strong

       (a) Mild: uterine wall easily indented

       (b) Moderate: uterine wall demonstrates resistance to pressure, though some indentation occurs

       (c) Strong: uterine wall cannot be indented

   b. External monitoring of contractions: tocotransducer

     (1) The tocotransducer reflects increased intra-abdominal pressure

     (2) Placement of the tocotransducer influences accuracy of information

     (3) Intra-abdominal pressure does not directly correlate with intrauterine pressure; therefore, it does not measure the actual intensity of contractions

     (4) There are no known risks of using the tocotransducer, but some women feel confined and uncomfortable

   c. Internal monitoring of contractions: intrauterine pressure catheter

     (1) Allows direct measurement of intrauterine pressure

     (2) Provides accurate measurement of actual intensity of uterine contraction

     (3) Associated risks

       (a) Introduction of infection into uterine cavity

       (b) Uterine rupture caused by traumatic insertion

   d. Montevideo units

     (1) Developed by Calderyo-Barcia to measure and quantify uterine work

     (2) Calculated by multiplying the frequency of contractions (as expressed by the number of contractions in 10 minutes) by their intensity

     (3) Expressed as millimeters of mercury per 10 minutes

     (4) Example

       (a) The client is contracting every 3 minutes; therefore, there are three contractions in 10 minutes

       (b) The intensity of the contraction at its peak is 35 mm Hg

       (c) $\dfrac{3 \text{ contractions}}{10 \text{ minutes}} \times \dfrac{35 \text{ mm Hg}}{\text{contractions}} = 105 \text{ mm Hg/10 minutes}$

LABOR PASSAGE

A. Assessment

1. History

   a. Musculoskeletal deformities and diseases

     (1) A contracted pelvis may lead to disproportion between the pelvis and the fetus

     (2) Uterine neoplasms (e.g., fibromyomas, ovarian cysts) may block the birth canal, impeding the passage

     (3) Bicornuate uterus

       (a) May lead to abortion, premature labor, or premature rupture of membranes

       (b) Has been implicated in incompetent cervix

       (c) May be causative factor of breech or transverse lie

(d) Vaginal delivery is possible, but may be accompanied by uterine inertia or obstruction of descent

(4) Maternal dwarfism
  (a) Defined as height of less than 147.3 cm (4 ft, 10 in) at maturity
  (b) Pelvic dimensions may be favorable if dwarfism is proportionate

(5) Kyphoscoliosis
  (a) If thoracic area is involved, there is little or no reduction of pelvic capacity
  (b) If dorsolumbar or lumbosacral area is involved, marked pelvic deformity is common

(6) Bony disease of femurs or acetabula may result in abnormal pressures on pelvis during development, leading to pelvic asymmetry and reduced pelvic capacity

(7) Nutritional deficiencies and diseases (e.g., rickets) may contribute to bone deformities that impede the passage

b. Pelvic trauma or injury may lead to asymmetry and reduced capacity

c. Cervical trauma or injury
  (1) Includes accidental insults as well as those resulting from surgical procedures (e.g., dilatation and curettage [D&C], cone biopsy, uterine aspiration)
  (2) May result in loss of cervical integrity with resultant incompetence
  (3) May result in cervical scarring and adhesions, with resultant failure to dilate
  (4) Cervical abnormalities are frequently found among women exposed in utero to diethylstilbestrol (DES)

2. Physical examination
  a. Pelvic shapes (Fig. 14–2)
    (1) Rigid classification is not possible
      (a) Name is assigned based on classification of inlet
      (b) Nonconforming characteristics are then described
    (2) Gynecoid: normal female
      (a) Uterine function is good
      (b) Early and complete internal rotation occurs
      (c) Labor prognosis is good
      (d) This shape offers the optimal diameters in all three planes of the pelvis
      (e) Approximate incidence is 50%
    (3) Android: male
      (a) Posterior segments are reduced in all the pelvic planes
      (b) Deep transverse arrest is common
      (c) Failure of rotation is common
      (d) Labor prognosis is poor
      (e) Approximate incidence is 20%, but it occurs more frequently among white women (30%) than nonwhite women (15%)
    (4) Anthropoid: apelike
      (a) Reduced transverse measurements are compensated by large anteroposterior diameters
      (b) Prognosis is generally more favorable than android or platypelloid
      (c) This shape may deliver occiput posterior
      (d) Approximate incidence is 25%, but it occurs more frequently among nonwhite women (50%) than white women (25%)
    (5) Platypelloid: flat female
      (a) Arrest at inlet is common
      (b) Labor prognosis is poor
      (c) Approximate incidence is 5%
  b. Pelvic dimension
    (1) The measurements that define the obstetric capacity of the pelvis

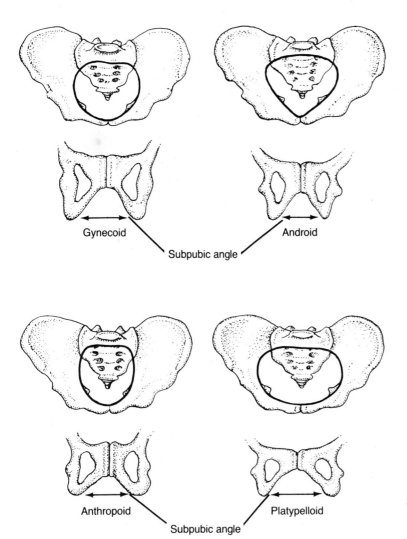

Figure 14–2
Caldwell-Moloy classification of pelves. (Reproduced by permission from *Biology of women* [2nd ed., p. 24] by Ethel Sloane. Albany, NY: Delmar Publishers Inc., Copyright 1985.)

(2) Important measurements
    (a) Obstetric conjugate of the inlet (Fig. 14–3)
       (i) Is the shortest diameter through which the baby must pass
      (ii) Extends from the middle of the sacral promontory to the posterior superior margin of the symphysis pubis
     (iii) Can be approximated by manually measuring the diagonal conjugate, extending from the subpubic angle to the middle of the sacral promontory, then subtracting 1.5 cm (0.6 in)
     (iv) Adequate measurement: 11.0 cm (4.4 in)
    (b) Transverse diameter between the ischial spines
       (i) The spines form the lateral boundaries of the pelvic cavity plane of least dimension (Fig. 14–4)
      (ii) Adequate measurement: 10.5 cm (4.2 in)
    (c) Subpubic angle (see Fig. 14–2)
       (i) Forms the apex of the anterior triangle of the pelvic outlet
      (ii) Adequate measurement: 90° or more
    (d) Bituberous diameter

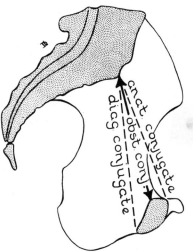

Figure 14–3
Obstetric conjugate. (From Oxorn, H. [1986]. *Oxorn-Foote human labor and birth* [5th ed., p. 29]. New York: Appleton & Lange.)

  (i) Transverse diameter of the pelvic outlet
  (ii) Adequate measurement: 11 cm (4.4 in)
(e) Posterior sagittal diameters (Fig. 14–5)
  (i) Extend from the intersection of the transverse and anteroposterior diameters to the posterior limit of the latter
  (ii) Represent the back portion of the anteroposterior diameters:
    ● Inlet: 4.5 cm (1.8 in)
    ● Cavity: 4.5 to 5.0 cm (1.8 to 2.0 in)
    ● Outlet: 9.0 cm (3.6 in)
(f) Curve and length of the sacrum
  (i) The sacrum forms the curved canal of the pelvic cavity
  (ii) Posterior wall should be deep and concave
  (iii) Sacrum should measure 10 to 15 cm (4 to 6 in)
(3) Maternal position
  (a) Posture influences pelvic size and contours
  (b) There is no correct position; each offers advantages and disadvantages

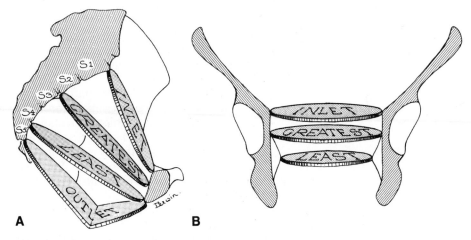

A   **B**

Figure 14–4
Pelvic cavity planes. (From Oxorn, H. [1986]. *Oxorn-Foote human labor and birth* [5th ed., p. 27]. New York: Appleton & Lange.)

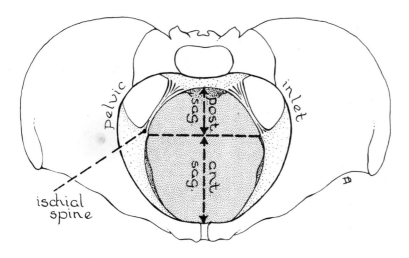

Figure 14–5
Posterior sagittal diameter. (From Oxorn, H. [1986]. *Oxorn-Foote human labor and birth* [5th ed., p. 29]. New York: Appleton & Lange.)

    (c) Dorsal or supine position
      (i) Position contributes to vena caval syndrome
      (ii) Position decreases intensity of uterine contractions
      (iii) Expulsive forces must work against gravity
      (iv) Lithotomy
        • Client is on her back, with her legs in stirrups
        • Mirror is required for client to see
        • Intervention by attendant is facilitated
      (v) Recumbent
        • Legs may be extended or knees flexed
        • Position decreases the ability of the client to push voluntarily
        • Position provides for ease of attendant
        • Position impedes the client's ability to see
    (d) Upright position
      (i) Position permits abdominal wall relaxation, which helps the fundus fall forward because of the force of gravity, causing straightening of the longitudinal axis of the birth canal
      (ii) Fetal head is directed to enter the pelvis in anterior position, which allows good application of the head to the cervix
      (iii) Fetal descent is enhanced
      (iv) Abdominal muscles work in synchrony with uterine contractions, maximizing expulsive forces
      (v) Client's ability to see the birth process is enhanced
      (vi) Position is technically more difficult for some attendants
      (vii) Squatting
        • Position enlarges the pelvic outlet by approximately 28%
        • Position induces a slight separation of the lower symphysis pubis, resulting in an enlarged outlet
        • Thighs are flexed and abducted, creating leverage on the innominate bones, thereby opening the bony outlet
        • Without the pressure of a bed, the sacrum and coccyx are easily pushed back by the descending fetus, thereby enlarging the outlet
        • Intra-abdominal pressure is increased by the pressure of the thighs on the abdomen
        • Pressure is evenly distributed to the perineum, reducing the need for episiotomy
        • Position may be tiring for the client to maintain
        • Position reduces visibility of perineum for the attendant

(viii) Sitting
- Position increases the pelvic diameters but not as much as squatting
- Position may increase edema of perineum

(ix) Standing
- Position is tiring for the client
- Position requires the assistance of two attendants or support persons

(e) Lateral position
(i) Relaxation of the pelvic muscles facilitates descent and rotation of the presenting part
(ii) Position avoids vena caval syndrome
(iii) Position is less efficient for expulsion
(iv) Position requires a support person to hold the anterior leg
(v) Position may impede interaction with the attendant or infant, since the delivery occurs at the woman's back

(f) Kneeling
(i) Position avoids vena caval syndrome
(ii) Kneeling assists rotation of a fetus in a posterior position
(iii) Position is tiring for the client
(iv) Position may reduce interaction with the infant, since the woman may be using her arms and hands to support herself

c. Cervical changes
(1) Effacement
(a) Shortening of the cervix
(b) Passive reduction in the length of the cervical canal from 2 cm (0.8 in) to a paper-thin orifice
(c) Internal os disappears as cervical canal is drawn up into the lower uterine segment
(d) In nulliparas, effacement generally begins before the onset of labor
(e) In multiparas, effacement may not begin until labor ensues
(2) Dilatation (Fig. 14–6)
(a) Opening of the external os
(b) Caused by two forces
(i) Pressure of the presenting part
(ii) Contraction and retraction of the uterine muscle

3. Diagnostic studies and techniques
a. Vaginal examination to assess cervical changes
(1) Effacement
(a) 0%: cervical canal is 2 cm (0.8 in) long
(b) 50%: cervical canal is 1 cm (0.4 in) long
(c) 100%: cervical canal is obliterated
(2) Dilatation
(a) 0 cm: external os is closed
(b) 10 cm (4 in): external os is fully dilated and will permit passage of the fetus
b. Manual determination of pelvic capacity
(1) Measurement of the diagonal conjugate permits calculation or estimation of the obstetric conjugate
(2) Engagement of the presenting part signals adequacy of the inlet but does not predict adequacy of the midpelvis or the pelvic outlet

PASSENGER

A. Assessment

1. History
a. Previous pregnancies
(1) Birth weight of previous children

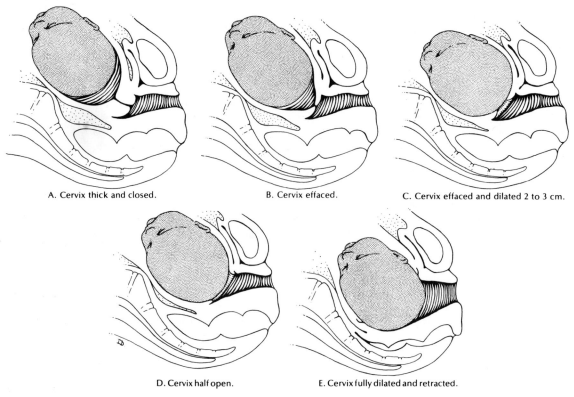

A. Cervix thick and closed.

B. Cervix effaced.

C. Cervix effaced and dilated 2 to 3 cm.

D. Cervix half open.

E. Cervix fully dilated and retracted.

Figure 14–6
Dilatation of the cervix. (From Oxorn, H. [1986]. *Oxorn-Foote human labor and birth* [5th ed., p. 119]. New York: Appleton & Lange.)

    (2) Malpresentation or disproportion encountered during previous labors
  b. Current pregnancy: unusual perceptions by the client that suggest a large infant or atypical positioning
2. Physical examination
  a. Fetal lie: relation of the long axis of the fetus to the long axis of the mother
    (1) Longitudinal lie: the long axes of the fetus and of the mother are parallel
    (2) Transverse or oblique lie: the long axis of the fetus is perpendicular to the long axis of the mother
  b. Fetal attitude: the relation of fetal parts to one another
    (1) Flexion: the typical fetal attitude in utero
    (2) Extension: tends to present larger fetal diameters
  c. Presentation: determined by the pole of the fetus that first enters the pelvic inlet
    (1) Cephalic: head first (95% of term deliveries)
    (2) Breech: pelvis first (3% of term deliveries)
    (3) Shoulder: shoulder first (2% of term deliveries)
  d. Presenting part
    (1) The specific fetal structure lying nearest to the cervix
    (2) Determined by the attitude of the fetus
    (3) Each presenting part has an identified denominator that is used to describe the fetal position in the pelvis
    (4) Cephalic presentations (Fig. 14–7)
      (a) Vertex (denominator is occiput)
        (i) Flexion
          • Normal fetal position, with baby's chin resting on its chest
          • Presents optimal fetal dimensions during labor
          • At term, the position of 95% of fetuses

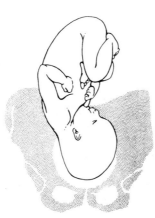

Vertex
(full flexion)

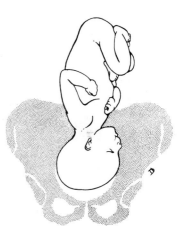

Vertex/"military"
(no flexion/no extension)

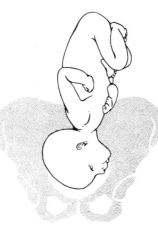

Frontum
(partial extension)

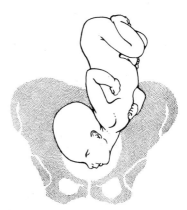

Face
(full extension)

Figure 14–7
Cephalic presentations. (From Oxorn, H. [1986]. *Oxorn-Foote human labor and birth* [5th ed., p. 55]. New York: Appleton & Lange.)

 (ii) No flexion and no extension
   ● Known as a "military attitude"
   ● Presents slightly larger diameters than full flexion
   ● Usually converts to flexion or full extension
   ● Prognosis for labor and delivery is generally favorable
(b) Frontum or brow (denominator is frontum)
 (i) Partial extension
 (ii) Incidence is less than 1%
 (iii) May be related to fetal anomaly
 (iv) May be associated with polyhydramnios or a small fetus
 (v) Presents relatively larger fetal diameters to pelvis
 (vi) Spontaneous delivery is possible if pelvis is large, contractions are adequate, and baby is small
 (vii) Delivery is expedited by conversion to vertex or face presentation
(c) Face (denominator is mentum/chin)
 (i) Full extension

(ii) Incidence is less than 1%

(iii) More frequent in multiparas

(iv) May be secondary to fetal factors that cause hyperextension, such as enlarged thyroid or multiple nuchal cords, for example

(v) Fetal diameters are essentially the same as a vertex presentation

(vi) Vaginal delivery is possible only if mentum is anterior

(5) Breech presentations (denominator is sacrum) (Fig. 14–8)

(a) Complete breech: flexion at hips, flexion at knees

(b) Frank breech: flexion at hips, extension at knees

(c) Footling breech: extension at one or both hips, extension at one or both knees

(d) Kneeling breech: extension at hips, flexion at knees

(e) Passage of meconium may occur secondary to pressure changes and does not necessarily indicate fetal stress or distress

(f) Associated with prematurity, placenta previa, multiparity, pelvic abnormality, and some congenital anomalies, such as hydrocephaly

(g) Associated with increased fetal mortality and morbidity

(i) Prematurity

(ii) Malformations

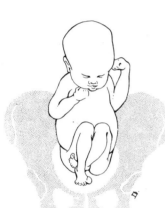

Complete
(hips flexed/knees flexed)

Frank
(hips flexed/knees extended)

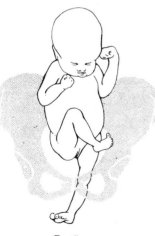

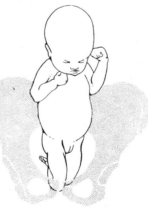

Footling
(hip extended/knee extended)

Kneeling
(hips extended/knees flexed)

Figure 14–8

Breech presentations. (From Oxorn, H. [1986]. *Oxorn-Foote human labor and birth* [5th ed., p. 57]. New York: Appleton & Lange.)

(iii) Asphyxia caused by prolonged compression of cord, prolapse of cord, or trauma to after-coming head, which does not have the opportunity to undergo molding

(iv) Injury to brain and skull, resulting in minute hemorrhages or fractures

(v) Trauma of manipulation during delivery, leading to cervical fractures, brachial plexus paralysis, liver rupture, and spinal cord traction

(h) Associated with protracted and dysfunctional labor

(6) Transverse presentation (Fig. 14–9)

    (a) Shoulder is the usual presenting part (denominator is scapula)

    (b) May be caused by anything that prevents descent of the head or the breech into the lower pelvis

        (i) Placenta previa

        (ii) Neoplasm

        (iii) Anomalies of the lower uterine segment

        (iv) Multiple gestation

        (v) Fetal anomalies

    (c) Associated with multigravidas, possibly secondary to increased relaxation of uterine and abdominal muscles

    (d) Vaginal delivery impossible without injury to mother and fetus

(7) Compound presentation

    (a) The infant assumes a unique posture, usually with the arm or the hand presenting alongside the presenting part

    (b) Presents increased fetal diameters

    (c) May interfere with the cardinal movements of labor

e. Fetal position

(1) The relation of the denominator to the maternal pelvis

(2) In practice, eight points are demarcated

(3) The denominator is assigned right or left, depending on which side of the maternal pelvis it is in

(4) The denominator is assigned anterior, posterior, or transverse according to maternal front, back, or side (Fig. 14–10)

(5) The occiput anterior position is most facilitative of vaginal delivery

(6) The occiput transverse position typically requires rotation to anterior or posterior position for delivery

(7) The occiput posterior position presents slightly larger diameters to pelvis

    (a) May slow progress of descent

    (b) Usually converts to anterior position during descent for delivery

    (c) An increased degree of internal rotation is required to align occiput beneath the maternal symphysis

    (d) Typically causes increased back pain during labor

f. Fetal station

(1) The relation of the presenting part to an imaginary line drawn between the ischial spines

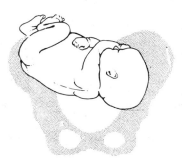

Figure 14–9
Transverse presentation. (From Oxorn, H. [1986]. *Oxorn-Foote human labor and birth* [5th ed., p. 57]. New York: Appleton & Lange.)

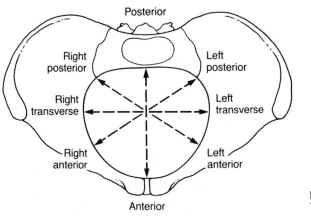

Figure 14–10
The pelvic diameters.

      (a) The ischial spines are 0 station
      (b) Above the spines is a negative value
      (c) Below the spines is a positive value
    (2) Engagement: when the widest diameter of the presenting part has passed the inlet
      (a) Usually corresponds to a 0 station
      (b) Actual station at engagement is influenced by the depth of the pelvis and the amount of caput succedaneum present
      (c) In primigravidas
        (i) Often occurs before labor
        (ii) When the fetus is unengaged at the outset of labor, disproportion is suggested
      (d) May occur anytime in multigravidas
    (3) Floating: when the presenting part is entirely out of the pelvis and freely movable in the inlet
    (4) Synclitism: when the biparietal diameter (BPD) of the fetal head is parallel to the planes of the maternal pelvis (Fig. 14–11)
    (5) Asynclitism: when the biparietal diameter is not parallel to the maternal pelvis (i.e., the fetal head appears tilted); may lead to a disproportion or delayed descent (see Fig. 14–11)
  g. Fetal size
    (1) Size alone is less significant than the relation between fetal size and pelvic dimensions
    (2) Macrosomia
      (a) Defined as birth weight above 4500 g (10 lb)
      (b) Incidence between 0.5% and 1.8%
      (c) Associated variables
        (i) Family history
        (ii) Multiparity
        (iii) Advanced maternal age
        (iv) Excessive maternal weight gain
        (v) Maternal diabetes
        (vi) Post-term gestation
        (vii) Male fetus
        (viii) Father of baby at least 10 years older than mother
      (d) Associated complications
        (i) Prolonged second stage of labor
        (ii) Maternal genital tract injury
        (iii) Postpartum hemorrhage related to atony
        (iv) Separation of pubic symphysis
        (v) Birth trauma

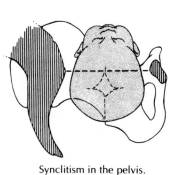
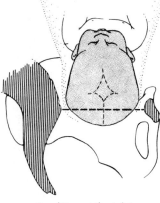

Synclitism in the pelvis.   Synclitism at the inlet.

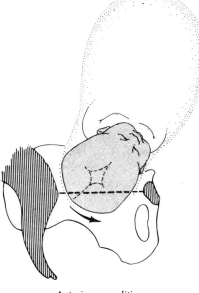

Anterior asynclitism.   Posterior asynclitism.

Figure 14–11
Synclitism and asynclitism. (From Oxorn, H. [1986]. *Oxorn-Foote human labor and birth* [5th ed., p. 71]. New York: Appleton & Lange.)

- Skull fracture
- Brachial plexus damage
- Clavicle fracture
- Asphyxia or depression

(3) Microsomia
　　(a) Typically occurs in the preterm gestation but may be associated with intrauterine growth retardation

(b) Associated with shortened second stage of labor

(c) May be possible to deliver the infant through an incompletely dilated cervix, predisposing to entrapment of the placenta or after-coming fetal parts and cervical lacerations or injury

(4) Fetal anomalies influencing fetal size

(a) Hydrocephalus

(b) Thyroid hypertrophy

(c) Abdominal distension secondary to kidney disease

(d) Omphalocele

(e) Myelocele

h. Fetal skull

(1) Is the most important structure, because it is the largest and least compressible

(2) Landmarks

(a) Cranial bones

(i) At birth, they are thin, poorly ossified, and easily compressible

(ii) Occipital: located posteriorly

(iii) Parietal (two): located laterally

(iv) Temporal (two): located anteriorly

(v) Frontal (two): located anteriorly

(b) Sutures

(i) The membranous tissue between the bones

(ii) Sagittal: lies between the parietal bones, in an anteroposterior direction

(iii) Lambdoidal: separates the occipital bone from the two parietal bones, and runs in a transverse direction

(iv) Coronal: separates the parietal bones from the frontal bones and runs in a transverse direction

(v) Frontal: lies between the frontal bones and is a continuation of the sagittal suture

(c) Fontanelles

(i) The intersections of the sutures

(ii) Anterior (bregma)

- Junction of the sagittal, frontal, and coronal sutures
- Diamond shaped, 3 × 2 cm (1 × 1 in)

(iii) Posterior (lambda)

- Junction of the sagittal and lambdoidal sutures
- Triangular shaped 1 × 2 cm (0.5 × 1 in)

(3) Molding

(a) The ability of the fetal head to change shape to accommodate the maternal pelvis

(b) Accomplished because of the lack of fusion of the cranial bones

(c) May decrease dimensions by 0.5 to 1.0 cm (0.2 to 0.4 in)

(4) Caput succedaneum

(a) Soft tissue edema caused by cervical pressure against the presenting head

(b) If severe, may obscure the suture lines, making determination of fetal position difficult

(c) May make determination of fetal station difficult

i. Cardinal movements

(1) The manner in which the baby moves and rotates to accommodate to the maternal pelvis

(2) Although often conceptualized as separate and sequential, the movements more typically occur concurrently

(3) Engagement and descent

(a) In nulliparas, engagement usually precedes the onset of labor, with additional descent occurring during labor

(b) In multiparas, engagement and descent may not occur before labor

   (c) Absence of descent in a primigravida may signal disproportion or malpresentation

   (d) The fetal head typically enters the pelvis with the sagittal suture aligned in the transverse diameter

   (e) Responsible for the subjective sensation felt by the mother as the fetus settles into the lower uterine segment—lightening; more commonly perceived by primigravidas

  (4) Flexion

   (a) Relative flexion is the natural posture of the fetus and is enhanced as the descending part encounters pelvic resistance

   (b) Flexion achieves the smallest fetal diameters presenting to the maternal pelvic dimensions

  (5) Internal rotation

   (a) Aligns the long axis of the fetal head with the long axis of the maternal pelvis (see Fig. 14–13)

   (b) The sagittal suture aligns in the anteroposterior diameter (see Fig. 14–5)

   (c) Occurs mainly during the second stage of labor

  (6) Extension

   (a) Resistance of the pelvic floor causes the presenting part to pivot beneath the symphysis pubis

   (b) Delivery is accomplished through extension of the head beneath the symphysis pubis

  (7) Restitution

   (a) The sagittal suture returns to an oblique diameter (see Fig. 14–5)

   (b) The oblique position realigns the sagittal suture with the fetal trunk axis

  (8) External rotation

   (a) Continuation of restitution, with the sagittal suture moving to a transverse diameter and the shoulders aligning in the anteroposterior diameter

   (b) The sagittal suture maintains alignment with the fetal trunk as the trunk navigates through the pelvis

  (9) Expulsion: after the delivery of the presenting part, the trunk typically follows easily

3. Diagnostic studies and techniques

 a. Leopold's maneuvers (Fig. 14–12)

  (1) Inspection and palpation of the maternal abdomen to determine the fetal position, station, and size

  (2) First maneuver: what is in the fundus?

   (a) Stand at the client's side and palpate the fundus

   (b) The head feels hard and smooth

   (c) The breech feels more irregular

  (3) Second maneuver: where is the back?

   (a) Face the client and place hands on the sides of her abdomen

   (b) The back feels firm and smooth

   (c) The small parts feel irregular

  (4) Third maneuver: what is the presenting part?

   (a) Move hands down the sides of the abdomen to grasp the lower uterine segment

   (b) The breech feels soft and irregular

   (c) The head feels globular and firm

  (5) Fourth maneuver: where is the cephalic prominence?

   (a) Face the client's feet and slide hands down the sides of the uterus to locate the side of greater resistance; this is the prominence

 b. Vaginal examination (Fig. 14–13)

  (1) Determine presentation

   (a) Cephalic

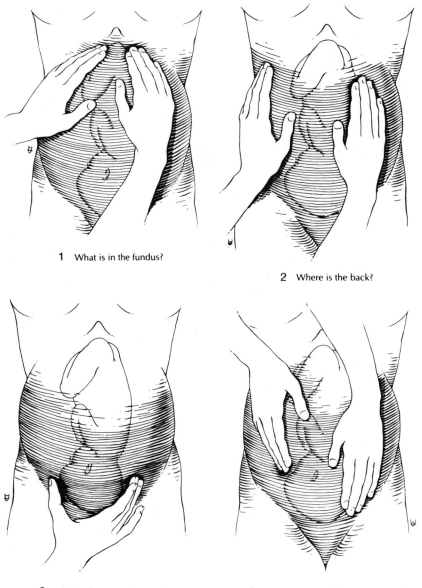

1 What is in the fundus?

2 Where is the back?

3 What is the presenting part?

4 Where is the cephalic prominence?

Figure 14–12
Leopold's maneuvers. (From Oxorn, H. [1986]. *Oxorn-Foote human labor and birth* [5th ed., pp. 77–79]. New York: Appleton & Lange.)

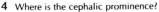

          (b) Breech
          (c) Shoulder
     (2) Determine station
          (a) Presenting part at level of ischial spines: 0 station
          (b) Presenting part above level of ischial spines: −1, −2, −3 cm station
          (c) Presenting part below level of ischial spines: +1, +2, +3 cm station
     (3) Determine position
          (a) Locate denominator by palpating sutures, facial features, or anatomical landmarks

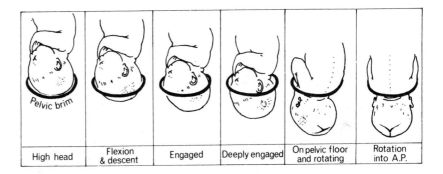

| High head | Flexion & descent | Engaged | Deeply engaged | On pelvic floor and rotating | Rotation into A.P. |

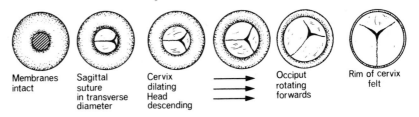

Membranes intact

Sagittal suture in transverse diameter

Cervix dilating Head descending

Occiput rotating forwards

Rim of cervix felt

Figure 14–13
Fetal head progressing through pelvis and changes in cervix. (From Myles, M.F. [1975]. *Textbook for nurse midwives* [p. 503]. Edinburgh: Churchill Livingstone.)

   (b) Define denominator in relation to the maternal pelvis (see Fig. 14–10)
c. Ultrasonography
   (1) Size
      (a) BPD measured with accuracy beginning at 13 weeks
      (b) BPD predictive of fetal age and fetal weight
   (2) Presentation: contents in lower pelvis identified
   (3) Morphology
      (a) Anencephaly demonstrated by lack of cerebral formation
      (b) Hydrocephaly suggested if BPD is greater than 11 cm (4.4 in)
      (c) Microcephaly may be suspected but can be difficult to diagnose
      (d) Anatomical structural defects may be recognizable

PSYCHE

A. Assessment

1. History
   a. Previous birth experiences
      (1) Complications of pregnancy, labor, and birth that occurred in previous pregnancies
      (2) Birth outcome of previous pregnancies
      (3) The degree to which the client's personal expectations for birth were achieved in previous pregnancies
   b. Current pregnancy experience
      (1) Planned versus unplanned pregnancy
         (a) A planned pregnancy imparts increased feelings of acceptance
         (b) An unplanned pregnancy may be accompanied by anger and rejection
      (2) Client age
         (a) Adolescent women must complete the developmental tasks of both adolescence and pregnancy

(b) Mature women are more accustomed to being in control of their lives and may be easily frustrated by the loss of control during pregnancy and birth

  (3) Difficulty in conceiving

    (a) Relative infertility may result in increased anxiety about the well-being of a "premium" pregnancy

    (b) Technology to assist conception and maintenance of the pregnancy may reduce a client's sense of involvement and control

  (4) Pregnancy discomforts may increase the client's anticipation of discomfort and difficulty during labor and birth

  (5) High-risk pregnancy

    (a) The client may experience increased anxiety and fears about her own well-being and the well-being of the fetus

    (b) The need for technology may interfere with the client's expectations for a natural birth

  (6) Completion of the developmental tasks of pregnancy: failure to complete the developmental tasks of pregnancy may result in increased fears and anxiety about the birth experience

c. Cultural considerations

  (1) Establish values and beliefs about sickness and health

  (2) Define the childbirth experience

    (a) Shameful versus joyful experience

    (b) Superstitions about pregnancy and birth

    (c) Prescribed behaviors and taboos influencing activities, food, and drink

  (3) Define kinship structure and relationships

    (a) Interaction between the couple

    (b) Parent–infant interactions

    (c) Role expectations of mother, father, and grandparents, for example

    (d) Involvement of support persons

    (e) Intergenerational behaviors

  (4) Define pain

    (a) Identifies the meaning and context of pain

    (b) Determines the acceptable response to pain (perceived pain is not always expressed as pain)

  (5) Determine the significance of touch

    (a) Soothing versus intruding

    (b) May be viewed as a symbol of intimacy

d. Expectations for birth experience

  (1) Childbirth can be viewed as either a meaningful or a stressful event

  (2) Goals can be realistic and attainable or too idealistic and in conflict with reality, thus leading to disappointment

  (3) Acceptable behavior for self and others is defined by cultural as well as other influences

  (4) Labor may be viewed as a test

e. Preparation for birth

  (1) Type of childbirth preparation

  (2) Familiarity with the institution and its policies and procedures

  (3) Type of relaxation techniques learned and practiced

f. Support system

  (1) The presence and support of a valued companion during birth is invaluable to most women

  (2) The woman's spouse or partner is the most frequently chosen labor companion

  (3) Additional support is often provided by the woman's mother and other female relatives

    (a) "Young" grandmothers may not be prepared to assume the grandparent role and thus may subconsciously withhold support

        (b) Grandparents may have misinformation and misperceptions, and may need knowledge of current practices

    (4) Religious values and spiritual faith also provide a supportive structure

2. Psychosocial responses

  a. Emotions of labor

    (1) Latent phase

      (a) Is excited

      (b) Is ready for anything

      (c) Experiences anxiety and fear

    (2) Active phase

      (a) Has decreased energy

      (b) Experiences fatigue

      (c) Turns attention to internal sensations

      (d) Feels serious

    (3) Transition

      (a) Is discouraged

      (b) Is irritable, nasty

      (c) Is panicky, overwhelmed by fears of death

      (d) Is impatient

      (e) Feels out of control

    (4) Second stage

      (a) Is focused

      (b) Has increased energy, though still fatigued

      (c) May have subconscious desire to hold on to the pregnancy that can lead to decreased pushing efforts

      (d) Is gratified that she can actively participate to bring about birth

    (5) Immediate postpartum period

      (a) Experiences joy and relief

        (i) Is able to see and hold baby

        (ii) Is eager to share the news with others

      (b) Begins grief work

        (i) Experiences loss of valued object (the pregnancy)

        (ii) Experiences loss of valued status (as a pregnant woman)

        (iii) May feel sense of failure at not achieving own expectations for labor and birth

        (iv) Experiences loss of some aspect of self

- Altered body image
- Changed self-esteem
- Changed self-concept
- Loss of former role

      (c) Fatigue: finally able to sleep after hours of work

  b. Psychological reactions to labor

    (1) Anxiety

      (a) Anxiety is defined as an uneasiness in response to a vague, nonspecific threat

      (b) At mild-to-moderate levels, anxiety is an effective stimulant to action

      (c) Excessive anxiety interferes with labor

      (d) Somatic cues

        (i) Muscular pain and stiffness (especially in neck and back)

        (ii) Chest pain or tightness

        (iii) Nausea

        (iv) Flushing

        (v) Numbness in hands and face

      (e) Behavioral cues

        (i) Crying, tearfulness

        (ii) Tremulous voice

        (iii) Inability to focus or concentrate

        (iv) Jitteriness

      (f) Physiological cues
        (i) Elevated blood pressure
        (ii) Elevated heart rate
        (iii) Dilated pupils
        (iv) Diarrhea
   (2) Fear
      (a) Fear is defined as a painful, uneasy feeling in response to an identifiable threat
      (b) Possible intrapartum threats
        (i) Labor is an unknown despite the best of preparations
        (ii) Maternal or fetal injury during labor and birth
        (iii) Pain
        (iv) Institutional procedures (e.g., IVs, shave preparation, enema, fetal monitor)
        (v) Impending irreversible lifestyle changes created by the birth of a baby
      (c) Fear causes peripheral vasoconstriction that may decrease uterine blood flow, decreasing uterine contractility
      (d) Fear typically enhances pain perception, leading to increased fear
   (3) Loss of control and sense of helplessness
      (a) For many, childbirth is first hospitalization
      (b) Personal belongings and clothing are removed
      (c) Routine procedures are unfamiliar and intimidating
      (d) Most clients recognize that, at some point in the labor process, they must depend on others for assistance
   (4) Feelings of aloneness or abandonment
      (a) Removal from familiar home environment
      (b) Restriction of support system
      (c) Changing patterns of communication
        (i) Increased reliance on nonverbal messages
          • Vision
          • Touch
          • Facial expression
          • Body movements
          • Vocal quality
        (ii) When verbal and nonverbal messages are out of synchrony, nonverbal communications are usually more accurate
        (iii) As labor progresses, most women turn inward, which may lead to distorted message reception
      (d) Isolation may decrease reality orientation, leading to increased anxiety and fear
   (5) Fatigue and weariness
      (a) Etiological factors
        (i) Sleep deprivation
        (ii) Sensory overload
        (iii) Generalized fatigue, which is common in late pregnancy
        (iv) Energy expended during labor
      (b) Fatigue generally leads to reduced energy and inability to focus and concentrate
      (c) Fatigue may decrease myometrial activity
 c. Coping strategies
   (1) There is no one correct style or technique
   (2) Controlling
      (a) The client seeks the opportunity to have influence in the decisions regarding her care
      (b) The client explores the options and alternatives in a given situation
      (c) The client relies on her knowledge base and relaxation skills

(d) The client's belief that she will succeed is affirmed

(e) Inability to participate in decision making leads to conflict

(3) Optimistic

    (a) The client freely releases the surge of energy that is generated by her emotions and feelings

    (b) The client smiles, laughs, cries, and demonstrates increased activity levels

    (c) The client accepts the expertise and assistance of those around her

    (d) The client demonstrates basic trust in the outcome

(4) Fatalistic

    (a) The client focuses on her perceived loss of control

    (b) The client avoids choosing options and participating in decision making

    (c) The client becomes preoccupied with details

    (d) The client has a heightened perception of danger, leading to increased fears

    (e) The client displays hostility, aggression, and withdrawal

    (f) The client demonstrates generalized distrust in the outcome and therefore views her own actions and those of others as meaningless

B. Nursing Diagnoses

1. Anxiety realted to
   a. Possible fetal conditions that are hindering labor
   b. A strange environment
   c. The disruption of normal routines and support systems
   d. The situational crisis of labor
2. Ineffective individual coping related to
   a. The situational crisis of labor
   b. Inadequate support systems or the absence of a support person
   c. Conflict between personal and cultural expectations and the health care system's practices
3. Fear related to
   a. The unknown of labor
   b. The threat of potential harm to self or fetus
   c. The anticipation of pain during labor
4. High risk for infection related to the use of an intrauterine pressure catheter (IUPC)
5. High risk for injury (fetal trauma, uterine trauma, cervical trauma, fetal distress or asphyxia) related to malpresentation
6. Knowledge deficit about the birthing process related to
   a. Inadequate preparation
   b. Unanticipated circumstances
7. Alteration in self-esteem related to
   a. Ineffective uterine contraction pattern
   b. Possible reduced pelvic capacity
   c. Impairment of the cardinal movements
8. Sensory perceptual alteration related to
   a. The physiological process of labor
   b. Invasive technology
   c. Multiple environmental distractors
9. Social isolation related to
   a. Changing patterns of communication
   b. An unfamiliar environment
   c. Inadequate support systems

C. Interventions/Evaluations

1. Anxiety related to possible fetal conditions that are hindering labor; a strange

environment; the disruption of normal routines and support systems; and the situational crisis of labor

a. Interventions
   (1) Therapeutic interventions
      (a) Provide the client with factual information about the baby's condition
         (i) Fetal heart rate
         (ii) Information regarding size and morphology gained from ultrasound examination
      (b) Reassure the client that cephalopelvic disproportion is not necessarily caused by fetal abnormalities
      (c) Encourage the client to avoid engaging in unrealistic fantasies about the baby
      (d) Explain all procedures and interventions to the client
      (e) Provide a quiet, restful environment with minimal stimulation
      (f) Remain with the client as much as possible
      (g) Be direct and specific in communicating with the client, offering her a limited number of options
      (h) Speak and behave calmly
      (i) Do not communicate one's own problems and concerns to the client
      (j) Encourage the client to remain focused on now and to avoid a past or future orientation
   (2) Diagnostic interventions
      (a) Obtain blood pressure, pulse, and respiration readings every 4 hours or as appropriate for the stage of labor
      (b) On an ongoing basis, evaluate the client's concerns about her fetus's well-being
      (c) On an ongoing basis, evaluate the client's ability to focus and concentrate
      (d) On an ongoing basis, evaluate the client's ability to respond to messages
      (e) On an ongoing basis, determine the synchrony between the client's verbal and nonverbal communications
b. Evaluations
   (1) The client demonstrates minimal anxiety as evidenced by
      (a) Having vital signs within normal limits
      (b) Verbalizing realistic expectations about the baby's condition
      (c) Using relaxation techniques
      (d) Verbalizing confidence in the health care providers
      (e) Understanding and responding correctly to messages
      (f) Demonstrating logical thought processes

2. Ineffective individual coping related to the situational crisis of labor; inadequate support systems or absence of a support person; conflict between personal and cultural expectations; and the health care system's practices
a. Interventions
   (1) Therapeutic interventions
      (a) Reinforce or teach relaxation techniques
      (b) Keep the client informed about her condition and her progress
      (c) Explain all procedures and interventions
      (d) Assist the client in identifying her strengths, and praise her for her demonstration of adaptive coping skills
      (e) Provide physical comfort measures
         (i) Cool cloth
         (ii) Mouthwash
         (iii) Back rub
         (iv) Sponge bath
         (v) Pillows

(f) Control the environment to minimize sensory overload and intrusion

(g) Remain with the client as much as possible

(h) Identify things within the client's control and encourage her to be involved

(i) Be direct in communicating with the client

(j) Support the support person

(i) Provide nourishment

(ii) Provide episodic relief from responsibility

(iii) Provide praise and encouragement

(k) Discuss with the client her expectations and values and integrate them into the labor experience as much as possible

(2) Diagnostic interventions

(a) On an ongoing basis, evaluate the client's use of relaxation techniques

(b) On an ongoing basis, evaluate the client's patterns of communication

(c) On an ongoing basis, evaluate the client's ability to receive and use information that is provided

(d) On an ongoing basis, evaluate the client's degree of satisfaction with the experience

b. Evaluations

(1) The client demonstrates effective coping as evidenced by

(a) Verbalizing her perception that she is coping with the labor process

(b) Participating in decision making about her own basic needs

(c) Using relaxation techniques in response to painful stimuli

(d) Communicating effectively with her support person and health care personnel

3. Fear related to the unknown of labor; the threat of potential harm to self or the fetus; and the anticipation of the pain of labor

a. Interventions

(1) Therapeutic interventions

(a) Orient the client to the surroundings

(b) Familiarize the client with the usual routines and procedures, and keep her informed about what to expect

(c) Remain with the client as much as possible

(d) Inform the client of her status and progress, offering reassurance when everything is normal

(2) Diagnostic interventions

(a) Obtain blood pressure, pulse, and respiration readings every 4 hours, or as appropriate for the state of labor and the client's labor progress

(b) On an ongoing basis, identify the client's concerns and expectations

(c) On an ongoing basis, determine the client's understanding of what is happening

b. Evaluations

(1) The client demonstrates minimal fear as evidenced by

(a) Having vital signs within normal limits

(b) Verbalizing a realistic and accurate perception of the labor experience

(c) Verbalizing a perception of being in a comforting environment

(d) Verbalizing confidence in the health care providers' ability to safeguard her well-being

4. High risk for infection related to the use of an intrauterine pressure catheter

a. Interventions

(1) Therapeutic interventions

(a) Use aseptic technique when assembling the pressure catheter

(b) Maintain asepsis during insertion of the pressure catheter

(c) Use aseptic technique during vaginal examinations

(d) Limit vaginal examinations to those necessary for clinical decision making

(2) Diagnostic interventions

(a) Every 2 to 4 hours, or as indicated by the stage of labor and the client's clinical status, obtain temperature

(b) As appropriate to the client's stage of labor and clinical status, assess fetal heart rate

(c) On an ongoing basis, assess characteristics of amniotic fluid

(d) On an ongoing basis, assess for uterine tenderness

(e) On an ongoing basis, monitor laboratory results

b. Evaluations

(1) The client does not develop chorioamnionitis as evidenced by

(a) Temperature is within normal limits for parturition

(b) Fetal heart rate is within normal limits

(c) Amniotic fluid is not foul smelling

(d) Uterus is relaxed and nontender between contractions

(e) White blood count is within normal limits for parturition

5. High risk for injury (fetal trauma, uterine trauma, cervical trauma, fetal asphyxia) related to malpresentation

a. Interventions

(1) Therapeutic interventions

(a) Report breech, transverse, and compound presentations promptly to the physician or nurse midwife

(b) Report arrest of the cardinal movements to the physician or nurse midwife

(c) Prepare the client for cesarean delivery as directed by the physician

(2) Diagnostic interventions

(a) As appropriate to the client's stage of labor and clinical status, perform a vaginal examination to assess presentation, station, and position

(b) As appropriate to the client's stage of labor and clinical status, assess fetal heart rate

(c) On an ongoing basis, assess for uterine tenderness

b. Evaluations

(1) The client and her baby are not injured as evidenced by

(a) No uterine rupture

(b) No cervical or vaginal lacerations

(c) No newborn birth trauma

(d) Newborn 5-minute Apgar score is greater than 7

6. Knowledge deficit about the birthing process related to inadequate preparation and unanticipated circumstances

a. Interventions

(1) Therapeutic interventions

(a) Explain the principles of labor and birth as related to the client's specific circumstances

(b) Explain all procedures

(c) Encourage the client to ask questions

(d) Answer questions honestly and promptly

(e) Identify changes in the client's status that might be misunderstood and offer anticipatory education

(2) Diagnostic interventions: on an ongoing basis, determine the client's level of comprehension

b. Evaluations

(1) The client understands the birthing process as evidenced by

(a) Describing accurately what is happening and what is expected to happen

(b) Asking questions which are reality oriented
7. Alteration in self-esteem related to ineffective uterine contraction pattern; possible reduced pelvic capacity; and impairment of the cardinal movements
  a. Interventions
    (1) Therapeutic interventions
      (a) Facilitate effective uterine contractions
        (i) Encourage the client to walk about as much as possible
        (ii) When the client is in bed, assist her to a lateral position with the head of the bed slightly elevated, using pillows and other supports
      (b) Promote maximum pelvic capacity and fetal descent and rotation
        (i) Assist the client to assume adaptive positions
- Upright
- Squatting
- Sitting
- Modified knee–chest
        (ii) Encourage the client to change position frequently
      (c) Provide the client with encouragement and support
        (i) Review the normal variations in labor patterns
        (ii) Provide positive feedback regarding
- Improved contraction strength
- Increasing frequency of contractions
- Increasing duration of contractions
- Fetal descent and rotation
        (iii) Provide positive feedback for the client's attempts to use alternate positions
        (iv) Remind the client that absolute pelvic measurements are less important than the relation between the pelvis and the baby
      (d) Permit the client to exercise autonomy by allowing her to determine positions of comfort
    (2) Diagnostic interventions
      (a) On an ongoing basis, assess the client's level of satisfaction with her labor
      (b) On an ongoing basis, assess the client's feelings of self-worth
  b. Evaluations
    (1) The client demonstrates positive self-esteem as evidenced by
      (a) Verbalizing satisfaction and contentment with the progress of her labor
      (b) Verbalizing statements of self-worth
8. Sensory perceptual alteration related to the physiological process of labor; invasive technology; and multiple environmental distractors
  a. Interventions
    (1) Therapeutic interventions
      (a) Eliminate unnecessary lights and noises
      (b) Remove unnecessary equipment and supplies from the bedside
      (c) Avoid unnecessary conversation at the bedside
      (d) Speak calmly, quietly, and slowly to the client
      (e) Provide a single source of sensory input
        (i) Music through earphones (in some clients, the use of earphones may contribute to isolation from her support system and health care providers)
        (ii) A focus point
    (2) Diagnostic interventions
      (a) On an ongoing basis, determine the client's reaction to the environment
      (b) On an ongoing basis, determine the client's patterns of communication

(c) On an ongoing basis, determine the client's problem-solving abilities
  b. Evaluations
    (1) The client does not suffer sensory overload as evidenced by
        (a) Describing self and situation accurately
        (b) Resting quietly between contractions, without restlessness, withdrawal, or agitation
        (c) Participating in decision making about her own basic needs
 9. Social isolation related to changing patterns of communication; an unfamiliar environment; and inadequate support systems
  a. Interventions
    (1) Therapeutic interventions
        (a) Encourage the client to express her thoughts and feelings
        (b) Respond to both verbal and nonverbal communications
        (c) Validate the messages being received
        (d) Decrease environmental distractions
        (e) Speak in a simple, focused manner
        (f) Communicate with the client in her own communication mode
            (i) Return eye contact
            (ii) Return touch
            (iii) Answer questions
    (2) Diagnostic interventions
        (a) On an ongoing basis, determine the client's patterns of communication
        (b) On an ongoing basis, determine the client's degree of satisfaction with the experience
  b. Evaluations
    (1) The client experiences adequate interaction with support persons and health care providers as evidenced by verbalizing that her messages are being understood and her needs being met

Health Education

A. Optimizing labor power

1. Encourage normal activity and exercise patterns throughout pregnancy
   a. Women with generally well-toned musculature tend to have more efficient uterine contractions
   b. Good abdominal musculature assists during the second stage of labor
   c. Women who exercise are generally more aware of their bodies and can more effectively control pushing efforts
2. Instruct the client in exercises specific to pregnancy and childbearing
   a. Kegel exercise to tone perineal floor
   b. Pelvic tilt to tone abdominal muscles and relieve backache (Fig. 14–14)
   c. Adductor stretching to tone thighs (tailor sitting)
3. Instruct the client in intrapartum activities that strengthen uterine effort
   a. Walking and remaining active as long as possible
   b. Lateral positions and an elevated head of the bed improve regularity and intensity of contractions
   c. Avoid supine hypotension, which leads to decreased uterine blood flow and decreased muscle strength

B. Maximizing labor passage

1. Instruct the client in postures that increase pelvic capacity
2. Instruct support person in techniques to achieve alternative postures
3. Encourage the client to change positions frequently during labor
   a. Provides dynamic pelvic capacity, which facilitates fetal passage
   b. Avoids excessive stress and tension on a single muscle group

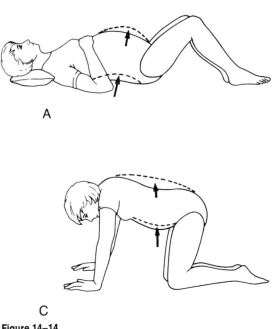

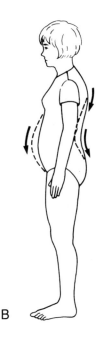

Figure 14–14
Pelvic tilt.

C. Emotional preparation for birth
1. Encourage attendance at childbirth preparation classes
2. Support self-study efforts, such as books and videos
3. Encourage rehearsal of coping strategies and relaxation techniques
4. Encourage guidance and support of family members

CASE STUDIES AND STUDY QUESTIONS

Primigravida in Early Labor

Sarah Williams is a 37-year-old G1 who began experiencing irregular contractions late Tuesday afternoon. Throughout Tuesday evening, she and her husband, Tom, diligently timed each contraction. They were very excited that labor had begun. They were equally excited that the baby's arrival had waited until the end of the academic year. Sarah had recently been promoted to associate professor, and she took great pride in personally reviewing all of her students' papers before issuing final grades.

Near midnight, the contractions were 3 to 4 minutes apart and lasted 45 to 50 seconds. Sarah's discomfort was increasing, although she remained able to focus on the relaxation breathing techniques she had learned. Tom was becoming tired, but he remained excited and eager to time each new contraction. When her membranes ruptured at 12:30 A.M.,

she phoned her physician, confident that her baby would be born soon.

Sarah and Tom arrived in labor and delivery at 1:10 A.M. Wednesday morning. On arrival, Sarah provided the nurse with a detailed summary of the previous 8 hours. She also shared with the nurse her goals for the birth experience, which included being permitted to breastfeed immediately after birth and going home as soon as possible. She was obviously uncomfortable with contractions, but she used her breathing techniques well.

The nurse escorted the couple to a labor/delivery/recovery (LDR) room, oriented them to the hospital environment, and assisted Sarah's changing into a hospital gown. Her initial assessment findings included
a. Maternal vital signs within normal limits.
b. Fetal heart rate of 136.
c. Contractions every 4 to 5 minutes, lasting 45 to 50 seconds, and of moderate intensity.

d. Cervix 100% effaced and 3 to 4 cm dilated.

e. Baby at 0 station, in the ROA position.

When the nurse informed Sarah and Tom of her findings, Sarah was obviously distressed and disappointed, "How can I be only 3 cm? I've been in labor for hours. I should be almost finished by now." As she spoke, she became increasingly agitated, and each new contraction heightened her frustration. She became restless and had difficulty in implementing her breathing techniques.

1. What factor is most responsible for Sarah's reaction to the nurse's information?

a. Maternal age.

b. The frequency and duration of her contractions.

c. Unrealistic expectations.

d. Her unfamiliarity with the hospital environment.

2. How should the nurse respond to Sarah?

a. Remind Sarah that first babies usually take 18 to 24 hours.

b. Assist Sarah in resuming the relaxation techniques she had been using on admission.

c. Inform Sarah that the physician will be contacted to obtain something to help her relax.

d. Obtain additional information about Sarah's birth plans.

3. How can the nurse assist Sarah to cope adaptively with her labor and birth?

a. Provide Sarah with information and support.

b. Leave Sarah and Tom alone as much as possible.

c. Share with Sarah her own birth experience.

d. Teach Sarah how to time her contractions.

4. What immediate intervention does Tom require?

a. Provision of scrub attire.

b. Information about the early discharge procedure.

c. Instruction about how to time contractions.

d. Information about how best to support Sarah.

Primigravida, Multiple Gestation

Joe and Judy Cannon, a couple in their mid-twenties, were thrilled when they first learned that Judy was pregnant. They had been married for more than a year, and Judy had quit her job at the local bookstore shortly after their marriage in anticipation of raising a family. Both came from large families, and they hoped to continue the tradition. Despite their desire for children and plans for a large family, they were shocked when the physician informed them that they were expecting twins.

As the shock faded, Judy began to revel in the specialness of her pregnancy and enjoyed the extra attention that her friends and family paid her. She was unprepared, however, for the increased discomfort she experienced. Her physician reassured her that both fetuses were healthy and that everything was normal, yet with each new sensation she worried that something was wrong.

At 37 weeks of gestation, Judy began having contractions. She phoned her physician immediately and went to the hospital.

On admission to labor and delivery, Judy was quiet and reserved. She told the nurse that her contractions had begun 2 hours earlier. Joe drove a delivery truck, and the company was trying to contact him to meet her at the hospital. She had tried to phone her mother but was unable to reach her at home. The nurse also learned that Judy and Joe had not attended childbirth preparation classes. According to Judy, "My husband's schedule is very unpredictable, and I couldn't go alone. Besides, most of the time I didn't have the energy to do much of anything."

The nurse's assessment revealed

a. Blood pressure 144/86, pulse 88, respirations 20.

b. Fetal heart tones, 124 in right lower quadrant (RLQ) and 136 in right upper quadrant (RUQ).

c. Contractions every 10 minutes, lasting 20 seconds, and of mild intensity.

d. Cervix 80% effaced and 4 cm dilated.

e. Fetus A presented vertex, at 0 station; fetus B also was vertex.

5. What factors should the nurse identify that may be contributing to Judy's anxiety level?

   (1) Her lack of attendance at childbirth preparation classes.

   (2) Multiple gestation.

   (3) Maternal age.

   (4) Inadequate support system.

   a. 1, 3.

   b. 1, 2, 4.

   c. 1, 3, 4.

   d. All of the above.

6. What should the nurse do first to minimize Judy's anxiety?

   a. Notify the physician, and obtain an order for medication.

   b. Instruct Judy in childbirth preparation information.

   c. Permit Judy to listen to the fetal hearts, and reassure her that the fetuses are doing well.

   d. Remain with Judy.

7. What is the significance of fetus A's station?

   a. Suggestive of pelvic adequacy.

   b. Indicative of malpresentation.

   c. Suggestive of a short labor.

   d. Indicative of the need to prepare for cesarean delivery.

8. What actions can the nurse take to increase the likelihood of a vaginal delivery?

   (1) Encourage Judy to walk around during the early stage of labor.

   (2) Keep Judy in bed, with the head of the bed slightly elevated.

   (3) Assist Judy in assuming upright positions.

   (4) Assist Judy with relaxation breathing techniques.

   a. 1, 3.

   b. 2, 3, 4.

   c. 2, 4.

   d. All of the above.

9. At the outset of her labor, what information would best assist Judy in coping adaptively?

   (1) An explanation of the procedures she should expect.

   (2) A discussion of the anatomy and physiology of labor.

   (3) A description of the institution's policies about support persons' attendance at cesarean birth

   (4) Instruction in relaxation techniques.

   a. 1, 3.

   b. 1, 2, 4.

   c. 1, 3, 4.

   d. All of the above.

Multigravida, Active Labor

Carol Anderson is a 34-year-old, 41-week-gestation, gravida 3, para 2 (G3,P2) who arrived in labor and delivery on Friday morning at 10:20 A.M. She states that when she awoke she noticed some pelvic heaviness, but that she ignored it as she got her 9-year-old and 6-year-old off to school. Once the house was quiet, she became aware that she was contracting regularly, though she describes the contractions as mild and cramplike. Because her previous labors were quick (first pregnancy, 11 hours; second pregnancy, 4 hours), Carol went right to the hospital without notifying her physician or husband: "The last time, it was over almost before it had begun."

Throughout the admission process, Carol remained calm. When the nurse was finished, she remarked, "Well, I guess I should call my husband if I expect him to get here in time."

Admission assessment includes

a. Maternal vital signs within normal limits.

b. Fetal heart tones 148/RLQ.

c. Contractions every 5 to 6 minutes, 30 to 45 seconds, and of mild-to-moderate intensity.

d. Cervix 70% effaced and 2 cm dilated.

e. Fetal position in right occiput posterior (ROP), at a −1 station.

10. What additional findings would reassure the nurse that Carol was in true labor?

    (1) The presence of a bloody show.

    (2) Bulging membranes.

(3) A progressive increase in the length of time between contractions.

(4) A progressive increase in the duration of the contractions.

a. 1, 3.

b. 1, 3, 4.

c. 1, 2, 4.

d. All of the above.

11. What is the significance of the baby's station and position?

a. Of little significance at this time.

b. Suggestive of cephalopelvic disproportion.

c. Suggestive of a prolonged labor.

d. Indicative of the need to prepare for cesarean delivery.

12. What additional assessments would be helpful to the nurse in planning care for the family?

(1) The gestational age and birth weight of Carol's previous deliveries.

(2) The time and amount of Carol's last oral intake.

(3) Carol's preparation for this birth experience.

(4) Carol's expectations about pain management.

a. 1, 3.

b. 1, 2, 4.

c. 1, 3, 4.

d. All of the above.

13. Which cardinal movement is most affected when a baby is occiput posterior?

a. Flexion.

b. Internal rotation.

c. Extension.

d. External rotation.

14. Which factors may contribute to the baby's presenting occiput posterior?

(1) Maternal pelvic shape.

(2) Maternal age.

(3) Fetal size.

(4) Postmaturity.

a. 1, 3.

b. 2, 3, 4.

c. 2, 4.

d. All of the above.

ADDITIONAL STUDY QUESTIONS

15. Which of the following are characteristic of the powers of the first stage of labor?

(1) Controlled by the involuntary nervous system.

(2) Responsible for cervical effacement and dilatation.

(3) Responsive to nursing interventions.

(4) Quantified by calculating frequency times intensity.

a. 1, 3.

b. 1, 2, 4.

c. 1, 3, 4.

d. All of the above.

16. True or false: Women should be encouraged to go through labor in the upright position because this is the most correct posture for childbirth.

17. Which of the following describe the delivery of a macrosomic baby?

(1) The infant is at increased risk of birth trauma.

(2) Prolonged labor is likely.

(3) The mother is at increased risk of birth trauma.

(4) Postpartum hemorrhage is likely.

a. 1, 3.

b. 1, 2, 4.

c. 1, 3, 4.

d. All of the above.

18. Which of the following are characteristic of the anxiety and fear experienced during labor?

    (1) Results in an elevated blood pressure and pulse rate.

    (2) Results in an improved ability to concentrate.

    (3) Results in increased pain perception.

    (4) May prolong labor.

    a. 1, 3.

    b. 1, 2, 4.

    c. 1, 3, 4.

    d. All of the above.

19. Which of the following nursing interventions are indicated to reduce sensory overload?

(1) Keep the room's lighting subdued.

(2) Speak quietly and calmly to the client and her support person.

(3) Provide music in the room.

(4) Avoid doing a procedure during a contraction.

a. 1, 3.

b. 1, 2, 4.

c. 1, 3, 4.

d. All of the above.

Answers to Study Questions

1. c	2. b	3. a
4. d	5. b	6. d
7. a	8. d	9. b
10. c	11. c	12. c
13. b	14. a	15. d
16. True	17. d	18. c
19. b		

REFERENCES

Anderson, C. (1976). Operational definition of "support." *Journal of Obstetric, Gynecologic, and Neonatal Nursing, 5*(1), 17–18.

Angelini, D. (1978). Body boundaries: Concerns of laboring women. *Maternal-Child Nursing Journal, 7*(1), 41–46.

Bates, B., & Turner, A.N. (1985). Imagery and symbolism in the birth practices of traditional cultures. *Birth, 12*(1), 29–35.

Block, C., & Block, R. (1975). The effect of support of the husband and obstetrician on pain perception and control in childbirth. *Birth and the Family Journal, 2*(2), 43–47.

Bobak, I., & Jensen, M.D. (1991). *Essentials of maternity nursing* (3rd ed). St. Louis: Mosby.

Chiota, B.J., Goolkasian, P., & Ladewig, P. (1976). Effects of separation from spouse on pregnancy, labor and delivery, and the postpartum period. *Journal of Obstetric, Gynecologic, and Neonatal Nursing, 5*(1), 21–23.

Clark, A. (1978). *Culture, childbearing, health professionals.* Philadelphia: Davis.

Clark, A., & Affonso, D. (Eds.). (1979). *Childbearing: A nursing perspective* (2nd ed.). Philadelphia: Davis.

Coleman, A., & Coleman, L. (1978). *Pregnancy: The psychological experience* (2nd ed.). New York: Bantam.

Fenwick, L., & Simkin, P. (1987). Maternal positioning to prevent or alleviate dystocia in labor. *Clinical Obstetrics and Gynecology, 30*(1), 83–89.

Friedman, E.A. (1978). *Labor: Clinical evaluation and management* (2nd ed.). New York: Appleton-Century-Crofts.

Gay, J. (1978). Theories regarding endocrine contributions to the onset of labor. *Journal of Obstetric, Gynecologic, and Neonatal Nursing, 7*(5), 42–47.

Harris, C.J. (1985). Rheumatoid arthritis and the pregnant woman. *American Journal of Nursing, 85*(4), 414–417.

Horn, M., & Manion, J. (1985). Creative grandparenting: Bonding the generations. *Journal of Obstetric, Gynecologic, and Neonatal Nursing, 14*(3), 233–236.

Jordan, B. (1978). The hut and the hospital: Information, power, and symbolism in the artifacts of birth. *Birth, 14*(1), 36–40.

Lehrman, E. (1985). Birth in the left lateral position: An alternative to the traditional delivery position. *Journal of Nurse-Midwifery, 30*(4), 193–197.

Liu, Y.C. (1989). The effects of the upright position during childbirth. *Image, 21*(1), 14–18.

Mackey, M.C., & Lock, S.E. (1989). Women's expectations of the labor and delivery nurse. *Journal of Obstetric, Gynecologic, and Neonatal Nursing, 18*(6), 505–512.

McKay, S. (1984). Squatting: An alternative position for the second stage of labor. *MCN: American Journal of Maternal Child Nursing, 9*(3), 181–183.

McKay, S., & Mahan, C. (1980). Laboring patients need more freedom to move. *Contemporary Obstetrics and Gynecology, 18*(7), 90–116.

Meissner, J.E. (1980). Predicting a patient's anxiety level during labor: A two-part assessment tool. *Nursing '80, 10*(7), 50–51.

Meleis, A., & Sorrell, L. (1981). Arab-American women and their birth experience. *MCN: American Journal of Maternal Child Nursing, 6*(5), 171–176.

Olds, S., London, M., & Ladewig, P. (1988). *Maternal-newborn nursing.* Menlo Park, CA: Addison-Wesley.

Oxorn, H. (1986). *Human labor and birth* (5th ed.). New York: Appleton-Century-Crofts.

Paciornik, M. (1990). Commentary: Arguments against episiotomy and in favor of squatting for birth. *Birth, 17*(2), 104–105.

Pillitteri, A. (1985). Maternal-newborn nursing: Care of the growing family (3rd ed.). Boston: Little, Brown.

Pritchard, J., MacDonald, P., & Gant, M. (1985). *Williams obstetrics* (17th ed.). New York: Appleton-Century-Crofts.

Roberts, J. (1980). Alternative positions for childbirth. Part I: First stage of labor. *Journal of Nurse-Midwifery, 25*(4), 11–18.

Roberts, J. (1980). Alternative positions for childbirth. Part II: Second stage of labor. *Journal of Nurse-Midwifery, 25*(5), 13–19.

Roberts, J., & Van Lier, D. (1984, Spring). Debate: Which position for the second stage? *Childbirth Educator,* pp. 33–38.

Roberts, J.E., Goldstein, S.A., Gruener, J.S., Maggio, M., & Mendez-Bauer, C. (1987). A descriptive analysis of involuntary bearing-down efforts during the expulsive phase of labor. *Journal of Obstetric, Gynecologic, and Neonatal Nursing, 16*(1), 48–55.

Romond, J., & Baker, I. (1985). Squatting in childbirth. *Journal of Obstetric, Gynecologic, and Neonatal Nursing, 14*(5), 406–411.

Stern, E.W., Glazer, G.L., & Sanduleak, N. (1988). Influence of the full and new moon on onset of labor and spontaneous rupture of membranes. *Journal of Nurse-Midwifery, 33*(2), 57–61.

Winslow, W. (1987). First pregnancy after 35: What's the experience? *MCN: American Journal of Maternal Child Nursing, 12*(2), 92–96.

Kathleen V. Smith

Normal Childbirth

Objectives

1. Determine the potential for alteration in health status during the intrapartum period

2. Recognize the signs and symptoms of labor

3. Identify phases of the first stage of labor

4. Describe the normal physiological changes occurring in all four stages of labor

5. Discuss methods of pain relief used during labor

6. Use nursing interventions that reflect knowledge of standards of care

7. Accurately record documentation of nursing care

8. Identify variables that may alter the course of labor and delivery

9. Modify the nursing plan of care to changes in patient status

10. Recognize the variables that influence the normal progress of labor

11. Practice the concept of family-centered care during the intrapartum period

Introduction

A. The intrapartum period of pregnancy or labor begins with the first stage's uterine contractions and the progressive dilatation of the cervix

B. From complete dilatation of the cervix to the infant's delivery is the second stage of labor

C. The third stage of labor is completed with the expulsion of the placenta and membranes

D. The fourth stage of labor is the first hour postpartum

Clinical Practice

PREMONITORY SIGNS

A. Assessment

1. History
   a. Lightening
      (1) On the average, lightening occurs 10 days before onset of labor in a primigravida
      (2) Increased pressure of presenting part leads to
         (a) Urinary frequency
         (b) Backache and leg pain
         (c) Increased vaginal discharge
         (d) Dependent edema
      (3) Lightening results in easier respirations
   b. Braxton Hicks contractions
      (1) Referred to as false labor
      (2) Walking lessens discomfort
      (3) Usually irregular in occurrence
      (4) No progressive shortening of interval between contractions
   c. Show
      (1) Late sign: occurs after the beginning of cervical changes and increased pressure of presenting part
      (2) Blood-tinged cervical mucus
   d. Spontaneous rupture of amniotic sac; leakage of clear or cloudy amniotic fluid
   e. Burst of energy: often 24 to 48 hours before labor onset
   f. Gastrointestinal (GI) symptoms
      (1) Diarrhea
      (2) Indigestion
      (3) Nausea and vomiting
   g. Sleep disturbances
      (1) Change in sleep pattern
      (2) Restlessness
2. Physical findings
   a. Lightening
      (1) The uterus and presenting part descend into pelvis
      (2) Occurrence is determined by abdominal and pelvic examination
   b. Braxton Hicks contractions
      (1) Movement of the cervix from a posterior position to an anterior position
      (2) Primes, or softens, cervix
   c. Cervical changes
      (1) Ripening and softening of cervix due to hormonal changes
      (2) Effacement: thinning of the cervix
      (3) Dilatation: opening of the cervix
   d. Spontaneous rupture of the amniotic sac
      (1) Barrier to infection is gone
      (2) There is danger of cord prolapse
   e. Burst of energy: increased epinephrine release caused by decreased progesterone release
   f. Weight loss: client may have a 0.9 to 1.36 kg (2- to 3-pound) weight loss 24 to 48 hours before onset of labor
3. Psychosocial: burst of energy may result in nesting urge
4. Diagnostic procedures
   a. Spontaneous rupture of amniotic sac
      (1) Visible pooling of fluid is observed

    (2) pH is tested with nitrazine
    (3) Sterile speculum examination is performed to obtain specimen for microscopic ferning pattern
  b. Vaginal examination for cervical status

B. Nursing Diagnoses

1. Anxiety related to uncertainty about onset of labor and ability to cope
2. Fear of pain related to impending labor
3. High risk for infection related to spontaneous rupture of membranes

C. Interventions/Evaluations

1. Anxiety related to uncertainty about onset of labor and ability to cope
  a. Interventions
    (1) Listen attentively to concerns
    (2) Allow verbalization of feelings
    (3) Provide information and support
    (4) Reinforce prenatal education
    (5) Provide an awareness of changes as labor begins
    (6) Give clear, concise explanations and repeat as necessary
    (7) Use anxiety-reduction techniques
        (a) Relaxation techniques
        (b) Guided imagery
    (8) Provide for the presence of a support person
  b. Evaluations
    (1) Client's anxiety is reduced
        (a) Relaxation techniques are demonstrated
        (b) Early signs of labor are verbalized
    (2) Client attended prenatal classes
2. Fear of pain related to impending labor
  a. Intervention
    (1) Encourage prenatal preparation for active labor participation
    (2) Review and demonstrate relaxation techniques
    (3) Discuss pain-relief methods
    (4) Explain all nursing activities
    (5) Answer questions presented
  b. Evaluation
    (1) Client verbalizes her fears
    (2) Client attended childbirth education classes
    (3) Client discusses the methods of pain relief available during labor
3. High risk for infection related to spontaneous rupture of membranes
  a. Intervention
    (1) Instruct the client and her family to notify medical personnel immediately after spontaneous rupture of membranes (SROM)
    (2) Instruct the client to refrain from sexual intercourse after SROM (if client is at home)
    (3) Monitor the client's temperature every 2 hours for elevation
    (4) Observe for foul-smelling vaginal discharge or amniotic fluid
    (5) Educate the client about the need for perineal cleanliness
        (a) Handwashing after voiding or defecation
        (b) Cleansing of perineal area from front to back
  b. Evaluations
    (1) Prompt medical notification occurs after SROM
    (2) Temperature remains within normal limits
    (3) Client washes hands and cleans perineum correctly

FIRST STAGE OF LABOR: DILATATION

A. Assessment

1. Physiological changes during first stage of labor
   a. Cardiovascular changes
      (1) Cardiac output increases
      (2) Slight pulse changes: may increase to more than 100 beats/min as a result of exhaustion or dehydration
      (3) Blood pressure (BP) changes very little
         (a) Increases are noted if monitored during a contraction
         (b) Hypotension may be seen: vena caval syndrome or supine hypotension due to pressure of pregnant uterus on inferior vena cava
      (4) White blood cell (WBC) count increases up to 20,000/mm^3 with strenuous labor
   b. GI changes
      (1) Motility and absorption are decreased
      (2) Gastric emptying time is decreased
      (3) Nausea and vomiting are common
   c. Renal changes
      (1) The tendency to concentrate urine results in specific gravity above 1.025
      (2) Pressure of full bladder is felt
         (a) Increased discomfort
         (b) Impedes labor
      (3) Pressure of presenting part on urethra may require catheterization to empty the urinary bladder
      (4) Proteinuria
         (a) Caused by increased metabolic activity
         (b) May be sign of pregnancy-induced hypertension (PIH)
2. Phases of labor
   a. Latent phase
      (1) Admission history
         (a) Identification of client
         (b) Prenatal history of physical
            (i) Estimated date of confinement (EDC)
            (ii) Pregnancies, births, abortions, living children
            (iii) Allergies
            (iv) Medications taken during pregnancy
               • Time and amount of last dose
               • Frequency of use during pregnancy
            (v) Chronic conditions and medical–surgical history
            (vi) Illness during pregnancy and recent exposures
            (vii) Results of laboratory work done during pregnancy
               • Complete blood count (CBC) and hemoglobin and hematocrit (H&H)
               • Blood type and Rh factor
               • Urinalysis
               • VDRL and serologic testing
               • Gonorrhea (GC) culture
               • *Chlamydia* culture
               • Rubella titer
               • Papanicolaou's stain test
            (viii) Special tests
               • Glucose screen
               • Sickle cell screen
               • Ultrasonography
               • Chorionic villi sampling (CVS), amniocentesis, percutaneous umbilical blood sampling (PUBS)

- Genetic studies
- Lecithin/sphingomyelin ratio (L/S), phosphatidylglycerol (PG)
- Maternal serum alpha-feto-protein (MSAFP)
- Human immunodeficiency virus (HIV) titer
- Hepatitis B surface antigen (HbsAg) titer for hepatitis screening
- Rh antibody screen
- Nonstress test (NST), oxytocin challenge test (OCT)
- Biophysical profile

  (ix) Childbirth preparation
- Birth plan
- Support system
- Previous experience
- Cultural influences
- Coping skills

(2) Physical findings

  (a) Vital signs: fetal heart tones (FHT), BP, temperature, pulse, respirations

  (b) Contraction status

    (i) Onset of contractions

    (ii) Present contraction status
- Frequency of contractions
  - Contractions may be irregular
  - Contractions occur every 5 to 10 minutes
- Duration: 30 to 45 seconds
- Contraction strength
  - Mild by palpation
  - 25 to 40 mm Hg by intrauterine pressure catheter (IUPC)

  (c) Vaginal examination

    (i) Cervix location (posterior, moving to anterior)

    (ii) Dilatation: 0 to 3 cm

    (iii) Effacement: 0 to 40%

    (iv) Fetal presentation or position

  (d) Vaginal discharge

    (i) Amniotic fluid
- Time of rupture
- Color, amount, and odor
- Consistency

    (ii) Bloody show
- Characteristics
- Amount

  (e) Abdominal examination

    (i) Fundal height

    (ii) Leopold's maneuvers to determine fetal lie

    (iii) Scars, ridges, or masses

  (f) Chest examination: heart and lung sounds

  (g) Deep tendon reflexes

    (i) Patellar or brachial

    (ii) Clonus

(3) Psychosocial

  (a) Emotional status

    (i) Confident, low anxiety level

    (ii) Excited, talkative

    (iii) Anticipatory, apprehensive

  (b) Support systems

  (c) Fears and concerns

   (d) Nonverbal clues

  (4) Diagnostic procedures

   (a) Urine screen

    (i) Specific gravity

    (ii) Protein

    (iii) Glucose

   (b) Routine blood screen

    (i) CBC (especially H&H)

    (ii) Serological testing

    (iii) Blood type and Rh factor

 b. Active phase

  (1) Physical findings

   (a) Contraction pattern (by electronic fetal monitoring [EFM] or by palpation) should be evaluated every 30 minutes

    (i) Frequency: every 2 to 5 minutes

    (ii) Duration: 45 to 60 seconds

    (iii) Intensity

     • Moderate to strong by palpation

     • 50 to 70 mm Hg by IUPC

   (b) Vaginal examination

    (i) Dilatation: 4 to 7 cm

    (ii) Effacement: 40 to 80%

    (iii) Station: -2 to 0

    (iv) Presenting part and position

    (v) Status of membranes

     • Intact

     • If ruptured

      ■ Color

      ■ Consistency

      ■ Odor

    (vi) Progression of labor: suggested dilatation rate

     • 1.2 cm/hr for primipara

     • 1.5 cm/hr for multipara

    (vii) Cervix location: anterior

   (c) Intake and output (I&O)

    (i) Hydration status

     • Last oral intake

     • IV fluid intake monitored

    (ii) Edema

    (iii) Nausea and vomiting

  (2) Psychosocial findings

   (a) Absorbed in serious work of labor

   (b) Intense and quieter

   (c) Dependency increases

   (d) Self-confidence wavers

 c. Transition phase

  (1) History

   (a) Childbirth preparation is important

   (b) Time for relaxation between contractions decreases

  (2) Physical findings

   (a) Dilatation: 8 to 10 cm

   (b) Effacement: 80 to 100%

   (c) Station: -1 to $+1$

   (d) Contractions

    (i) Frequency: every 2 to 3 minutes

    (ii) Duration: 60 to 90 seconds

    (iii) Intensity

- Strong by palpation
- 70 to 90 mm Hg by IUPC
(e) Strong urge to push if station is low
(f) Backache
(g) Nausea and vomiting
(h) Trembling limbs
(i) Vaginal discharge: bloody show increases
(j) I&O
   (i) Monitor oral and IV intake
   (ii) Frequent bladder emptying is important to allow descent of fetus
   (3) Psychosocial findings
      (a) Supportive needs increase, but client is agitated and irritable
      (b) Client is increasingly discouraged because of fatigue and may want to give up
      (c) Client's coping ability decreases as she feels overwhelmed
      (d) Client relaxation is almost impossible
3. Analgesia or anesthesia for first stage of labor
   a. Goal: change perception through
      (1) Relaxation to decrease tension
      (2) Medication to increase pain threshold
   b. Pain receptors are stimulated by uterine contractions that result in
      (1) Myometrial anoxia
      (2) Cervical stretching
      (3) Pressure on pelvic nerves
      (4) Traction on supporting and nearby structures
      (5) Distension of pelvic floor
   c. Pain perception is affected by
      (1) Past experience
      (2) Cultural expectations
      (3) Psychosexual development
      (4) Fatigue, anemia
      (5) Fear, anxiety, emotional stress
      (6) Environment
      (7) Support system
   d. Medications
      (1) Barbiturates (phenobarbital [Nembutal], secobarbital [Seconal])
         (a) Provide sedation or sleep
         (b) Reduce tension and fear
         (c) Used for rest
      (2) Tranquilizers (hydroxyzine [Vistaril], promethazine [Phenergan])
         (a) Are antianxiety agents
         (b) Provide muscle relaxation
         (c) Contain antiemetic properties
         (d) May potentiate narcotics
      (3) Narcotics (meperidine [Demoral], morphine, butorphanol [Stadol], nalbuphine [Nubain])
         (a) Increase pain threshold: client's ability to tolerate or cope with discomfort increases
         (b) May increase or decrease uterine activity
         (c) May cause drowsiness
   e. Regional anesthesia
      (1) Paracervical block (*Note:* This anesthesia is rarely used anymore and is described here only for historical purposes)
         (a) Local anesthesia is injected transvaginally lateral to cervix at dilatation of 4 to 6 cm
         (b) Lower uterine segment, cervix, and upper vagina are affected
         (c) Effect on fetus is transient bradycardia

(1) Epidural or caudal
  (a) Local anesthesia is injected into epidural or caudal space
  (b) Nerves leaving the spinal cord are blocked
  (c) Entire pelvis and lower extremities are affected so that the client perceives touch but not pain
  (d) Fetal effect: uterine blood flow is decreased if maternal hypotension occurs, leading to potential fetal distress
f. Nonpharmacological methods
  (1) Transcutaneous electrical nerve stimulation (TENS)
    (a) Electrodes are placed on either side of client's lower spine
    (b) Electrical stimulation provided by client during contractions
    (c) Provides alternate sensation to decrease perception of pain from contractions
  (2) Touch
    (a) Acupressure: increases endorphine release and reduces sensation
    (b) Cutaneous stimulation: effleurage provides an alternative sensation
    (c) Massage
    (d) Hot or cold application
  (3) Relaxation techniques
    (a) Biofeedback
    (b) Visual imagery
    (c) Controlled breathing patterns
    (d) Shower or jacuzzi

B. Nursing Diagnoses

1. High risk for altered maternal tissue perfusion related to position in labor
2. Altered urinary elimination pattern related to progression of labor
3. Anxiety related to labor and birth
4. Fatigue related to prolonged labor
5. Fear related to discomfort of labor
6. Ineffective individual coping related to progress of labor
7. Pain due to uterine contractions and cervical dilatation
8. High risk for fluid volume deficit related to decreased intake or abnormal loss
9. High risk for infection related to vaginal examinations following SROM

C. Interventions/Evaluations

1. High risk for altered tissue perfusion related to position in labor
  a. Interventions
    (1) Discourage supine position: preventing supine hypotension or vena caval syndrome
    (2) Assess BP between contractions for an accurate reading
    (3) Encourage frequent position changes
  b. Evaluations
    (1) Vital signs and fetal heart rate (FHR) remain stable
    (2) No supine hypotension is seen
2. Altered urinary elimination pattern related to progression of labor
  a. Interventions
    (1) Maintain an accurate I&O record
    (2) Encourage adequate intake of oral fluids
    (3) Monitor IV fluid intake
    (4) Encourage bladder elimination every 2 hours
  b. Evaluations
    (1) I&O is balanced
    (2) Bladder is emptied regularly
    (3) Bladder is not palpable
3. Anxiety related to labor and birth
  a. Interventions
    (1) Orient the client to her environment

      (2) Call the client by her name

      (3) Encourage verbalization of feelings

      (4) Listen attentively

      (5) Provide information about routine procedures

      (6) Monitor vital signs and labor status, and keep the client and her family informed

      (7) Encourage participation of support system

      (8) Encourage relaxation techniques

      (9) Respect the client's privacy

  b. Evaluations

      (1) Client identifies stressors

      (2) Client remains in control and relaxed

      (3) Support system is stable and present

4. Fatigue related to prolonged labor

  a. Interventions

      (1) Encourage rest in latent phase: promote relaxation

      (2) Encourage rest between contractions in active phase and transition

      (3) Minimize environmental stimuli

      (4) Offer comfort measures

      (5) Offer and explain analgesia or anesthesia, if indicated and desired

  b. Evaluations

      (1) Client rests and relaxes

      (2) Analgesia or anesthesia is accepted by client

      (3) No adverse effects of medication are seen in mother or fetus

5. Fear related to discomfort of labor

  a. Interventions

      (1) Offer anticipatory guidance

      (2) Orient the client to her surroundings

      (3) Give clear explanations of what is to come (the labor process and possible interventions)

      (4) Maintain support system

      (5) Allow and encourage verbalization of source of fear

  b. Evaluations

      (1) Confidence and control are exhibited

      (2) Support system is strong

6. Ineffective individual coping related to progress of labor

  a. Interventions

      (1) Encourage expression of feelings

      (2) Reinforce previously learned coping methods

      (3) Maintain and assist support system

      (4) Present new methods of coping with the situation

      (5) Provide comfort measures

  b. Evaluations

      (1) Client communicates feelings about situation

      (2) Client's confidence is restored

      (3) Client uses learned coping skills

7. Pain due to uterine contractions and cervical dilatation

  a. Interventions

      (1) Document uterine activity and labor progress

      (2) Provide comfort measures

         (a) Encourage breathing and relaxation techniques

         (b) Encourage bladder emptying

         (c) Encourage frequent position changes

         (d) Provide back rubs

      (3) Use nonpharmacological measures of pain relief

      (4) Administer analgesia as ordered

      (5) Assist with anesthesia as needed

  b. Evaluations

(1) Discomfort is decreased
(2) No adverse side effects are observed from analgesia or anesthesia in mother or baby
8. High risk for fluid volume deficit related to decreased intake or abnormal loss
   a. Interventions
      (1) Monitor hydration status
      (2) Monitor vital signs for deviations from normal
         (a) Monitor BP, pulse, and respirations every 30 to 60 minutes
         (b) Signs may indicate bleeding: elevated pulse, decreased BP
         (c) Monitor temperature every 4 hours (every 2 hours after ROM) for elevation, which may indicate dehydration
      (3) Monitor FHR for signs of distress caused by decreased uteroplacental perfusion (see Chapter 16 for further discussion of fetal assessment)
         (a) May be done continuously with EFM
         (b) Monitor every 15 minutes if no EFM
      (4) Monitor I&O
         (a) Encourage voiding every 2 hours
         (b) Test urine for specific gravity (normal is 1.010 to 1.025)
         (c) Administer oral or IV fluids as indicated
      (5) Observe for obvious vaginal bleeding
   b. Evaluations
      (1) Vital signs and FHR remain stable
      (2) Adequate hydration is maintained
      (3) No obvious signs of bleeding are observed
9. High risk for infection related to vaginal examination after ROM
   a. Interventions
      (1) Maintain good perineal hygiene
      (2) Document time of ROM and characteristics of amniotic fluid
      (3) Monitor temperature every 2 hours after ROM
      (4) Monitor laboratory data as indicated
      (5) Perform vaginal examinations only when necessary
      (6) Ensure aseptic technique during procedures
      (7) Observe FHR for tachycardia, often an early indication of maternal infection
   b. Evaluations
      (1) There is no evidence of infection
         (a) Vital signs and FHR remain normal
         (b) Laboratory data are within normal limits
      (2) Time and date of ROM are documented
      (3) Character of amniotic fluid is documented
      (4) No foul-smelling fluid is observed

SECOND STAGE OF LABOR: INFANT EXPULSION

A. Assessment

1. Physical findings
   a. Vaginal examination
      (1) Dilatation: 10 cm (complete dilation)
      (2) Effacement: 100%
      (3) Station: 0 to +2
   b. Contractions
      (1) Frequency: every 2 to 3 minutes
      (2) Duration: 60 to 90 seconds
      (3) Intensity
         (a) Strong by palpation
         (b) 80 to 100 mm Hg by IUPC

c. Diaphoresis
d. Signs of descent or presenting part
  (1) The urge to push becomes uncontrollable
    (a) Traditionally, women have been taught to push in the following manner
      (i) Hold the breath
      (ii) Bear down on the rectum for a count of 10
      (iii) Inhale again, push again, and repeat the process three or four times for each contraction
      (iv) Assume a C-shaped position around the fetus, with the chin on the chest
    (b) Pushing in this fashion leads to hemodynamic changes in the mother from the resultant Valsalva maneuver and may also produce abnormalities in the FHR
    (c) Suggestions for alternative pushing efforts
      (i) The open-glottis method, in which air is released during pushing, so no intrathoracic pressure builds up
      (ii) The urge-to-push method, in which the mother bears down as she feels the urge and in a manner that feels right to her
        ● Most women make three to five brief (4- to 6-second) pushes with each contraction
        ● Most pushes are accompanied by the release of air
    (d) Alternative pushing methods would be helpful for women with cardiac or hypertensive conditions, in which a prolonged Valsalva effect is contraindicated
  (2) Bulging of perineum occurs
  (3) Anal changes occur
    (a) Passing of flatus or stool
    (b) Rectal mucosa exposed
  (4) Opening of the vaginal introitus occurs
  (5) The presenting part is visible: crowning
  (6) Burning or stretching sensation is felt in the perineal area
  (7) Urine is expressed during pushing
e. Anesthesia for delivery
  (1) Continuation of caudal or epidural anesthesia
  (2) Pudendal anesthesia
    (a) Is transvaginal block of pudendal nerve near ischial spines
    (b) Affects vaginal and perineal area
    (c) Has little or no fetal effect
  (3) Saddle block: low spinal anesthesia
    (a) Local anesthesia is introduced into the subarachnoid space
    (b) Motor and sensory nerves are blocked
    (c) Effect on fetus is decreased blood flow with maternal hypotension secondary to peripheral vasodilation
  (4) Local infiltration
    (a) Perineal body is injected with local anesthesia
    (b) Done just before delivery at site of episiotomy
    (c) Has no fetal effect
f. Episiotomy: incision in perineum to provide more space for presenting part
  (1) Indications
    (a) To prevent tearing
    (b) To prevent undue stretching of bladder and rectal supports
    (c) To reduce time and stress of second stage
    (d) To allow for ease in manipulation with a forceps or breech delivery
  (2) Types
    (a) Median or midline
      (i) Advantages

- Heals quickly
- Easily repaired
- Less discomfort
- Less dyspareunia

(ii) Disadvantage: extension can involve rectal area

(b) Mediolateral: 45-degree angle to left or right

  (i) Advantages

- Used for large infant
- No rectal involvement

  (ii) Disadvantages

- Heals more slowly
- Is more painful
- Causes greater blood loss

g. Lacerations

(1) First degree: involves perineal skin and vaginal mucous membrane

(2) Second degree: involves skin and mucous membrane plus fascia of perineal body

(3) Third degree: involves skin, mucous membrane, and muscle of perineal body; extends into rectal sphincter

(4) Fourth degree: extends into rectal mucosa to expose the lumen of the rectum

2. Psychosocial

a. Client is less irritable and agitated

b. Client is more cooperative

c. Client's modesty not a priority

d. Client may doze off between contractions

e. Client is intent on work of pushing

3. Diagnostic procedures

a. Method for controlled vaginal vertex delivery

(1) Maintain gentle pressure on presenting part

(2) Provide perineal support

(3) Support fetal head as it delivers

(4) Check for nuchal cord

(5) Suction infant's mouth, then nose

(6) Deliver anterior shoulder under symphysis

(7) Deliver posterior shoulder over coccyx

(8) Rest of infant delivers easily

(9) Note time of delivery; the point at which the entire infant body is free of the mother

b. Assisted delivery

(1) Indications for forceps or vacuum use

(a) Maternal

  (i) Progress of second stage stops as the result of

- Inadequate contraction strength
- Poor pushing efforts
- Excessive infant size
- Fetal position: posterior or asynclitic

  (ii) Maternal condition that warrants a shortened second stage (e.g., cardiac problems)

  (iii) Extreme fatigue of mother after prolonged labor, particularly second stage

(b) Fetal

  (i) Preterm infant (potential for cranial damage with prolonged pushing)

  (ii) Distress that warrants a shortened second stage

(2) Prerequisites

(a) There is no cephalopelvic disproportion (CPD)

(b) Head is engaged
(c) Membranes are ruptured
(d) Cervix is completely dilated
(e) Bladder is empty
(3) Types of assisted deliveries
(a) Low/outlet forceps: used when the head is visible at the perineum
(b) Midforceps
(i) Head is at the ischial spines
(ii) Often needed for rotation to anteroposterior position
(c) Vacuum
(i) Head is visible
(ii) Silastic suction cup is applied to presenting part and gentle traction is exerted while the mother pushes
(4) After any assisted delivery, the infant should be examined thoroughly for possible injuries
(a) Bruising
(b) Cephalhematoma (area of edema of scalp at location of Silastic cup is usual with vacuum extractions)
(c) Facial nerve damage
(5) Use of forceps or vacuum may predispose the client to lacerations of the vagina or perineum

B. Nursing Diagnoses

1. Altered urinary elimination related to pressure of presenting part
2. Altered tissue perfusion related to expulsive efforts
3. Impaired tissue integrity related to delivery process
4. Ineffective individual coping during second stage
5. Pain related to descent of fetus and perineal stretching
6. High risk for infection related to prolonged second stage

C. Interventions/Evaluations

1. Altered urinary elimination related to pressure of presenting part
   a. Interventions
   (1) Encourage emptying of bladder
   (2) Catheterize distended bladder if the client is unable to void
   (3) Monitor the client's I and O
   b. Evaluations
   (1) Bladder does not become distended
   (2) I&O is adequate
   (3) Complications are avoided or minimized
2. Altered tissue perfusion related to expulsive efforts
   a. Interventions
   (1) Encourage side-lying or pillow-propped position because dorsal recumbent position occludes the inferior vena cava
   (2) Closely monitor vital signs after analgesia or anesthesia
   (3) Discourage prolonged Valsalva maneuvers while pushing
   (4) Administer oxygen as indicated
   (5) Maintain adequate fluid intake
   b. Evaluations
   (1) Vital signs and FHR remain within normal limits
   (2) Gentle pushing is used
   (3) No signs of dizziness or syncope are noted
3. Impaired skin integrity related to delivery process
   a. Interventions
   (1) Encourage upright rather than recumbent position for pushing
   (2) Encourage gentle pushing efforts to allow for gradual stretching of tissue
   (3) Avoid precipitous or uncontrolled delivery when possible

          (4) Position the client to facilitate perineal floor relaxation and increased pelvic diameters (see Chapter 14 for complete discussion of optimal positions for expulsion)

    b. Evaluation: no lacerations occur

  4. Ineffective individual coping during second stage

    a. Interventions

      (1) Support and direct coach during second stage of labor

      (2) Encourage rest periods between pushing contractions

      (3) Provide comfort measures

      (4) Provide mirror to observe progress of pushing

      (5) Provide encouragement

    b. Evaluations

      (1) Client uses effective coping skills

      (2) Client is actively involved in her care

      (3) Client uses effective breathing and expulsive methods

  5. Pain related to descent of fetus and perineal stretching

    a. Interventions

      (1) Assist with nonpharmacological techniques

        (a) Breathing patterns

        (b) TENS

      (2) Provide information and analgesia or anesthesia, as necessary

      (3) Monitor response to medications used

      (4) Put side rails up after analgesia or anesthesia has been administered

    b. Evaluation: comfort is attained

  6. High risk for infection

    a. Interventions

      (1) Use clean or aseptic technique as appropriate

        (a) Keep the perineal area clean

        (b) Using institution's designated solutions, cleanse perineal area before delivery

      (2) Monitor temperature and pulse for deviations

    b. Evaluations

      (1) Clean, aseptic conditions are maintained

      (2) No evidence of infection is observed

THIRD STAGE OF LABOR: PLACENTAL EXPULSION

A. Assessment

1. Physical findings

    a. Signs of separation of placenta

      (1) Gush of blood occurs

      (2) Cord lengthens at vaginal opening

      (3) Fundus rises in abdomen

      (4) Uterine shape changes from flat to firm and globular as placenta drops into lower uterine segment

    b. Types of placental delivery

      (1) Spontaneous

        (a) Schultz's mechanism: fetal side delivers first

        (b) Duncan's mechanism: maternal side delivers first

      (2) Manual extraction: placental separation and removal are assisted by delivery attendant

    c. Placental abnormalities (Fig. 15–1)

      (1) Battledore: cord is inserted at or near the placental margin, rather than in the center

      (2) Circumvellate: the fetal surface of the placenta is exposed through a ring of chorion and amnion opening around the umbilical cord

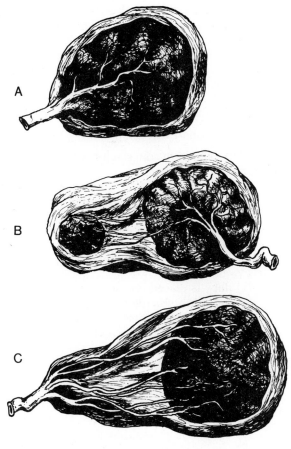

Figure 15–1
Placental variations: *A*, battledore placenta; *B*, placenta succenturiate; and *C*, velamentous insertion of the umbilical cord. (From Bobak, I., Jensen, M., & Zallar, M. [1989]. *Maternity and gynecologic care* [4th ed., p. 767]. St. Louis: Mosby.)

(3) Succenturiate: one or more accessory lobes of fetal villi have developed
    (a) Vessels from the major to the minor lobe are supported only by membranes, increasing the risk of the minor lobe's being retained during the third stage
    (b) There may also be blood loss if these vessels are nicked during intrauterine procedures
(4) Velamentous insertion of cord: fetal vessels separate in the membranes before reaching the placenta
    (a) If bleeding is seen, it should be tested for fetal hemoglobin by means of Kleihauer-Betke test to determine if fetal or maternal blood
    (b) Fetus may become hypovolemic
    (c) Fetus is most vulnerable during labor and delivery
    (d) Condition is more common with
       (i) Multiple gestation
       (ii) Fetal anomalies (Neeson & May, 1986)
(5) Vasa previa: associated with velamentous insertion of the cord
    (a) The umbilical vessels in the membranes cross the region of the internal os and present ahead of the fetus
    (b) Potential danger to the fetus is considerable if rupture of the membranes is accompanied by rupture of a fetal vessel
    (c) In severe cases, vasa previa can lead to exsanguination of the fetus (Pritchard, MacDonald, & Gant, 1985)
    (d) Vasa previa may be diagnosed by
       (i) Vaginal examination
       (ii) Amnioscopy

(iii) Palpation of a vessel pulsating synchronously with the FHR in the membranes in front of the fetus
(e) Cesarean delivery may be indicated if the health care provider believes the risk of hemorrhage to be great

B. Nursing Diagnoses

1. Anxiety related to concern for the newborn
2. High risk for fluid volume deficit related to blood loss

C. Interventions/Evaluations

1. Anxiety related to concern for well-being of newborn
   a. Interventions
      (1) Provide early infant contact as soon as possible: place the infant on the mother's abdomen after delivery if not contraindicated
      (2) Encourage touching and holding of the infant
      (3) Explain any procedures for stimulation or resuscitation of the baby to allay anxiety
      (4) Reassure the mother about the baby's status and well-being
   b. Evaluations
      (1) Baby is placed on the mother's abdomen
      (2) Mother holds the baby
      (3) Mother reports assurance of the infant's well-being
2. High risk for fluid volume deficit related to blood loss
   a. Interventions
      (1) Ensure that placenta is delivered within 30 minutes
      (2) Monitor vaginal bleeding with delivery of the placenta
      (3) Monitor firmness of the uterus
      (4) Administer oxytocin as indicated
   b. Evaluations
      (1) Blood loss is less than 500 ml
      (2) Uterus is firm after placental delivery

FOURTH STAGE OF LABOR: IMMEDIATE POSTPARTUM PERIOD

A. Assessment

1. Physical findings
   a. Vital signs
      (1) Blood pressure is taken every 15 minutes
         (a) Transient changes are secondary to decreased blood volume after delivery
         (b) Excitement may elevate BP
         (c) Low reading is often a late sign of blood loss
      (2) Pulse is checked every 15 minutes
         (a) Low readings often compensate for decreased vascular bed and decreased intra-abdominal pressure
         (b) Rapid pulse may indicate an increase in blood loss or a temperature elevation
      (3) Temperature: slight elevation is normal (100°F) (37.8°C) as the result of dehydration and the fatigue of labor
   b. Fundal checks: every 15 minutes
      (1) Fundus is firm and well contracted
      (2) Fundus is midway between umbilicus and symphysis after delivery of placenta
      (3) Fundus rises slowly to the level of umbilicus during the first hour after placental delivery
   c. Lochia estimation: every 15 minutes

        (1) Nature of flow
            (a) Intermittent
            (b) Trickle
            (c) Clots
        (2) Amount of flow: greater than 500 ml indicates postpartum hemorrhage
        (3) Character and odor of flow
    d. Perineal inspection
        (1) Episiotomy, lacerations, or both
            (a) Intact: edges approximated
            (b) No hematomas, redness, or edema
        (2) Clean
2. Psychosocial
    a. Joy: sense of peace and excitement
    b. Excitement: wide awake, talkative, hungry, and thirsty
    c. Attachment process begins
        (1) Mother inspects the newborn
        (2) Mother wants to cuddle the infant and begin breastfeeding
        (3) Mother feels the need to "let the world know"

B. Nursing Diagnoses

1. High risk for altered family process related to acceptance of newborn
2. Altered urinary elimination related to process of labor and delivery
3. Pain related to early uterine involution
4. High risk for fluid volume deficit related to fluid shift in early postpartum period
5. High risk for infection related to labor and delivery

C. Interventions/Evaluations

1. High risk for altered family process related to acceptance of newborn
    a. Interventions
        (1) Provide for early infant contact
        (2) Assist with early breastfeeding
        (3) Call attention to quiet, alert state of infant
        (4) Provide information about infant's ability to see and hear
        (5) Postpone eye prophylaxis
    b. Evaluations
        (1) Parental exploration of infant
        (2) Infant is cuddled and breastfed if desired
2. Altered urinary elimination related to process of labor and delivery
    a. Interventions
        (1) Encourage emptying of the bladder
        (2) Monitor fundal height
        (3) Catheterize distended bladder if the client is unable to void
        (4) Monitor I and O
    b. Evaluations
        (1) Bladder does not become distended
        (2) No displacement of uterus is seen
        (3) I&O adequate
        (4) Complications are avoided or minimized
3. Pain related to early uterine involution
    a. Interventions
        (1) Assist with nonpharmacological methods of relief
            (a) Apply an ice bag to soothe perineum
            (b) Supply a warm blanket if client is chilled
        (2) Provide medication as ordered
    b. Evaluations
        (1) Comfort is attained

(2) Client verbalizes pain reduction
4. High risk for fluid volume deficit related to fluid shift in early postpartum period
   a. Interventions
      (1) Monitor vital signs
      (2) Administer IV and oral fluids as indicated
      (3) Monitor vaginal discharge for excessive bleeding
      (4) Monitor fundal height and firmness
   b. Evaluations
      (1) Vital signs are within normal limits
      (2) Hydration is maintained
      (3) Blood loss is less than 500 ml
      (4) Uterus remains firmly contracted
5. High risk for infection related to labor and delivery
   a. Interventions
      (1) Use clean or aseptic technique, as appropriate
         (a) Apply a sterile perineal pad after delivery
         (b) Clean the perineal area from front to back
      (2) Inspect the perineal area for breakdown
      (3) Emphasize good handwashing technique to client
      (4) Monitor client's pulse and temperature for deviations
   b. Evaluations
      (1) Clean and aseptic conditions are maintained
      (2) Skin condition is documented
      (3) No evidence of infection is seen
      (4) Client washes her hands

VARIABLES INFLUENCING LABOR AND DELIVERY

Induction/Augmentation

Initiation or augmentation of uterine contractions will accomplish delivery

A. Assessment

1. History
   a. Relative indications for induction or augmentation
      (1) Maternal
         (a) Diabetes
         (b) PIH
         (c) Slowed progress of labor
         (d) History of precipitate labor
         (e) Chorioamnionitis
      (2) Fetal
         (a) Prolonged rupture of membranes
         (b) Postmaturity
         (c) Rh sensitization
         (d) Fetal death
   b. Relative contraindications for induction or augmentation
      (1) Maternal
         (a) Previous classic uterine incision
         (b) Placenta previa
         (c) Grand multipara
         (d) Overdistended uterus
         (e) Active genital herpes
      (2) Fetal
         (a) Cephalopelvic disproportion
         (b) Severe fetal distress

(c) Fetal malposition
(d) Fetal immaturity
2. Physical findings: the Bishop score measures physiological readiness of cervix (Table 15–1)
   a. Dilatation
   b. Effacement
   c. Station
   d. Cervical consistency
   e. Cervical position
3. Diagnostic findings
   a. Maternal readiness
      (1) Informed consent
      (2) Bishop score of 5 to 7 indicative of probable induction success
   b. Fetal readiness
      (1) Gestational age established by early ultrasound test or measurement of appropriate parameters
      (2) Acceptable L/S ratio (usually 2:1 or higher)
      (3) Presence of phosphatidylglycerol in amniotic fluid
4. Methods of induction or augmentation
   a. Amniotomy: mechanical
      (1) Allows for pressure of presenting part on cervix
      (2) Side effects
         (a) Increased risk of infection
         (b) Increased risk of prolapsed cord
   b. Prostaglandin
      (1) Used as suppository or gel to ripen cervix
      (2) Side effects
         (a) Nausea and vomiting
         (b) Diarrhea
         (c) Fever
   c. Oxytocin: goal is to mimic natural labor
      (1) Given IV in secondary line with an infusion pump
      (2) Side effects
         (a) Tetanic contractions
         (b) Maternal hypotension
         (c) Antidiuretic effect
         (d) Neonatal hyperbilirubinemia has been reported

Table 15–1
BISHOP SCORE

	0	1	2	3
Dilatation	Closed	1–2 cm	3–4 cm	≥5 cm
Effacement	30%	40–50%	60–70%	≥80%
Station	−3	−2	−1/0	+1
Cervical consistency	Firm	Medium	Soft	
Cervical position	Posterior	Middle	Anterior	

Total possible score is 13. High score indicates a greater chance for successful outcome. With a score of 9, successful induction is likely; with 7, success is likely for a primigravida; and with 5, success is likely for a multipara. However, a high score at early gestation forewarns of possible premature labor.

From NAACOG. (1991). *Inpatient obstetrics certification review manual.* Washington, DC: NAACOG.

B. Nursing Diagnoses

1. Anxiety related to induction or augmentation
2. Pain related to uterine contractions
3. High risk for fluid volume excess related to use of oxytocin
4. High risk for injury related to induction

C. Interventions/Evaluations

1. Anxiety related to induction or augmentation
   a. Interventions
      (1) Present procedure with clear explanations
      (2) Maintain frequent presence, with continuous EFM for fetus and maternal contractions
      (3) Reassure the client of fetal status and progress of labor
   b. Evaluations
      (1) Client verbalizes understanding of situation and plan of care
      (2) Client is involved in alternative birth plan
      (3) Client uses effective coping methods
2. Pain due to uterine contractions
   a. Interventions
      (1) Anticipate that the client will feel the pain from contractions sooner than with naturally occurring labor
      (2) Provide comfort measures
      (3) Promote the use of breathing and relaxation techniques
      (4) Support the birthing coach
      (5) Provide and monitor analgesia or anesthesia, as appropriate
      (6) Use nonpharmacological means of pain control
   b. Evaluations
      (1) Client reports increased comfort
      (2) Support person is actively participating
      (3) No adverse effects of medication are seen in mother or infant
3. High risk for fluid volume excess related to use of oxytocin
   a. Interventions
      (1) Monitor I&O strictly
      (2) Maintain an accurate record of the amount of oxytocin administered
      (3) Observe for signs of water intoxication
         (a) Altered consciousness
         (b) Excessive fluid intake compared with output
         (c) Edema
   b. Evaluations
      (1) Adequate I and O is maintained
      (2) Water intoxication is avoided
4. High risk for injury related to induction
   a. Interventions
      (1) Observe institution's written policy or protocol for oxytocin use; a suggested protocol follows
         (a) Dilute 10 U of oxytocin in 1000 ml of lactated Ringer's solution or other physiological electrolyte solution, so that each milliliter contains 10 mU of oxytocin
         (b) Administer by means of infusion pump as secondary line, connected as close as possible to the primary IV site
         (c) Initial dose is usually 0.5 to 1.0 mU/min
         (d) Dose may be gradually increased in increments of 1 to 2 mU/min every 30 to 60 minutes
         (e) Once the desired frequency of contractions is reached (usually every 3 minutes), the rate may be maintained (a patient seldom requires more than 20 to 40 mU/min)
      (2) Nurse to patient ratio should be 1:1 or 1:2

      (3) During administration, accurate monitoring is required of
         (a) Uterine contractions for frequency, duration, and intensity
         (b) Uterine resting tone
         (c) FHR response to contractions
         (d) Maternal vital signs
      (4) Discontinue oxytocin infusion
         (a) With a tetanic contraction (one lasting longer than 90 seconds)
         (b) With uterine hyperstimulation (contractions occurring less than 2 minutes apart)
         (c) With elevated uterine resting tone
         (d) With nonreassuring FHR patterns (see Chapter 16 for complete discussion of FHR patterns)
   b. Evaluation
      (1) Oxytocin is administered via infusion pump
      (2) Accurate documentation is made of dosage
      (3) No adverse effects of oxytocin are seen in mother or fetus

Dysfunctional Labor

A. Assessment

1. History
   a. Abnormal progress of labor (some overlapping exists between classifications)
      (1) Nulliparous women are more subject to conditions that occur in early labor
         (a) Hypertonic uterine dysfunction
         (b) Primary inertia
         (c) Prolonged latent phase
      (2) Multiparous women more often demonstrate problems that occur in the active phase
         (a) Hypotonic uterine dysfunction
         (b) Secondary inertia
         (c) Protraction or arrest of the active phase
   b. Altered Friedman curve (Fig. 15–2)
      (1) Friedman demonstrated a normal labor pattern by plotting, on a graph, cervical dilatation and degree of descent against lapsed time
      (2) Categories of delayed progression according to his terminology
         (a) Prolonged latent phase
         (b) Protraction disorders
         (c) Arrest disorders

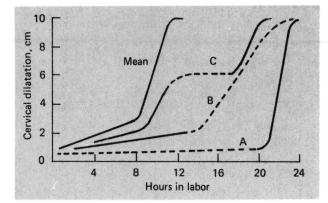

Figure 15–2
The major labor aberrations are shown in comparison with the mean cervical dilatation time curve for nulliparous women: *A,* prolonged latent phase; *B,* protracted active phase dilatation; and *C,* secondary arrest of dilatation. (From Friedman, E. [1965]. In J. P. Greenhill [Ed.], *Obstetrics* [13th ed.]. Philadelphia, Saunders.)

2. Physical findings
   a. Hypertonia (primary inertia)
      (1) Uncoordinated uterine activity: no normal resting phase
      (2) More than one uterine pacemaker sending signals
      (3) Frequent contractions
      (4) Occurs in latent phase (protracted latent phase)
      (5) Painful because of uterine anoxia
   b. Hypotonia (secondary inertia)
      (1) Ineffective tightening and pressure
      (2) Contractions insufficient to dilate cervix
      (3) Poor contraction intensity
      (4) Occurs in active phase (protracted active phase)
   c. Precipitate labor
      (1) Labor of less than 3 hours
      (2) Low maternal tissue resistance
      (3) Often rapid transit of fetus through birth canal
3. Diagnostic findings
   a. Pathological retraction ring (Bandl's ring) (Fig. 15–3)
      (1) A normal physiological retraction ring develops at the junction of the active upper and passive lower segments of the uterus
      (2) A pathological ring is an exaggeration of this physiological ring; it grips the fetus, preventing descent
      (3) Labor is arrested at this point
      (4) The uterus above the ring becomes thicker, and the lower segment thins out and ruptures unless the obstruction is relieved
      (5) Drugs to relax the uterus are used
      (6) If drug therapy is not successful, delivery must be made by cesarean birth
   b. Fetus in occiput posterior position
      (1) A larger diameter presents to the pelvis
      (2) The degree of flexion is altered
      (3) Cervical dilatation and fetal descent are slowed

B. Nursing Diagnoses

1. Anxiety related to abnormal progress of labor
2. Knowledge deficit related to dysfunctional labor
3. Pain related to abnormal labor pattern
4. High risk for infection related to prolonged labor

C. Interventions/Evaluations

1. Anxiety related to abnormal progress of labor

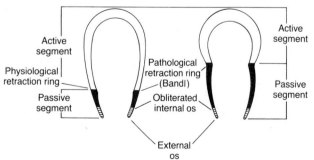

Figure 15–3
Pathological retraction ring in uterus during labor: A, normal second stage; and B, abnormal second stage—dystocia. (Redrawn from Cunningham, G., MacDonald, P., & Gant, N. [1988]. *Williams obstetrics* [18th ed., p. 214]. Norwalk, CT: Appleton & Lange.)

a. Interventions
  (1) Monitor progress of labor
    (a) Document contraction pattern
    (b) Perform vaginal examinations to determine cervical dilatation and fetal descent
    (c) Communicate deviations from normal to physician or midwife
  (2) Explain unknown or unplanned situations in an easily understood manner
  (3) Identify how this situation may alter birth plan
  (4) Maintain a positive attitude about ability to cope
  (5) Reassure the client as to the status of the fetus
b. Evaluations
  (1) Client verbalizes understanding of the situation and the options available
  (2) Client has a positive attitude and realistic expectations about outcome

2. Knowledge deficit related to dysfunctional labor
  a. Interventions
    (1) Provide factual information about dysfunctional labor
    (2) Explain expected treatment and outcome
      (a) Oxytocin use for hypotonic labor
      (b) Sedation
      (c) Regional anesthesia for hypertonic labor
    (3) Encourage questions and expression of feelings
  b. Evaluations
    (1) Client verbalizes understanding of dysfunctional labor
    (2) Client is cooperative and involved in alternative to birth plan
    (3) Informed consent has been given

3. Pain related to abnormal labor pattern
  a. Interventions
    (1) Provide analgesia or anesthesia as appropriate
    (2) Use counterpressure with low back pain or other nonpharmacological techniques
    (3) Document contractions and response and coping ability
  b. Evaluations
    (1) Reduction of client's tension and anxiety provides comfort
    (2) Client verbalizes decreased discomfort
    (3) No adverse effects of medications are seen in mother or fetus

4. High risk for infection due to prolonged labor
  a. Interventions
    (1) Monitor and document vital signs and FHR
    (2) Maintain good aseptic technique
      (a) Minimize vaginal examinations
      (b) Perineal cleanliness
    (3) Monitor characteristics and odor of amniotic fluid
    (4) Administer antibiotics as indicated
  b. Evaluations
    (1) Temperature, FHR, and WBC count are within normal limits
    (2) There is no sign of infection

Cesarean Birth

Delivery is through incisions in abdominal and uterine walls

A. Assessment

1. History
  a. Previous uterine surgery
  b. Maternal condition: hemorrhage, for example

   c. Maternal illness
  2. Physical findings
   a. Indications for cesarean birth
    (1) Fetal distress, disease, or anomaly
    (2) Fetal malposition or malpresentation
    (3) Fetal macrosomia
    (4) Active herpes genitalis
    (5) Cephalopelvic disproportion
    (6) Placental abnormality
     (a) Placenta previa
     (b) Abruptio placentae
   b. Vaginal birth after cesarean (VBAC)
    (1) Decision making
     (a) Nonrepeating condition
     (b) Desire to avoid cesarean birth
     (c) Ability to do emergency cesarean birth
     (d) Benefits mother by shortening recovery time
    (2) Risks
     (a) Small possibility of uterine rupture
     (b) Need for close monitoring during labor
  3. Psychosocial
   a. Relief after long labor with failure to progress
   b. Fear if fetus or mother is stressed
   c. Helplessness if birth plan is altered
   d. Disappointment if vaginal delivery is not achieved
  4. Diagnostic findings
   a. Preoperative CBC, urinalysis, blood typed and crossmatched
   b. Fetal lung maturity and gestational age if elective
   c. Ultrasound for fetal position and placental placement
  5. Anesthesia
   a. General
    (1) General anesthesia usually is used only in emergency situations or when regional anesthesia is contraindicated
    (2) General anesthesia leads to central nervous system (CNS) depression of mother and fetus
    (3) Mother must take nothing by mouth
    (4) Antacids are given before surgery
    (5) Because of the resulting hypoxia in the baby, it is recommended that induction time to birth be less than 8 minutes
   b. Regional
    (1) Spinal
     (a) Local anesthesia is injected into the subarachnoid space
     (b) Motor and sensory block ensues
     (c) Spinal anesthesia has the potential for causing severe headaches during recovery period
    (2) Epidural
     (a) Local anesthesia is injected into epidural space
     (b) Sensory block of entire pelvis and legs ensues
     (c) Epidural block has the potential for hypotensive episode if the mother is not well hydrated first
     (d) If hypotension occurs, fetus may suffer distress

B. **Nursing Diagnoses**

1. Anxiety related to surgical delivery
2. Knowledge deficit related to cesarean birth
3. Pain related to surgical intervention
4. High risk for fluid volume deficit related to surgical procedure and blood loss

5. High risk for infection related to surgical procedure
6. Self-esteem disturbance related to change in birth plan

C. Interventions/Evaluations

1. Anxiety related to surgical delivery
   a. Interventions
      (1) Assist client with appropriate coping techniques
      (2) Encourage active participation in decision making
      (3) Provide clear explanations of all proposed treatment options
      (4) Facilitate involvement of support person
      (5) Reassure client about infant if surgery is performed for fetal distress
   b. Evaluation
      (1) Client uses effective coping methods
      (2) Client verbalizes understanding of the situation and the options available
2. Knowledge deficit related to cesarean birth
   a. Interventions
      (1) Provide factual information about cesarean birth and informed consent
      (2) Explain expected procedures
         (a) Anesthesia preparation
            (i) IV fluid
            (ii) Client takes nothing by mouth
            (iii) Antacid administered if general anesthesia planned
         (b) Foley catheter
         (c) Skin preparation
      (3) Encourage questions and verbalization of situation
   b. Evaluations
      (1) Client verbalizes understanding and acceptance of situation not a part of birth plan
      (2) Client is cooperative and involved in preparation for cesarean birth
3. Pain related to surgical intervention
   a. Interventions
      (1) Use nonpharmacological methods for relief as appropriate
      (2) Provide analgesia or anesthesia as appropriate
      (3) Position for comfort
   b. Evaluations
      (1) Reduction of tension and anxiety provides comfort
      (2) Client reports decreased discomfort
      (3) No adverse effects from medication are seen
4. High risk for fluid volume deficit related to surgical procedure and blood loss
   a. Interventions
      (1) Monitor I and O and hydration status
      (2) Observe and document blood loss
      (3) Monitor vital signs for impending shock
   b. Evaluations
      (1) Hydration is maintained
      (2) No excessive blood loss is seen
      (3) Vital signs remain within normal limits
5. High risk for infection due to cesarean birth
   a. Interventions
      (1) Monitor and document vital signs and FHR
      (2) Monitor characteristics and odor of amniotic fluid
      (3) Maintain good aseptic technique during
         (a) Vaginal examinations
         (b) Catheterization
         (c) Preoperative skin preparation
      (4) Monitor blood loss

(5) Administer antibiotics as indicated
b. Evaluations
(1) Temperature and WBC count within normal limits
(2) Client has no infection
6. Self-esteem disturbance related to change in birth plan
a. Interventions
(1) Discuss changes in birth plan
(2) Encourage verbalization of feelings about a cesarean birth rather than a vaginal delivery
(3) Involve the client in decision making
(4) Provide positive reassurances
b. Evaluations
(1) Client verbalizes self-confidence
(2) Client verbalizes positive attitude and realistic expectations

Health Education

A. **Intrapartum health education should provide the following**

1. Information about the process of labor
2. Clear explanations about the procedures (risk versus benefits) performed during the process of labor and delivery
3. Information about the available pain-relief methods
4. Methods of involvement and participation during the intrapartum period
5. Preoperative teaching for cesarean birth
6. Information about variables that may alter or influence a birth plan

---

CASE STUDY AND STUDY QUESTIONS

Donna Verlo, a 24-year-old gravida 2, para 1 (G2,P1), is admitted to labor and delivery at 39 weeks' gestation. A vaginal examination indicates her cervix is 80% effaced and 3 cm dilated. The presenting vertex is at −1 station. The amniotic sac is not palpated, and Donna says she thinks it has ruptured.

1. What should the nurse ask about the amniotic sac?

   a. The time the membranes ruptured.

   b. The frequency of contractions.

   c. The presence of back pain.

   d. The presence of bloody show.

2. During this early phase of labor, how often should the FHR be evaluated?

   a. At least every 15 minutes.

   b. Every 5 to 10 minutes, depending on the technique.

   c. At least every 30 minutes.

   d. At least every hour.

3. To promote comfort, Donna is encouraged to assume certain positions while in labor and to avoid others. Which of the following should not be used during labor?

   a. Lateral position.

   b. Squatting position.

   c. Standing position.

   d. Supine position.

4. As Donna's labor progresses to 5 cm, she becomes increasingly uncomfortable and requests an epidural anesthetic. After this is in place, what should the nurse be particularly alert to?

   a. Possible hypertensive rebound.

   b. Possible hypotensive episode.

   c. Increased thirst.

   d. Signs of water intoxication.

When Donna is comfortable from the epidural, it is observed that her contractions have spaced out to a frequency of every 5 to 6 minutes and are only mild to palpation. An oxytocin infusion is started to augment her labor.

5. What would be the most likely classification for the dysfunctional labor?

 a. Pathologic retraction ring.

 b. Hypertonic labor.

 c. Protracted active phase.

 d. Prolonged latent phase.

6. All of the following are possible side effects of oxytocin administration except:

 a. Fetal hyperglycemia.

 b. Fetal hyperbilirubinemia.

 c. Hyperstimulation of the uterus.

 d. Water intoxication.

7. When should the oxytocin infusion be discontinued?

 a. When the client is comfortable with her contractions.

 b. When signs of fetal distress are seen on the fetal monitor.

 c. When the contractions are 3 minutes apart.

 d. When the client is ready to push.

8. On assessment, Donna is found to be completely dilated and effaced and at a +1 station. Which of the following findings suggest transition to the second stage of labor?

 a. Decreased urge to push.

 b. Decreased bloody show.

 c. FHR accelerations.

 d. Bulging of the perineum.

Because of the epidural anesthetic, Donna is not able to push as effectively. She pushes the baby to a +3 station but cannot bring it under the symphysis to effect delivery. It is decided to assist her by use of the vacuum extractor.

9. Which of the following are prerequisites for use of the vacuum?

 (1) Membranes intact.

 (2) Presenting part engaged.

 (3) Cervix completely dilated.

 (4) Documentation of gestational age.

 (5) Empty bladder.

 a. 1, 2, 3.

 b. 2, 4, 5.

 c. 2, 3, 5.

 d. 3, 5.

10. What should the infant be carefully examined for after this procedure?

 a. Brachial plexus injury.

 b. Respiratory distress.

 c. Facial bruising.

 d. Cephalhematoma.

11. Which of the following structures are involved when an episiotomy is performed?

 (1) Vaginal mucosa.

 (2) Levator ani muscle.

 (3) Glans clitoris.

 (4) Cardinal ligament.

 (5) Fourchette.

 a. 1.

 b. 1, 2.

 c. 1, 2, 5.

 d. All of the above.

12. Obstetrical forceps are often used to facilitate delivery. In which of the following conditions might such a delivery be indicated?

 (1) The cervix fails to dilate completely.

 (2) The mother has cardiovascular disease.

 (3) The mother has a contracted pelvis.

 (4) The umbilical cord is prolapsed.

 (5) Meconium-stained amniotic fluid is passed with a vertex presentation at full dilatation.

 a. 1, 2.

 b. 3, 5.

 c. 2, 5.

 d. 2, 3, 4.

13. Which of the following signs would indicate that delivery is imminent?

    (1) The mother has the desire to defecate.

    (2) An increase in frequency, duration, and intensity of uterine contractions.

    (3) The mother begins to bear down spontaneously with uterine contractions.

    (4) Bulging of the perineum occurs.

    (5) There is an increase in the amount of blood-stained mucus flowing from the vagina.

    a. 4.

    b. 1, 3, 4.

    c. 2, 4, 5.

    d. 2.

    e. All of the above.

14. The nurse caring for the mother and baby in the fourth stage of labor would do which of the following?

    (1) Keep the mother warm and out of drafts.

    (2) Massage the uterus every 15 minutes, or more often, if needed.

    (3) Massage the uterus continuously.

    (4) Check maternal vital signs every 15 minutes.

    (5) Administer oxytocin as ordered.

    a. 1, 2, 4.

    b. 2, 4, 5.

    c. 3, 4.

    d. 2, 4.

    e. 1, 4, 5.

15. Identify and match the most important risks of the various methods of obstetrical anesthesia listed below.

    (1) General anesthesia   a. Fetal brady-cardia

    (2) Regional conduction anesthesia   b. Aspiration of stomach contents

    (3) Paracervical block   c. Maternal hypo-tension

16. Match each term or phrase with the definition that best fits it.

    (1) Enlargement of the external os to 10 cm in diameter   a. Uterine atony

    (2) Maximum shortening of the cervical canal   b. Complete dilatation

    (3) A condition caused by failure of the uterine muscle to stay contracted after delivery   c. Lightening

    (4) Surgical incision of the perineum during the second stage of labor   d. Complete effacement

    (5) Settling of the baby's head into the brim of the pelvis   e. Episiotomy

Answers to Study Questions

1. a	2. c	3. d
4. b	5. c	6. a
7. b	8. d	9. c
10. d	11. a	12. c
13. e	14. b	

15. (1) b   (2) c   (3) a

16. (1) b   (2) d   (3) a   (4) e   (5) c

REFERENCES

Allen-Farley, A. (1987). Vaginal birth after cesarean section. *NAACOG Update Series #5.* Washington, DC: NAACOG.

Barnett, M.M., & Humerick, S.S. (1982). Infant outcome in relation to second stage labor pushing method. *Birth, 9*(4), 221–229.

Bloom, K. (1984). Assisting the unprepared woman during labor. *Journal of Obstetric, Gynecologic, and Neonatal Nursing, 13*(5), 303–306.

Brucher, M.C. (1986). Once a section, not always a section. *NAACOG Update Series #4.* Washington, DC: NAACOG.

Butnarescu, G.F., & Tillotson, D.M. (1983). *Maternity nursing theory to practice.* New York: Wiley.

Carr, K.C. (1987). Management of the second stage of labor. *NAACOG Update Series #1.* Washington, DC: NAACOG.

Cogan, R. (1987). Labor support. *NAACOG Update Series #5*. Washington, DC: NAACOG.

Cohen, S.M., Kenner, C.A., & Hollingsworth, A.O. (1991). *Maternal, neonatal, and women's health nursing*. Springhouse, PA: Springhouse.

Cunningham, G., MacDonald, P., & Gant, N. (1988). *Williams obstetrics* (18th ed.). Norwalk, CT: Appleton & Lange.

Doeges, M.E., Kenty, J.R., & Moorhouse, M.F. (1988). *Maternal newborn careplans*. Philadelphia: Davis.

Hazle, N.R. (1986). Hydration in labor: Is routine intravenous hydration necessary? *Journal of Nurse–Midwifery, 31*(4), 171–176.

Jones, E.J. (1986). The nurse's role in induction/augmentation of labor. *NAACOG Update Series #4*. Washington, DC: NAACOG.

Kirby-McDonnel, A. (1989). Epidural anesthesia for labor & delivery. *NAACOG Update Series #6*. Washington, DC: NAACOG.

Knuppel, R.A., & Drukker, J.E. (1986). *High-risk pregnancy: A team approach*. Philadelphia: Saunders.

Long, P.J. (1984). Emergency delivery. *NAACOG Update Series #1*. Washington, DC: NAACOG.

Malinowski, J.S., Pedigo, C.G., & Phillips, C.R. (1989). *Nursing care during the delivery process* (3rd ed.). Philadelphia: Davis.

Marshall, C. (1985). The art of induction/augmentation of labor. *Journal of Obstetric, Gynecologic, and Neonatal Nursing, 14*(1), 22–28.

May, K.A., & Mahmeister, L.R. (1990). *Comprehensive maternity nursing process and the childbearing family*. Philadelphia: Lippincott.

McKay, S. (1981). Second stage labor: Has tradition replaced safety? *American Journal of Nursing, 81*(5), 1016–1019.

NAACOG. (1991). *Standards for the nursing care of women and newborns* (4th ed). Washington, DC: NAACOG.

NAACOG. (1988). *Practice competencies and educational guidelines for nurse providers of intrapartum care*. Washington, DC: NAACOG.

NAACOG. (1988). *The nurse's role in induction/augmentation of labor*. Washington, DC: NAACOG.

NANDA. (1990). *Taxonomy I revised*. St. Louis: North American Nursing Diagnosis Association.

Neeson, J., & May, K. (1986). *Comprehensive maternity nursing*. Philadelphia: Lippincott.

Olds, S., London, M., & Ladwig, M. (1992). *Maternity newborn nursing: A family-centered approach* (4th ed.). Redwood City, CA: Addison-Wesley.

Reeder, S., & Martin, L., (1987). *Maternity nursing: family, newborn and women's health care* (16th ed.). Philadelphia: Lippincott.

Simkin, P. (1987). The normal first and second stages of labor. *NAACOG Update Series #5*. Washington, DC: NAACOG.

Varney, H. (1980). *Nurse-midwifery*. Boston: Blackwell.

Judy Schmidt

Fetal Assessment

Objectives

1. Identify and interpret fetal heart rate (FHR) patterns of variable, late, and early decelerations and accelerations

2. Identify baseline (BL) features, including rate, long-term variability (LTV), and short-term variability (STV)

3. Explain the difference between LTV and STV and their significance in the interpretation of FHR tracings

4. Assess the status of the fetus as shown by periodic patterns, rate, and variability

5. State and write accurate and complete descriptions of FHR events for the patient record

6. Reiterate the critical values of fetal blood gases and pH and relate these to the probable status

7. Discuss the probable etiology of FHR pattern changes

8. State appropriate interventions for deceleration patterns and altered variability

9. Explain the physiology of interventions used to improve FHR

Introduction

Electronic fetal monitoring (EFM) uses electronic techniques to continuously monitor FHR and uterine contractions (UCs). The technique provides a permanent record that can be observed and discussed instantaneously or retrospectively by professional care providers. Events that cannot be heard or measured by auscultation, such as variability, or other methods are available through EFM. Therefore, EFM is another tool available to the care provider to easily provide information that would otherwise consume many hours of care and yield less complete data.

A. Instrumental methods of FHR assessment
1. Fetoscope
    a. Assesses rate and significant rate changes of accelerations and decelerations
    b. Evaluates FHR and rhythm intermittently
    c. Provides no permanent record

   d. Is difficult to use with inexperience, maternal movement, and UCs
   e. Does not allow the assessment of variability or subtle changes in FHR from baseline (BL)
2. Doppler methods: hand held
   a. Assesses rate and significant accelerations and decelerations
   b. Evaluates FHR intermittently
   c. Provides no permanent record
   d. Is easier to use than a fetoscope
   e. Is more difficult to use with maternal movement
   f. Does not allow the assessment of variability or subtle changes in FHR from BL
3. Ultrasound tests using an electronic fetal monitor
   a. Assesses rate, accelerations, decelerations, and LTV; some monitors may partially evaluate STV on the ultrasound mode
   b. Provides a continuous assessment of FHR (if adequate application is possible)
   c. Provides a permanent record
   d. Can be observed from many locations when visual screens are used as a central display or as a bedside monitor that can show any or all clients in the labor unit
4. Spiral electrode via EFM
   a. Assesses FHR, accelerations, decelerations, LTV, and STV with optimal accuracy
   b. Provides a continuous assessment (if adequate application is possible)
   c. Provides a permanent record
   d. Can be observed from many locations when visual screens are used
5. Fetal scalp sampling (see later)

B. **Fetal factors influencing the FHR**
1. Parasympathetic nervous system
   a. Slows the FHR and variability
   b. Provides variability
   c. Is of vagal origin
2. Sympathetic nervous system
   a. Increases the rate
   b. Influences epinephrine and norepinephrine
3. Baroreceptors
   a. Are located in carotid artery and aortic arch
   b. Respond to fetal blood pressure changes and transfer information to sympathetic and parasympathetic systems
4. Chemoreceptors
   a. Are located in aortic arch and carotid artery
   b. Consist of peripheral receptors in the central nervous system (CNS)
   c. Respond to fetal oxygen and carbon dioxide changes and transfer the information to sympathetic and parasympathetic systems
   d. Are the least-understood factor influencing FHR
5. CNS states
   a. In fetal sleep cycles of 20 to 40 minutes, variability and reactivity decrease
   b. In alert states, FHR variability and reactivity increase

Clinical Practice

BASELINE VARIATIONS

Baseline Fetal Heart Rate

A. Assessment

Normal rate ranges from 120 to 160 beats per minute (bpm); usually 10 minutes or more is needed to establish an FHR BL (Fig. 16–1).

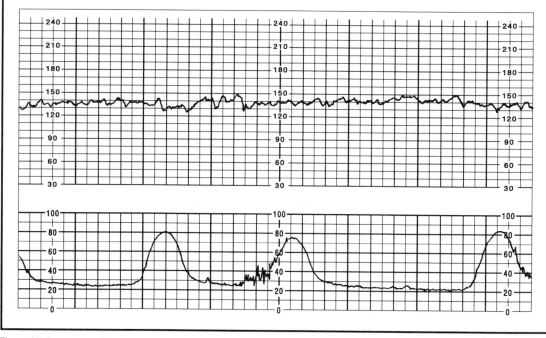

Figure 16–1
Normal baseline and variability.

1. Tachycardia
   a. History: possible etiology
      (1) Maternal fever
      (2) Infection
      (3) Beta-sympathetic drugs
      (4) Maternal endogenous epinephrine
      (5) Maternal or fetal cardiac abnormality
      (6) Chronic fetal hypoxemia
      (7) Thyrotoxicosis
      (8) Compensatory mechanism following hypoxic insult
   b. Physical findings (Fig. 16–2)
      (1) Persistent FHR that is of more than 160 bpm
      (2) Duration that is a minimum of 10 minutes and has no maximum (days or weeks are possible)
2. Bradycardia
   a. History: possible etiology
      (1) Decreased cord perfusion
      (2) Anesthetic agents
      (3) Medications, such as propranolol
      (4) Substance abuse
      (5) Hypothermia
      (6) Terminal fetal condition
   b. Physical findings (Fig. 16–3)
      (1) FHR below 120 bpm
      (2) Duration of at least 10 minutes

B. Nursing Diagnoses

1. Fetus at high risk for impaired gas exchange related to intrapartal reduction of oxygen levels

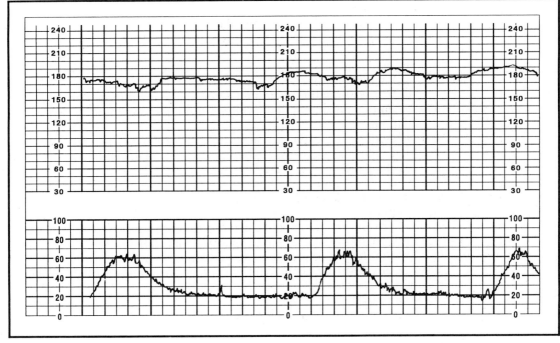

Figure 16–2
Tachycardia from maternal fever.

2. Maternal anxiety related to fetal status
3. Alteration in maternal comfort related to immobility

C. Interventions/Evaluations

1. Fetus at high risk of impaired gas exchange related to intrapartal reduction of oxygen levels
   a. Interventions
      (1) Increase hydration
      (2) Position the mother on her side

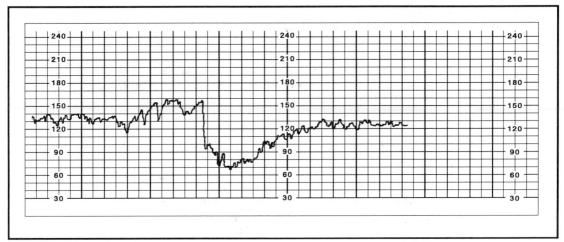

Figure 16–3
Transient bradycardia.

            (3) Administer oxygen

            (4) Monitor maternal vital signs and blood pressure

            (5) For tachycardia: administer antipyretic medications if ordered for maternal fever

            (6) For bradycardia

                (a) Vaginal examination for possible cord prolapse

                (b) Scalp stimulation if ordered according to institutional protocol

            (7) Accurately document FHR findings and interventions

        b. Evaluations

            (1) No evidence of fetal tachycardia or bradycardia on the fetal monitor

            (2) Maternal vital signs and blood pressure remain within or return to normal limits

            (3) No cord is felt on vaginal examination

  2. Maternal anxiety related to fetal status

        a. Interventions

            (1) Provide information about the possible causes of change in FHR BL

            (2) Provide information about the current fetal status

            (3) Explain the reasons for the interventions

            (4) Remain with the client, and encourage a significant other to remain when possible

        b. Evaluations

            (1) Client reports a decrease in anxiety

            (2) Support person remains at the bedside

  3. Alteration in maternal comfort related to immobility

        a. Interventions

            (1) Change her position frequently

            (2) Use measures such as pillows, blankets, and back rubs to maintain her position and promote comfort

            (3) Explain why certain positions may be necessary for fetal well-being

        b. Evaluations

            (1) Client changes positions when requested and for her own comfort

            (2) Client indicates an understanding of the necessity for certain position changes

Variability

A. Assessment

  1. LTV

        a. History

            (1) Amplitude of FHR described by the following terms

                (a) Normal: a change of more than 6 to 10 bpm from BL (see Fig. 16–1)

                (b) Increased: a change of more than 15 bpm from BL (Fig. 16–4)

                (c) Marked or saltatory: a change of more than 25 bpm from BL

                (d) Decreased: a change of more than 6 to 10 bpm from BL (Fig. 16–5)

                (e) Absent: a change of less than 2 bpm from BL

            (2) Cyclicity: 3 to 6 cycles per minute is normal

            (3) Undulating pattern: sinusoidal

                (a) Sine wave appears with an absent STV

                (b) Usually occurs spontaneously

                (c) Indicates fetal anemia, severe hypoxemia, or both

                (d) Is associated with Rh sensitization

                (e) Is associated with fetomaternal hemorrhage

            (4) Undulating pattern: pseudosinusoidal

                (a) Is preceded by a normal FHR

                (b) Follows the administration of analgesics or other drugs

                (c) Is temporary and self-limiting

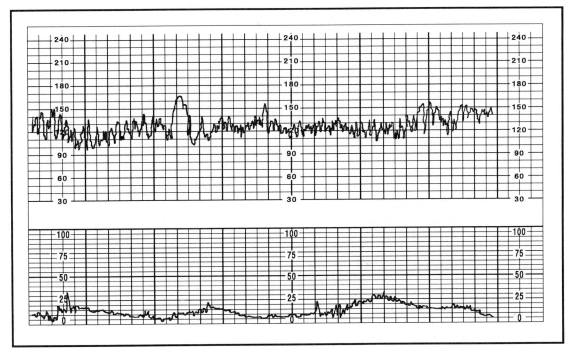

Figure 16–4
Increased LTV.

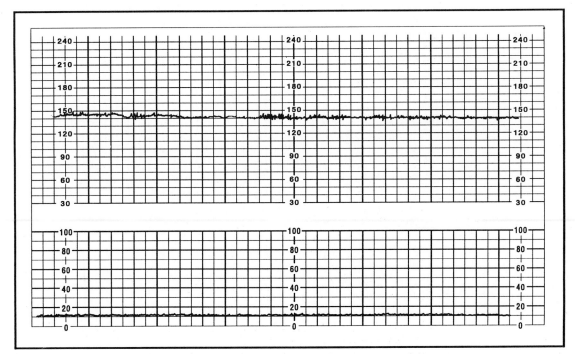

Figure 16–5
Decreased LTV on ultrasound.

        (d) STV is usually present

        (e) Has the sawtooth appearance of FHR

    b. Physical findings

        (1) LTV can be determined by fluctuations of the FHR or where the line (tracing the fetal heart) goes

        (2) An awake and active fetus has a normal or increased LTV

        (3) A sleeping fetus may have a decreased LTV during a typical sleep cycle, which lasts about 30 minutes

2. STV

    a. History: STV can be described by using the following terms

        (1) Present: FHR line is rough (see Fig. 16–1)

        (2) Absent: FHR line is smooth (Figs. 16–6 and 16–7)

        (3) Intermittent: FHR line has alternate periods of roughness and smoothness

    b. Physical findings

        (1) STV is determined by the time interval from one fetal heartbeat to the next, which is a short time interval measured in milliseconds; it is poorly defined by numerical values

        (2) STV is visualized by evaluating the actual line tracing the FHR

3. Arrhythmias or dysrhythmias

    a. History

        (1) Pattern appearance varies

        (2) Exact type of premature ventricular contraction or premature atrial contraction may be unknown

        (3) Are usually benign in the presence of variability and reactivity

        (4) Usually resolve after birth

    b. Physical findings (Fig. 16–8)

        (1) Irregular tracing shape and sound of the fetal heart occur

        (2) Irregularity of the pattern is persistent

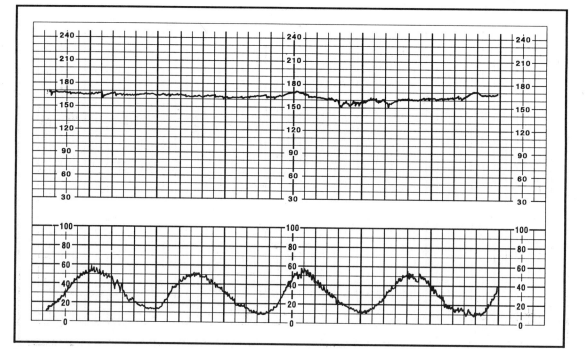

Figure 16–6
STV and LTV decreased related to hyperstimulation.

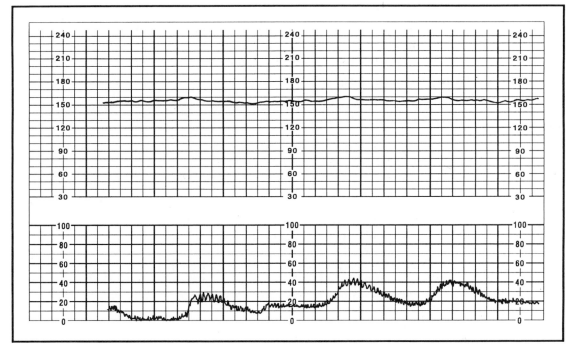

Figure 16–7
STV absent.

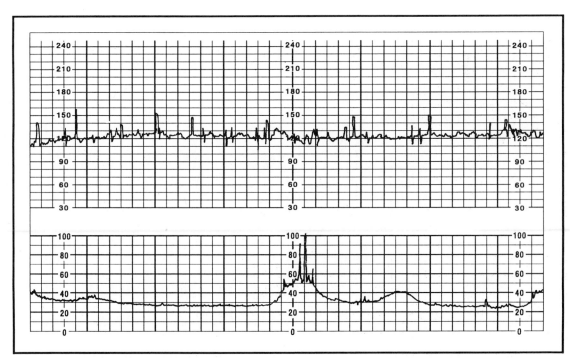

Figure 16–8
Arrhythmias or ectopic beats, LTV present, STV present.

B. Nursing Diagnoses

1. Fetus at high risk for impaired gas exchange related to intrapartal reduction of oxygen levels
2. Maternal anxiety related to fetal status

C. Interventions/Evaluations

1. Fetus at high risk for impaired gas exchange related to intrapartal reduction of oxygen levels
   a. Interventions
      (1) Investigate the possible causes of decreased variability
         (a) If hypoxia is suspected
            (i) Change maternal position (preferably to a lateral position)
            (ii) Administer oxygen
            (iii) Give fluids by bolus
            (iv) If oxytocin is being administered, discontinue the infusion
            (v) If hyperstimulation is observed, administer tocolytics, as ordered
         (b) Investigate a history of maternal drug intake (therapeutic and illicit)
         (c) Determine if the fetus is in a sleep cycle
      (2) Perform scalp stimulation as a test of fetal response to stimulus
   b. Evaluations
      (1) Possible cause of decreased variability is identified
      (2) Maternal position is changed
      (3) Oxygen is administered
      (4) Oxytocin is discontinued or tocolytics are administered
      (5) Fetus responds to scalp stimulation with accelerations in FHR
2. Maternal anxiety related to fetal status
   a. Interventions
      (1) Reassure about fetal condition
      (2) Explain the interventions in terms of improving fetal well-being
   b. Evaluations: client reports a decrease in anxiety

PERIODIC PATTERNS

Periodic patterns are FHR patterns that are associated with UCs.

Variable Decelerations

A. Assessment

1. History: probable etiology
   a. Umbilical cord compression
   b. Decreased umbilical cord perfusion
   c. Baroreceptor stimulation with vagal response
   d. Hypoxia and hypercarbic states
2. Physical findings
   a. Pattern characteristics
      (1) Variable shape: W, U, V shapes (Figs. 16–9, 16–10, and 16–11)
      (2) Variable onset
      (3) Often drops abruptly and significantly below the BL of the FHR
      (4) May or may not be associated with preaccelerations and postaccelerations (also called shoulders)
      (5) May resemble other periodic patterns, such as late and early decelerations
   b. Indicative of fetal well-being
      (1) STV is present
      (2) Quick fetal recovery

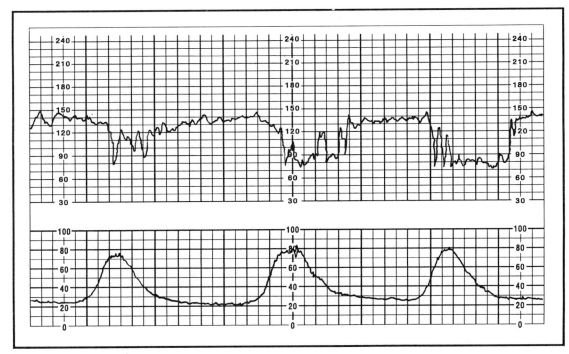

Figure 16–9
Variable decelerations tolerated well by fetus as evidenced by recovery and good LTV and STV.

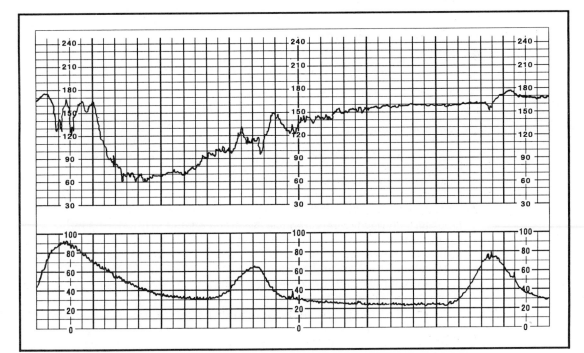

Figure 16–10
Variable deceleration, decreased LTV.

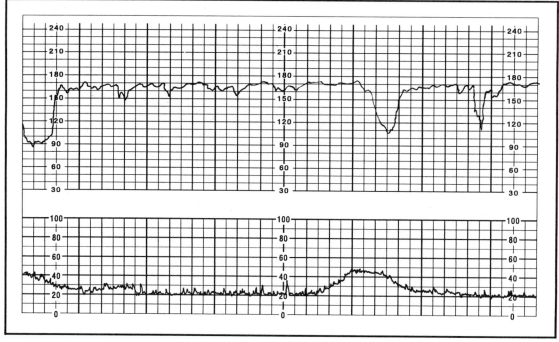

Figure 16–11
Variable decelerations, LTV present, STV absent.

   c. Indicative of fetal compromise
     (1) STV is absent
       (a) STV is usually lost first at the nadir of deceleration
       (b) STV is lost next during the recovery of deceleration
       (c) STV is lost last between decelerations (in BL rate)
     (2) Slow fetal recovery
     (3) Compensatory overshoots of FHR
       (a) Without variability and persistent
       (b) Of 20 to 30 bpm above FHR BL
       (c) Lasts more than 20 to 30 seconds
     (4) Change of BL with decreased variability

B. Nursing Diagnoses

1. Fetus at high risk for impaired gas exchange related to intrapartal reduction of oxygen levels
2. Maternal anxiety related to fetal status

C. Interventions/Evaluations

1. Fetus at high risk for impaired gas exchange related to intrapartal reduction of oxygen levels
   a. Interventions
     (1) Change of maternal position
       (a) Change pressure on umbilical cord
         (i) May abolish, improve, or worsen FHR pattern
         (ii) Change to lateral left or lateral right position or
         (iii) Hands-and-knees position or
         (iv) Lateral (15° to 20°) with slight Trendelenburg position
       (b) Avoid supine hypotension and maximize uteroplacental blood flow

      (2) Administer nondextrose IV fluid bolus

         (a) May improve blood volume and perfusion and, thereby, the FHR pattern, UC pattern, or both

         (b) May be contraindicated with cardiovascular or hypertensive maternal disease

      (3) Administer oxygen when STV is absent or intermittent

         (a) With rebreather bag on a face mask, use 10 to 12 l/min

         (b) Without rebreather bag on a face mask, use at least 6 to 8 l/min

         (c) To maximize oxygen therapy, ensure that an adequate blood volume is present

            (i) Oxygen is volume-dependent, as opposed to diffusion-dependent

            (ii) Position laterally, provide IV fluids, or both

      (4) Perform scalp stimulation

         (a) Sympathetic response may improve recovery and variability

         (b) Is useful for prolonged decelerations

         (c) Is useful for bradycardias

         (d) Is useful for slow recovery of variable decelerations

         (e) May improve BL variability

         (f) Note: fetal heart accelerations following scalp stimulation will usually rule out an acidotic fetus

      (5) Administer amnioinfusion according to hospital protocol

         (a) Cushions the cord and lessens its compression

         (b) Relieves or lessens variable decelerations

         (c) Dilutes meconium, if it is present

         (d) Sample protocol (see own institutional guidelines)

            (i) Infuse 15 to 20 ml of fluid per minute until the decelerations resolve

            (ii) Then administer an additional 250 ml

            (iii) Total infusion amount is approximately 500 to 800 ml

            (iv) Infusion may be discontinued when variables are abolished, the meconium is diluted, or 800 ml is infused

      (6) Document the client record (chart or computer chart)

         (a) Write the duration and depth of the deceleration

         (b) Recovery time: if it is slow, note the recovery time in seconds

         (c) Rate and variability: LTV and STV

         (d) Document the trend of the pattern, including UCs

         (e) Do not document each deceleration of a pattern or trend

         (f) Document interventions and the resulting change (favorable or unfavorable) or absence of change in the FHR pattern

         (g) Use hospital-approved abbreviations (see examples in Table 16–1)

  b. Evaluation

    (1) Absence of or improvement in variable decelerations

    (2) Improved variability during deceleration and in BL

    (3) Improved recovery time to BL, with variability

2. Maternal anxiety related to fetal status

  a. Interventions

    (1) Remain calm

    (2) Provide explanations to the client and family of the interventions and reasons for them

    (3) Explain that often some dramatic FHR patterns are seen that the fetus tolerates well

    (4) Explain that the inability to correct nonreassuring or distress patterns may result in rapid action or intervention on the part of several professionals

  b. Evaluations: client reports a decrease in anxiety

Table 16–1
ABBREVIATIONS FOR CHARTING ELECTRONIC FETAL MONITORING

EFM	Electronic fetal monitor(ing)
FHR	Fetal heart rate or rhythm
US	Ultrasonography (external)
TOCO	Tocodynamometer (external)
SE	Spiral electrode (internal)
IUPC	Intrauterine pressure catheter (internal)
UC	Uterine contraction
BL	Baseline (refers to FHR and sometimes to baseline tonus)
bpm	Beats per minute
LTV +	Long-term variability is present, >6 to 10 beats amplitude and 3 to 6 cycle changes/min
LTV 0	Long-term variability is absent, <2 bpm amplitude and 3 cycle changes
LTV ↓	Long-term variability is decreased <6 to 10 bpm amplitude and <3 cycle changes/min
LTV ↑	>15 beats amplitude
LTV marked	>25 beats amplitude
STV +	Short-term variability is present; roughness of tracing line is present
STV 0	Short-term variability is absent; tracing line is smooth
STV inter	Short-term variability is intermittent; + and 0 during a >10-minute observation
Late decel	Late deceleration
Early decel	Early deceleration
Var decel	Variable deceleration
Prolonged decel	Deceleration more than 2 minutes

Late Decelerations

A. Assessment

1. History
   a. Probable etiology is decreased uteroplacental blood flow related to one of the following
      (1) Uteroplacental insufficiency (anatomically deficient)
      (2) Impeded blood flow (also termed reflex late decelerations) resulting from
         (a) Supine position
         (b) Maternal hypotension from
            (i) Blood loss
            (ii) Anesthesia
            (iii) Medication
            (iv) Drug use
         (c) Uterine hyperstimulation, which significantly reduces placental blood flow
   b. Clinical conditions that contribute to uteroplacental insufficiency as evidenced by late decelerations
      (1) Pregnancy-induced hypertension
      (2) Chronic maternal disease (e.g., diabetes, lupus, or hypertension)
      (3) Intrauterine growth retardation
      (4) Uterine hyperstimulus, high BL resting tone, or both
      (5) Abruptio placentae
      (6) Maternal drug use
      (7) Maternal smoking
      (8) Poor maternal nutrition
      (9) Postdate pregnancy
      (10) Supine position maintained during labor or delivery
      (11) Hypotension associated with anesthesia
      (12) Placenta: frequently small, aged, calcified, or deteriorated
      (13) Trauma: associated with blood loss and hypotension

(14) Medication reactions

(15) Multiple gestation

2. Physical findings: pattern characteristics (Figs. 16–12 to 16–14)

   a. Shape is uniform

   b. Pattern is smooth and persistent

   c. Onset and offset occur late in a UC

     (1) Usually begin at or slightly after the peak (acme) of a UC; the onset may be 20 to 30 seconds after the UC begins

     (2) HR recovers to BL between UCs

   d. BL commonly has absent or decreased variability: LTV and STV

   e. Decelerations usually occur within the normal FHR range; a deviation of 10 to 30 bpm from BL is common

   f. The intensity of the client's UC is reflected in the depth of the deceleration; note also that

     (1) In the absence of hyperstimulation, numerical intrauterine pressure catheter values are not a diagnostic aid

     (2) Hyperstimulation is indicated when UCs have a frequency of less than every 2 minutes or a duration of longer than 90 seconds, or by a BL tonus of greater than 20 to 25 mm Hg, according to the type of intrauterine pressure catheter used

B. Nursing Diagnoses

1. Fetus at high risk for impaired gas exchange related to intrapartal reduction of oxygen levels

2. Maternal anxiety related to fetal status

C. Interventions/Evaluations

1. Fetus at high risk for impaired gas exchange related to intrapartal reduction of oxygen levels

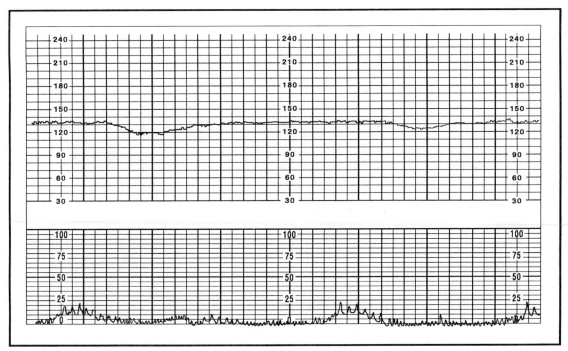

Figure 16–12
Late decelerations on ultrasound test, LTV absent.

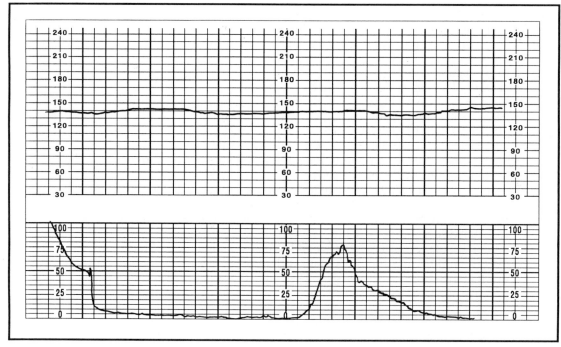

Figure 16–13
Late decelerations, LTV and STV absent.

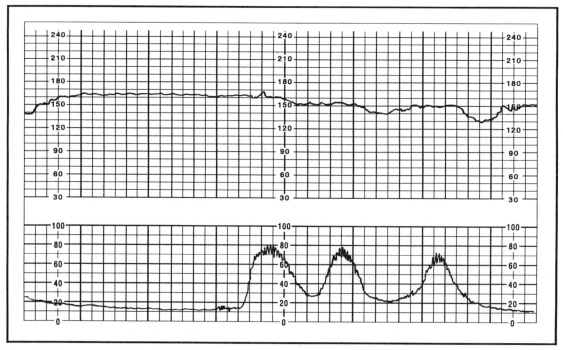

Figure 16–14
Late decelerations, occurring with double and triple UCs.

a. Interventions
   (1) Position the client in an extreme lateral position, which
      (a) Maximizes the uteroplacental blood flow
      (b) Avoids the supine hypotension effect
   (2) Administer a nondextrose IV fluid bolus, which
      (a) Corrects hypotension
      (b) Increases volume for improved oxygen saturation
   (3) Hyperoxygenate the client to maximize fetal oxygenation
      (a) Administer 8 l/min with snug-fitting face mask, or 10 to 12 l/min, if a face mask with rebreather bag is used
      (b) Maintain oxygen when absent or decreased STV persists
      (c) Reduce physiological stress, such as hyperstimulation and supine hypotension, which can decrease oxygenation
   (4) Discontinue uterine stimulation
      (a) Oxytocin (Pitocin) and other uterine stimulants are contraindicated
      (b) Nipple stimulation is contraindicated
      (c) Administer tocolytics, such as terbutaline, ritodrine, or magnesium sulfate, as ordered
   (5) Communicate the irreversibility or worsening pattern of late decelerations
      (a) The likelihood of hypoxia, acidosis, and asphyxia increases with the duration of late deceleration patterns
      (b) Fetal compromise may have occurred before admission
   (6) Documentation (Tables 16–2 and 16–3)
      (a) Document the depth, duration, and persistence of the deceleration pattern and their timing in relationship to UCs
      (b) Document variability during decelerations and of the BL of the FHR
      (c) Document interventions and resulting changes, if any, in the FHR pattern
      (d) Document that primary care provider was notified and the action that was taken
      (e) Use hospital-approved abbreviations (see Table 16–1)

Table 16–2
INFORMATION INCLUDED IN DOCUMENTATION

BL FHR
LTV
STV (if possible)
Accels
Decels
Type or shape
Depth (nadir)
Duration
Recovery pattern and time
UC pattern

Table 16–3
DOCUMENTATION EXAMPLES OF EFM EVENTS

1. Var decel to 80 bpm × 30 seconds; to BL of 130 bpm after decel LTV +, STV +
2. Late decels to 110 bpm × 40 seconds; to BL of 130 bpm after decel STV 0, LTV ↓
3. Var decel to 50 to 60 bpm × 60 to 70 seconds, recovery × 30 seconds to BL of 140 bpm after decel, BL STV inter, LTV ↓

If any one of the examples above continues as written, the subsequent note would state, *pattern continues.*

b. Evaluations
   (1) Late deceleration pattern is corrected by
      (a) Maternal position change
      (b) Oxygen therapy
      (c) Cessation of uterine stimulation
      (d) Fluid therapy
   (2) STV and LTV are restored
2. Maternal anxiety related to fetal status
   a. Interventions
      (1) Explain interventions to the client
      (2) Reassure about fetal status
      (3) Reassure about the intervention's ability to correct patterns and restore fetal well-being
      (4) Anticipate events and explain possible treatment options
   b. Evaluation: client reports a decrease in anxiety

Early Decelerations

A. Assessment

1. History: probable etiology
   a. Head compression
   b. Vagal stimulation
   c. True existence of early decelerations is questionable and poorly understood
2. Physical findings: pattern characteristics (Fig. 16–15)
   a. Decelerations begin and end with the UC
   b. Are mild and have a uniform shape
   c. Rarely occur below 110 bpm (or more than 20 bpm below the BL)
   d. Are usually associated with the presence of LTV or STV
   e. Are rarely nonreassuring

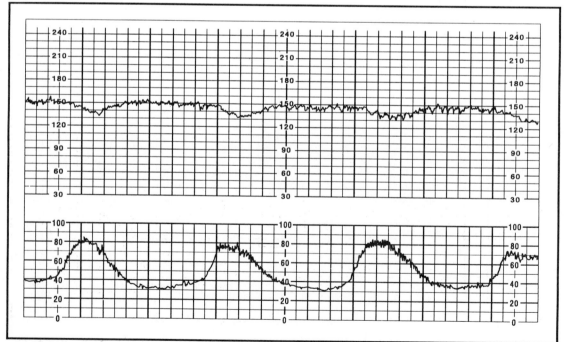

Figure 16–15
Early deceleration.

    f. Are rarely seen

    g. Occur more frequently in primigravidas

    h. Occur more frequently with cephalopelvic disproportion, especially with minimal dilation and high station

B. Nursing Diagnosis

1. Maternal anxiety related to fetal status

C. Interventions/Evaluations

1. Maternal anxiety related to fetal status
   a. Interventions
      (1) Vaginal examination for dilation, fetal position, and station
      (2) Explain that the fetus is usually not in distress with this pattern
      (3) Explain what possible treatment options may exist if the pattern continues without a progressive change of labor status
      (4) Documentation
         (a) Document the depth, duration, and timing of deceleration
         (b) Document variability of the deceleration and BL
         (c) Document the maternal position
         (d) Document the fetal station and presenting part, if possible
         (e) Use hospital-approved abbreviations (see Table 16–1 for examples)
   b. Evaluations
      (1) Pattern resolves
      (2) Client reports a decrease in anxiety

Accelerations

A. Assessment

1. History: probable etiology
   a. Fetal stimulation or movement
   b. Sympathetic stimulation
   c. Partial umbilical cord compression with mild hypotension
2. Physical findings (Figs. 16–16 and 16–17)
   a. Pattern characteristics
      (1) FHR increases above BL
      (2) Variability is usually present

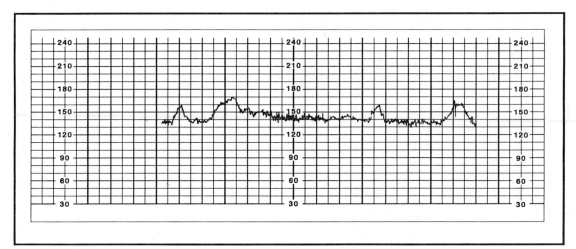

Figure 16–16
Accelerations with fetal movement.

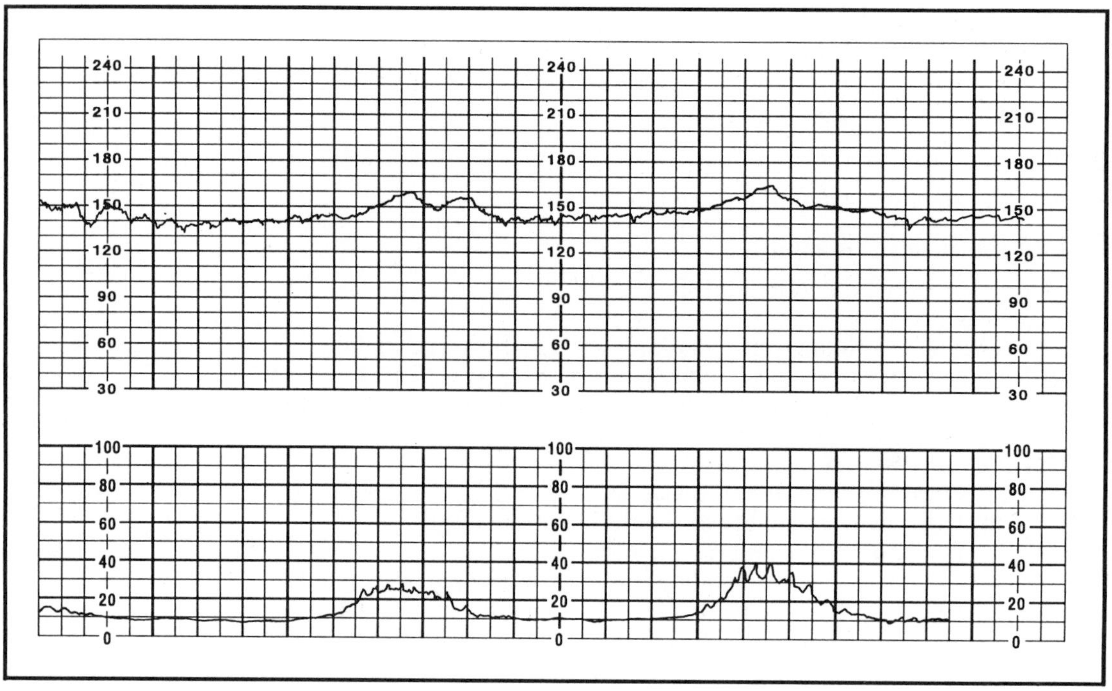

Figure 16–17
Acceleration with UCs.

(3) Increased FHR indicates fetal well-being when the amplitude is more than 15 bpm and the duration is longer than 15 seconds' reactivity
(4) May occur before or after variable decelerations, or both
(5) Occur with UCs
(6) Overshoots are approximately 20 to 30 bpm above BL of the FHR, lasting 20 to 30 seconds or more
    (a) Variability is absent or decreased
    (b) Are a probable compensatory mechanism
    (c) Are more common following fetal hypoxic insults
  b. Clinical findings
    (1) When associated with fetal activity or stimuli that meet established criteria, accelerations are called reactivity
      (a) Observed in an active fetus or a stimulated fetus
      (b) Observed in a fetus of more than 28 to 30 weeks' gestation
    (2) When associated with UCs, they are called periodic accelerations
    (3) When associated with variable decelerations, they are called preaccelerations and postaccelerations or shoulders (note the previous definition of overshoots)

B. Nursing Diagnosis

1. Maternal anxiety related to fetal status

C. Interventions/Evaluations

1. Maternal anxiety related to fetal status
  a. Interventions
    (1) Decrease or increase fetal stimuli, as needed
    (2) For compensatory accelerations, such as overshoots
      (a) Position the client laterally
      (b) Observe variability

(c) Notify the physician, as needed

(d) Provide fluid bolus and oxygen, if needed

(3) Reassure client and explain the presence or absence of fetal well-being

(4) Document information on the chart (or computer chart)

(a) Document reactivity of FHR

(b) Document altered variability, which is

(i) Often associated with persistent overshoots

(ii) Less frequently associated with variable decelerations and periodic accelerations

(c) Use hospital-approved abbreviations (see Table 16–1)

b. Evaluations

(1) Reactivity and variability are present

(a) FHR increases to more than 15 bpm above BL, which is reassuring

(b) Periodic accelerations (occurring with UCs) are not a sign of fetal compromise

(2) Client has decreased anxiety

FETAL SCALP SAMPLING

A. Introduction

1. A sample of fetal scalp blood is obtained to measure the acid and base levels of the fetus

a. pH is measured

b. Evaluates fetal status when intrapartum compromise is suspected

2. Samples must be obtained correctly during BL of the FHR rather than at the nadir of a deceleration

3. Scalp sampling is a supplement to EFM and is not meant to replace it

4. BL values for acidemia determination vary with institutions and agreement is not universal

B. Assessment

1. Fetal scalp sample with a pH greater than 7.15 to 7.20 is nonacidotic and reassuring of the fetal status; pH of fetal arteriole blood sampling range is 7.15 to 7.43, with a mean of 7.28

2. However, a fetal scalp sample pH of 7.15 to 7.25 is preacidotic, and other factors of fetal status, such as variability of the FHR, should also be considered

3. A fetal scalp sample pH of less than 7.15 to 7.20 is acidotic, and there is an 80% chance of fetal compromise

4. Intermittent scalp sampling: uses blood pH; several samples show the trend and verify the accuracy

5. Continuous tissue pH monitoring uses a fiberoptic electrode to measure the pH; it can be used with fetal spiral electrode of electronic fetal monitor; the future use of this technology is uncertain

6. Maternal alkalosis and acidosis influence quality of blood available to the fetus; fetal pH values and comparison values of fetal and maternal pH may be helpful in situations when the acid-base balance of the mother is in question

C. Nursing Diagnoses

1. Fetus at high risk for impaired gas exchange related to intrapartal reduction of oxygen levels

2. Maternal anxiety related to fetal status and procedure

D. Interventions/Evaluations

1. Fetus at high risk for impaired gas exchange related to intrapartal reduction of oxygen levels

a. Interventions

          (1) Provide optimal intrauterine environment with position, fluids, oxygen, and other treatments and medications, as needed

          (2) Continue to interpret FHR tracing

          (3) Prepare for and assist with sampling procedure according to protocol

          (4) Assist with the accurate assessment of blood pH evaluation according to hospital protocol

      b. Evaluation: fetal oxygenation is assessed by scalp sampling

    2. Maternal anxiety related to fetal status and procedure

      a. Interventions

          (1) Explain the necessity for the procedure in terms of the assessment of fetal well-being

          (2) Explain the procedure, step by step

          (3) Provide support by significant other or another nurse during the procedure

          (4) Anticipate future events and explain the possible treatment options based on results of scalp sampling

      b. Evaluations

          (1) Client reports decreased anxiety

          (2) Support person is at bedside

          (3) Client can explain reasons for the procedure and possible outcomes

Health Education

A. Use a holistic approach for maternal support and education throughout the pregnancy and prenatal period
1. Assess the client's family and support system
2. Assess the educational level and educational needs of the client

B. Use the minimal standards of care, as identified by NAACOG

C. Evaluate predelivery instruction about fetal assessment techniques

D. Evaluate previous experience with fetal assessment results

E. Explain the technique used, its purpose, and the appropriate client compliance needed

F. Answer questions and explain the data obtained, as appropriate, at the client's level of understanding
1. Anxiety level and educational needs have an impact on outcome
2. Catecholamine release and physiological stress response are associated with an observable change in FHR

CASE STUDIES AND STUDY QUESTIONS

J.S., a 30-year-old gravida 6, para 3 arrives at the labor and delivery room of a local hospital, which performs approximately 125 to 150 deliveries per month. J.S. states she has had one previous cesarean section for fetal distress, has had no prenatal care, and believes that she is due in 2 weeks, which, according to her last menstrual period, appears to be accurate. Her FHR is 144 by Doppler ultrasound; she has intact membranes and is 3 cm dilated, 80% effaced, −1 station, vertex presentation; blood pressure, 120/80; pulse, 76; respirations, 18; temperature, 36.6°C (97.8°F). An EFM was applied by using the tocodynamometer and ultrasonography.

1. According to the EFM tracing A, the BL FHR is the following (Fig. 16–18)

    (1) 130 to 150 bpm.

    (2) About 140/bpm.

    (3) LTV is present (LTV +).

    (4) LTV is absent (LTV 0).

    a. 2, 3.

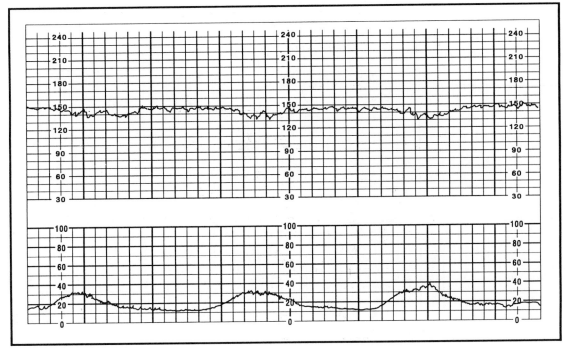

Figure 16–18
Tracing A.

b. 1, 3.

c. 1, 4.

d. 2, 4.

2. The periodic pattern of tracing A is

a. No periodic pattern is shown.

b. Normal BL tracing.

c. Late decelerations.

d. Early decelerations.

3. The UCs are

a. Every 1 to 1½ minutes × 50 seconds.

b. Every 2½ minutes × 50 to 60 seconds.

c. Hypotonic.

d. Hypertonic.

4. During tracing B (Fig. 16–19), J.S. suddenly says, "I have to push," and that she feels that "something is wrong." The nurse finds that J.S. is 3 cm dilated and notes that her tracing shows

  (1) A BL rate of about 140, reactivity, and LTV+.

  (2) A BL rate of about 150, and LTV 0.

  (3) UCs every 1 to 1½ minutes × 40 to 50 seconds.

  (4) UCs every 30 seconds × 30 to 40 seconds.

a. 1, 3.

b. 1, 4.

c. 2, 3.

d. 2, 4.

5. In tracing B (Fig. 16–19), the FHR pattern shows

a. LTV + and late decelerations.

b. LTV 0 and variable decelerations.

c. LTV + and variable decelerations.

d. LTV 0 and early decelerations.

6. In tracing C (Fig. 16–20), 9 minutes later, an abrupt change in the FHR occurs; J.S.'s nurse applies oxygen, changes the maternal position, gives a fluid bolus, and applies a spiral electrode. Also, preparations for a cesarean section are begun. These interventions occur

a. To treat an FHR of 70 to 80 bpm with STV 0.

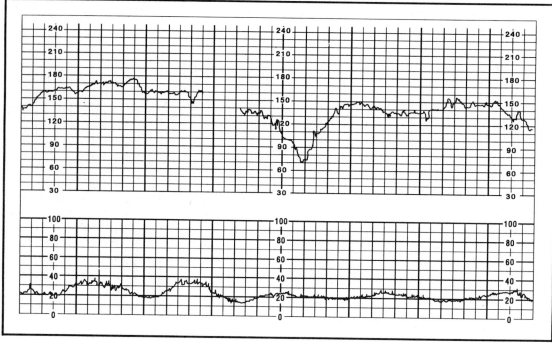

Figure 16–19
Tracing B.

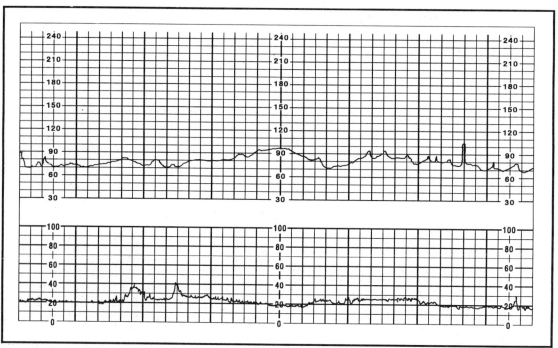

Figure 16–20
Tracing C.

b. To attempt to improve the fetal environment.

c. Because the nurse suspects an abruptio placentae or uterine rupture.

d. All of the above.

7. In tracing D (Fig. 16–21), the surgery team is preparing for a cesarean section while the physician is en route to the delivery room. The pattern is said to be terminal. This means

a. The fetus will die no matter what occurs.

b. The fetus is dying, but immediate intervention may produce a viable newborn.

c. The fetus will have permanent compromise if it lives.

d. The fetus will be depressed at birth.

The physician arrived a few minutes after this tracing (see Fig. 16–21) had been made and delivered a nonviable fetus that was floating in the abdomen. The entire lower uterine segment had ruptured and the placenta was wedged against the remaining segment of the uterus. The maternal toxicology report was positive for amphetamines and negative for cocaine.

R.K., a 27-year-old gravida 1, para 0 who is 5 days postdates, is admitted in spontaneous labor. R.K.'s vital signs at admission are FHR, 160 bpm; blood pressure, 124/84; pulse, 112; respirations, 20; and temperature, 38.2°C (100.8°F). Her vaginal examination at admission shows a 2- to 3-cm posterior cervix, 50% effacement, −1 station, and a light meconium-stained amniotic fluid. At admission, an IV solution of lactated Ringer's was started and opened for a fluid bolus. Tracing E (Fig. 16–22) was begun about 1 hours after admission and showed which of the following?

8. (1) LTV +, UCs every 3 minutes × 50 to 60 seconds.

(2) LTV 0, UCs every 3 minutes × 50 to 60 seconds.

(3) STV 0 absent.

(4) STV + present.

(5) Late decelerations.

a. 1, 4.

b. 2, 3.

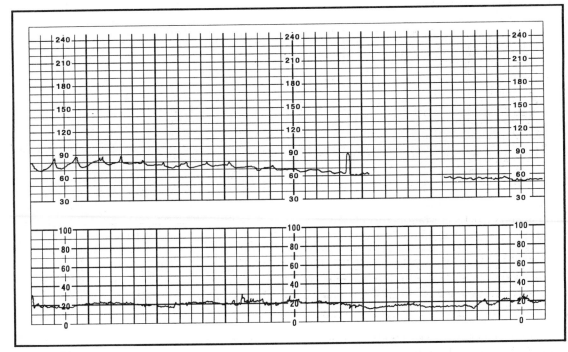

Figure 16–21
Tracing D.

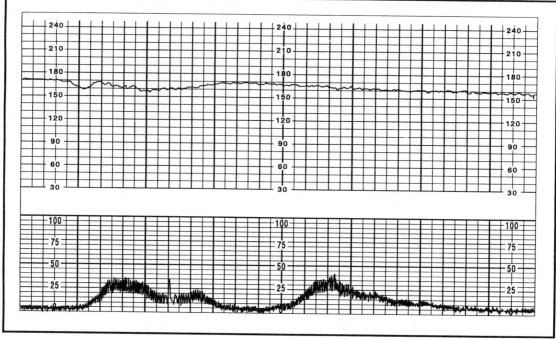

Figure 16–22
Tracing E.

c. 2, 4.

d. 2, 3, and 5.

9. In tracing F (Fig. 16–23), an arrow indicates scalp stimulation of the fetus. This action implies

   a. That an adequate fetal acceleration indicates an intact autonomic nervous system.

   b. Fetal well-being.

   c. A nonacidotic fetus.

   d. An acidotic fetus.

   e. Only a, b, and c.

D.H. is a 35-year-old gravida 2, para 1 diabetic who is at 38 weeks' gestation and planning a vaginal birth after cesarean (VBAC). D.H.'s vital signs at admission were FHR, 130 bpm; BP, 158/72; pulse, 80; respirations, 20; and temperature, 36.8°C (98.2°F). Her vaginal examination shows a thick cervix, ballottable vertex, and intact membranes.

10. Tracing G (Fig. 16–24) began within minutes of her admission to the labor and delivery room. The tracing shows which of the following?

(1) LTV 0, BL FHR 130 bpm.

(2) LTV +, BL FHR 120 to 130 bpm.

(3) Late decelerations.

(4) Variable decelerations.

(5) Fetal distress.

a. 2, 3.

b. 2, 4.

c. 1, 3, and 5.

d. 1, 4, and 5.

11. Because tracing G (Fig. 16–24) did not show improvement with interventions, epidural anesthesia was initiated and another cesarean section was performed to deliver a male infant weighing 3997 g (8 lb, 13 oz). The Apgar score and blood gases would be expected to be

   a. Normal blood gases, Apgar score above 7.

   b. Normal blood gases, Apgar score below 7.

   c. Acidotic blood gases, Apgar score below 7.

   d. Acidotic blood gases, Apgar score above 7.

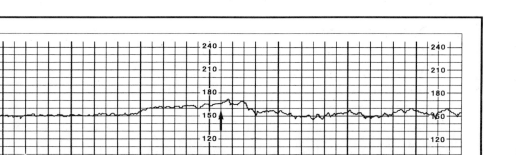
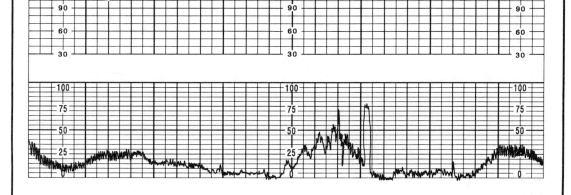

Figure 16–23
Tracing F.

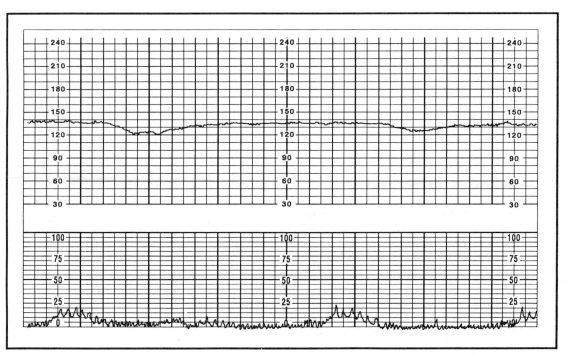

Figure 16–24
Tracing G.

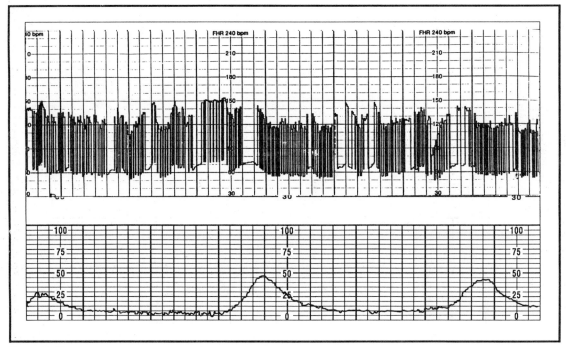

Figure 16–25
Tracing H.

12. Tracing H (Fig. 16–25) represents which of the following?

    a. Machine malfunction.

    b. Fetal arrhythmia.

    c. Fetal demise.

    d. Maternal heart rate.

13. Tracing I (Fig. 16–26) occurred approximately 1 hour after an amniocentesis, while the fetus was receiving routine ob-

servation. Interpretation of the tracing is

    a. Reactive nonstress test.

    b. Increased LTV.

    c. Variable decelerations.

    d. Sinusoidal pattern.

Tracing J (Fig. 16–27) is of a gravida 1, para 0 who is receiving oxytocin at 4 mU/min. She is 5 to 6 cm dilated, −1 station, and 90% effaced.

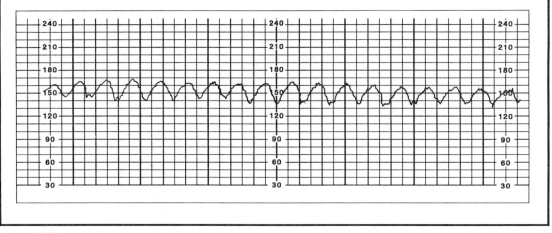

Figure 16–26
Tracing I.

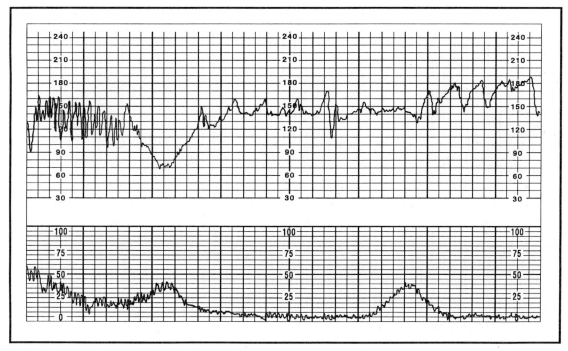

Figure 16–27
Tracing J.

14. At the start of the strip, which of the following interpretations can be made?

    (1) LTV + and STV +.

    (2) LTV ↑ and STV +.

    (3) Variable deceleration.

    (4) Early deceleration.

    a. 1, 4.

    b. 2, 3.

    c. 1, 3.

    d. 2, 4.

15. In tracing J (Fig. 16–27), at the end of the strip the FHR is 180 bpm. This represents

    a. Accelerations of the FHR.

    b. Overshoots of the FHR.

    c. Variable decelerations with overshoots.

    d. A normal FHR response.

M.A. is a gravida 1, para 0 in labor at 6 to 7 cm of dilatation, 90% effaced, and −1 station.

16. Tracing K (Fig. 16–28) shows her to have which of the following?

    (1) LTV +, STV +.

    (2) LTV ↓.

    (3) Accelerations.

    (4) Variable decelerations.

    (5) UCs every 2½ to 3 minutes × 50 seconds.

    (6) Subnormal UCs.

    a. 1, 3, 5.

    b. 1, 3, 6.

    c. 2, 3, 4, 5.

    d. 2, 4, 6.

Answers to Study Questions

1. a	2. d	3. b
4. a	5. c	6. d
7. b	8. c ·	9. d ·
10. c ·	11. c ·	12. b ·
13. d ⌣	14. b	15. a
16. a		

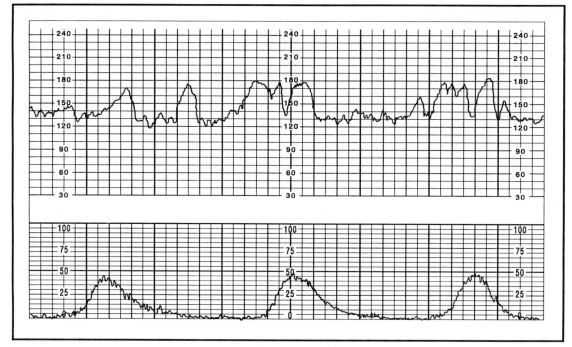

Figure 16–28
Tracing K.

REFERENCES

Clark, S., & Miller, F. (1984, January). Scalp blood sampling—FHR patterns tell you when to do it. *Contemporary Ob/Gyn, 47–58.*

Hon, E. (1975). *An introduction to FHR monitoring* (2nd ed.). Los Angeles: University of Southern California.

Martin, C. (1978). Regulation of the FHR and genesis of FHR patterns. *Seminars in Perinatology, 2*(2):131–144.

Murray, M. (1988). *Antepartal and intrapartal monitoring.* Washington, DC: NAACOG.

NAACOG. (1989). *Critical concepts in fetal heart rate monitoring: A videotape presentation of five videos.* Baltimore: Williams & Wilkins/Washington, DC: NAACOG.

NAACOG. (1988). *Essentials of electronic fetal monitoring: A videotape presentation of three videos.* Washington, DC: NAACOG.

NAACOG. (1989). *Statement: Nursing responsibilities in implementing intrapartum fetal heart rate monitoring.* Washington, DC: NAACOG.

Parer, J. (1989). Fetal heart rate. In R.K. Creasy & R. Resnik (Eds.), *Maternal-fetal medicine: Principles and practice* (pp. 314–343). Philadelphia: Saunders.

Petrie, R. (1986). Intrapartum fetal monitoring. *Clinical Obstetrics and Gynecology, 29*(1):146–152.

Schifrin, B. (1985). *Exercises in fetal monitoring* (Vol. 1). Los Angeles: BPM.

Schmidt, J. (1987). Documenting EFM events. *Perinatal Press, 10*(6): 79–81.

Wagner, P. (1990). FHR auscultation, NAACOG OGN nursing practice resource. Washington DC: NAACOG.

Other

NAACOG. (1990, March). Fetal heart rate auscultation. *OGN Nursing Practice Resource.*

THE POSTPARTUM PERIOD

Linda Bond

Physiological Changes

Objectives

1. Identify normal physiological changes in the reproductive system after childbirth

2. Describe systemic physiological changes after childbirth

3. Estimate the date of the return of the menstrual cycle

4. Design an individualized client educational plan based on data obtained from the nursing assessment

5. Predict postpartum complications based on assessment data

6. Formulate nursing interventions to prevent anticipated problems identified from the nursing assessment

Introduction

A. The postpartum period (puerperium)

1. Begins after delivery of the placenta (the immediate postpartum period, the first 2 hours after delivery, are termed the fourth stage of labor, and the 3 months after delivery are termed the fourth trimester)
2. Delivery of the uterine contents initiates a series of physiological and physical changes that return the woman's body to a nonpregnant state of function

B. Maternal system changes

1. Reproductive system
   a. Uterus
      (1) Involution (retrogressive return to normal condition after pregnancy)
         (a) Immediately after delivery
            (i) Weight is 1000 g (2 lb, 4 oz)
            (ii) Fundal height is measured midway between symphysis and umbilicus (12 cm (4.7 in) above symphysis pubis) in midline
            (iii) Afterpains (contractions) are common, especially for multiparas and breastfeeding mothers
         (b) At 1 hour post partum
            (i) Fundal height at the umbilicus is 20 cm (7.9 in) in midline

        (ii) Consistency is firm and contracted
- (c) At day 2 and after
  - (i) Fundal height decreases by 1 cm (0.4 in)/day and is no longer palpable by day 10
  - (ii) Afterpains decrease in frequency after the first few days, and usually are associated with
    - Breastfeeding
    - Multiparity
    - Multiple fetuses
    - Conditions producing overdistension of the uterus
- (d) Postpartum hemorrhage is the leading cause of maternal morbidity and mortality (see Chapter 35 for a complete discussion)
- (2) Lochia
  - (a) Composition
    - (i) Endometrial tissue
    - (ii) Blood
    - (iii) Lymph
  - (b) Stages
    - (i) Rubra (red): 1 to 3 days
      - Scant: less than 2.5 cm (1 in) on menstrual pad in 1 hour
      - Light: less than 10 cm (4 in) on menstrual pad in 1 hour
      - Moderate: less than 15 cm (6 in) on menstrual pad in 1 hour
      - Heavy: saturated menstrual pad in 1 hour
      - Excessive: menstrual pad saturated in 15 minutes
    - (ii) Serosa (pink, brown tinged): 3 to 10 days
    - (iii) Alba (yellowish-white): 10 to 14 days but can last 3 weeks and remain normal
  - (c) Danger sign is the reappearance of bright red blood after lochia rubra has stopped
  - (d) Odor is normally that of fresh blood
  - (e) Amount may increase temporarily on standing because of pooling in uterus and vagina
  - (f) Amount of lochia may be less after cesarean section but stages remain unchanged
- (3) Return of the menstrual cycle
  - (a) Nonlactating women
    - (i) At 6 to 8 weeks (40 to 45%)
    - (ii) At 12 weeks (75%)
    - (iii) Within 6 months (100%)
  - (b) Lactating women: most resume menstruation within 12 weeks although some may not resume menstruation for as long as 18 months and still be normal
- (4) Ovulation: resumes in 12 to 18 weeks, and is dependent upon prolactin levels
  - (a) For lactating women, 80% of the first few cycles are anovulatory
  - (b) For nonlactating women, 50% of the first few cycles are anovulatory
- b. Cervix
  - (1) Cervix is edematous immediately postdelivery
  - (2) Cervix is easily distensible for 4 to 6 days after delivery
  - (3) Internal os is closed by 2 weeks
  - (4) External os widens and appears as a slit
- c. Vagina
  - (1) Rugae reappear in 4 weeks
  - (2) Vagina returns to near prepregnant size at 6 to 8 weeks postdelivery but will always remain slightly larger
  - (3) Normal mucus production usually returns with ovulation

    d. Perineum
       (1) Episiotomy is normally without redness, discharge or edema; most healing takes place within the first 2 weeks
       (2) Intact perineum may have ecchymosis, edema, or both
       (3) Hemorrhoids may be present
       (4) Lacerations may be present
          (a) First degree: through skin and structures that are superficial to muscle
          (b) Second degree: extends through perineal muscles
          (c) Third degree: continues through anal sphincter muscle
          (d) Fourth degree: also involves anterior rectal wall

2. Breasts
    a. Changes of pregnancy regress in 1 to 2 weeks of postpartum period if mother is not breastfeeding
    b. Nipples are erectile when stimulated
    c. Breasts increase in vascularity, and swell in response to presence of prolactin at the second or third postpartum day (engorgement)
    d. Nonbreastfeeding engorgement will subside in 24 to 36 hours (see Chapter 19 for complete discussion of lactation)

3. Endocrine system
    a. Placental hormones
       (1) Human chorionic gonadotropin levels are nonexistent at the end of the first postpartum week
       (2) Human chorionic somatomammotropin is undetectable by 24 hours postdelivery
       (3) Plasma progesterone levels are undetectable by 72 hours postdelivery; production is reestablished with the first menstrual cycle
       (4) Plasma estrogen levels decrease to 10% of the prenatal value within 3 hours after delivery and reach the lowest levels by day 7
    b. Pituitary hormones
       (1) Serum prolactin levels rise significantly during the first 2 weeks and rapidly decline to prepregnant levels in the absence of breastfeeding
       (2) Follicle-stimulating hormone (FSH) and luteinizing hormone (LH) are absent during the first few weeks of the postpartum period

4. Cardiovascular system
    a. Heart
       (1) Returns to normal position because of shift in diaphragm and abdominal contents
       (2) Cardiac output increases during first and second stages of labor and declines rapidly after delivery, returning to normal within 2 to 3 weeks
       (3) Cardiac load is increased because of uterine blood flow being redirected into the general circulation
    b. Blood volume
       (1) There is an immediate decrease at delivery related to blood loss (normal blood loss at delivery is 300 to 400 ml for a vaginal delivery and 600 to 800 ml for a cesarean delivery)
       (2) Reduction to normal prepregnant volume takes 3 to 4 weeks
    c. Hematological changes
       (1) Hematocrit
          (a) Rises immediately after delivery and is related to a decrease in plasma volume and to dehydration
          (b) Returns to prepregnant value (37 to 47%) in 4 to 5 weeks
       (2) WBC count
          (a) May increase to 20,000 per mm^3 or more during the first 10 days postpartum (average is 14,000 to 16,000 per mm^3)
          (b) Increase is primarily in neutrophils

(c) May increase without the presence of infection; however, an increase of more than 30% over a 6-hour period is suggestive of infection

(3) Coagulation system

(a) Clotting factor levels remain elevated during the early postpartum period; uterine clots may form at the placental attachment location or from pooled blood in the uterine cavity

(b) During the remainder of puerperium, uterine clots that measure more than 1 cm are considered to be abnormal

(c) Return of clotting factors to normal levels occurs at 4 to 5 weeks postdelivery

d. Vital signs

(1) Blood pressure readings immediately postdelivery should be the same as those taken during labor

(a) Increased blood pressure might suggest pregnancy-induced hypertension

(b) Decreased blood pressure might suggest orthostatic hypotension or uterine hemorrhage

(2) Temperature may be slightly elevated because of dehydration: 36.2° to 38°C (98° to 100.4°F)

(3) Pulse rate: bradycardia is normal in early postpartum period

(a) Normal range is 40 to 80 beats/min

(b) Tachycardia is abnormal and may indicate uterine hemorrhage or infection

5. Respiratory system

a. Pulmonary function

(1) Is affected primarily by change in thoracic cage cavity

(a) Diaphragm descends

(b) Organs revert to normal positions

(2) Returns to prepregnant levels by 6 to 8 weeks of the postpartum period

(3) Respirations are usually in the range of 16 to 24/min

b. Acid-base balance returns to prepregnant levels by 3 weeks postdelivery

c. Basal metabolic rate remains elevated for as long as 14 days of the postpartum period

6. Gastrointestinal system

a. Appetite returns to normal immediately postdelivery

b. Gastric motility may remain decreased, leading to constipation

c. Normal bowel elimination resumes at 2 to 3 days postdelivery

7. Urinary system

a. Postdelivery edema of bladder, urethra, and urinary meatus is common because of delivery trauma

(1) Urinary retention may occur

(2) An elevated or laterally displaced uterus is a common sign of urinary retention after delivery

b. Kidney function

(1) Mild proteinuria may persist related to catabolism in early postpartum period

(2) Diuresis begins within 12 hours postdelivery and continues throughout the first week of the postpartum period

(3) Normal function returns by 6 to 7 weeks after delivery

8. Musculoskeletal system

a. Abdominal musculature

(1) Fibers shorten

(2) Wall weakness remains for 6 to 8 weeks and may contribute to problem of constipation

b. Joint stabilization returns after 6 to 8 weeks of the postpartum period

9. Integumentary system

a. Hyperpigmentation usually disappears with termination of pregnancy
b. Diaphoresis is common, especially at night, for the first week
   (1) Can become profuse at times
   (2) Is a mechanism to reduce the retained fluids associated with pregnancy
10. Immune system
   a. For women with Rh incompatibility, antiRh₀D immune globulin is administered within 72 hours after delivery to prevent antibody formation if the mother is nonsensitized
   b. Blood group incompatibility: ABO incompatibility should be detected early to prevent neonatal complications
   c. If the rubella titer is 1 : 8 or less, the woman should receive a rubella virus vaccine and instructions to avoid pregnancy for the next 3 months

Clinical Practice

A. Assessment

1. Frequency of postpartum checks according to protocol or as follows
   a. First hour: every 15 minutes; second hour: every 30 minutes
   b. First 24 hours: every 4 hours
   c. After 24 hours: every 8 hours
2. Vital signs and blood pressure
3. Breasts
   a. Soft, filling, or firm
   b. Engorged, reddened, or painful
   c. Nipples: erectility, possible cracks and redness
4. Uterus
   a. Consistency and tone
   b. Position
   c. Height
   d. Size
5. Cesarean section incision site, if appropriate
   a. Dressing and incision
   b. Drainage
   c. Edema, color changes, or both (redness or ecchymosis)
6. Bladder and urinary output
   a. Voiding pattern and amounts voided
   b. Distension
   c. Pain
7. Bowel
   a. Bowel movements
   b. Hemorrhoids
   c. Bowel sounds: auscultate all four quadrants, especially postcesarean section
8. Lochia
   a. Type and amount
   b. Presence of odor
   c. Presence of clots
9. Perineum
   a. Episiotomy, lacerations, and hemorrhoids
   b. Bruising, hematoma, edema, discharge, and loss of approximation
   c. Reddened areas indicative of infection
10. Extremities for thrombophlebitis
   a. Homans's sign (calf pain from passive dorsiflexion of foot)
   b. Check for redness, tenderness, and warmth
11. Diagnostic studies commonly ordered: complete blood count (CBC), hemoglobin and hematocrit (Hgb/HCT) levels, and urinalysis (UA)

B. Nursing Diagnoses

1. Impaired tissue integrity related to episiotomy or laceration
2. Altered urinary elimination: high risk for retention related to perineal edema
3. Altered bowel elimination: high risk for constipation related to perineal discomfort and slowed peristalsis
4. Alteration in comfort: pain related to episiotomy, hemorrhoids, or cesarean section incision

C. Interventions/Evaluations

1. Impaired tissue integrity related to episiotomy or laceration
   a. Interventions
      (1) Monitor episiotomy for redness, edema, bruising, hematoma, intact sutures, and bleeding
      (2) Apply ice packs for 2 hours to decrease edema (can be used later for analgesic effect for up to 24 hours)
      (3) Apply heat three or four times daily after 24 hours postdelivery
         (a) Dry: heat lamp
         (b) Moist: sitz bath
      (4) Pain relief
         (a) Analgesia: oral
         (b) Analgesia: topical
   b. Evaluations: improved tissue integrity as indicated by
      (1) Signs that episiotomy is healing
      (2) Signs of infection are absent
      (3) Discomfort is kept at tolerable levels
2. Altered urinary elimination: high risk for retention related to perineal edema
   a. Interventions
      (1) Check for bladder distension, avoid overdistension, and catheterize, if indicated
      (2) Monitor voiding patterns and amount, and catheterize for residual, if indicated
      (3) Encourage regular voiding
      (4) Encourage early ambulation
      (5) Ensure adequate fluid intake
      (6) Offer warm sitz bath, if needed
   b. Evaluations: urinary elimination reestablished as indicated by
      (1) First void within 4 to 8 hours after delivery
      (2) Nondistended bladder
      (3) Voidings more than 200 ml in first two voids
         (a) Less than 100 ml/void suggests retention with overflow, and thus, catheterization for residual is suggested
         (b) No complaints of still feeling urge to void immediately after voiding
      (4) No pain or discomfort with voiding
3. Altered bowel elimination: high risk for constipation related to perineal discomfort and slowed peristalsis
   a. Interventions
      (1) Encourage adequate intake of fluids (maximum intake of 2000 ml/day)
      (2) Encourage diet high in fiber and roughage
      (3) Encourage ambulation
      (4) Administer stool softener, laxative, enema, or suppository, as ordered
      (5) Encourage warm sitz baths
      (6) Apply topical anesthetics, as ordered
      (7) Teach methods to avoid constipation, and importance of bowel movement within 2 to 3 days (especially important with early discharge practices)
      (8) Acknowledge client's fear associated with first postdelivery bowel movement

      (9) Monitor bowel sounds postcesarean section

  b. Evaluations: bowel elimination reestablished as indicated by

    (1) Bowel movement (soft, formed stool) by second or third postpartum day

    (2) Return of bowel sounds in postcesarean section client

    (3) Reports of minimal discomfort

4. Alteration in comfort: pain related to episiotomy, hemorrhoids, or cesarean section incision

  a. Interventions

    (1) Inspect condition of perineum

    (2) Administer cold or hot perineal treatment

    (3) Administer analgesic medication, as ordered

    (4) Monitor cesarean section delivery clients for incisional pain

      (a) Morphine epidurals

        (i) Narcotic receptors exist along the pain pathway in spinal cord and base of brain

        (ii) Because receptors are specific for narcotics, small quantities of morphine (0.5 mg) can produce marked analgesia that lasts 12 to 24 hours postdelivery

        (iii) Side effects: respiratory depression, pruritus, nausea or vomiting, and urinary retention

      (b) Patient-controlled analgesia (PCA)

        (i) An electronic demand system that permits client to activate a timing device connected to an infusion pump containing analgesia

        (ii) Client pushes a button to receive a small IV dose of analgesia

        (iii) Device prevents overdosing by "locking out" for a specified amount of time

        (iv) Dose and time intervals can be adjusted by care providers

    (5) Explain cause of pain and how long pain will last

    (6) Explore various methods of nonpharmaceutical pain relief, (e.g., relaxation techniques)

  b. Evaluations: minimal pain is experienced when client

    (1) Reports only tolerable discomfort

    (2) Does not demonstrate signs of discomfort

    (3) Communicates need for pain relief

Health Education

A. **Physiological changes**

1. Involution of uterus and stages of lochia
2. Diaphoresis
3. Weight loss

  a. Usual loss of 10 to 12 lb occurs after delivery

  b. Additional 5 to 8 lb loss occurs from diuresis and involution

4. Breast changes occur, whether nursing or not nursing
5. Discomforts and measures to provide comfort

  a. Incisional healing (use ice packs, sitz bath, local or topical anesthetic or analgesic)

  b. After pains (administer analgesic)

  c. Breast engorgement (provide supportive brassiere or binder, ice packs, or analgesic)

  d. Hemorrhoids (use ice packs, sitz baths, heat lamp, or topical anesthetic; avoid constipation)

B. **Return of menstruation and ovulation**

C. **Self-care measures**

1. Personal hygiene, including perineal care

2. Postpartum exercises, including Kegel's exercises
3. Activities scheduled to avoid fatigue
4. Diet instructions
5. Special instructions
   a. Breast and nipple care; nursing or nonnursing instructions
   b. Incisional care; postcesarean section care

D. **Signs and symptoms of infection**
1. Elevated temperature, foul-smelling lochia, redness or swelling of incisions
2. Instruct when to notify health care provider

E. **Routine postpartum checkup with health care provider for self and infant has been scheduled**

F. **Resumption of sexual intercourse**
1. May be safely resumed when there is no active bleeding and episiotomy has healed (approximately 3 weeks)
2. Comfort level may be assessed by placing two fingers in vagina and rotating

G. **Family planning and birth control**
1. Provide information about various methods
2. Methods to use with intercourse before postpartum check (condoms or foam, for example) (see Chapter 20 for a complete discussion of contraception)

CASE STUDIES AND STUDY QUESTIONS

Sue Black, aged 15 years, was delivered of her first infant 1 hour ago. It was a normal vaginal delivery. She plans to bottlefeed her baby.

1. What progression can Sue expect in the stages of the lochia?

   a. Rubra, alba, serosa.

   b. Alba, rubra, serosa.

   c. Serosa, alba, rubra.

   d. Rubra, serosa, alba.

2. On examination, where would the uterus normally be located?

   a. At the level of the symphysis pubis.

   b. Midway between the umbilicus and symphysis.

   c. At the level of the umbilicus.

   d. At the level of xyphoid process.

3. Sue may experience diaphoresis for the first few days of the postpartum period. Diaphoresis occurs because of which of the following?

   a. An infection in the reproductive tract.

   b. The restoration of prepregnant body fluid levels.

   c. The establishment of lactation.

   d. The toxic side effects of certain pain medications.

4. Since Sue is not breastfeeding, what breast changes can she expect during the postpartum period?

   a. The breasts will immediately return to the prepregnant state.

   b. Engorgement may occur for 24 to 36 hours.

   c. Engorgement occurs only with breastfeeding.

   d. The breasts will return to the prepregnant state in 1 week.

Patricia Song, aged 31 years, was delivered of her third child by planned cesarean section 3 hours ago. She will breastfeed this infant as she has her other children.

5. Afterpains are caused by which of the following?

   a. Analgesic drugs.

   b. Surgical incision into the uterus.

   c. Contractions of the uterus.

   d. Multiparity.

6. Which answer best describes the routine postpartum assessment for Patricia?

a. Should be the same as that for any multipara.

b. Should be unnecessary because Patricia already knows what to expect.

c. Should be expanded to include a postoperative check.

d. Should be limited to a postoperative check.

ADDITIONAL QUESTIONS

7. On day 2 after an uncomplicated vaginal delivery, the nursing assessment indicated the following findings. Which finding is considered abnormal?

   a. Uterus firmly contracted at the level of the umbilicus and shifted to the right.

   b. Lochia rubra and a moderate flow without clots.

   c. Diaphoretic state.

   d. Breast discharge that is clear and yellowish.

8. For how many weeks after birth does the lochia normally last?

   a. 1 week.

   b. 3 weeks.

   c. 6 weeks.

   d. 8 weeks.

9. What effect does involution have on the uterus?

   a. Slightly reduces the size of the uterus.

   b. Has no effect on the uterus.

   c. Has a dramatic reduction effect.

   d. Causes a gradual reduction in size that takes up to 8 weeks.

10. Which of the following physiological changes of the postpartum period does not occur?

    a. Repositioning of anatomical organs.

    b. Return of ovulation and the menstrual cycle.

    c. Increase in blood volume.

    d. Closing of internal and external cervical os.

11. A slight temperature elevation (37.6°C [99.6°F]) at 12 hours after delivery is most likely caused by which of the following?

    a. Infection

    b. Hemorrhage

    c. Exhaustion

    d. Dehydration

Answers to Study Questions

1. d	2. c	3. b
4. b	5. c	6. c
7. a	8. b	9. d
10. c	11. d	

REFERENCES

Auvenshine, M.A., & Enriquez, M.G. (1990). *Comprehensive maternity nursing: Perinatal and women's health* (2nd ed.). Boston: Jones & Bartlett.

Bobak, I.M., Jensen, M.D., & Zalar, M.K. (1989). *Maternity and gynecologic care* (4th ed.). St. Louis: Mosby.

Carpenito, L.J. (1989). *Nursing diagnosis* (3rd ed.). Philadelphia: Lippincott.

Davis, J.H., Brucker, M.C., & Macmullen, N.J. (1988). A study of mothers' postpartum teaching priorities. *Maternal-Child Nursing Journal, 17*(1), 41–50.

Doenges, M.E., Kenty, J.R., & Moorhouse, M.F. (1988). *Maternal/newborn care plans.* Philadelphia: Davis.

Ferguson, H. (1987). Planning letter-perfect postpartum care. *Nursing 87, 17*(5), 50–51.

Fischman, S.H., Rankin, E.A., Doeken, K.L., & Lenz, E.R. (1986). Changes in sexual relationships in postpartum couples. *Journal of Obstetric, Gynecologic, and Neonatal Nursing, 15*(1), 58–63.

Fuller, S.A. (1986). Care of the postpartum adolescent. *Maternal-Child Nursing, 11*(6), 398–403.

Gorrie, T.M. (1986). Postpartal nursing diagnosis. *Journal of Obstetric, Gynecologic, and Neonatal Nursing, 15*(1), 52–56.

Greene, G.W., Smiciklas-Wright, H., School, T.O., & Karp, R.J. (1988). Postpartum weight change: How much of the weight gained in pregnancy will be lost after delivery? *Obstetrics and Gynecology, 71*(5), 701–707.

Hampson, S.J. (1989). Nursing interventions for the first three postpartum months. *Journal of Obstetric, Gynecologic, and Neonatal Nursing, 18*(2), 116–122.

Jacobson, H. (1985). A standard for assessing lochia volume. *Maternal-Child Nursing, 10*(3), 174–175.

LaFoy, J., & Geden, E.A. (1989). Postepisiotomy pain: Warm versus cold sitz bath. *Journal of Obstetric, Gynecologic, and Neonatal Nursing, 18*(5), 399–403.

Loveman, A., Colburn, V., & Dobin, A. (1986). AIDS in pregnancy. *Journal of Obstetric, Gynecologic, and Neonatal Nursing, 15*(2), 91–93.

Malinowski, J. (1978). Bladder assessment in the postpartum patient. *Journal of Obstetric, Gynecologic, and Neonatal Nursing, 7*(4), 14–16.

NAACOG. (1987). *Competencies and program guidelines for nurse providers of childbirth education.* Washington, DC: NAACOG.

OGN Nursing Practice Resource. (1986, October). *Postpartum follow-up: A nursing practice guide (R25).* Washington, DC: NAACOG.

OGN Nursing Practice Resource. (1989, December). *Nursing diagnosis.* Washington, DC: NAACOG.

Olds, S.B., London, M.L., & Ladewig, P.A. (1988). *Maternal-newborn nursing* (3rd ed.). Menlo Park, CA: Addison-Wesley.

Polden, M. (1985). Teaching postnatal exercises. *Midwives' Chronicle, 98*(1173), 271–274.

Ramler, D., & Roberts, J. (1986). A comparison of cold and warm sitz baths for relief of postpartum perineal pain. *Journal of Obstetric, Gynecologic, and Neonatal Nursing, 15*(6), 471–474.

Samples, J.T., Dougherty, M.C., Abrams, R.M., & Batich, C.D. (1988, May/June). The dynamic characteristics of the circumvaginal muscles. *Journal of Obstetric, Gynecologic, and Neonatal Nursing, 17*(3), 194–201.

Sherwen, L.N., Scoloveno, M.A., & Weingarten, C.T. (1991). *Nursing care of the childbearing family.* Norwalk, CT: Appleton & Lange.

Sleep, J., & Grant, A. (1987, December). Pelvic floor exercises in postnatal care. *Midwifery, 3*(4), 158–164.

Tribotti, S., Lyons, N., Blackburn, S., Stein, M., & Withers, J. (1988). Nursing diagnoses for the postpartum woman. *Journal of Obstetric, Gynecologic, and Neonatal Nursing, 17*(6), 410–416.

Weiner, S.M. (1989). *Clinical manual of maternity and gynecologic nursing.* St. Louis: Mosby.

Other

NAACOG (1991, June). Postpartum nursing care: Vaginal delivery. *OGN Nursing Practice Resource.*

NAACOG (1989, March). Mother-baby care. *OGN Nursing Practice Resource.*

Linda C. Johnson

Psychological Changes

Objectives

1. Define parent-infant attachment

2. Name factors that can have a significant impact on the nature of attachment for the infant, mother, and father

3. List attachment behaviors that can be observed in parents and infants

4. Define phases in the development of attachment

5. Identify tools that can be used to assess optimal maternal-infant attachment

6. Name interventions available to the nurse for the promotion of parent-infant attachment

7. List factors that have an impact on the acquisition of the maternal role

8. Name phases that are an observable part of the process of transition into the maternal role

9. Identify common emotional responses of fathers, siblings, and grandparents during the postpartum period

10. Recognize parental behaviors that deviate from normal adjustment during the postpartum period

11. Differentiate between "baby blues" and postpartum depression

12. Develop a discharge teaching plan designed to facilitate parent-infant attachment and assumption of the parenting role

Introduction

There are a number of critical psychosocial adaptations to be made during the immediate postpartum period if the highest quality parent-infant relationship is to be attained.

A. One of the most important adaptations is parent-infant attachment

B. All family members undergo a series of emotional adjustments after birth

C. The mother experiences body image changes, role changes, and a degree of emotional upheaval

D. One common maternal emotional response during the immediate postpartum period is known as baby blues: baby blues are defined and differentiated from postpartum depression

E. Fathers, siblings, and grandparents also experience role changes and exhibit observable behavior changes; factors having an impact on role transitions of all family members are described

Clinical Practice

Attachment

A. Introduction

1. Attachment is defined as the enduring emotional bond between a parent (or parent figure) and an infant (Klaus & Kennell, 1976)
2. Attachment is essential to the infant's physical and psychological growth and, in fact, to his or her very survival
3. The mother-infant bond is the basis on which all subsequent attachments are formed and plays a major formative role in the infant's developing sense of self (Bowlby, 1969)
4. The infant's first and most significant attachment is to the mother figure; however, it is important to note that the infant attaches to more than one person; infants also attach to the father, siblings, and other significant caregivers
5. Major theorists and researchers in the field of parent-infant attachment include Bowlby (1959, 1969) Ainsworth (1978), Brazelton (1974), Klaus & Kennell (1976), and Rubin (1963, 1975)

B. Assessment

1. History: factors influencing attachment
   a. Maternal factors
      (1) Past experience with one's own mother
      (2) Cultural and ethnic background
      (3) Socioeconomic status
      (4) Wanted versus unwanted status of infant
      (5) Quality of relationship with infant's father
      (6) Degree of paternal support
      (7) Age and maturity level
      (8) Circumstances surrounding delivery
         (a) High-risk versus low-risk delivery
         (b) Type of delivery
         (c) Prolonged separation from infant after delivery
      (9) Physical health and intelligence
   b. Infant factors
      (1) Sex
      (2) Appearance
      (3) Presence or absence of abnormalities
      (4) Temperament
      (5) Degree of alertness
   c. Paternal factors
      (1) Age
      (2) Maturity
      (3) Past experiences with infants

(4) Degree to which infant matches expectations

(5) Quality of the relationship with infant's mother

(6) Degree to which father has been included in prenatal and birth experiences

2. Observable behaviors

  a. Attachment

    (1) Definition: social signals designed to increase proximity of parent and child

    (2) Observable behaviors in mother toward infant

      (a) Touching and fondling

      (b) Holding

      (c) Gazing

      (d) Cuddling

      (e) Kissing

    (3) Behaviors observable in infant

      (a) Signaling behaviors (nondiscriminatory before 8 weeks)

        (i) Crying

        (ii) Smiling

        (iii) Babbling

        (iv) Grasping

        (v) Following with eyes and gazing

      (b) Approach behaviors (require locomotion and are not observed before age of 6 months)

        (i) Clinging

        (ii) Moving toward mother

        (iii) Following mother

  b. Malattachment: maternal behaviors indicating high risk for malattachment follow

    (1) Prenatally

      (a) Excessive mood swings

      (b) Emotional withdrawal

      (c) Excessive preoccupation with appearance

      (d) Numerous physical complaints

      (e) Failure during last trimester to prepare for infant's birth

    (2) Postnatally

      (a) Negative comments about infant's appearance

      (b) Disappointment about infant's sex

      (c) Failure to look at infant

      (d) Failure to touch or stroke infant

      (e) Failure to respond to infant's signaling behaviors

      (f) Failure to name infant

      (g) Limited handling of infant

      (h) Failure to meet infant's physical needs

3. Psychosocial responses related to attachment

  a. Phases in the development of attachment

    (1) Introductory phase

      (a) Initial maternal contact with infant

        (i) Touches infant with finger tips

        (ii) Explores infant's extremities

        (iii) Touches infant with palms of hands

        (iv) Touches larger body areas of infant

        (v) Enfolds infant with whole hand and arm

        (vi) Positions self to have eye-to-eye contact with infant (en face position)

    (2) Acquaintance phase

      (a) Early postpartum period: first few days

             (i) Process of maternal identification of infant as her own: mother identifies infant's behaviors and appearance as similar to those of other family members

             (ii) Attachment behaviors in infant facilitate acquaintance process by eliciting caretaking responses from mother

         (3) Mutual regulation phase

           (a) Initial postpartum period (first few weeks)

             (i) Mutual regulation of behaviors

             (ii) Infant expresses needs, mother responds to needs

             (iii) Goal of phase is reciprocity

           (b) Reciprocity

             (i) Interactional cycle between mother and infant that occurs simultaneously, based on mutual cueing behaviors

             (ii) Rhythms of interaction form basis of communication

             (iii) Evidence that formation of attachment has occurred

     b. Significance of attachment

       (1) Malattachment positively correlated to

         (a) Problems in parenting

         (b) Failure to thrive in infant

         (c) Child neglect and abuse

     c. Cultural variation in patterns of attachment

       (1) Patterns of attachment vary with culture

       (2) Observable behavior should be compared with norms for cultural group

  4. Several tools for assessment of attachment are available

     a. Attachment assessment form (Perry, 1988)

       (1) Provides cues for observing mother-infant or father-infant interactions

       (2) Assesses process of attachment from prenatal period through 6 weeks postpartum period

     b. Mother-Infant Screening Tool (MIST) (Reiser, 1981)

       (1) Scores mother and infant on tactile, visual, auditory, and feeding behaviors

C. Nursing diagnosis

1. High risk for psychological injury, related to failure to achieve parent-infant attachment

D. Interventions/Evaluations

1. Interventions

     a. Provide time for parent-infant interaction as soon after birth as mother's and infant's conditions permit

     b. Provide sufficient time for nurse to give information to parents about their infant's condition and to assist them in caretaking

     c. Encourage parents to participate in infant's care

     d. Provide environment that encourages questions and expression of feelings

     e. Encourage early and frequent skin-to-skin and eye-to-eye contact between mother and infant (touching, unwrapping, examining infant)

     f. Develop a team approach for support and encouragement of positive parent-infant interactions

     g. Provide daily information about infant's condition if infant is admitted to the neonatal intensive care unit (NICU) or transferred to another institution

2. Evaluations

     a. Positive parent-infant attachment indicated by observed positive reciprocal relationship between parents and infant

     b. Community health follow-up ensured at posthospitalization if problems related to parent-infant attachment are observed

MATERNAL EMOTIONAL ADJUSTMENTS DURING THE POSTPARTUM PERIOD

A. Introduction

1. The most important psychological adjustment for the mother during the postpartum period is the relinquishing of the role of pregnant woman and the taking on of the role of the mother
2. Role change involves loss of and grieving for roles and expectations that must be abandoned and the acquisition of skills and behaviors related to the new role of mother
3. New mothers typically progress through a series of developmental stages; the rate of progression through these stages is unique to each mother

B. Assessment

1. History: factors influencing transition to the maternal role
   a. Condition of mother
      (1) Prolonged labor
      (2) Use of drugs during labor
      (3) Type of delivery (e.g., cesarean section birth)
      (4) Other complications at time of delivery
   b. Condition of infant
      (1) Prematurity
      (2) Admission to NICU for other reasons
      (3) Physical anomalies
   c. Socioeconomic factors
      (1) Maternal fear related to ability to economically care for infant
      (2) Degree of maternal social support
   d. Familial factors
      (1) Demands of infant's other siblings
      (2) Quality of maternal relationship with partner
   e. Maternal age or parity
      (1) Previous experience with maternal role
         (a) Very young mothers may lack information about infant care
         (b) Older mothers may face conflicts related to meeting demands of all family members
   f. Role conflict related to career demands: active career women may have difficulty in adjusting to role changes and conflicting demands of infant, family, and job
2. Observable stages in acquiring the role of mother
   a. Dependent and "taking-in" phase of mother (Rubin, 1975)
      (1) Increase in dependent behavior of mother
         (a) Is physically exhausted after delivery
         (b) Focuses on her own physical needs
         (c) Wants to be cared for
      (2) Mother asks many questions and talks a great deal about delivery experience
      (3) Phase typically lasts 1 to 2 days
      (4) May be the only phase observed by nurse during hospitalization because of a trend toward a shortened inpatient stay for uncomplicated obstetrical clients
   b. Dependent-independent or "taking-hold" phase of mother
      (1) Begins to focus on needs of infant
      (2) Relinquishes pregnant role
      (3) Takes on maternal role
      (4) Is interested in learning to care for infant
      (5) Experiences a period of high fatigue and increased demands by infant

(6) May experience baby blues
(7) Is typically in this phase 4 to 5 weeks
c. Interdependent or letting go phase of mother
(1) Lets go of perception of infant as extension of herself and views infant as separate
(2) Refocuses on relationship with partner
(3) May return to work and relinquish part of childcare to other caretakers
d. Assessment tool: the Funke-Irbe Mother-Infant Interactional Assessment ([FIMI] Dickason, Schult, & Silverman, 1990) provides criteria for assessment of mother-infant interactions in areas of feeding, moving and holding, cleaning and diapering, and verbal and nonverbal communication

C. Nursing Diagnosis
1. High risk for alteration in parenting related to failure to take on role of mother

D. Interventions/Evaluations
1. Interventions
a. Allow mother to participate in infant's care and have infant in room with mother, if conditions permit
b. Provide nursing care for infant if mother is too exhausted to participate
c. Provide teaching related to physical caretaking skills
(1) Teach mother techniques of infant feeding
(2) Demonstrate and supervise mother's physical care activities (e.g., diapering and bathing)
(3) Discuss with mother normal infant rhythm and ways in which infant communicates needs
d. Provide community health follow-up for mother identified to be at risk for failure to assume maternal role, for example, mothers who
(1) Are adolescents
(2) Have inadequate social support
(3) Fail to demonstrate interest in caring for infant
e. Followup with a phone call 2 days postdischarge for clarification of any of mother's questions
2. Evaluations
a. Mother demonstrates ability to feed infant successfully
b. Mother demonstrates competence in caregiving activities
c. Mother verbalizes awareness of infant's rhythms and cues related to
(1) Hunger
(2) Sleep
(3) Stimulation
(4) Socialization
(5) Discomfort and pain

BABY BLUES

A. Introduction
1. Baby blues are also known as postpartum blues or third-day blues (Dickason, Schult, & Silverman, 1990)
2. Postpartum blues are described as a mild, transient, mood disturbance and frequently begin on approximately the third postpartum day and last 2 or 3 days (Selby, 1980); some mothers studied experienced postpartum blues for several weeks, and most of these experienced a peak of negative emotions at 4 to 5 weeks (Gennaro, 1988)
3. Approximately 50 to 70% of women experience baby blues during the postpartum period
4. The onset of postpartum blues coincides with the normal physiological drop in

estrogen and progesterone; this change in hormonal level has been suggested as a possible cause of baby blues

5. The experience of baby blues may be intensified in the breastfeeding mother

B. Assessment

1. History: onset typically occurs on the third postpartum day
2. Observable symptoms
   a. Irritability
   b. Restlessness
   c. Crying spells
   d. Sleeplessness
   e. Anger toward family members, including infant
   f. Anxiety
   g. Moodiness
3. Psychosocial responses seen in postpartum depression and psychosis include
   a. Exaggerated and prolonged irritability
   b. Labile behavior
   c. Withdrawal
   d. Inability to cope
   e. Inappropriate responses to infant and family
   f. Psychotic (out of touch with reality) behavior

C. Nursing Diagnosis

1. High risk for ineffective coping, related to mood alteration

D. Interventions/Evaluations

1. Interventions
   a. Observe and document alteration in maternal mood.
   b. Provide supportive environment
   c. Provide adequate opportunities for mother to rest and sleep
   d. Provide mother with relief from infant care
   e. Educate client's partner or significant other about expected behavior
   f. Reassure mother that negative emotions are normal
2. Evaluations
   a. Symptoms are determined to be typical of baby blues
   b. Mother verbalizes ability to cope with mood swings and provide appropriate infant care
   c. Appropriate psychiatric referrals have been made if symptoms have progressed to postpartum depression or psychosis

PATERNAL ADJUSTMENT DURING THE POSTPARTUM PERIOD

A. Introduction

1. During the past 2 decades, fathers have taken an increasingly active role in parenting in U.S. society
2. In many families, fathers now provide a significant amount of infant care and are active participants in all aspects of parenting; researchers have begun to investigate father-neonate interactions more frequently
3. Early involvement of fathers in prenatal classes and infant care has been shown to facilitate adaptation to parenting and to strengthen father-infant attachment
4. It is important for the nurse to be able to assess the degree to which fathers are successfully adjusting to the new role of parent

B. Assessment

1. History: factors influencing acquisition of role of father

    a. Paternal factors
- (1) Age
- (2) Marital status
- (3) Cultural background
- (4) Socioeconomic status
- (5) Educational level
- (6) Previous experience
- (7) Attitudes and expectations about fatherhood
- (8) Level of knowledge about needs of mother prenatally and postnatally
- (9) Level of knowledge about infant care

2. Observable behavior in acquiring role of father
   - a. Early contact with infant
     - (1) May be engrossed with infant
     - (2) Similar progression in touching patterns to those for mother
   - b. May actively participate in care
   - c. Initiates play more frequently than does mother

C. Nursing Diagnosis

1. High risk for alteration in parenting related to failure to take on role of father

D. Interventions/Evaluations

1. Interventions
   - a. Provide information and support about role of father
   - b. Encourage active participation in all phases of maternity experience
   - c. Provide teaching as needed about needs of mother and infant
     - (1) Teach infant-feeding techniques
     - (2) Demonstrate and supervise physical care activities (e.g., bathing and diapering)
     - (3) Discuss normal rhythms and ways in which infant communicates needs
     - (4) Discuss typical emotional and physical needs of mother during postpartum period
   - d. Encourage active participation of father in infant care if infant requires admission to NICU
2. Evaluations
   - a. Father verbalizes satisfaction with new paternal role
   - b. Father provides evidence of active participation in caretaking of infant
   - c. Father demonstrates competence in caregiving activities
   - d. Father verbalizes awareness of infant's rhythms and cues related to
     - (1) Hunger
     - (2) Sleep
     - (3) Stimulation
     - (4) Socialization
     - (5) Discomfort or pain
   - e. Father provides evidence of a supportive relationship with mother and other children in the family

SIBLING RESPONSE TO THE BIRTH EXPERIENCE

A. Introduction

1. The birth of additional children requires role changes for siblings
2. Needs for love and attention are strong in children, and they frequently need help in learning to share their parents' love with a new sibling
3. Many prenatal programs now include a sibling class as a part of their preparation-for-childbirth series to more fully assist parents in preparing their children for the new baby
4. Role negotiations are necessary on the part of siblings for continued smooth functioning of the family unit

B. Assessment

1. History: factors influencing sibling response to new family member
   a. Age: cognitive and emotional development of sibling may have an impact on his or her ability to accept a new family member
   b. Gender: if gender of new infant does not match expectations of sibling, acceptance of new sibling may be delayed
   c. Spacing of siblings: closely spaced siblings may exhibit more aggressive behavior toward new sibling
   d. Relationship with parents: degree of security in relationship with parents has a positive impact on sibling's ability to accept new family member
   e. Self-esteem: poor self-esteem can magnify feelings of insecurity and result in a negative response to new sibling
   f. Amount of preparation: lack of preparation or involvement may delay sibling's acceptance of new family member
2. Observable behaviors indicating adaptation
   a. Is excited about new sibling
   b. Is able to participate positively in care of infant (as appropriate for age)
   c. Relates positively to parent
   d. Transient, regressive behavior disappears within a few days to weeks of birth of new sibling
3. Observable behavior indicating problems in adaptation
   a. Regressive behavior that does not disappear within a few weeks of new sibling's arrival home
   b. Continued expressions of anger toward infant or other siblings (occasional expressions of anger are a normal adaptive response)
   c. Physical mistreatment of infant
   d. Refusal to eat
   e. Persistent sleep disturbances
   f. Persistent clinging to parents

C. Nursing Diagnosis

1. High risk for ineffective coping, related to failure to accept new brother or sister

D. Interventions/Evaluations

1. Interventions
   a. Explain to parents need for sibling involvement in birth experience
   b. Allow siblings to be present during birth, if parent requests it, and if there has been appropriate preparation
   c. Provide teaching related to infant care and allow siblings to participate in supervised care of infant during hospitalization
2. Evaluations
   a. Siblings demonstrate behaviors indicating adaptation
   b. Appropriate community referrals are made if signs of maladjustment are observed

ADAPTATION OF GRANDPARENTS DURING THE POSTPARTUM PERIOD

A. Introduction

1. Birth of the first grandchild is usually an occasion of joy for the parents of the infant's mother and father
2. However, this event requires the acquisition of a new role and necessitates changes in the new grandparents' relationship with their children
3. When grandparents are involved in the birth experience and are present during part of the postpartum stay, family-centered care requires incorporation of grandparents into the nursing plan of care for the new family unit

B. Assessment

1. History: factors influencing transition to the role of grandparent
   a. Marital status of son or daughter
   b. Age of son or daughter
   c. Acceptance of pregnancy
   d. Positive interaction and acceptance of neonate
   e. Age of grandparent
   f. Desire or lack of desire to become grandparent
   g. Fear of aging
2. Observable behaviors related to role acceptance
   a. Excitement about new infant
   b. Desire to be actively involved in care of infant
   c. Providing of emotional support for birth parents and other family members
3. Observable behaviors indicating failure to accept role of grandparent
   a. Lack of acceptance of infant
   b. Failure to provide emotional support to birth parents and to siblings of their new grandchild

C. Nursing Diagnosis

1. High risk for anxiety related to stress of changing family structure and the transition to role of grandparent

D. Interventions/Evaluations

1. Interventions
   a. Allow grandparents to participate in infant caregiving, when desired
   b. Teach grandparents current concepts of infant care
   c. Encourage new parents to include grandparents in new family life
   d. Incorporate extended family issues into parenting classes
   e. Encourage grandparents to provide extra attention and support to their new grandchild's siblings
2. Evaluations
   a. Grandparents express acceptance of new infant
   b. Grandparents actively support emotional needs of their son or daughter and other grandchildren

Health Education

A. Introduction

1. As economic constraints for families and decreased reimbursement for hospitals from third-party payors continue the national trend toward shortened in-hospital stays for uncomplicated obstetrical care, discharge planning and patient teaching become even more vital components of the nurse's role
2. These economic factors also increase the need for the hospital-based nurse to provide postdischarge follow-up
3. Communication with community agencies for referral and follow-up of identified problems is essential for the health and welfare of the new family unit

B. Family education plan

1. Develop a teaching plan with new family based on individually stated or observed needs; the teaching plan should include the following components
   a. Description of characteristics of a normal newborn
   b. Explanation of hospital routines
   c. Description of infant-feeding techniques
   d. Demonstration and supervision of physical care
      (1) Bathing

      (2) Changing
      (3) Holding
      (4) Feeding
  e. Discussion of normal rhythms and cues of infant related to
      (1) Hunger
      (2) Sleep
      (3) Socialization
      (4) Discomfort
  f. Discussion of signs and symptoms of illness
  g. Discussion of balance of maternal and infant needs, as well as those of other household members
  h. Discussion of normal growth and development and appropriate approaches to encourage development
  i. Discussion of role changes experienced by all family members
  j. Discussion of plans for maternal reentry into the work force (if applicable) and provision of criteria for evaluation of day-care centers

CASE STUDIES AND STUDY QUESTIONS

Mary J., a 16-year-old primigravida has given birth to a 3005-g (6-lb, 10-oz) infant girl 15 hours ago. Mary delivered her daughter vaginally with no complications after a 12-hour labor. Mary is unmarried and has been living with her father since her parents' divorce. Mary did not receive prenatal care until the last trimester of her pregnancy because she was attempting to conceal her pregnancy from her father. She attended no preparation-for-childbirth classes. Until delivery, Mary was ambivalent about keeping her baby; however, she has now decided she wants to take responsibility for her baby and is planning to keep the child. Mary has had no previous experience in caring for children and is expressing concern about her ability to care for her child.

STUDY QUESTIONS

1. Which of the following factors predispose Mary to problems in the area of maternal-infant attachment?

   a. Mary's marital status.

   b. Mary's lack of prenatal care.

   c. Mary's ambivalence about keeping her baby.

   d. Mary's age.

   e. All of the above.

2. A plan of care designed to assist Mary in taking on the maternal role would include which one of the following?

   a. Allowing Mary periods of rest when she feels unable to care for her infant.

   b. Insisting that Mary breastfeed her infant on demand.

   c. Allowing Mary to observe the nurse as she provides physical care for her infant.

   d. Questioning Mary about whether she is sure she wants to keep her baby.

3. During Mary's first contact with her infant, the nurse observes a number of behaviors. Circle all of the behaviors that are commonly observed during the introductory phase of attachment.

   a. Describing the infant as looking just like her mother.

   b. Touching the infant with her finger tips.

   c. Examining the infant's fingers and toes.

   d. Looking directly at the infant's eyes.

4. While Mary is holding her infant, the nurse observes their interaction. Circle all of the observed behaviors on the part of the infant that are designed to strengthen mother-infant attachment.

   a. Crying.

   b. Sleeping.

c. Gazing.

d. Grasping.

5. Circle all of the following observed behaviors on the part of Mary that are designed to strengthen mother-infant attachment.

a. Touching.

b. Gazing.

c. Kissing.

d. Rocking.

6. Which behavior is an indication that Mary will successfully attach emotionally to her infant and be able to provide appropriate care for the infant?

a. Allowing the nurse to tell her what she needs to do for the baby.

b. Talking with the social worker about placement for the baby if she is unable to handle the situation.

c. Responding to the infant's cry by picking up the baby and attempting to determine why the baby is crying.

d. Feeding the infant each time it cries.

7. Which of the following describes the process whereby a neonate gives cues and the parent or other caretaker interprets these cues?

a. Communication cueing.

b. Synchrony.

c. Reciprocity.

d. Attachment.

8. Which of the following is significantly correlated with malattachment?

a. Cesarean delivery.

b. Multiparity.

c. Child abuse.

d. Age of mother.

Mrs. C. is a 34-year-old multipara being cared for in your labor delivery postpartum recovery (LDRP) unit. She was delivered of a 3969-g (8-lb, 12-oz) boy 10 hours ago. She and her infant are in stable condition after an uncomplicated delivery. Mrs. C. has requested rooming-in and you have been assigned the care of this mother and infant. Mr. C. has also been present while you are caring for Mrs. C.

9. In thinking about your priorities for caring for Mrs. C. and her infant, in which of the following stages of the parenting role would you expect her to be?

a. Taking in.

b. Taking hold.

c. Interdependent.

d. Independent-dependent.

10. Circle the typical behaviors included during this phase.

a. Focusing on relationship with partner.

b. Expressing a desire to be cared for physically.

c. Focusing on needs of infant.

d. Focusing on one's own physical needs.

11. During your care of Mrs. C. and her infant, which of the following interventions would most likely facilitate maternal role taking?

a. Allowing her to rest after delivery by caring for her infant in the well-baby nursery.

b. Scheduling a film for the mother to view on infant cardiopulmonary resuscitation (CPR).

c. Allowing the mother to participate in the supervised physical care of the infant.

d. Allowing unlimited visiting of family members and friends.

12. Mrs. C. is very happy about her successful delivery of a healthy baby. On the second day you care for her, she begins to ask you many questions about infant care. Circle the important content areas to be included in your discharge teaching plan.

a. Physical care of infant.

b. Infant-feeding techniques.

c. Ways in which infants communicate needs.

d. Need for proper rest and nutrition for the mother.

e. All of the above.

13. Which of the following is the most effective way of facilitating Mr. C.'s taking on of the role of father?

   a. Encouraging Mr. C. to care for other siblings at home while Mrs. C. is hospitalized.

   b. Allowing Mr. C. to observe demonstrations of infant care.

   c. Allowing Mr. C. to be involved in the physical care of the infant during hospitalization.

   d. Allowing Mr. C. to carry the infant when the mother is being discharged.

14. After Mrs. C.'s discharge from the hospital, you receive a call from her. She is very upset and worried. She was so happy when she left the hospital and cannot understand why she is feeling anxious and sad, crying frequently, and having difficulty in sleeping. Which of the following problems is most likely the explanation of Mrs. C.'s behavior?

   a. Postpartum depression.

   b. Marital problems.

   c. Baby blues.

   d. Exhaustion.

15. Which of the following would you include in your advice to Mrs. C.?

   a. Advise that she seek marital counseling.

   b. Advise that she seek personal counseling.

   c. Advise her that her emotional response is common in the early postpartum period and should be self-limiting.

   d. Advise that she arrange for additional help with infant care until she is less exhausted.

16. Mrs. C. also shares her concern that her $2\frac{1}{2}$ year-old son has been difficult to manage since her return home. She is not sure whether or not his behavior is normal. Which of the following observable behaviors are indicative of problems in sibling adaptation?

   a. Regression.

   b. Occasional expressions of anger toward the infant.

   c. Expressions of need for reassurance of love from the parents.

   d. Physical mistreatment of the infant.

Answers to Study Questions

1. e	2. a	3. b, c, d
4. a, c, d	5. a, b, c	6. c
7. c	8. c	9. a
10. b, d	11. c	12. e
13. c	14. c	15. c
16. d		

REFERENCES

Ainsworth, M.D.S., Bleher, M.C., Waters, E., & Wall, S. (1978). *Patterns of attachment*. Hillsdale, NJ: Erlbaum.

Ament, L.A. (1990). Maternal tasks of the puerperium reidentified. *Journal of Obstetric, Gynecologic, and Neonatal Nursing, 19*, 330–335.

Anderberg, G.J. (1988). Initial acquaintance and attachment behavior of siblings with the newborn. *Journal of Obstetric, Gynecologic, and Neonatal Nursing, 17*(1), 49–54.

Bobak, I.M., Jensen, M.D., & Zalar, M.K. (1989). *Maternity and gynecologic care. The nurse and the family*. St. Louis: Mosby.

Bowlby, J. (1969). *Attachment and loss: Vol. I. Attachment*. New York: Basic.

Bowlby, J. (1959). The nature of the child's tie to his mother. *International Journal of Psychoanalysis, 39*, 350.

Brazelton, T. B. (1974). The origins of reciprocity: The early mother-infant interaction. In M. Lewis & L.A. Rosenblum (Eds.), *The effect of the infant on its caregiver*. New York: Wiley.

Brouse, A.J. (1988). Easing the transition to the maternal role. *Journal of Advanced Nursing, 13*, 167–172.

Craft, M.J., & Denehey, J.A. (Eds.). (1990). *Nursing interventions for infants and children*. Philadelphia: Saunders.

Dickason, E.J., Schult, M.O., & Silverman, B.L. (1990). *Maternal-infant nursing care*. St. Louis, Mosby.

Gay, J.T., Edgil, A.E., & Douglas, A.B. (1988). Reva Rubin revisited. *Journal of Obstetric, Gynecologic, and Neonatal Nursing, 17*(6), 394–399.

Gennaro, S. (1988). Postpartal anxiety and depression in mothers of term and preterm infants. *Nursing Research, 37*(2), 82–84.

Helfer, R.E., & Kempe, C.H. (1976). *Child abuse and neglect.* Cambridge, MA: Ballinger.

Kenner, C., Conrad, L., & Tscheschlog, B. (1991). *Maternal, neonatal, and women's health nursing.* Springhouse, PA: Springhouse.

Klaus, M.H. (1970). Human maternal behavior at first contact with her young. *Pediatrics, 46,* 187.

Klaus, M., & Kennell, J. (1976). *Maternal-infant bonding.* St. Louis: Mosby.

Mercer, R. (1981). The nurse and maternal tasks of early postpartum. *Maternal Child Nursing 6(5),* 341–345.

NAACOG (1987). *Competencies and program guidelines for nurse providers of CBE.*

Olds, S.B., London, M.L., & Ladewig, P.A. (Eds.). (1988). *Maternal-newborn nursing: A family-centered approach.* Menlo Park, CA: Addison-Wesley.

Perry, S. (1988). Attachment. In S.B. Olds, M.L. London, & P.A. Ladewig (Eds.), *Maternal-newborn nursing: A family-centered approach.* Menlo Park, CA: Addison-Wesley.

Reiser, S.L. (1981). A tool to facilitate mother-infant attachment. *Journal of Obstetric, Gynecologic, and Neonatal Nursing, 10,* 294–297.

Rubin, R. (1975). Maternal tasks in pregnancy. *Maternal-Child Nursing Journal, 4,* 143–153.

Rubin, R. (1963). Maternal touch. *Nursing Outlook, 11,* 828.

Selby, J.W. (1980). *Psychology and human reproduction.* New York: Free Press.

Svejda, M.J., Campos, J.J., & Emde, R.N. (1980). Mother-infant "bonding": Failure to generalize. *Child Development, 51,* 775.

Other

NAACOG (1991, June). Postpartum nursing care: Vaginal delivery. *OGN Nursing Practice Resource.*

NAACOG (1989, March). Mother-baby care. *OGN Nursing Practice Resource.*

Mary Katherine Bourgeois Harris

Breastfeeding

Objectives

1. Identify the two hormones necessary for the synthesis of milk and the milk ejection reflex

2. List two strategies to correct flat or inverted nipples

3. State two subjective findings that can contribute to a poor initial feeding

4. Demonstrate criteria for correct positioning of the infant at the breast

5. List three objective findings that contribute to poor "latching on"

6. List four strategies to decrease breast and nipple pain related to engorgement, plugged ducts, mastitis, or all three

7. Describe two interventions to assist a lactating mother in each of the following special circumstances: infant of a cesarean birth; reluctant or sleepy infant; irritable or fussy infant; infant with physiological jaundice; preterm or hospitalized infant; multiple birth infants; or handicapped infant

8. List three suggestions to increase an inadequate milk supply

9. State expected nutritional needs of the lactating woman

10. Identify which infants may benefit from supplemental lactation aids

11. Participate as a team member in planning care for infants and mothers with special needs in collaboration with a lactation specialist or consultant, physical therapist, occupational therapist, and other healthcare professionals

12. Develop a source of referrals for families with special needs

13. Pursue advanced education and training specialization in lactation services according to individual interest

Introduction

An understanding of anatomy and physiology of breastfeeding is essential for the nurse assisting families during the immediate newborn period. The knowledge the nurse imparts provides the foundation for long-term success with lactation.

The encouragement and practical skills shared assist the mother and infant in establishing a positive basis for their breastfeeding experience. The encouraging of frequent feedings every 2½ to 3 hours of unlimited length (minimum of 10 to 15 minutes at each breast) with the infant correctly positioned and latched on ensures an adequate supply of breast milk.

Clinical Practice

A. Physiology (Fig. 19–1)

1. Hormonal influences during pregnancy begin in the first trimester related to the following
   a. Ductal sprouting (estrogen)
   b. Ductal branching (estrogen)
   c. Lobular formation (progesterone)
2. Initiation of milk production (Fig. 19–2)
   a. Prolactin level increases (at term, 200 to 500 ng/ml)
   b. Estrogen and progesterone levels decrease after delivery
   c. Suckling provides continued stimulus for prolactin and oxytocin release
   d. Prolactin and oxytocin are essential for synthesis and release of milk
   e. Let-down reflex (milk ejection reflex) is triggered by the infant suckling at the nipple, the mother's emotional response to the infant, or both; alveoli contract, eject milk into the ducts, and then into sinuses and out through the nipple; there are several let-downs during a feeding; most mothers notice only the first one; the first let-down occurs during the first 1 to 3 minutes of a feeding
3. Stages of human milk
   a. Colostrum: present at first postpartum week; thick and yellow; increased volume in parous women
   b. Transitional milk: present 7 to 10 days to 2 weeks of postpartum period; not as yellow as colostrum

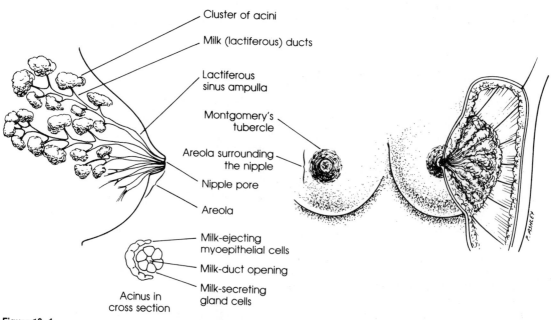

Figure 19–1
Anatomy of the breast. (From Burroughs, A. [1992]. *Maternity nursing: An introductory text.* Philadelphia: Saunders, p. 15.)

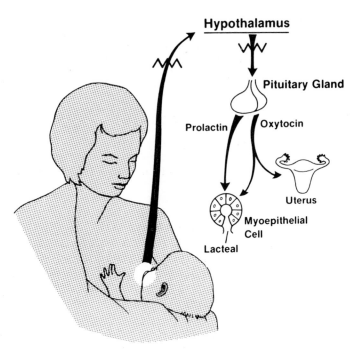

Figure 19-2
Ejection reflex arc. (From Lawrence, R.A. [1989]. *Breastfeeding: A guide for the medical profession.* [3rd ed.]. St. Louis: The C.V. Mosby Co., p. 112.)

c. Mature milk: present after first 2 weeks; whiter and thinner than transitional milk
d. Fore milk: immediate milk received in feeding; satisfies infant's initial thirst
e. Hind milk: later milk received in feeding; higher in fat content (4 times higher than fore milk); may come 10 minutes or later into feeding; satisfies hunger and promotes infant weight gain

B. Assessment

1. History
   a. Previous maternal breastfeeding experience
   b. Desire of mother to breastfeed and anticipated duration of breastfeeding
   c. Exposure of mother to breastfeeding education
   d. Cultural influences on mother
   e. Maternal support system
   f. Previous and current maternal infections and sexually transmitted diseases
   g. Previous and current maternal exposures to environmental hazards
   h. Previous and current maternal use and abuse of tobacco, alcohol, and drugs (recreational, prescription, or over-the-counter)
   i. Difficult birth, cesarean section, or both
   j. Fetal distress
   k. Preterm infant or multiple births
   l. Hospitalized or handicapped infant, or both
   m. Infant with poor sucking reflex
   n. Infant with poor latching on
   o. Maternal complaints of pain
      (1) Nipple
      (2) Breast
      (3) Related to incision, episiotomy, or position
   p. Any pre-existing maternal health condition
2. Physical findings
   a. Inspect nipples for the following
      (1) Protracted: protrude slightly at rest; when stimulated become erect and easy for infant to grasp

        (2) Flat: are difficult for baby to grasp and unchanged with stimulation

        (3) Inverted: are rare; retract at rest and when stimulated

        (4) Traumatized: are cracked, blistered, fissured, or bleeding; are painful when infant nurses

  b. Inspect breast for the following

    (1) Previous surgery

      (a) Augmentation: client has the ability to breastfeed as long as milk ducts have not been severed (need to consult with surgeon about specific procedure performed; mother with poor milk production may benefit from supplemental lactation device); caution should be observed until safety of breast implants has been established

      (b) Reduction: results in variable success and dependent on extent of tissue removed; if nipple has been relocated, ducts usually have been severed (check with surgeon); client may need supplemental lactation device

      (c) Mastectomy: infant can feed from remaining breast

    (2) Size and condition of breast

      (a) Size of breast not related to ability to produce milk; large-breasted mother may need to hold breast back so infant can grasp nipple

      (b) Fibrocystic breasts: may go into remission during lactation; may improve with decrease in caffeine intake and ingestion of vitamin E (600 IU daily)

      (c) Engorgement: breasts are tender, swollen, firm, and warm to the touch; mother may have fever

      (d) Plugged duct: blocked milk duct; may have palpable lump and localized tenderness, swelling, and redness in area; mother may have headache

      (e) Breast infection or mastitis: may be associated with unresolved plugged duct, cracked nipple, or both; mother may have more severe symptoms similar to those of influenza (fever, chills, joint pain, headache, nausea, and vomiting); usually only one breast with localized redness is involved

  c. Observe maternal positioning of infant; three positions are possible

    (1) Cradle-hold position

    (2) Football-hold position

    (3) Side-lying position

  d. Observe suckling infant

    (1) Check placement of lips, gums, and tongue

    (2) Listen for infant's swallowing pattern

C. Nursing Diagnoses

1. Knowledge and skill deficit related to maternal inexperience in positioning infant

2. High risk for maternal discomfort related to incorrect latching on secondary to flat or inverted nipples, nipple confusion, or both

3. High risk for maternal anxiety related to initial feeding secondary to inexperience

4. Alteration in maternal comfort related to breast or nipple pain because of nipple trauma, engorgement, plugged ducts, mastitis, or all of these conditions

5. Anxiety about breastfeeding ability related to unexpected childbearing experience secondary to infant of a cesarean section, irritable or fussy infant, sleepy or reluctant infant, infant with physiological jaundice, preterm or hospitalized infant, multiple birth infants; or handicapped infant

6. High risk for disturbances in maternal self-concept and self-esteem related to inability to provide an adequate milk supply for infant

7. Alteration in nutrition secondary to increased nutritional demands during lactation

8. High risk for maternal anxiety related to altered role change and sexual identity as a lactating mother

D. Interventions/Evaluations

1. Knowledge or skill deficit related to maternal inexperience in positioning infant
    a. Interventions for positioning (mother needs to be in a relaxed position; as she supports her infant, the infant must grasp the nipple and areola while keeping it correctly latched on in his or her mouth; the combination of proper positioning and correct latching on prevents or decreases incidence of sore nipples; when choosing a position for nursing, first ensure mother is comfortable and well supported with pillows before attempting to position the infant)
        (1) Cradle-hold position (Fig. 19–3)
            (a) Roll infant's body toward mother
            (b) Grasp infant's thigh with hand and tuck infant's lower arm around mother's waist
            (c) Bring baby to breast, not breast to baby (pillows positioned under infant are helpful)
            (d) Support breast with opposite hand (Fig. 19–4) (no cigarette or scissor hold)
        (2) Football-hold position offers a good control of infant's head and is helpful after cesarean birth (Fig. 19–5)
            (a) Place infant on pillow at mother's side
            (b) Have mother support infant's upper back with arm and support head in hand
            (c) Have mother place hand that is holding infant's head level with the breast
            (d) Have mother use opposite hand to support breast
        (3) Side-lying position (Fig. 19–6)
            (a) Place infant on side, facing mother's abdomen
            (b) Have mother support breast with opposite hand

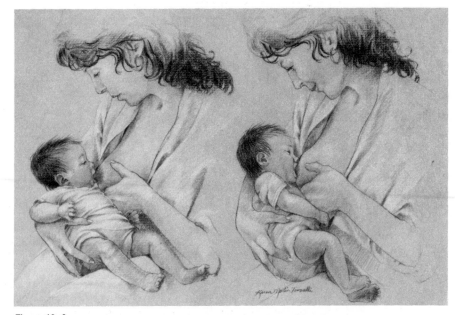

Figure 19–3
Poor body position is shown on the left; good baby position is shown on the right (© 1991 Childbirth Graphics Ltd., Rochester, NY.)

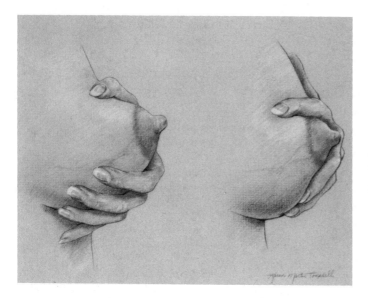

Figure 19–4
Hand position on the left helps direct the nipple and areola into the baby's mouth as she latches on. The hand position on the right, the scissors or cigarette position, flattens the nipple and makes it more difficult for the baby to latch on. (© 1991 Childbirth Graphics Ltd., Rochester, NY.)

b. Evaluations
    (1) Mother reports absence of shoulder, neck, or back pain
    (2) Nipple shows no evidence of trauma
    (3) Mother appears relaxed and verbalizes confidence with positioning infant
2. High risk for maternal discomfort related to incorrect latching on secondary to flat or inverted nipples, nipple confusion, or both (Fig. 19–7)
    a. Interventions for latching on (correct placement of the infant's mouth on the nipple ensures good stimulation for adequate milk supply and decreases or prevents sore nipples)
        (1) Have mother tickle infant's lips with breast
        (2) Allow mouth to open wide and center breast in mouth

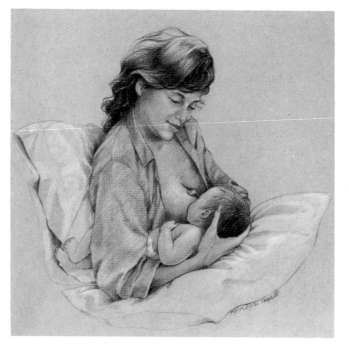

Figure 19–5
Football hold. (© 1991 Childbirth Graphics Ltd., Rochester, NY.)

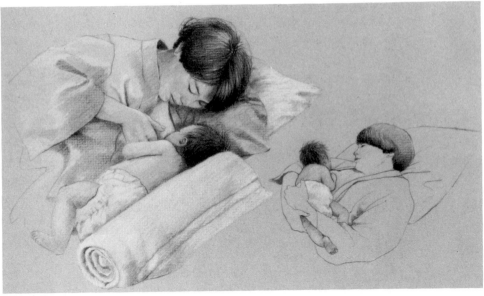

Figure 19-6
Side-lying position. (© 1991 Childbirth Graphics Ltd., Rochester, NY.)

(3) Have mother pull infant in close, place jaw behind nipple on areola with lips flanged
(4) Mother can remove infant from breast by breaking the suction: insert a finger gently into the corner of baby's mouth or press finger against breast near corner of baby's mouth

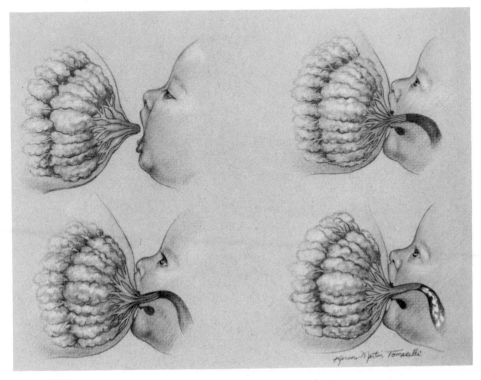

Figure 19-7
Latch-on and sucking sequence. (© 1991 Childbirth Graphics, Ltd., Rochester, NY.)

b. Evaluations
   (1) Infant's mouth is opened wide; lips are not tucked or curled
   (2) Lips are placed behind nipple on areola
   (3) Tongue is placed under breast
   (4) Infant is not chewing on own tongue
   (5) Few or no complaints of sore nipples occur
c. Interventions for flat or inverted nipples (Fig. 19–8)
   (1) Have mother wear Netsy cup/breast cup during third trimester: gentle pressure stretches and encourages nipple to protrude; can also be worn during postpartum period
   (2) Have mother apply ice to nipple a few minutes before feeding to increase nipple protractability
   (3) Have mother use breast pump a few minutes before feeding to increase nipple protractability
   (4) Do not use rubber nipple shield because infant can use shield as a pacifier, which does not stimulate sinuses and frequently results in an inadequate milk supply
d. Evaluations
   (1) There is improved protrusion of nipples, when stimulated
   (2) There is improved ability of infant to grasp nipple
   (3) There are few or no complaints of sore nipples
e. Interventions for nipple confusion (associated with infant's being fed supplements from rubber nipples; the placement and action of feeding from rubber nipples require the tongue to be up and forward; when suckling at the breast, the tongue thrusts forward over the lower gum to grasp the nipple, the lips flange around the areola and the gums compress the milk sinuses; the tongue then creates a wavelike backward motion to extract milk)
   (1) Have mother avoid the use of rubber nipples during the first 4 to 6 weeks
   (2) Have mother use a supplemental lactation device if additional fluids are medically necessary
f. Evaluations
   (1) Infant accepts breast without pulling away and appears content and satisfied
   (2) There is an adequate milk supply
   (3) There is little or no nipple pain

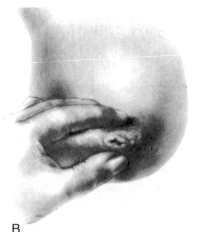

A   B

Figure 19–8
Normal nipple compared with inverted nipple. *A,* Normal nipple everts with gentle pressure; *B,* inverted nipple inverts with gentle pressure. (From Lawrence, R.A. [1989]. *Breastfeeding: A guide for the medical profession* [3rd ed.]. St. Louis: The C.V. Mosby Co., p. 126.)

3. High risk for maternal anxiety related to initial feeding secondary to inexperience
    a. Interventions for initial feeding
       (1) Evaluate maternal discomfort and institute relief measures (medicate as per physician's order) for source of pain (incision, episiotomy, or uterus)
       (2) Initiate feeding as soon as possible with alert mother and infant (is ideal to initiate in delivery or recovery room)
       (3) Position mother for comfort and provide back, neck, and arm support according to choice of position
       (4) Initiate correct latching on and positioning
       (5) Reassure mother if infant appears disinterested; some newborns are not immediately ready to nurse; encourage her to snuggle, hold, and enjoy her infant instead
       (6) Support and encourage mother to verbalize any feelings of disappointment or rejection, or expectations related to initial feeding
    b. Evaluations
       (1) There is an increase in length of time infant is interested at breast (minimum of 10 to 15 minutes) with both breasts being offered, thereby encouraging the release of hind milk
       (2) There are frequent feedings; most infants nurse between 8 and 12 times a day during the first month
       (3) Mother states she has little or no nipple pain
       (4) Infant seems satisfied
       (5) Mother verbalizes confidence and increased breastfeeding skill is observed
4. Alteration in maternal comfort related to nipple or breast pain because of nipple trauma, engorgement, plugged ducts, mastitis, or all of these conditions
    a. Intervention for sore nipples: usually associated with nursing incorrectly; waiting too long between feedings, poor positioning, and poor latching on all are contributing factors; limiting of feeding times does not prevent sore nipples
       (1) Inspect nipple tissue for redness, fissures, or blisters
       (2) Have mother apply ice immediately before feeding to allow easier grasping of nipple and to produce a numbing effect
       (3) Have mother express a few drops of milk before feeding so that infant does not need to nurse as vigorously
       (4) Have mother change positions with each feeding so that area of tissue breakdown does not have repeated mechanical trauma (football-hold position is especially helpful in encouraging infant to open mouth wide)
       (5) Check correct positioning of infant
       (6) Check latching on and placement of tongue, lips, and gums
       (7) Correct and prevent engorgement
       (8) Offer mother a mild analgesic 30 minutes before feeding (per physician's order)
       (9) Have mother use only cotton breastpads; plastic-lined breastpads retain moisture
       (10) Discontinue use of soap; rinse breast with water
       (11) Discontinue feeding before mother falls asleep
       (12) Discontinue use of lanolin if mother is allergic to wool
       (13) Short (10 minute) and more frequent feedings (every 1½ to 2 hours) may be helpful
       (14) Detach infant by breaking suction with finger
       (15) After feeding, apply a few drops of breast milk to nipple and let dry (breast milk is very healing)

(16) Keep brassiere down to allow air to reach nipple between feedings (or use hair dryer on low setting, or 100-watt light bulb for 1 minute)

b. Evaluations

(1) Mother reports decrease in pain

(2) Nipple area decreases in redness, cracking, bleeding, blisters, or fissures

c. Interventions for engorgement (a normal fullness is expected in the first days of breastfeeding, but engorgement is an exaggerated response related to rigid feeding schedules, delayed first feeding, and use of supplements or limited time at each feeding; mother's breasts are painful, swollen, and firm and the nipple is difficult for the infant to grasp because of areolar fullness)

(1) Encourage early feedings

(2) Encourage frequent feedings (every 2 to 3 hours, with a minimum of 10 to 15 minutes at each breast)

(3) Discontinue use of supplements unless medically indicated per physician's order

(4) Administer a mild analgesic 30 minutes before feeding (per physician's order)

(5) Apply warm compress to breast or offer shower before feeding

(6) Offer gentle massage of breast to encourage let-down and soften areolar tissue

(7) Use breast pump to soften areolar tissue (excessive pumping aggravates the problem)

(8) Apply ice packs, 5 to 10 minutes after feeding

d. Evaluations

(1) There is a decrease and resolution of pain, swelling, and tenderness within 12 to 24 hours

(2) Areolar tissue softens and nipple is easier to grasp

e. Interventions for plugged ducts (a decrease in the flow of milk results in a localized obstruction; area may be palpable and reddened)

(1) Administer a mild analgesic, per physician's order

(2) Apply a warm compress to breast before feeding

(3) Offer gentle breast massage before feeding

(4) Have infant feed at involved breast first

(5) Have mother use gravity to facilitate emptying by leaning over; football-hold position is helpful

(6) Ensure frequent feedings (every 2 to 3 hours, with 10 to 15 minutes at each breast)

(7) Offer pumping, which may be necessary if infant is ill or reluctant to nurse

(8) Caution mother to check that her brassiere is not too tight or that underwires are contributing to the problem

f. Evaluations

(1) Pain, tenderness, and swelling decrease

(2) Resolution of palpable lump

g. Interventions for mastitis (reddened and painful area of the breast accompanied by any or all of the following: fever, symptoms similar to those of influenza, joint pain, headache, and nausea)

(1) Ensure bed rest for 24 to 48 hours

(2) Administer antibiotics, per physician's order

(3) Increase fluid intake and ensure adequate nutrition

(4) Administer an analgesic, per physician's order

(5) Evaluate hygiene and encourage good handwashing

(6) Reassure mother that she can continue breastfeeding

(7) Apply warm compress to breast or offer gentle massage before feeding

(8) Ensure frequent feedings (every 2 to 3 hours, with 10 to 15 minutes at each breast)

(9) Vary infant's positions

(10) Express milk with pump or hand if breast is not emptied by infant

h. Evaluations

(1) Pain, swelling, and tenderness decrease

(2) Fever decreases

(3) Inflammation and infection process resolve

5. Anxiety about breastfeeding ability related to unexpected childbearing experience secondary to infant of a cesarean section, irritable or fussy infant, sleepy or reluctant infant, infant with physiological jaundice, preterm or hospitalized infant, multiple birth infants, or handicapped infant

a. Interventions for infant of a cesarean section

(1) Reassure mothers who have had cesarean sections that they can and do breastfeed as successfully as mothers who have had vaginal births

(2) Medicate mother 15 to 30 minutes before feedings to minimize transmission of medication in milk to infant

(3) Encourage mobility and self-care for mother

(4) Position infant in football hold to avoid incisional discomfort

(5) Encourage night feedings to increase milk supply and decrease engorgement

(6) Encourage good nutrition as essential for healing needs

(7) Allow mother to express any feelings of disappointment

b. Evaluations

(1) Mother demonstrates increasing competence with self-care and asks for assistance as needed

(2) Mother demonstrates knowledge of nutritional needs by diet choices

(3) Mother verbalizes confidence with breastfeeding ability

(4) Mother has a plan for assistance at discharge

c. Interventions for a sleepy or reluctant infant (difficult to awaken, loses interest quickly, and does not nurse vigorously)

(1) Wake infant after 3½ to 4 hours

(2) Encourage at least eight feedings per day

(3) Use arousing techniques: unwrap blankets, apply cool cloth to infant's body, change diapers, burp frequently

(4) Express or pump milk so it is readily available

(5) Avoid use of rubber nipple and pacifiers

(6) Encourage rooming-in so that when infant is awake, mother is available

d. Evaluations

(1) There are increasing interest and time spent at breast

(2) Infant weight gain follows expected curve

(3) There is increasing maternal confidence in meeting infant needs

e. Interventions for a fussy or irritable infant: may have strong sucking need, may become frantic when beginning feeding, or may want to nurse more often than every 2 hours

(1) Use slow, gentle movements

(2) Provide a quiet environment: (e.g., audio taped music, dim lights, rocking chair, or cradle)

(3) Use infant massage and skin-to-skin contact

(4) Use soft, cloth infant carriers

(5) Follow infant's preference for swaddling

(6) Express or pump milk so it is readily available

(7) Burp infant frequently (may swallow air when fussing)

(8) Allow infant's non-nutritive sucking needs to be met with pacifier or sucking of own fingers

(9) Have mother keep diet history (irritable behavior may be associated with an offending food)

(10) Avoid using supplements with rubber nipples: this will reinforce impatience and increase the risk of nipple confusion
f. Evaluations
(1) There is a decrease in irritability and fussiness
(2) Infant is able to wait at least 2 hours between feedings
(3) There is an increase in awareness of mother to infant cues
g. Interventions for physiological jaundice (a healthy newborn may show signs of physiological jaundice [increased bilirubin values, yellowing of the skin and sclera are objective findings] on the second or third day of life; treatment with sunlight or phototherapy assists in decreasing bilirubin levels; the encouraging of water supplements does not facilitate a decrease in bilirubin levels; bilirubin can be reabsorbed in the intestines; frequent breastfeeding promotes increased bowel movements and decreased reabsorption)
(1) Encourage frequent feedings (every 2 to 3 hours)
(2) Have mother use techniques to arouse infant, if sleepy or disinterested
(3) Discourage use of rubber nipples for supplements (causes increased nipple confusion, decreased interest in breastfeeding, and may decrease the number of infant stools)
(4) Explore use of phototherapy in mother's hospital room or home use of phototherapy
(5) Encourage mother to verbalize concerns
h. Evaluations
(1) There is a decrease in bilirubin levels
(2) There is an increase in infant's interest in feedings
i. Interventions for preterm or hospitalized infant (can be an overwhelming experience for most parents; the concern about immediate needs, financial costs, and long-term outcomes is of most importance; the immunological advantages, nutritional components, and digestibility of breast milk are of great value to a preterm or hospitalized infant)
(1) Encourage and praise mother's decision to breastfeed
(2) Provide an electric breast pump while infant is hospitalized
(3) Begin pumping as soon as possible
(4) Have mother use relaxation techniques, warm compresses, and visualize (or gaze at a picture of) her infant before beginning to pump
(5) Provide mother with time to touch infant before pumping: as infant's condition improves and stabilizes, just holding the infant helps with let-down
(6) Pump at least eight times daily (with a minimum of 10 minutes for each breast); pump at least once during the night (use of a pump that can be used on both breasts at once is especially helpful when long-term pumping is necessary)
(7) Provide mother with written instructions for pumping and milk collection at discharge
(8) Give mother referral for electric pump rental
(9) Refer mother to lactation specialists or consultant when necessary for help with an immature suck reflex when infant is put to breast
(10) Use supplemental lactation device to increase caloric volume without using rubber nipple
j. Evaluations
(1) There is increasing volume of collected breast milk
(2) Mother has increasing confidence and skill when infant is put to breast
k. Interventions for multiple births (the mother may have to cope with the challenges of a cesarean section, preterm infants, and providing for long-term follow-up of more than one newborn; breastfeeding assists in bonding and meeting the individual needs of each baby)
(1) Reassure mother that milk supply is determined by milk demand and that the supply adjusts to infants' demand

     (2) Assist mother with positioning of two infants (both in cradle position, legs crossing; both in football position; or one in football position and one in cradle position)

     (3) Assist mother in anticipatory planning for rest and nutritional needs

     (4) Provide mother with a referral to a local chapter of Mother of Twins or Mother of Multiples

     (5) Provide mother with a feeding schedule to help her get needed rest

  l. Evaluations

     (1) Mother reports satisfaction with breastfeeding

     (2) Infant's weight follows growth curve

  m. Interventions for a handicapped infant (when a family's dream of having a so-called perfect baby does not materialize, a period of grieving is appropriate and expected; breastfeeding enhances the bond between mother and child; providing breast milk may increase a mother's ability to nurture and comfort her infant)

     (1) Encourage and listen to mother's feelings of disappointment, disbelief, and anger

     (2) Provide flexibility in hospital routine for family support

     (3) Provide information for support groups specific to disability (e.g., cleft palate, Down's syndrome, and spina bifida)

     (4) Initiate a collaborative care plan and include a lactation specialist or consultant, occupational therapist, physical therapist, and any other pertinent health care providers to provide consistent, optimal care for specific maternal and infant needs

  n. Evaluations

     (1) Mother has a realistic approach to infant's ability to nurse and to maternal time and effort needed to explore alternatives (e.g., long-term pumping with supplemental nursing device)

     (2) Mother has an increasing acceptance and understanding of infant's disability

     (3) Mother has increasing confidence and ability with breastfeeding skills

6. High risk for disturbances in maternal self-concept and self-esteem related to inability to provide an adequate milk supply for infant

  a. Interventions related to milk supply (the amount of breast milk produced is related to nipple stimulation, adequate let-down, and nutritional intake)

     (1) Ensure sufficient stimulation with frequent feedings (every 2 to 3 hours, with 10 to 15 minutes at each breast)

     (2) Encourage rooming-in

     (3) Evaluate for any missed or supplemented feedings

     (4) Wake infant if asleep longer than 3 hours

     (5) Avoid use of pacifier

     (6) Use lactation supplemental device if it is medically indicated that infant needs additional calories

     (7) Evaluate for poor latching on

     (8) Listen for infant swallowing

     (9) Ensure adequate maternal fluid intake of 1920 ml (2 qt) daily

     (10) Evaluate maternal activity level and encourage rest

     (11) Consider underlying maternal health condition if poor milk supply continues

  b. Evaluations

     (1) Mother notices a sense of fullness before feeding

     (2) Mother notices a let-down and softening of breast after feeding

     (3) There are six to eight wet diapers a day

     (4) Infant has regular patterns of wakefulness, sleep, and feeding

     (5) Infant's weight loss is not more than 5 to 10% during the first week

     (6) Infant's weight follows a normal growth curve

7. Alteration in nutrition secondary to increased nutritional demands during lactation

a. Interventions related to the following: *Nutrition:* a wide selection of foods can be offered, according to a mother's individual tastes and preferences; any food, in moderation, can be part of a diet during lactation; foods that produce gastrointestinal irritation in a mother probably also produce it in the infant; the average diet during lactation consists of 2200 calories daily; it takes between 500 and 700 calories to produce milk; fat stores from pregnancy help provide some of these additional calories; 1920 ml (2 qt) of liquids and the following servings from all food groups are to be encouraged: protein, three or four; dairy, four to six; fruit, four; grains, four; vegetables, four; *Alcohol:* a safe level of alcohol has not been determined; even moderate amounts of alcohol may slow brain growth in the infant; *Drugs and Medications:* multiple factors affect excretion of maternal medications in breast milk (solubility, route of administration, accumulation of substance, duration of use, weight of infant, and amount and number of times that infant breastfeeds); for specific prescription and over-the-counter medications, see Lauwers and Woessner (1990); *Tobacco:* smoking of 20 cigarettes/day or more may cause nausea and vomiting in the infant and cause a decrease in milk supply; any exposure to second-hand smoke is detrimental; parents should be encouraged not to allow smoking when infant is present; *Caffeine:* may be taken in moderate amounts; infants who are frequently colicky, wakeful, or hyperactive may be consuming excessive amounts of caffeine in their breast milk and maternal consumption of caffeine needs to be decreased
  (1) Review dietary choices
  (2) Provide consultation with a dietitian as needed
  (3) Offer sample menus
  (4) Plan menus according to cultural or religious preferences
  (5) Inform mother of Women, Infants, and Children (WIC) program, a supplemental food and nutritional counseling program for pregnant, postpartum, and lactating mothers with children (income and risk qualifications need to be met)
  (6) Eliminate foods suspected of aggravating colic
  (7) Encourage the decrease or elimination of maternal use of tobacco, and of infant's exposure to second-hand smoke
b. Evaluations
  (1) Mother makes good dietary choices from menu and maintains an adequate level of fluids
  (2) There is an increase in maternal energy levels
  (3) There is adequate healing of episiotomy or other incisions
  (4) Mother has an adequate milk supply
  (5) There is a decrease in tobacco use
8. High risk for maternal anxiety related to altered role change and sexual identity as lactating mother
a. Interventions related to sexuality (new parents need time to adjust to each other sexually after the birth of their child; time schedules, responsibilities, and role changes are all factors that may affect sexual desires and needs)
  (1) Allow client to express her concerns and feelings
  (2) Use of a water-soluble lubricant may be helpful for decreased vaginal lubrication related to lowered estrogen levels during lactation
  (3) Reassure client that many women notice a let-down reflex during intercourse
  (4) Reassure client that some women find their breasts are very sensitive while lactating. Reassure client that an erotic response to breastfeeding can occur and has no significance.
  (5) Reassure client that some women feel overwhelmed by partner's touch after caring for a baby all day
  (6) Encourage parents to find time for themselves as a couple

(7) Reaffirm that menstruation may be delayed during lactation, but pregnancy can occur

(8) Provide client with information on barrier methods of contraception

b. Evaluations

(1) Parents express realistic expectations for coping with individual sexual needs

(2) Parents have a plan for contraception, if an immediate pregnancy is not desired

Health Education

A. The health care provider offers educational assistance about the following topics through the written word, audio-visual materials, and individual or group instruction

1. Preparation for breastfeeding
   a. Normal physiology
   b. Correction of flat or inverted nipples
   c. Production of milk
   d. Let-down (milk ejection reflex)
   e. Stages of human milk
2. Initial Feeding
   a. Correct positioning
   b. Correct latching on
3. Correction and prevention of common breastfeeding problems
   a. Sore nipples
   b. Engorgement
   c. Plugged ducts
   d. Mastitis
   e. Building and maintaining of a milk supply
4. Resource and referral information available for special situations
   a. Cesarean birth
   b. Irritable or fussy infant
   c. Sleepy or reluctant infant
   d. Infant with physiological jaundice
   e. Preterm or hospitalized infant
   f. Infants of a multiple birth
   g. Handicapped infant
5. Nutritional guidelines for lactation
6. Sexuality and contraception during lactation

B. Evaluations: the mother is able to do the following

1. Demonstrate correct latching on and positioning for breastfeeding before discharge
2. State measures to correct common breastfeeding problems (with the help of written material)
3. Provide information about resources available that are appropriate for special circumstances
4. Make good nutritional choices
5. Begin discussions with partner for planning contraceptive needs

---

CASE STUDY AND STUDY QUESTIONS

Molly Champlin is a 27-year-old gravida 2, para 1 (G2,P1) woman. She had an uncomplicated spontaneous vaginal delivery at 39 weeks' gestation and her daughter weighed (3629 g) 8 lb and had Apgar scores of 9 to 10. Molly had previously attempted to breastfeed her first daughter, but quit after 2 weeks because of cracked nipples and a poor milk supply. She states, "I really want to breastfeed this baby at least 6 months."

1. What additional information is needed to help plan for Molly's care?

   (1) Previous breastfeeding experience.

   (2) Previous use of drugs, tobacco, and alcohol.

   (3) Maternal support systems.

   (4) Previous breast surgery.

   a. 1, 2.

   b. 2, 4.

   c. 3, 4.

   d. 1, 4.

   e. All of the above.

2. On physical examination you observe that the mother's nipples are inverted; what would be helpful to make the nipples easier for the infant to grasp?

   (1) Application of ice before feeding.

   (2) Use of breast or Netsy cups.

   (3) Use of rubber nipple shield.

   (4) Toughening with wash cloth.

   (5) Use of pump before feeding.

   a. 1, 2, 4.

   b. 1, 2, 3.

   c. 2, 3, 4.

   d. 1, 2, 5.

   e. All but 5.

3. How soon after delivery should Molly be encouraged to attempt to nurse her daughter?

   a. Immediately after delivery.

   b. Between 3 and 6 hours after delivery.

   c. Between 6 and 12 hours after delivery.

   d. At 12 hours after delivery.

4. Molly expresses concern about how to prevent sore nipples: which of the following is helpful?

   (1) Limiting of feedings to 5 minutes each breast.

   (2) Checking for correct latching on.

   (3) Checking for positioning of infant.

   (4) Use of a supplemental bottle.

   (5) Air-drying nipples after feeding.

   a. All of the above.

   b. 1, 2, 3, 5.

   c. 2, 3.

   d. 2, 4, 5.

   e. 2, 3, 5.

5. What two hormones most affect milk synthesis and the milk ejection/let-down reflex?

   (1) Progesterone.

   (2) Estrogen.

   (3) Oxytocin.

   (4) Follicle-stimulating hormone (FSH).

   (5) Prolactin.

   a. 1, 2.

   b. 2, 5.

   c. 3, 4.

   d. 4, 5.

   e. 3, 5.

6. List three strategies to prevent and decrease engorgement.

7. List five comfort measures to resolve engorgement.

8. List three strategies to increase milk supply.

9. What two breastfeeding aids may be helpful to a mother with a preterm or hospitalized infant?

10. Which of the following are true about a cesarean-section birth mother and breastfeeding?

    (1) Usually cannot breastfeed until the fourth postpartum day.

    (2) Needs help positioning infant during first few days.

(3) May find football-hold position comfortable.

(4) Should pump milk while taking pain medication.

a. All of the above.

b. All but 1.

c. 2, 3.

d. 1, 3.

e. 1, 3, 4.

Answers to Study Questions

1. e
2. d
3. a

4. e
5. e
6. Frequent feedings, every 2 to 3 hours; sufficient length, with 10 to 15 minutes at each breast; avoidance of supplements.
7. Analgesia, per doctor's order; warm compresses before feeding; hand express/pump to soften areolar tissue; frequent feedings, every 2 to 3 hours; sufficient length, with 10 to 15 minutes at each breast; avoidance of supplements; application of ice, after feeding.
8. Frequent feedings, every 2 to 3 hours; sufficient length, with 10 to 15 minutes at each breast; adequate maternal nutrition and fluid intake; adequate maternal rest.
9. Electric or hand breast pump; supplemental lactation device.
10. c

REFERENCES

Coreil, J., & Murphy, J. (1988). Maternal commitment, lactation practices, and breastfeeding duration. *Journal of Obstetric, Gynecologic, and Neonatal Nursing, 17*(4), 273–278.

de Cavalho, M., Klaus, M., & Merkatz, R. (1981). Frequency of breastfeeding and serum bilirubin concentrations. *American Journal of Diseases in Children, 136,* 737–738.

de Cavalho, M., Robertson, S., & Klaus, M. (1984). Does the duration and frequency of early breastfeeding affect nipple pain? *Birth, 11*(2), 81–84.

Dilts, C. (1985). Nursing management of mastitis due to breastfeeding. *Journal of Obstetric, Gynecologic, and Neonatal Nursing, 14*(4), 286–288.

Evans, C., Lyons, N., & Kellien, M. (1986). The effects of infant formula samples on breastfeeding practice. *Journal of Obstetric, Gynecologic, and Neonatal Nursing, 15*(5), 401–405.

Frantz, K., & Kalman, M. (1979). Breastfeeding works for Cesarean moms, too. *RN, 42*(12), 39–45.

Hayes, B. (1981). Inconsistencies among nurses in breastfeeding knowledge and counseling. *Journal of Obstetric, Gynecologic, and Neonatal Nursing, 10*(6), 430–433.

Huggins, K. (1986). The nursing mother's companion. Boston: Harvard Common Press.

Kaughman, K., & Hall, L. (1989). Influences of the social network on the choice and duration of breastfeeding in mothers of preterm infants. *Research in Nursing and Health, 12,* 149–159.

Le Leche League International. (1987). *The womanly art of breastfeeding.* Franklin Park, IL: La Leche International.

Lawrence, R. (1989). *Breastfeeding: A guide for the medical profession.* (3rd ed.) St. Louis: Mosby.

Lawrence, R. (1982). Practices and attitudes toward breastfeeding among medical professionals. *Pediatrics, 70*(6), 912–920.

Lauwers, J., & Woessner, C. (1990). *Counseling the nursing mother: A reference guide for health care providers and lay counselors.* Wayne, NJ: Avery.

Minchin, M.K. (1989). Positioning for breastfeeding. *Birth, 16*(2), 67–73.

NAACOG (1991, Nov.). Facilitating breastfeeding. *OGN Nursing Practice Resource.*

Riordan, J. (1983). *A practical guide to breastfeeding.* St. Louis: Mosby.

Shrago, L., & Bocar, D. (1990). The infant's contribution to breastfeeding. *Journal of Obstetric, Gynecologic, and Neonatal Nursing, 19*(3), 209–215.

Simpoulous, A.P., & Grove, G.D. (1984). Factors associated with the choice and duration of infant feeding practices. *Pediatrics, 74,* 603–614.

Taylor, P., Maloni, J., & Brown, D. (1986). Early suckling and prolonged breastfeeding. *American Journal of Diseases in Children, 140,* 151–154.

Tellalian, L. (1986). Breastfeeding educator: A companion role for childbirth educators. *Genesis, 83*(4), 27–35.

Tully, M.R., & Overfield, M.J. (1989). *Breastfeeding: A handbook for hospitals.* Evansville, IN: Mead Johnson.

Wiles, L.S. (1984). The effect of prenatal breastfeeding education on breastfeeding success and maternal perception of the infant. *Journal of Obstetric, Gynecologic, and Neonatal Nursing, 13*(4), 253–257.

ADVANCED BREASTFEEDING EDUCATION FOR HEALTH PROFESSIONALS

Health Education Associates, 211 Easton Road, Glenside, PA 19038.

Human Lactation Center, 666 Sturges Highway, Westport, CT 06880.

International Lactation Consultant Association, PO Box 4031, University of Virginia Station, Charlottesville, VA 22903.

La Leche League International, 9616 Minneapolis Avenue, Franklin Park, IL 60131.

Lactation Associates, 123 Aldrich Street, Boston, MA 02131.

The Lactation Institute and Breastfeeding Clinic, 16161 Ventura Boulevard, Suite 223, Encino, CA 91436.

UCLA Extension, Department of Health Sciences, Room 614, 10995 Le Conte Avenue, Los Angeles, CA 90024.

PRINTED AND AUDIO-VISUAL BREASTFEEDING MATERIALS

Childbirth Graphics, PO Box 17025, Rochester, NY 14617.

La Leche League International, 9616 Minneapolis Avenue, Franklin Park, IL 60131.

Lifecircle, 2378 Cornell Drive, Costa Mesa, CA 92626.

BREAST PUMPS, HAND

Kaneson Breast Pump, 341 Jefferson Avenue, Downingtown, PA 19335.

Happy Family Breast Pump, 12300 Venice Boulevard, Los Angeles, CA 90066.

Mary Jane Breast Pump, 5510 Cleon Avenue, North Hollywood, CA 91609.

BREAST PUMPS, ELECTRIC

Egnell, 412 Park Avenue, Cary, IL 60013.

Medela, PO Box 386, Crystal Lake, IL 60814.

Whiteriver, 23010 Lake Forest Drive, Suite 10, Laguna Hills, CA 92653.

MILK CUPS

Netsy Swedish Milk Cups, 34 Sunrise Avenue, Mill Valley, CA 94941.

O-Cal-Ette, 1818 S. Redwood, Salt Lake City, UT 84104.

Woolwich Breast Cup, La Leche League, 9616 Minneapolis Avenue, Franklin Park, IL 60131.

SUPPLEMENTAL LACTATION TRAINER

Lact-Aid, PO Box 6861, Denver, CO 80206.

Supplemental Nursing System, Medela, Inc, PO Box 386, Crystal Lake, IL 60814.

Kathryn V. Deitch

Family Planning

Objectives

1. Describe the various methods of birth control

2. Compare the effectiveness ratings of the various methods of birth control

3. Obtain a contraceptive history from a woman

4. Describe the risks and benefits of each method of birth control

5. Rank the various contraceptives in order of their appropriateness for a woman who has just been delivered of a baby

6. Explain how the postpartum state affects the choice of contraception

7. Identify ethnocultural considerations that affect the choice of contraception for a woman in a postpartum state

8. Identify social and psychological considerations that help determine the appropriate choice of a contraceptive method after childbirth

Introduction

Helping women make decisions about family planning is an important role for the nurse who cares for women during the postpartum period. The increasing practice of shortening hospital stays for women after childbirth means that they may have limited contact with healthcare providers during the weeks after childbirth. If decisions are not made early in the postpartum period, women may find themselves using contraceptive methods that are inappropriate for the postpartum period. Nursing practice must include assessment of contraceptive knowledge, attitudes toward contraception, attitudes toward future pregnancies, and the need for family planning methods before the woman's next contact with the healthcare provider.

Clinical Practice

A. Assessment

1. Contraceptive history
   a. Previous contraceptive use
      (1) Identify dissatisfaction with any of the methods
      (2) Identify satisfaction with any of the methods
      (3) Identify the method of choice
2. Obstetrical and gynecological history
   a. Previous contraceptive complications
   b. Problems with current pregnancy or delivery that affect the choice of contraception
      (1) Hypertension
      (2) Thrombophlebitis
      (3) Diabetes
   c. Problems with current delivery that affect the timing of resumption of sexual intercourse
      (1) Operative delivery
      (2) Episiotomy/lacerations
      (3) Infection
3. Breastfeeding plans
   a. Planned length
   b. Perceived importance
4. Psychosocial responses
   a. Attitude toward timing of resumption of sexual activities
   b. Religious or cultural views about contraception
      (1) Identify religious or cultural barriers to contraception or to the use of particular contraceptive methods
      (2) Identify differences in beliefs or values between the woman and her partner
      (3) Identify conflicts between a desire to avoid conception and religious or cultural values that affect choice
   c. Attitudes toward future pregnancies and their appropriate timing
   d. Motivation to avoid future pregnancy
5. Contraceptive knowledge
   a. Postpartum fertility
   b. Various methods and their uses
   c. Method of choice
   d. Partner's method of choice

B. Nursing Diagnoses

1. Knowledge deficit related to postpartum fertility
2. Knowledge deficit related to proper use of contraceptive method of choice
3. High risk for noncompliance related to selected contraceptive method
4. Alteration in family relationships related to value differences between the woman and her partner about contraceptive choices

C. Interventions/Evaluations

1. Knowledge deficit related to postpartum fertility
   a. Interventions
      (1) Explain the timing of the return of ovulation and menses during the postpartum period
      (2) Explain the lack of effectiveness of lactation in preventing conception during the postpartum period
      (3) Explain the possibility that pregnancy can occur without the resumption of menses

   b. Evaluations
- (1) The woman states that 4 to 6 weeks after delivery is the usual time for the return of menses in the nonlactating woman
- (2) The woman explains that breastfeeding on demand (at least six to seven times daily) without supplementing the infant's diet with formula or other food delays the resumption of ovulation and menses for some, but not all, women
- (3) The woman acknowledges that pregnancy can occur with the first postdelivery ovulation even though no menses have occurred
- (4) The woman states an understanding of the risk of pregnancy during the postpartum period and the need to use contraception if pregnancy is not desired

2. Knowledge deficit related to the proper use of contraceptive method of choice
   a. Interventions (Table 20–1)
- (1) Assess the woman's knowledge of selected method
- (2) Identify the appropriateness of selected method for the postpartum period
- (3) Describe the proper use of the method
- (4) Identify advantages and disadvantages of selected method
- (5) Determine the woman's access to selected method
- (6) Review complications of selected method and their signs and symptoms
- (7) Explain the steps the woman is to take if complications occur
- (8) Explain the importance of consistent use
- (9) Evaluate the woman's comfort with use and confidence in selected method after teaching

   b. Evaluations
- (1) The woman explains how her method of choice is to be used
- (2) The woman identifies advantages and disadvantages of her method
- (3) The woman states how she plans to obtain her method of choice
- (4) The woman identifies signs and symptoms of complications of her method of choice
- (5) The woman states her planned action if problems occur with her method of choice
- (6) The woman states her understanding of the importance of consistent use of her method of choice to prevent pregnancy
- (7) The woman states that she feels capable of comfortable use of the selected method

3. High risk for noncompliance related to selected contraceptive method
   a. Interventions
- (1) Identify the woman's level of commitment to avoiding pregnancy
- (2) Identify the woman's attitude toward contraception and her selected method
- (3) Identify partner's acceptance of the selected method

   b. Evaluations
- (1) The woman identifies how highly she values avoiding pregnancy
- (2) The woman describes how she feels about contraception
- (3) The woman describes the use of her selected method of contraception
- (4) The woman's partner describes his willingness to accept the use of her selected method

4. Alteration in family relationships related to value differences between the woman and her partner about contraceptive choices
   a. Interventions
- (1) Discuss the partner's reaction to contraceptive plans
- (2) Encourage discussion of contraceptive goals between the woman and her partner
- (3) Encourage active participation of the partner in contraceptive planning

Table 20–1
METHODS OF CONTRACEPTION

Method	Failure Rate: Accidental Pregnancy Rate (Typical Use: First Year) (%)	Postpartum Use	Risks/Disadvantages	Benefits
Abstinence	0	Is the method of choice for first 4–6 weeks, especially for operative deliveries, complications, and lacerations	May be unacceptable to woman or partner; may cause relationship problems when there is disagreement	Promotes healing and involution
Vasectomy or male sterilization	0.15	Has no contraindications	Is permanent; requires minor surgery	No further monitoring required after verification that all sperm in system have been ejaculated
Bilateral tubal ligation or female sterilization	0.4	May be performed during cesarean section; may be performed soon after vaginal delivery	Is permanent; may present surgical complications	Requires no further monitoring
Oral contraceptives Two types 1. Regular pill: combined estrogen plus progestin 2. Mini pill: progestin only	3	May interfere with lactation by decreasing milk supply; if lactating, use mini pill or wait until lactation is well established	Minor side effects are breast tenderness, nausea, irregular bleeding (especially with mini pill); major risks are rare in women age 36 and below who do not smoke; blood clots, liver tumor, cerebrovascular accident (CVA), myocardial infarction (MI), gallbladder disease; requires regular monitoring by healthcare provider	May be acceptable for healthy women aged 36–50 years who do not smoke; menses are lighter and shorter, and there are fewer cramps; may protect against breast, ovarian, and uterine disease
Foams with condoms, used together	3	Has no contraindications	Irritation and allergic reactions are rare; must be inserted/put on just before intercourse; is messy; may decrease sensation	As effective as the pill when used together; foam is lubricant; available over the counter; provides protection against sexually transmitted diseases

Diaphragm with spermicide	18	Is not recommended; decreased levels of estrogen make the vagina thinner and drier than normal and insertion difficult; must be refitted after a pregnancy; proper fitting is not possible until involution is complete	Causes irritation, allergic reactions, bladder irritation; must be inserted before intercourse and left in place for 6 hours; some positions may dislodge	Not appropriate during the early postpartum period
Cervical cap with spermicide	18	Same as diaphragm	Are same as for diaphragm except may leave in place longer; may increase risk of cervical neoplasia; few healthcare providers fit caps	Not recommended during the postpartum period
IUD	3	Is not recommended during the postpartum period	Must be inserted by a healthcare provider during menses; has an increased risk of pelvic infection; may increase menstrual flow and cramps	Once in place, requires little monitoring by woman; for suitable candidate, may be inserted during first menses after childbirth
Sponge	28	May cause irritation related to decreased levels of estrogen; may increase risk of pelvic infection	Is difficult to remove; causes irritation and allergic reactions; linked to toxic shock syndrome	Is available over the counter; may be left in place longer than diaphragm; is disposable
Spermicide alone	21	May cause irritation because of decreased levels of estrogen	May cause allergic reactions; is messy; insert just before intercourse	Available over the counter; affords some protection against sexually transmitted diseases
Condoms alone	12	Have no contraindications	Irritation and allergic reactions are rare; may break or leak; may decrease sensation; must use correctly	Available over the counter; affords protection against sexually transmitted diseases
Natural family planning, fertility awareness, periodic abstinence	20	Are not recommended; require signs and symptoms of hormone fluctuation during normal cycling; this cycling does not occur during the postpartum period, especially during lactation	No risks; requires practice and education from trained professional; require self-monitoring and recordkeeping as well as varying periods of abstinence	Require no devices or chemicals; may be acceptable for couples who do not wish to use other methods because of religious or other reasons

Table continued on following page

Table 20–1
METHODS OF CONTRACEPTION (*Continued*)

Method	Failure Rate: Accidental Pregnancy Rate (Typical Use: First Year) (%)	Postpartum Use	Risks/Disadvantages	Benefits
Withdrawal	18	Has no contraindications	Requires interruption of sexual response cycle; fluid with sperm is often released before ejaculation	Requires no devices or chemicals
Norplant	0.04	No studies are available of use during first 6 weeks; lactating concerns same as those for the birth control pill	Requires insertion and removal of implants in arm by trained healthcare provider; change in bleeding pattern common; risks similar to mini pill; expensive	Contains progestin only; circulating hormone level less than that with mini pill; lasts 5 years; little monitoring required after insertion

Data from Hatcher, R., Stewart, F., Trussell, J., Kowal, D., Guest, F., & Cates, W. (1990). *Contraceptive Technology; 1990–1992* (15th ed.). New York: Irvington.

(4) Recognize that conflict in this area between the woman and her partner leads to increased risk of noncompliance and increases the stress of adjustment during the postpartum period

b. Evaluations

(1) The woman and her partner discuss contraceptive goals

(2) The woman's partner discusses his reaction to her contraceptive plans

(3) The woman's partner actively participates in decisions for contraception

(4) The woman and her partner identify areas of conflict and their potentially negative effects on contraceptive use and family adjustment

Health Education

The health education component of family planning is shown in Table 20–1.

CASE STUDIES AND STUDY QUESTIONS

Tina, age 36, was delivered of her first child 12 hours ago. She will be discharged after an overnight stay. Her delivery was uncomplicated, and she has no serious medical problems except that her social history reveals a habit of smoking two packs of cigarettes per day. She tells you that she is anxious to resume sexual relations and plans to begin taking birth control pills immediately.

1. What additional information would you need to help Tina determine whether or not her plans to use the pill are appropriate?

   a. Her breastfeeding plans.

   b. Family history of breast or uterine cancer.

   c. The type of pill she used before.

   d. Presence of lacerations or episiotomy.

2. Tina tells you that she plans to nurse her baby for at least a year and that the breastfeeding experience is very important to her. What would be her *best* option in using birth control pills?

   a. Begin taking the same pill she used before pregnancy.

   b. Change to a different brand of birth control pill.

   c. Use an alternative method until lactation is well established.

   d. Use abstinence until lactation is well established.

3. Additional teaching will be planned for Tina based on your knowledge that

   a. Her risk of developing serious side effects from birth control pills is greater because she is over the age of 35 years and she smokes.

   b. It is unknown whether she is motivated to avoid an immediate pregnancy.

   c. Her delivery experience makes a minimum 6-week period of abstinence essential to avoid postdelivery complications.

   d. She is unwilling to consider other methods of contraception.

4. Which of the following groups of contraceptive methods are the most effective?

   a. Intrauterine device (IUD), fertility awareness, or cervical cap.

   b. Abstinence, birth control pills, or foam and condoms used together.

   c. Sterilization, diaphragm, or birth control pills.

   d. Condoms, abstinence, or sterilization.

5. Which of the following risks is not associated with oral contraceptive use?

   a. Clotting disorders.

   b. Benign liver tumor.

   c. Breast cancer.

   d. Gallbladder disease.

6. Which one of the following risks is not associated with the IUD?

   a. Pelvic inflammatory disease.

   b. Increased menstrual cramping.

   c. Increased flow and duration of menses.

   d. Clotting disorders.

7. Which of the following methods of contraception has the highest rate of accidental pregnancies during the first year of use?

   a. Fertility awareness.

   b. Withdrawal.

   c. Condoms only.

   d. Sterilization.

8. Which one of the following contraceptive methods is available only with a prescription?

   a. Condoms.

   b. Spermicide.

   c. Cervical cap.

   d. Natural family planning.

Nancy, age 28 years, has just been delivered of her third child without difficulty. She plans a long breastfeeding experience. She states that after a 3 to 4 week period of sexual abstinence, she plans to use a diaphragm that she has had for several years.

9. Which of the following is correct?

   a. Contraception is not necessary as long as she breastfeeds because she cannot become pregnant while nursing.

   b. It is appropriate to use the current diaphragm unless it is torn or has obvious holes.

   c. A diaphragm is difficult to use during involution, especially while nursing, because of problems with fit and irritation.

   d. An IUD is a better choice because Nancy is in a monogamous relationship.

Jane, age 24 years, has given birth to her second daughter in 12 months. Jane is crying and tells you that her husband "cannot wait to try again for a boy" and "is glad he does not have to wait any longer for sex." She says she doesn't feel "like a real woman anymore" because she feels "too tired and sore to even think about making love," and she doesn't want another baby right away.

10. Which of the following should you not encourage Jane to do?

    a. Talk honestly with her partner about her feelings.

    b. Discuss her concerns about family planning with her partner.

    c. Continue to practice abstinence until she feels ready to resume sexual activities.

    d. Sign a consent for bilateral tubal ligation.

Answers to Study Questions

1. a	2. c	3. a
4. b	5. c	6. d
7. a	8. c	9. c
10. d		

REFERENCES

Bobak, I., Jensen, M., & Zalar, M. (1989). *Maternity and gynecologic care: The nurse and the family* (4th ed.). St. Louis: Mosby.

Dickey, R. (1987). *Managing contraceptive pill patients* (5th ed.). Durant, OK: Creative Informatics.

Fogel, C., & Woods, N. (1981). *Health care of women: A nursing perspective.* St. Louis: Mosby.

Hatcher, R., Stewart, F., Trussel, J., Kowal, D., Guest, F., Stewart, G., & Cates, W. (1990). *Contraceptive technology, 1990–1992* (15th ed.). New York: Irvington.

NAACOG (1991, Sept.). Contraceptive options. *OGN Nursing Practice Resource.*

Pritchard, A., MacDonald, P., & Gant, N. (1985). *Williams obstetrics* (17th ed.). Norwalk, CT: Appleton-Century-Crofts.

Willson, J., Carrington, E., & Ledger, W. (1987). *Obstetrics and gynecology* (8th ed.). St. Louis: Mosby.

THE NORMAL NEWBORN

Linda Howard Glenn

Adaptation to Extrauterine Life

Objectives

1. Describe cardiopulmonary changes that occur with birth

2. Identify signs indicating a need for resuscitation

3. Identify parameters used in the Apgar scoring of a newborn

4. Assess newborn's ability to adapt to extrauterine life

5. Apply the Apgar scoring scale to a particular situation

6. Apply principles of neonatal resuscitation to a particular situation

Introduction

Adaptation to extrauterine life requires profound physiological changes, the most critical of which is independent respiration.

A. Transition from fetus to neonate

1. Respiratory changes
   a. Physical stimuli: compression of the fetal chest during vaginal delivery forces lung fluid out and allows for recoil of the thorax to its original size when the fetus exits from the mother's body; this compression creates a negative pressure by which air is sucked back into the lung fields, replacing fetal lung fluid
   b. Chemical stimuli: decreases in blood oxygen concentration and cessation of placental blood flow stimulate the medulla to trigger respiratory efforts; surfactant, a phospholipid coating the alveolar epithelium, reduces the surface tension of the lung mucosa and allows exhalation without lung collapse
   c. Thermal stimuli: sudden chilling of the moist infant stimulates skin sensory receptors to transmit impulses to the respiratory center
   d. Tactile stimuli: normal handling after delivery (e.g., drying the newborn) may have an effect on respiration; however, if the infant's respirations are depressed, time should not be spent on continued attempts to stimulate the infant by slapping the heels or buttocks

2. Circulatory changes
    a. With expansion of lung fields, pulmonary capillary resistance falls and pulmonary blood flow increases; the remaining lung fluid is removed by the pulmonary capillaries and lymphatic vessels
    b. As pulmonary blood flow and systemic vascular resistance increase from lack of placental blood flow, pressure changes occur within the heart chambers
        (1) The resulting increase in pressure in the left side of the heart begins to functionally close the two remaining fetal circulatory shunts
        (2) The foramen ovale closes almost immediately
        (3) An increase of blood oxygen concentrations causes the muscular walls of the ductus arteriosus to functionally close in about 12 hours

B. **Other physiological changes**

1. Thermoregulation: the neonate's body must balance heat generation and heat loss; heat is generated by metabolism of brown fat
2. Gastrointestinal system: the newborn's digestive tract becomes functional by processing foodstuff by using digestion, absorption, and metabolism
3. Hematopoietic and renal systems
    a. The newborn must maintain and regulate
        (1) Blood volume
        (2) Fluid and electrolyte balance
        (3) Metabolite excretion
    b. The newborn must replace fetal red blood cells with normal red blood cells
4. Endocrine system: although functioning, the endocrine system is immature at term, and consequently, antidiuretic hormone (ADH) may not be produced in quantities adequate to prevent diuresis and dehydration in the neonate
5. Immune system: the newborn has several fragile defenses against infection: the integument, the reticuloendothelial system, and antibodies
    a. The skin is thin and easily disrupted, allowing for microbial entry
    b. The reticuloendothelial system has poor ability to localize infection and is easily overwhelmed by invading agents
    c. The antibody system is dependent on passive immunity gained from maternal circulation until the infant starts producing gamma globulin at about 2 months of age

Clinical Practice

A. **Assessment**

1. Physical findings
    a. Apgar scoring
        (1) Was developed by Virginia Apgar in 1952 to describe the five components related to immediate extrauterine adaptation
        (2) Components are listed in Table 21–1
        (3) Scoring is done at 1, 5, and sometimes 10 minutes of life; the newborn is given a score from 0 to 2 for each category, based on the elements described in Table 21–1
        (4) This system was initially developed to provide physicians with a standardized approach to the evaluation of newborns; studies have shown that 5-minute scores correlate with mortality in neonates and morbidity in surviving children
    b. Delivery room assessment
        (1) Identifying the infant at risk
            (a) Review maternal history
            (b) Review prenatal course
            (c) Review fetal well-being during labor and delivery

Table 21–1
COMPONENTS OF APGAR SCORING

Sign	Score		
	0	1	2
Heart rate	Absent	Below 100 beats/min	Over 100 beats/min
Respiratory effort	Absent	Weak, irregular	Good crying
Muscle tone	Flaccid	Some flexion of extremities	Well flexed
Reflex irritability (catheter in nose or slap sole of foot)	No response	Grimace	Cry
Skin color	Pale	Blue	Completely pink

From Klaus, M.H., & Fanaroff, A.A. (1986). *Care of the high-risk neonate* (3rd ed). Philadelphia: Saunders.

    (2) Indications for resuscitation
      (a) Apnea
      (b) Heart rate (HR) less than 100 beats/min
      (c) Central cyanosis
    (3) Indications for intubation
      (a) Meconium-stained amniotic fluid
      (b) Ineffectiveness of bag and mask ventilation (bmv)
      (c) Need for prolonged ventilation (e.g., for an extremely small infant)
    (4) Techniques for chest compressions
      (a) Two-finger
      (b) Two-thumb (only when chest circumference is smaller than performer's hands and compression of rib cage can be avoided)
2. Equipment required for resuscitation in delivery room
  a. Radiant warmer with light source
  b. Oxygen
  c. Suction machine and suction catheters
  d. Bulb syringe
  e. Intubation equipment
    (1) Laryngoscope size 0 and 1 blades
    (2) Endotracheal tubes of 2.5 to 4.0 mm
  f. Resuscitation bag and masks
  g. Umbilical cannulation tray with 3.5 and 5.0 French catheters
  h. Medications
    (1) Epinephrine: 1 : 10,000 concentration
    (2) Volume expanders (e.g., 5% albumin, normal saline [NS], or Ringer's lactate)
    (3) Sodium bicarbonate: 4.2% solution (0.5 mEg/ml)
    (4) Naloxone hydrochloride (Narcan): 0.4 or 1.0 mg/ml vials
  i. Gloves (sterile and examination)
  j. Adhesive tape
  k. Tincture of benzoin

B. **Nursing Diagnoses**

1. High risk for alteration in thermoregulation, hypothermia, related to moist body surface
2. High risk for ineffective airway clearance related to inability to adequately clear secretions from airways
3. High risk for ineffective breathing patterns related to shallow or periodic breathing
4. High risk for alterations in respiratory function related to apnea
5. High risk for impaired gas exchange related to poor respiratory effort and retained lung fluid

6. High risk for alterations in cardiac output; decreased, related to bradycardia
7. High risk for alterations in tissue perfusion; decreased, related to decreased cardiac output

C. Interventions/Evaluations

Interventions build upon each other because a total resuscitative effort is necessary. Figure 21–1 details sequential steps for resuscitation interventions.

1. High risk for alteration in thermoregulation, hypothermia, related to moist body surface
   a. Interventions
      (1) Place infant under preheated radiant warmer
      (2) Dry infant thoroughly and quickly
      (3) Remove and replace wet linens
   b. Evaluation: skin temperature is 36.4 to 37°C (97.6 to 98.6°F)
2. High risk for ineffective airway clearance related to inability to adequately clear secretions from airways
   a. Interventions
      (1) Position infant's head in "sniff" position or slight extension
      (2) Suction mouth, then nose
   b. Evaluations
      (1) Respiratory effort is good and infant has lusty cry
      (2) Fluid in airways has been removed to allow for normal breathing
3. High risk for ineffective breathing patterns related to shallow or periodic breathing
   a. Interventions
      (1) Position head in "sniff" position or slight extension
      (2) Suction mouth, then nose
      (3) Assess respiratory effort and HR
      (4) Provide bmv for HR less than 100 beats/min (with oxygen 80 to 100%)
   b. Evaluations
      (1) Respiratory effort is free of retractions, grunting, and nasal flaring
      (2) HR is more than 100 beats/min after 30 seconds of bmv
      (3) Skin color is normal or acrocyanotic
4. High risk for alteration in respiratory function related to apnea
   a. Interventions
      (1) Position head in "sniff" position or slight extension
      (2) Suction mouth, then nose
      (3) Provide tactile stimulation (slap foot, flick heel with finger, rub back)
      (4) Assess respiratory effort
      (5) Use bmv (with oxygen of 80 to 100%)
      (6) Assess HR
   b. Evaluations
      (1) Respiratory effort is within normal limits after 30 seconds
      (2) HR is more than 100 beats/min
      (3) Skin color is normal or acrocyanotic
5. High risk for impaired gas exchange related to poor respiratory effort and retained lung fluid
   a. Interventions
      (1) Assess HR
      (2) Administer bmv with oxygen for HR less than 100 beats/min
      (3) Assess color
      (4) If oxygen is needed for cyanosis, should be free-flow oxygen by mask if HR more than 100 beats/min
   b. Evaluations
      (1) HR improves to more than 100 beats/min
      (2) Skin color becomes normal or acrocyanotic
6. High risk for alteration in cardiac output; decreased, related to bradycardia

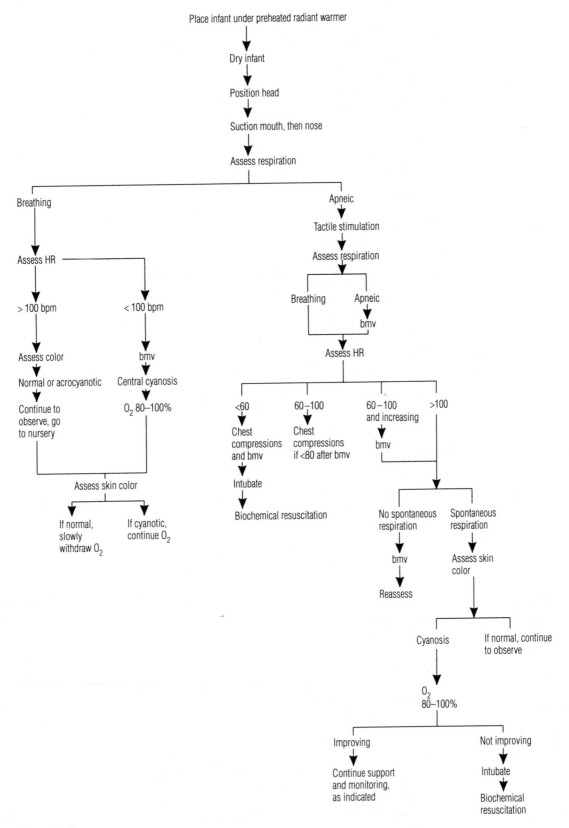

Figure 21–1
Summary of resuscitation steps

a. Interventions
(1) Assess HR
(2) Begin bmv with oxygen if HR less than 100 beats/min
(3) Begin chest compressions if HR less than 80 beats/min after 30 seconds of bmv
(4) Intubate if HR does not increase or bmv does not appear adequate
(5) Begin biochemical resuscitation if HR remains less than 80 beats/min after 30 seconds of bmv and chest compressions (drug dosages given in Table 21–2)
b. Evaluations
(1) Improvement in cardiac output will be evidenced by the following
(a) HR improving and more than 100 beats/min
(b) Skin color improving
7. High risk for alteration in tissue perfusion, decreased, related to decreased cardiac output
a. Interventions
(1) Assess HR
(2) Begin bmv with oxygen if HR is less than 100 beats/min
(3) Begin chest compressions if HR less than 80 beats/min
(4) Intubate if HR remains less than 100 beats/min
(5) Begin biochemical resuscitation if HR remains less than 80 beats/min after 30 seconds of bmv and chest compressions
b. Evaluations
(1) HR is more than 100 beats/min
(2) Skin color is within normal limits

Health Education

When resuscitative efforts occur in the delivery room, parents become concerned about the activity occurring around the infant.

A. **It is important to discuss the normal course of events of birth and care of the newborn infant with parents before delivery so that they are not alarmed by normal delivery room events**

B. **If there is a need for more in-depth resuscitation, provide parents with information as soon as possible**

CASE STUDY AND STUDY QUESTIONS

Baby Smith was born to a gravida 3, para 2 (G3,P2) woman, who was in labor for 24 hours and delivered of her son by emergency cesarean section for fetal distress. The infant was limp, had a weak cry, gasping respirations, an HR of 80 beats/min and was cyanotic at 1 minute of life. After 3 minutes of resuscitative efforts, the infant had spontaneous respirations and an HR of 120 beats/min, had regained some flexion, was crying with stimulation, and was acrocyanotic.

1. What was the initial 1-minute Apgar score for this infant?

a. 2

b. 3

c. 4

d. 5

2. In what sequence (1 to 5) should the activities occur for initial resuscitation of this infant?

_____Position infant's head.

_____Suction mouth.

_____Dry infant.

_____Place infant under preheated radiant warmer.

_____Suction nose.

3. If the infant has no respiratory movement

Table 21–2
MEDICATIONS FOR NEONATAL RESUSCITATION

Medication	Concentration to Administer	Preparation	Dosage/Route*		Total Dose/Infant		Rate/Precautions
Epinephrine	1 : 10,000	1 ml	0.1–0.3 ml/kg IV or IT	**Weight** 1 kg 2 kg 3 kg 4 kg	**Total ml** 0.1–0.3 ml 0.2–0.6 ml 0.3–0.9 ml 0.4–1.2 ml		Give rapidly
Volume expanders	Whole blood 5% albumin Normal saline Ringer's lactate	40 ml	10 ml/kg IV	**Weight** 1 kg 2 kg 3 kg 4 kg	**Total ml** 10 ml 20 ml 30 ml 40 ml		Give over 5–10 minutes
Sodium bicarbonate	0.5 mEq/ml (4.2% solution)	20 ml or two 10-ml prefilled syringes	2 mEq/kg IV	**Weight** 1 kg 2 kg 3 kg 4 kg	**Total dose** 2 mEq 4 mEq 6 mEq 8 mEq	**Total ml** 4 ml 8 ml 12 ml 16 ml	Give slowly, over at least 2 minutes Give only if infant being effectively ventilated
Naloxone	0.4 mg/ml	1 ml	0.25 ml/kg IV, IM, SQ, IT	**Weight** 1 kg 2 kg 3 kg 4 kg	**Total ml** 0.25 ml 0.50 ml 0.75 ml 1.00 ml		Give rapidly
	1.0 mg/ml	1 ml	0.1 ml/kg IV, IM, SQ, IT	**Weight** 1 kg 2 kg 3 kg 4 kg	0.1 ml 0.2 ml 0.3 ml 0.4 ml		
Dopamine	$6 \times \dfrac{\text{Weight} \times \text{Desired dose}}{\text{(kg)} \quad (\mu g/kg/min)}$ = Mg of dopamine per 100 ml of solution desired fluid (ml/hr)		Begin at 5 µg/kg/min (may increase to 20 µg/kg/min, if necessary) IV	**Weight** 1 kg 2 kg 3 kg 4 kg	**Total µg/min** 5–20 µg/minute 10–40 µg/minute 15–60 µg/minute 20–80 µg/minute		Give as a continuous infusion using an infusion pump Monitor HR and blood pressure closely Seek consultation

Reproduced with permission. © *Textbook of Neonatal Resuscitation*, 1987, 1989. Copyright American Heart Association.

* Abbreviations: IM, intramuscular; IT, intratracheal; IV, intravenous; SQ, subcutaneous.

after suctioning and tactile stimulation, what should be done next?

a. Check HR.

b. Give bmv with 60% oxygen.

c. Try tactile stimulation again.

d. Give bmv with 80 to 100% oxygen.

4. Under which of the following conditions should chest compressions begin on an infant?

(1) HR is less than 100 beats/min.

(2) HR is less than 60 beats/min.

(3) HR is between 60 and 80 beats/min and not increasing.

(4) HR is more than 80 beats/min and increasing

Which is the best combination?

a. 1, 2.

b. 1, 2, 3.

c. 2, 3, 4.

d. 2, 3.

5. What is baby Smith's 5-minute Apgar score?

a. 8

b. 7

c. 6

d. 10

6. At which of the following time intervals after birth has the Apgar score been shown to correlate with morbidity and mortality in newborns?

a. 1 minute.

b. 10 minutes.

c. 5 minutes.

d. None correlates.

Answers to Study Questions

1. b   2. 3,4,2,1,5   3. d
4. d   5. a   6. c

REFERENCES

Apgar, V. (1966). The newborn scoring system. *Pediatric Clinics of North America, 13*(3), 645–650.

Axton, S.E. (1989). *Nursing diagnosis pocket guide: Neonatal and pediatric care plans* (2nd ed.). Baltimore: Williams & Wilkins.

Bloom, R.S., & Cropley, C. (1987). Textbook of neonatal resuscitation. Dallas: American Heart Association.

Carpenito, L.J. (1991). *Handbook of nursing diagnosis* (4th ed.). Philadelphia: Lippincott.

Klaus, M.H., & Fanaroff, A.A. (1986). *Care of the high-risk neonate* (3rd ed.). Philadelphia: Saunders.

Whaley, L.E., & Wong, D.L. (1991). *Nursing care of infants and children* (4th ed.). St. Louis: Mosby.

CHAPTER 22

Linda Howard Glenn

Biological and Behavioral Characteristics

Objectives

1. Identify normal physical characteristics of the newborn

2. Compile data necessary to assess gestational age

3. List benefits of feeding with breast milk versus formula

4. Define sensory capabilities of the newborn

5. Distinguish sleep and wake cycles of the newborn

6. Identify considerations to be taken into account when examining infants of varying ethnic backgrounds

7. Relate health educational topics commonly needed for families of newborn infants

8. Determine a plan of action based on given physical parameters

9. Interpret physical and neurological findings for gestational age classification

10. Critique findings from a physical examination for departures from the norm

11. Devise a health educational plan for a particular situation

12. Relate sleep and wake cycles of the newborn to parents for purposes of parental education

Introduction

After immediate life-threatening conditions have been assessed and the infant begins to stabilize, a thorough and systematic assessment is necessary. Physical and neurobehavioral examinations, including gestational age classification, assist in determining nursing interventions and medical management.

Clinical Practice

A. Physical findings at term

1. Measurements: normal ranges

a. Weight is 2500 to 4000 g (5 lb, 8 oz to 8 lb, 13 oz)
b. Head circumference is 33 to 35.5 cm (13 to 14 in)
c. Chest circumference is 30.5 to 33 cm (12 to 13 in)
d. Length from head to heel is 48 to 53 cm (19 to 21 in)
e. Vital signs
  (1) Respirations are 30 to 60 breaths/min and may be irregular
  (2) Heart rate is 120 to 140 beats/min and regular
2. Physical examination: normal findings
  a. Posture
    (1) General flexion
    (2) Extremities flexed onto the chest and abdomen
  b. Skin
    (1) Smooth, pink to reddish (see also "n" on next page)
    (2) Possible flaking in areas of major creasing
    (3) Vernix caseosa between folds
    (4) Lanugo, especially on back, but may be absent or patchy
    (5) Acrocyanosis: cyanosis of hands and feet
    (6) Cutis marmorata: transient mottling, especially when exposed to cool temperatures
    (7) Erythema toxicum: pink, papular rash with vesicles on chest, abdomen, back, and buttocks
    (8) Physiologic jaundice (see Chapter 38 for a complete discussion of neonatal hyperbilirubinemia)
    (9) Discolorations
      (a) "Stork bite" birthmarks (telangiectatic nevi): flat, deep pink areas over eyelids or on forehead, especially at bridge of nose in infants with fair skin
      (b) Mongolian spots: bluish-black areas of pigmentation usually located on the back and buttocks in infants with dark skin
  c. Head: molding may occur because of delivery
    (1) Size, shape, and consistency of fontanels
      (a) Anterior: open, diamond shaped, 2 to 4 cm (1 to 2 in)
      (b) Posterior: small, triangular, 0.5 to 1 cm (0.25 to 0.5 in)
    (2) Bruising is common and cephalhematoma or caput succedaneum may also be present
  d. Eyes
    (1) Lids usually are edematous
    (2) Color of iris: slate gray, dark blue, or brown
    (3) Presence of red reflex
    (4) Absence of tears
    (5) Possible presence of scleral hemorrhages
    (6) May fix on objects and follow to midline
  e. Ears
    (1) Position: top of pinna is horizontal to outer canthus of eye
    (2) Pinna: is flexible and well formed with cartilage present
    (3) Loud noise: elicits startle reflex
  f. Nose
    (1) Nasal patency and discharge
    (2) Sneezing
  g. Mouth
    (1) Intact palate with midline uvula
    (2) Normal frenulum of tongue and upper lip
    (3) Minimal or absent salivation
    (4) Suck, root, and gag reflexes present
  h. Neck: short and thick
    (1) "Stork bite" birthmarks (telangiectatic nevi) that are flat, deep pink areas on back of neck

      (2) Tonic neck reflex present
      (3) Intact clavicles
      (4) Absence of webbing
  i. Chest: somewhat barrel shaped with anteroposterior and lateral diameters being equal
      (1) Slight sternal retractions
      (2) Breast enlargement and engorgement
      (3) Bilateral bronchial breath sounds
      (4) Apex or point of maximal impulse (PMI) at left third or fourth intercostal space
  j. Abdomen: cylindrical shape
      (1) Liver: 1 to 3 cm below right costal margin
      (2) Kidneys: 1 to 2 cm above and to both sides of umbilicus and felt with deep palpation
      (3) Bowel sounds present
      (4) Three vessels in cord
  k. Genitals
      (1) Female
         (a) Labia and clitoris: edematous
         (b) Hymenal tag: often present
         (c) Labia majora: larger than labia minora
         (d) Urethral meatus: located behind clitoris
         (e) Vaginal discharge: whitish or blood tinged
      (2) Male
         (a) Scrotum: large, edematous, and pendulous
         (b) Testes: palpable
         (c) Urethral opening: at tip of glans penis
         (d) Foreskin: tightly adhered (phimosis)
  l. Extremities
      (1) Symmetry of extremities
      (2) Full range of motion
      (3) All 10 fingers and toes present with an absence of webbing
      (4) Brachial and femoral pulses present and equal
      (5) Pink nail beds or acrocyanosis
      (6) Creases on anterior two-thirds of sole
      (7) Scarf sign present
      (8) Normal hip abduction without clicks
  m. Back
      (1) Spine intact without openings, masses, curves, dimples, or hairy tufts
      (2) Patent anal opening
      (3) Even gluteal folds
      (4) Trunk incurvation reflex present
  n. Factors to consider when assessing newborns of color
      (1) Skin color and determination of oxygenation: observe for pinkness of the mucous membranes, nail beds, palms of hands, and tongue
      (2) Mongolian spots: common in newborns with darker skin
      (3) Jaundice
         (a) May be determined by observing scleral color
         (b) Some ethnic groups, such as Hispanics and Asians, have a mustard or orange skin undertone
      (4) Ear level in Asians: determined by measuring from inner canthus through outer canthus to pinna
      (5) Genitals and nipples: usually darker than abdominal skin color in dark-skinned people
3. Neurological assessment
  a. Newborn reflexes

(1) Rooting: when cheek is touched or stroked, infant turns head toward stroked side and opens mouth to receive nipple

(2) Sucking: strong sucking movements of mouth can be elicited and may occur during sleep

(3) Swallow: follows sucking, usually at pauses, and can be seen at neck

(4) Palmar and plantar grasps: touching palms of hands or feet causes flexion of fingers or toes

(5) Moro reflex (startle): general body response to sudden stimulus that is a combination of full extension then abduction of limbs

(6) Babinski reflex: upward stroking of sole and across ball of foot causes great toes to hyperextend and foot to dorsiflex

b. Other neurological characteristics

(1) Posture: general flexed position similar to that maintained in utero

(2) Tone: extremities have brisk recoil to flexion; infant able to hold head erect momentarily while sitting

(3) Tremors or jitteriness: momentary quivering or tremors may occur as a result of immature nervous system; however, twitches, unstimulated tremors, and myoclonic jerking are not normal

4. Behavioral characteristics

a. Crying

(1) Strong and lusty

(2) Crying sounds vary in the same infant, based on level of discomfort

b. Sucking

(1) Sucking behavior is usually noted within the first hour of life

(2) May have sucking motions during sleep

(3) May suck on fingers, fist, or thumb between feedings

c. Sleep and activity patterns: neonates cannot be stereotyped by number of waking and sleeping hours per day

(1) Although all infants display the six major behavioral states outlined by Brazelton (1973), individual infants have cycles of sleep and activity that are unique

(2) Identifying infant's behavioral state is helpful in determining the infant's ability to perceive stimuli and interact with others; behavioral states follow

(a) Deep sleep: quiet sleep without movement except for sudden jerky movements; hard to awaken from this state

(b) Light sleep: eyes closed with some eye movement seen under lids, active body movements; sucking may be present

(c) Drowsy: eyes open or closed, lids usually heavy; active body movements with occasional fussing

(d) Quiet alert: alert with eyes open and attentive to close objects; little body movement

(e) Active alert: eyes open with a lot of active body movement, especially in response to stimuli

(f) Crying: eyes tightly closed at times with crying, thrashing, and movements of head and extremities

d. Sensory capabilities

(1) Hearing

(a) Ability to hear begins in utero during the last trimester and is well developed at birth

(b) Newborn will turn head toward familiar voices or noise

(2) Vision

(a) Newborn can focus on close-up objects about 7 to 12 in (17.8 to 30.5 cm) away (e.g., the mother's face when at breast)

(b) Because the retinal cones are not fully developed at birth, it is generally accepted that infants focus on dark and light contrasts rather than on colors

(3) Taste: can distinguish between sweet and sour at 3 days of age
(4) Smell or olfaction: can distinguish between mother's breasts and breast milk and those of another by fifth day of age
(5) Touch: sensitive to pain, usually responds to tactile stimuli

5. Gestational age assessment (see Chapter 36 for a complete discussion of gestational age significance/risks)
   a. Determination of gestational age is sometimes difficult because of inaccuracies in menstrual history and obstetrical phenomena
   b. Reliable assessment of gestational age is based on neurological development and physical characteristics found by direct examination of infant
   c. Classification of infant allows clinician to anticipate clinical problems and apply early diagnostic testing
      (1) Classifications: infant's weight and weeks of gestation are classified as follows
         (a) Appropriate for gestational age (AGA): characterizes about 80% of the neonatal population
         (b) Small for gestational age (SGA) (<2500 g [5 lb, 8 oz] for term neonate)
            (i) Less growth has occurred in utero than expected
            (ii) Associated risks include hypoglycemia, asphyxia, respiratory distress syndrome, meconium aspiration, intrauterine infection, and hyperbilirubinemia
         (c) Large for gestational age (LGA) (>4000 g [8 lb, 13 oz] for term neonate)
            (i) Growth is accelerated for length of gestation
            (ii) Associated risks include birth trauma, hypoglycemia, hypocalcemia, hyperbilirubinemia, meconium aspiration, and polycythemia
      (2) Assessing for gestational age (see Chapter 11 for a complete discussion of antepartum fetal assessment)
         (a) Calculating dates
            (i) Count the number of weeks from the first day of the last menstrual period
            (ii) Is subject to the woman's ability to correctly recall the date and regularity of her menses
         (b) Maternal examination
            (i) Height of uterine fundus has been found to correspond with length of gestation
            (ii) Is limited to normal pregnancies in which polyhydramnios or multiple gestation, for example, does not occur
         (c) Fetal examination: ultrasound evaluation of length and head size
         (d) Postnatal examination: most reliable measure
            (i) External physical characteristics of fetus progress in an orderly fashion during gestation, which makes determination of age possible
            (ii) Guides are frequently used in the nursery to determine neuromuscular and physical maturity (Tables 22–1, 22–2, and Fig. 22–1 are commonly used)
            (iii) Neurological characteristics (Fig. 22–2)
               • Although neurological characteristics also progress during pregnancy, these signs can be affected by illness, neurological damage, or other conditions leading to depression in the infant (including effects of labor and delivery)
               • Neurological examination is best performed when infant is 24 hours old

Table 22–1
SCORING SYSTEM OF EXTERNAL PHYSICAL CHARACTERISTICS*

External Sign	Score†				
	0	1	2	3	4
Edema	Obvious edema of hands and feet; pitting over tibia	No obvious edema of hands and feet; pitting over tibia	No edema		
Skin texture	Very thin, gelatinous	Thin and smooth	Smooth; medium thickness; rash or superficial peeling	Slight thickening; superficial cracking and peeling, especially of hands and feet	Thick and parchmentlike; superficial or deep cracking
Skin color	Dark red	Uniformly pink	Pale pink; variable over body	Pale; only pink over ears, lips, palms, or soles	
Skin opacity (trunk)	Numerous veins and venules clearly seen, especially over abdomen	Veins and tributaries seen	A few large vessels clearly seen over abdomen	A few large vessels seen indistinctly over abdomen	No blood vessels seen
Lanugo (over back)	No lanugo	Abundant; long and thick over whole back	Hair thinning, especially over lower back	Small amount of lanugo and bald areas	At least half of back devoid of lanugo
Plantar creases	No skin creases	Faint red marks over anterior half of sole	Definite red marks over >anterior half; indentations over < anterior third	Indentations over >anterior third	Definite deep indentations over >anterior third
Nipple formation	Nipple barely visible; no areola	Nipple well defined; areola smooth and flat, diameter <0.75 cm	Areola stippled, edge not raised, diameter < 0.75 cm	Areola stippled, edge raised, diameter >0.75 cm	
Breast size	No breast tissue palpable	Breast tissue on one or both sides, <0.5 cm	Breast tissue on both sides, one or both 0.5 to 1.0 cm	Breast tissue on both sides, one or both >1 cm	
Ear form	Pinna flat and shapeless; little or no incurving of edge	Incurving of part of edge of pinna	Partial incurving of whole of upper pinna	Well-defined incurving of whole of upper pinna	
Ear firmness	Pinna soft, easily folded, no recoil	Pinna soft, easily folded, slow recoil	Cartilage to edge of pinna but soft in places, ready recoil	Pinna firm, cartilage to edge, instant recoil	
Genitals: male	Neither testis in scrotum	At least one testis high in scrotum	At least one testis right down		
Genitals: female (with hips half abducted)	Labia majora widely separated, labia minora protruding	Labia majora almost cover labia minora	Labia majora completely cover labia minora		

* To be used in conjunction with Figure 22–2.
† If score differs on two sides, take the mean.
Adapted by Dubowitz, V., & Goldberg, C. (1970). Clinical assessment of gestational age in the newborn infant. *Journal of Pediatrics, 77,* 1–10.

Table 22–2
TECHNIQUES OF NEUROLOGICAL ASSESSMENT*

Posture
With the infant supine and quiet, score as follows
Arms and legs extended	=0
Slight or moderate flexion of hips and knees	=1
Moderate to strong flexion of hips and knees	=2
Legs flexed and abducted, arms slightly flexed	=3
Full flexion of arms and legs	=4

Square Window
Flex the hand at the wrist. Exert pressure sufficient to get as much flexion as possible. The angle between the hypothenar eminence and the anterior aspect of the forearm is measured and scored. Do not rotate the wrist.

Ankle Dorsiflexion
Flex the foot at the ankle with sufficient pressure to get maximum change. The angle between the dorsum of the foot and the anterior aspect of the leg is measured and scored.

Arm Recoil
With the infant supine, fully flex the forearm for 5 seconds, then fully extend by pulling the hands and release. Score the reaction as follows:
Remain extended or random movements	=0
Incomplete or partial flexion	=1
Brisk return to full flexion	=2

Leg Recoil
With the infant supine, the hips and knees are fully flexed for 5 seconds, then extended by traction on the feet and released. Score the reaction as follows:
No response or slight flexion	=0
Partial flexion	=1
Full flexion (less than 90° at knees and hips)	=2

Popliteal angle
With the infant supine and the pelvis flat on the examining surface, the leg is flexed on the thigh and the thigh fully flexed with the use of one hand. With the other hand the leg is then extended and the angle attained scored.

Heel-to-Ear Maneuver
With the infant supine, hold the infant's foot with one hand and move it as near to the head as possible without forcing it. Keep the pelvis flat on the examining surface. Score.

Scarf Sign
With the infant supine, take the infant's hand and draw it across the neck and as far across the opposite shoulder as possible. Assistance to the elbow is permissible by lifting it across the body. Score according to the location of the elbow:
Elbow reaches the opposite anterior axillary line	=0
Elbow between opposite anterior axillary line and midline of thorax	=1
Elbow at midline of thorax	=2
Elbow does not reach midline of thorax	=3

Head Lag
With the infant supine, grasp each forearm just proximal to the wrist and pull gently to bring the infant to a sitting position. Score according to the relationship of the head to the trunk during the maneuver:
No evidence of head support	=0
Some evidence of head support	=1
Maintains head in the same anteroposterior plane as the body	=2
Tends to hold the head forward	=3

Ventral Suspension
With the infant prone and the chest resting on the examiner's palm, lift the infant off the examining surface and score.

---

* To be used in conjunction with Figure 22–2.
† If score differs on two sides, take the mean.
Adapted by Dubowitz, V., & Goldberg, C. (1970). Clinical assessment of gestational age in the newborn infant. *Journal of Pediatrics, 77,* 1–10.

D. Nursing Diagnosis

1. Parental knowledge deficit related to lack of experience with newborn care and behavior

E. Interventions/Evaluations

1. Parental knowledge deficit related to lack of experience with newborn care and behavior
   a. Interventions
      (1) Assess prior knowledge and experience with newborn care and behavior
      (2) Instruct about and demonstrate general newborn care based on assessment of prior knowledge and experience and behavior to expect, including sleep and wake cycles

Neuromuscular Maturity

	0	1	2	3	4	5
Posture						
Square Window (wrist)	90°	60°	45°	30°	0°	
Arm Recoil	180°		100°-180°	90°-100°	<90°	
Popliteal Angle	180°	160°	130°	110°	90°	<90°
Scarf Sign						
Heel to Ear						

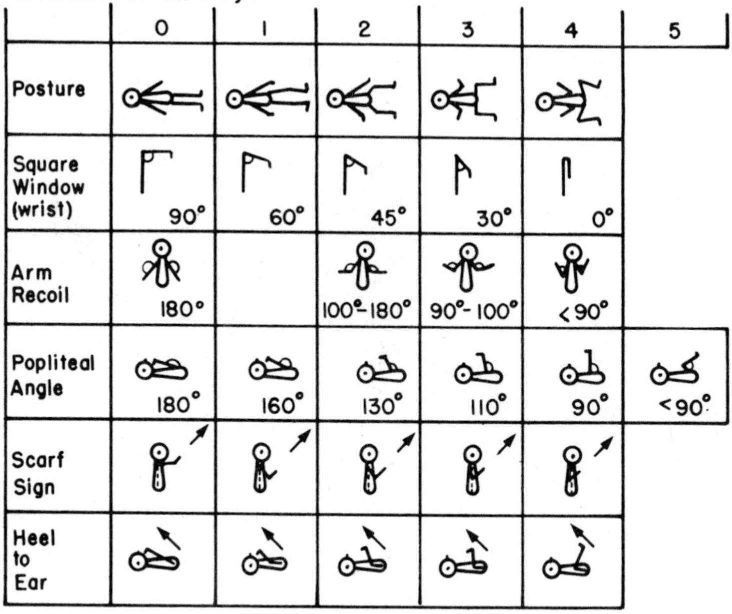

Apgars _____ 1 min _____ 5 min

Age at Exam _____ hrs

Race _____ Sex _____

B.D. _____

LMP _____

EDC _____

Gest. age by Dates _____ wks

Gest. age by Exam _____ wks

B.W. _____ gm. _____ %ile

Length _____ cm. _____ %ile

Head Circum. _____ cm. _____ %ile

Clin. Dist. None _____ Mild _____

Mod. _____ Severe _____

PHYSICAL MATURITY

Skin	gelatinous red, transparent	smooth pink, visible veins	superficial peeling &/or rash few veins	cracking pale area rare veins	parchment deep cracking no vessels	leathery cracked wrinkled
Lanugo	none	abundant	thinning	bald areas	mostly bald	
Plantar Creases	no crease	faint red marks	anterior transverse crease only	creases ant. 2/3	creases cover entire sole	
Breast	barely percept.	flat areola no bud	stippled areola 1–2 mm bud	raised areola 3–4 mm bud	full areola 5–10 mm bud	
Ear	pinna flat, stays folded	sl. curved pinna; soft with slow recoil	well-curv. pinna; soft but ready recoil	formed & firm with instant recoil	thick cartilage ear stiff	
Genitals ♂	scrotum empty no rugae		testes descending, few rugae	testes down good rugae	testes pendulous deep rugae	
Genitals ♀	prominent clitoris & labia minora		majora & minora equally prominent	majora large minora small	clitoris & minora completely covered	

MATURITY RATING

Score	Wks
5	26
10	28
15	30
20	32
25	34
30	36
35	38
40	40
45	42
50	44

Figure 22–1

Neuromuscular maturity and physical maturity. (Adapted by Dubowitz, V., & Goldberg, C. (1970). Clinical assessment of gestational age in the newborn infant. *Journal of Pediatrics*, 77(1), 1–10.)

NEUROLOGICAL SIGN	SCORE					
	0	1	2	3	4	5
POSTURE						
SQUARE WINDOW	90°	60°	45°	30°	0°	
ANKLE DORSIFLEXION	90°	75°	45°	20°	0°	
ARM RECOIL	180°	90–180°	<90°			
LEG RECOIL	180°	90–180°	<90°			
POPLITEAL ANGLE	180	160°	130°	110°	90°	<90°
HEEL TO EAR						
SCARF SIGN						
HEAD LAG						
VENTRAL SUSPENSION						

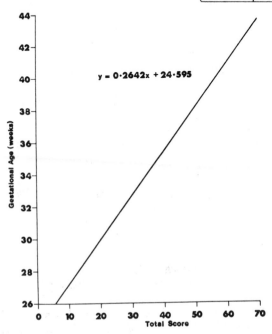

$$y = 0.2642x + 24.595$$

Gestational Age (weeks) — Total Score

Figure 22–2
Scoring of neurological findings in the infant and graph for ascertaining gestational age from the total score of physical and neurological development. (Modified from Klaus, M.H., & Fanaroff, A.A. (1986). *Care of the high-risk neonate* (3rd ed.). Philadelphia: Saunders, p. 81.)

(3) Review and demonstrate newborn's sensory capabilities
  b. Evaluations
      (1) Parent correctly demonstrates newborn care activities
      (2) Parent correctly states information about newborn behavior and sleep and wake cycles

Health Education

New parents have many questions about the appearance and behavior of their newborn infant. The nurse can use this curiosity to begin initial health teaching about skin discolorations, reflexive movements, and neurological characteristics during the physical examination, when performed in the presence of parents. Specific teaching points to include follow.

A. General newborn appearance

1. Weight and measurements
2. Physical appearance: norms and slight departures that may apply

B. Newborn behaviors

1. Reflexes and how they influence movements
2. Behavioral characteristics
3. Sleep and wake cycles to expect and opportunities for interaction
4. Sensory capabilities

CASE STUDY AND STUDY QUESTIONS

Baby Juarez was born to a 29-year-old, gravida 1, para 1 (G1, P1) Hispanic. She was born vaginally after a difficult delivery with shoulder dystocia. At admission, her weight was 4400 g (9 lbs, 11½ oz). Physical and neurological examination places her at 40 weeks gestation. Her physical examination reveals an unequal Moro reflex with decreased movement in the left arm and crepitus at the left neck area. Bluish marking was also noted across the lower back.

1. What is the correct diagnosis for this infant?

   a. LGA with a risk for hypoglycemia.

   b. AGA with a risk for hypothermia.

   c. SGA with a risk for hypoglycemia.

   d. Infant of diabetic mother (IDM) with a risk for respiratory distress.

2. Which of the following do the physical findings of an unequal Moro reflex, crepitus at the neck, and delivery history suggest?

   a. Torticollis.

   b. Cystic hygroma.

   c. Fractured clavicle.

   d. Erb's palsy.

3. What does the bluish marking across the lower back indicate?

   a. Purpura.

   b. Bruising from delivery.

   c. Blue nevi.

   d. Mongolian spots.

4. What is the significance of the bluish marking?

   a. Is a sign of disseminated intravascular coagulation (DIC) and hepatosplenomegaly.

   b. Indicates that hyperbilirubinemia may follow.

   c. Is a circumscribed vascular tumor of the skin.

   d. Is a typical marking in dark-skinned people that presents no health problem.

5. In view of the infant's size and gestational age, about which of the following would

you be most concerned for this infant in the transition nursery?

a. Hypothermia.

b. Hypoglycemia.

c. Respiratory distress.

d. Feeding difficulties.

Answers to Study Questions

1. a	2. c	3. d
4. d	5. b	

REFERENCES

Apgar, V. (1966). The newborn scoring system. *Pediatric Clinics of North America, 13*(3), 645–650.

Axton, S.E. (1989). *Nursing diagnosis pocket guide: Neonatal and pediatric care plans* (2nd ed.). Baltimore: Williams & Wilkins.

Battaglia, F., & Lubchenco, L. (1967). A practical classification of newborn infants by weight and gestational age. *Journal of Pediatrics, 71*(2), 159–163.

Benakappa, D.G., Raju, M., Shivananda, S., & Benakappa, A.D. (1989). Breast-feeding practices in rural Karnataka, India, with special reference to lactation failure. *Acta Paediatrica Japanese Overseas Education 31*(4), 391–398.

Blackburn, S. (1983). Fostering behavioral development of high-risk infants. *Journal of Obstetric, Gynecologic, and Neonatal Nursing, 12*(3), (Suppl.) 76–86.

Bloom, R.S., & Cropley, C. (1987). *Textbook of neonatal resuscitation.* Dallas: American Heart Association.

Brazelton, T.B. (1973). *Neonatal behavioral assessment scale.* London: Spastics International Medical.

Carpenito, L.J. (1991). *Handbook of nursing diagnosis* (4th ed.). Philadelphia: Lippincott.

Colangelo, C., Bergen, A., & Gottleib, L. (1976). *A normal baby: The sensory-motor process of the first year.* New York: Blythdale Children's Hospital.

Dubowitz, L., Dubowitz, V., & Goldberg, C. (1970). Clinical assessment of gestational age in the newborn infant. *Journal of Pediatrics, 77*(1), 1–10.

Hopkins, B., & Westra, T. (1989). Maternal expectations of their infant's development: Some cultural differences. *Developmental Medicine and Child Neurology, 31*(3), 384–390.

Johnson, S.H. (1979). *High-risk parenting: Nursing assessment and strategies for the family at risk.* Philadelphia: Lippincott.

Klaus, M.H., & Fanaroff, A.A. (1986). *Care of the high-risk neonate* (3rd ed.). Philadelphia: Saunders.

Klaus, M.H., & Kennell, J.H. (1982). *Parent-infant bonding* (2nd ed.). St. Louis: Mosby.

Romero-Gwynn, E. (1989). Breast-feeding pattern among Indochinese immigrants in northern California. *American Journal of Diseases in Childhood, 143*(7), 804–808.

Romero-Gwynn, E., & Carias, L. (1989). Breast-feeding intentions and practice among Hispanic mothers in southern California. *Pediatrics, 84*(4), 626–632.

Sardana, R. (1985). Examining for defects. *Nursing Mirror, 160*(2), 38–41.

Whaley, L.E., & Wong, D.L. (1991). *Nursing care of infants and children* (4th ed.). St. Louis: Mosby.

Other

NAACOG (1991, Aug.). Physical assessment of the neonate. *OGN Nursing Practice Resource.*

NAACOG (1991, April). Prevention, recognition, and management of neonatal pain. *OGN Nursing Practice Resource.*

Linda Howard Glenn

Immediate Nursing Care

Objectives

1. Recognize factors that contribute to hypothermia

2. Define nutritional needs of the normal newborn

3. Identify cultural factors that may influence infant feeding practices of major ethnic groups in the United States

4. Identify interventions for infant thermoregulation control

5. Relate health educational topics commonly needed for families of newborn infants

6. Devise a health educational plan for a particular situation

7. Assess readiness and ability of the newborn to feed orally

Introduction

A. Although observation of the infant's adaptation to extrauterine life and physical assessment begins in the delivery room, general observations and assessment of the infant are ongoing throughout the hospital stay

B. Admission to the nursery

1. Complete head-to-toe assessment
2. Eye care
3. Umbilical cord care
4. Vitamin K administration
5. Blood glucose determination (e.g., using Dextrostix or Chemstrip: 40 to 60 mg/dl)

C. Thermoregulation

1. This is the means by which a balance is maintained between the amount of body heat lost and the amount of body heat produced
2. A significant decrease in temperature ($<35.8°C$ [$<96.6°F$]) increases oxygen consumption
3. Temperature regulation is poor in the newborn because of the ratio of his or her large body surface to body mass and inability to generate heat from muscular movement

a. Heat production and conservation
  (1) Flexed fetal position decreases body surface, which minimizes heat loss
  (2) Peripheral vasoconstriction
  (3) Nonshivering heat production by brown fat metabolism is stimulated by norepinephrine, resulting in lipolysis and fatty acid oxidation, which releases heat to the perfusing blood
b. Means of heat loss
  (1) Convection: heat is lost to air or fluid around the infant that is cooler than infant's temperature (e.g., air as drafts on infant from an open door in the delivery room)
  (2) Radiation: heat lost to solid objects near infant that are cooler than infant's temperature (e.g., windows to the outside not covered by draperies)
  (3) Conduction: heat lost to cold surfaces or to objects with which infant comes in contact (e.g., x-ray plate or unheated mattress)
  (4) Evaporation: heat lost when water evaporates from the infant's skin surface or respiratory tract (e.g., infant not dried immediately after birth)
c. Providing and maintaining a neutral thermal environment (NTE)
  (1) Definition: an environment in which heat production and oxygen consumption are minimized
  (2) Devices used
    (a) Incubators: usually single-walled plastic boxes that warm the infant by convection
    (b) Radiant warmers
      (i) An unenclosed bed with radiant heat panels placed above the infant
      (ii) Although delivery of nursing care is more convenient, convective and evaporative heat losses and insensible water losses are increased
    (c) Nursing care
      (i) Keep infant dry by drying body parts as bathed
      (ii) Dress infant and wrap tightly in blankets
      (iii) Cover infant's head with cap or hat
      (iv) Assess infant's temperature every hour until stable

D. Nutritional needs

1. Infants born beyond 32 to 34 weeks' gestation have adequate suck-and-swallow coordination for oral feedings unless neurological damage has occurred or the infant is too ill to safely handle feedings
2. The goal of feedings is to provide energy for metabolic requirements and growth
3. Feeding and calorie requirements: 100 to 120 kcal (150 to 180 ml or 5 to 6 oz) /kg/day for a normal term infant
4. Types of nutrition and feeding methods
  a. Breastfeeding: considered the most perfect form of nutrition for the normal newborn (see Chapter 19 for a complete discussion of breastfeeding)
    (1) Provides 20 kcal/oz (30 ml)
    (2) Advantages of breast milk
      (a) Is more easily digested because of greater abundance of lactalbumin, higher percentage of amino acids, and softer curd formation than formula
      (b) Has a higher content of lactose, cystine, and monosaturated fatty acids than does formula
      (c) Has a higher calcium-to-phosphorus ratio than does formula
      (d) Is economical, always available, and ready for consumption
      (e) Contains antibodies
      (f) Decreases occurrence of allergic reactions, colic, and spitting up

(g) Breastfeeding provides opportunity for close maternal-infant relationship

(3) Disadvantages

(a) Empties more rapidly from infant's stomach, which necessitates more frequent feedings

(b) Has a lower mineral content than does formula

(c) May be inconvenient or limit activities outside the home for the mother

b. Bottlefeeding: commercially prepared formulas are based on cow's milk and have been modified to closely resemble human milk

(1) Provides 20 kcal/oz (30 ml)

(2) Advantages of formula

(a) Although controversial, may "stay with the infant longer" because it is harder to digest and, therefore, requires feeding the infant less frequently

(b) Allows "freedom" from infant, because other caretakers can feed infant

(3) Disadvantages of formula

(a) Is more costly, especially if purchased in ready-to-serve concentration

(b) Must be prepared, if not purchased in ready-to-serve concentration

(c) Is more difficult to digest and forms harder curds because of higher casein content

(d) Has increased risk for infection of infant if not properly prepared

c. General considerations about feeding the newborn

(1) When bottlefeeding, alternate holding from one arm to the other (one side to the other) to enhance infant stimulation

(2) Allow infant about 20 minutes of sucking per feeding

(3) Position infant on abdomen or right side after feedings to prevent regurgitation and possible aspiration

(4) Do not prop up bottles because this denies vital human contact and also can lead to aspiration and middle ear infections

(5) Discard all unused formula in bottles after the feeding

(6) Feeding schedules vary based on parental preference but are usually every 2 to 4 hours

(7) If bottlefeeding, commercial formula use is recommended for the first 9 to 12 months at its regular strength of 20 kcal/oz (30 ml)

d. Cultural and economic factors: role in feeding practices

(1) Although it is the practice of many cultural groups to breastfeed infants in their country of origin, changes in this practice have occurred as individuals from various cultural groups immigrate to the United States; reasons for this may be

(a) Availability and lower cost of formulas

(b) Free samples given to mothers at discharge from hospital

(c) Presence of formula bottles in crib when infant is brought to mother's room

(d) Prevalence of bottlefeeding in the media with little public display of breastfeeding

(2) Hispanic mothers

(a) Are likely to initiate breastfeeding and sustain feedings for longer periods than white mothers; this behavior tends to occur in Hispanic families who have close family ties in Mexico and who visit Mexico frequently

(b) Believe colostrum is bad for the baby, so will use formula until the milk comes in

(c) Continue to supplement breastfeeding with formula and begin offering infant solid food early

(3) Asian mothers
  (a) Most Asian women breastfeed their infants
  (b) Because of the belief that the body loses heat during delivery, they need time to recover the heat
  (c) With traditional Asian families, another relative cares for the baby during this time, except during feeding
  (d) Many Asian immigrants do not have extended family members present to take care of the infant during the first few days after birth
  (e) Lack of family members means that the mother is not traditionally relieved of normal household responsibilities so that breastfeeding can be established
(4) Economic factors may also play a part in the choice related to formula feeding among cultures that would breastfeed in the country of origin
  (a) There may be a change in socioeconomic status of women immigrating to the United States who frequently must work to support the family
  (b) Women have the opportunity of going to school and raising their economic status
  (c) Extended family members who have also immigrated to the United States may be available to help raise the child and provide child care while the mother works
(5) Regardless of the cultural origin, any family's behaviors may be influenced by the community norms and health care workers' actions
(6) Various ethnic groups may not have adequate knowledge about the economic or health benefits of breastfeeding

Clinical Practice

A. Assessment

1. History
   a. Ethnic background
   b. Length of labor
   c. Exposure to medications during labor
   d. Events surrounding delivery
   e. Maternal estimated date of confinement (EDC)
2. Physical findings
   a. Temperature assessment in the newborn
      (1) Axillary: easy to do, but may take up to 8 minutes to stabilize
      (2) Rectal: ascertains core temperature, but core temperature does not drop until infant fails to produce heat
      (3) Skin: thermistor probe is sensitive to early cold stress, but is not available in every hospital
   b. Assessment for beginning infant feedings
      (1) Respiratory stability: respiratory rate of 30 to 60 breaths/min, absence of retractions or distress
      (2) Appearance of abdomen: rounded, absence of discoloration or visible loops of bowel
      (3) Absence of emesis or inability to swallow
      (4) Presence of bowel sounds
      (5) Passage of stool: meconium should be passed within the first 24 hours
      (6) Muscle tone and activity within normal limits
      (7) Regulated temperature
      (8) Regulation of blood glucose: inability to maintain may necessitate more frequent feedings

B. Nursing Diagnoses

1. High risk for infection related to infant's poor physiological response to pathogens
2. High risk for hypothermia related to infant's poor ability to regulate own temperature
3. High risk for hyperthermia related to infant's poor ability to regulate own temperature
4. High risk for alteration in nutrition: less than body requirements, related to infant's poor suck-and-swallow coordination
5. Knowledge deficit in parents related to inexperience with newborn care and lack of parenting skills

C. Interventions/Evaluations

1. High risk for infection related to infant's poor physiological response to pathogens
   a. Interventions
      (1) Consider doing initial temperature assessment via axillary mode until infant has been bathed to reduce risk of exposure to human immunodeficiency virus (HIV) via rectal mucosa
      (2) Be certain traces of maternal blood have been removed from infant's skin surface before injections or invasion procedures
      (3) Clean injection sites with alcohol before injections
      (4) Clean and observe any scalp monitoring sites for abscesses, redness, or drainage
      (5) Use alcohol for umbilical stump care
      (6) Instill substance for eye prophylaxis as per protocol (1% silver nitrate, erythromycin, and tetracycline are most common)
      (7) Check circumcision site with every diaper change and remove petroleum jelly–covered gauze after 4 hours
   b. Evaluations
      (1) Infant has minimal exposure to pathogens
      (2) Temperature of infant remains within normal limits
      (3) Signs of infection are absent at any areas where skin integrity has been disturbed
      (4) Eyes remain free of any purulent drainage
      (5) Circumcision site remains free of swelling, redness, or drainage
2. High risk for hypothermia related to infant's poor ability to regulate own temperature
   a. Interventions
      (1) Prewarm incubators and radiant warmers, use temperature chart as guide (Table 23–1)
      (2) Dry infant immediately after delivery
      (3) Use and change warm blankets under and around infant frequently
      (4) Close door to delivery or surgical suite or nursery and place radiant warmer away from traffic patterns and air drafts
      (5) Maintain delivery room and nursery at temperature between 24° and 26.5°C (75° and 80°F)
      (6) Place hat on infant's head, to decrease heat loss (covers 12% of the body surface)
      (7) To warm infant set incubator temperature at 1.5°C (2.6°F) higher than infant's temperature until infant's temperature begins to stabilize
      (8) Check infant's temperature every 30 to 60 minutes until stable, then every 4 to 8 hours
   b. Evaluations
      (1) Infant regains normal temperature within range of 36.4° to 37°C (97.6° to 98.6°F)
      (2) Temperature stabilizes within 4 hours

3. High risk for hyperthermia related to infant's poor ability to regulate own temperature
   a. Interventions
      (1) Use warming devices, such as heat lamps, sparingly and for only 15-minute intervals
      (2) Use temperature charts to preset environmental temperature of incubators (see Table 23–1)
   b. Evaluation: Infant's temperature stabilizes within normal range
4. High risk for alteration in nutrition (less than body requirements) related to infant's poor suck-and-swallow coordination
   a. Interventions
      (1) Assess for ability to feed
      (2) Give first feeding using sterile water or assist with first breastfeeding
      (3) Select appropriate formula, if infant to be bottlefed
      (4) Begin feedings at breast or with bottle
   b. Evaluations
      (1) Infant is able to initiate and sustain suck-and-swallow coordination
      (2) Color and respiratory effort remain normal during feeding
      (3) Infant consumes 15 to 30 ml (1/2 to 1 oz) formula or nurses at breast 10 minutes/feeding

Table 23–1
NEUTRAL THERMAL ENVIRONMENTAL TEMPERATURES*

Age and Weight	Range of Temperature (°C)	Age and Weight	Range of Temperature (°C)
0–6 hours		72–96 hours	
Under 1200 g	34.0–35.4	Under 1200 g	34.0–35.0
1200–1500 g	33.9–34.4	1200–1500 g	33.0–34.0
1501–2500 g	32.8–33.8	1501–2500 g	31.1–33.2
Over 2500 (and >36 weeks)	32.0–33.8	Over 2500 (and >36 weeks)	29.8–32.8
6–12 hours		4–12 days	
Under 1200 g	34.0–35.4	Under 1500 g	33.0–34.0
1200–1500 g	33.5–34.4	1501–2500 g	31.0–33.2
1501–2500 g	32.2–33.8	Over 2500 (and >36 weeks)	
Over 2500 (and >36 weeks)	31.4–33.8	4–5 days	29.5–32.6
12–24 hours		5–6 days	29.4–32.3
Under 1200 g	34.0–35.4	6–8 days	29.0–32.2
1200–1500 g	33.3–34.3	8–10 days	29.0–31.8
1501–2500 g	31.8–33.8	10–12 days	29.0–31.4
Over 2500 (and >36 weeks)	31.0–33.7	12–14 days	
24–36 hours		Under 1500 g	32.6–34.0
Under 1200 g	34.0–35.0	1501–2500 g	31.0–33.2
1200–1500 g	33.1–34.2	Over 2500 (and >36 weeks)	29.0–30.8
1501–2500 g	31.6–33.6	2–3 weeks	
Over 2500 (and >36 weeks)	30.7–33.5	Under 1500 g	32.2–34.0
36–48 hours		1501–2500 g	30.5–33.0
Under 1200 g	34.0–35.0	3–4 weeks	
1200–1500 g	33.0–34.1	Under 1500 g	31.6–33.6
1501–2500 g	31.4–33.5	1501–2500 g	30.0–32.7
Over 2500 (and >36 weeks)	30.5–33.3	4–5 weeks	
48–72 hours		Under 1500 g	31.2–33.0
Under 1200 g	34.0–35.0	1501–2500 g	29.5–32.2
1501–2500 g	33.0–34.0	5–6 weeks	
1501–2500 g	31.2–33.4	Under 1500 g	30.6–32.3
Over 2500 (and >36 weeks)	30.1–33.2	1501–2500 g	29.0–31.8

* Adapted from Scopes and Ahmed. For his table, Scopes had the walls of the incubator 1° to 2° warmer than the ambient air temperatures.
   Generally speaking, the smaller infants in each weight group require a temperature in the higher portion of the temperature range. Within each time range, the younger the infant, the higher the temperature required.

(4) Infant has approximately eight wet diapers every 24 hours

(5) Infant has stools every day with color and consistency expected for age and type of feedings

5. Knowledge deficit in parents related to inexperience with newborn care and lack of parenting skills

   a. Interventions

      (1) Assess for prior parenting and infant care experiences

      (2) Instruct in and assess ability to establish breastfeeding or bottlefeeding pattern

      (3) Instruct in newborn nutrition

      (4) Instruct in use of bulb syringe and thermometer

      (5) Instruct in infant safety techniques

      (6) Provide information on community resources

      (7) Review follow-up plan for pediatric and well-baby care

   b. Evaluations

      (1) Parent-infant dyad is able to establish oral feedings to desired amount and frequency of intake

      (2) Parent verbalizes important factors to remember about nutrition

      (3) Parent demonstrates and verbalizes safety measures pertinent to the newborn's care

      (4) Parent demonstrates use of bulb syringe and thermometer

      (5) Parent verbalizes knowledge of resources as appropriate to needs

Health Education

Health education centers on the preparation of parents for care of their newborn infant. Educational topics include general newborn care, newborn nutrition, safety, and community resources to aid the family.

A. General newborn care

1. How to bathe while conserving heat and providing for safety
2. How to take a temperature reading
3. How to use bulb syringe
4. How to diaper
5. How to care for circumcision site: ordinary cleaning of the diaper area and inspection for bleeding, swelling, or decreased urine output; petroleum jelly gauze applied during the procedure can be removed after a few hours
6. How to clean genitalia
   a. Girls: separate labia and clean from front to back
   b. Boys: retract foreskin, clean, and replace; most boys have a tight foreskin at birth that loosens with time
7. How to care for cord: wipe the umbilical stump with rubbing alcohol on cotton gauze, allow to dry, then diaper with diaper folded down below stump to allow it to stay dry
8. How to detect signs of illness and when to contact the physician

B. Newborn safety and protection

1. Selection and use of car seat and safety straps
2. Prevention of choking, using prone or right-side-lying position
3. Safety measures when using changing tables and countertops for caregiving activities
4. First aid for choking
5. Use of purified water for preparation of formula
6. Avoidance of bottle propping
7. Use of handwashing and avoidance of exposure to others and to illness
8. Safety measures when bathing in sinks or bathing basins

C. Newborn nutrition

1. Preparation of formulas
2. Cleaning of bottles and nipples
3. Reasons to avoid honey and corn syrup
4. Feeding schedules versus on-demand feedings
5. Expected amounts of intake
6. Color, consistency, and frequency of stools
7. Initial weight loss and subsequent gain

D. Community resources

1. Local chapters of La Leche League
2. Home health supply companies (e.g., for breast pumps)

E. Pediatric health maintenance and follow-up

1. First pediatrician or well-baby clinic visit (usually within 7 to 14 days after birth)
2. Schedule and importance of immunizations

CASE STUDY AND STUDY QUESTIONS

A 38-week-gestation, 2800-g (6 lb, 3 oz) infant with nasal flaring and mild retractions has been admitted to the nursery for observation. Admitting vital signs were temperature 35.7°C (96.2°F); heart rate, 148 beats/min; and respirations, 68/min. After stabilization, the baby was taken to his mother, who had indicated that she wanted to breastfeed. You help her with positioning the infant and "latching on." When you return in 5 minutes, the infant is in the mother's lap and she asks you for a bottle of formula.

1. Given the vital signs, what is the most likely explanation for the respiratory distress?

   a. Prematurity.

   b. Hypothermia.

   c. Small for gestational age (SGA).

   d. Pneumonia.

2. Using Table 23–1, at what temperature would you set the incubator to provide a neutral thermal environment?

   a. At 34.0° to 35.4°C (93.9 to 95.7°F).

   b. At 33.9° to 34.4°C (93.2 to 93.9°F).

   c. At 32.0° to 33.8°C (89.6 to 92.8°F).

   d. At 29.8° to 32.8°C (85.6 to 91°F).

3. What is the most frequent mechanism of heat loss in the newborn infant?

   a. Radiation.

   b. Conduction.

   c. Convection.

   d. Evaporation.

4. Your response to the mother's request for a bottle of formula is which of the following?

   a. To return to the nursery and prepare a bottle of formula.

   b. To reinstruct the mother in breastfeeding techniques.

   c. To discuss the mother's request with her.

   d. To refuse to give her a bottle of formula because you have breastfed all of your children.

5. The mother believes she does not have enough milk and she wants to provide a supplement. Which of the following is the best response to her?

   a. The nutritional requirements of the infant are minimal at this time and she has enough milk.

   b. The infant should suck at the breast to stimulate milk production.

   c. Colostrum is beneficial to the infant's health.

   d. All of the above.

6. After the mother has fed her infant, you return to her room to check on their pro-

gress and find the infant lying flat on his back in his crib. Which of the following is false?

a. You know this practice may have a cultural base.

b. The infant should be lying on his right side or abdomen.

c. There is an increased risk of aspiration.

d. The infant's position is of no concern.

7. Which of the following is not true of breast milk?

a. A softer curd forms that is more easily digested.

b. Breast milk contains high mineral levels.

c. Breast milk has a higher calcium-to-phosphorus ratio.

d. Breast milk is economical.

Answers to Study Questions

1. b	2. c	3. d
4. c	5. d	6. d
7. b		

REFERENCES

Axton, S.E. (1989). *Nursing diagnosis pocket guide: Neonatal and pediatric care plans* (2nd ed.). Baltimore: Williams & Wilkins.

Carpenito, L.J. (1991). *Handbook of nursing diagnosis* (4th ed.). Philadelphia: Lippincott.

Dodman, N. (1987). Newborn temperature control. *Neonatal Network, 6*(16), 19–22.

Klaus, M.H., & Fanaroff, A.A. (1986). *Care of the high-risk neonate* (3rd ed.). Philadelphia: Saunders.

Romero-Gwynn, E. (1989). Breast-feeding pattern among Indochinese immigrants in northern California. *American Journal of Diseases in Childhood, 143*(7), 804–808.

Romero-Gwynn, E., & Carias, L. (1989). Breast-feeding intentions and practice among Hispanic mothers in Southern California. *Pediatrics, 84*(4), 626–632.

Scopes, J., & Ahmed, I. (1966). Range of critical temperatures in sick and premature newborn babies. *Archives of Diseases in Childhood, 41,* 417–419.

Whaley, L.E., & Wong, D.L. (1991). *Nursing care of infants and children* (4th ed.). St. Louis: Mosby.

Other

NAACOG (1992, Jan.). Neonatal skin care *OGN Nursing Practice Resource.*

Linda Howard Glenn

Psychosocial Adaptations

Objectives

1. Identify infant-related factors affecting the attachment process

2. State interventions for consoling the crying infant

3. Identify cultural influences to consider when addressing parenting skills and beliefs

4. Relate education topics commonly needed for families of newborn infants

5. Determine risk factors that may affect the attachment process

6. Interpret parenting skills that may be culturally based, but that are not necessarily considered safe practices in the U.S. culture and philosophy of medical care

Introduction

Newborns demonstrate that they can purposefully react to stimuli, thereby greatly affecting how others act toward them

A. Behavioral patterns

1. Initial period of reactivity within the first hour of life is characterized by
   a. Alert eyes that fixate on objects
   b. Attentiveness to sounds
   c. Bodily movements that appear to respond to noises, such as the mother's voice
2. These activities, combined with the infant's appearance, evoke responses in the parents that help facilitate the attachment process
3. Social behaviors during the newborn period are predominantly crying, reflexive movements, and visual attentiveness; these behaviors are also cues for engagement of the parents to respond to the infant's needs
   a. Reflex responses: grasping with hand when palm is touched and roots to nipple or finger when cheek is brushed
   b. Visual attention: gazes or is alert to objects within 17.8 to 30.5 cm (7 to 12 in) and appears to prefer the human face to look at, as well as objects with dark and light contrasts
   c. Crying: crying sounds usually are not specific to the type of discomfort in

the newborn, as they are in older infants; the newborn tends to cry in response to any discomfort that needs to be remedied

B. **Infant behavior and parental attachment: the personality of an individual infant is as unique as the personality of an individual adult**

1. The formation of a relationship between the parent and infant is based on reciprocal cues
2. An infant responds to the care given by the parent and, in turn, the parent's attitudes toward the infant and perception about parenting skills are shaped by the infant's responses
3. Infants have individual temperaments; some may be fussy, calm, awake all of the time, or asleep a lot; these are individual characteristics that are unique to each infant and should not be confused with abnormal behavior, such as drug withdrawal or neurological problems, for example

Clinical Practice

A. Assessment

1. Infant risk factors affecting the attachment process
   a. Feeding difficulties
   b. Sleeping problems (e.g., days and nights reversed)
   c. Neurological problems related to asphyxia, congenital anomalies, or medications
   d. Withdrawal from drugs
   e. Recovery from maternal sedatives, analgesics, and anesthetics
   f. Being one newborn of multiple births
   g. Physical anomalies
2. Cultural influences on parenting skills, child-care beliefs, and parental teaching come from a core of native theories developed in each culture
   a. Parental expectations and parenting actions are shaped from these beliefs or theories
   b. Unlike infant feeding behaviors, parenting beliefs and behaviors do not change as readily when families immigrate.
   c. Specific assessments when dealing with the newborn's family should focus on feeding behaviors, safety practices, and parental expectations for the infant's behavior
      (1) Feeding behaviors
         (a) Use of nonmilk formula preparations when feeding the newborn (e.g., rice water, bean curd water, and teas)
         (b) Use of bottles to feed infant table food
         (c) Propping of bottle
         (d) Length of bottlefeeding in relation to dentition
      (2) Safety practices
         (a) Burping and proper positioning of the infant after feeding to reduce aspiration; many cultures believe the infant will suffocate if placed in a prone position
         (b) Use of household remedies to manage common newborn problems (e.g., diarrhea and colic)
         (c) Willingness to seek medical care and to consent to immunizations
      (3) Parental expectations
         (a) Expectations about achievement of developmental milestones
         (b) Activities to aid the infant in reaching developmental milestones (e.g., selection of toys, books, etc.)
      (4) Circumcision

(a) Many families in the United States have infant boys circumcised
(b) Circumcision is traditional in the Jewish culture and is performed on the eighth day of life during a ceremony
(c) Hispanic cultures usually do not circumcise boys

B. Nursing Diagnoses

1. High risk for alteration in family process related to addition of family member and lack of knowledge about infant behaviors
2. Parental knowledge deficit related to cultural differences
3. High risk for alteration in parenting related to unrealistic expectations of infant and lack of attachment behaviors

C. Interventions/Evaluations

1. High risk for alteration in family process related to addition of family member and lack of knowledge about infant behaviors
   a. Interventions
      (1) Assess parents' level of knowledge, cultural values, and prior parenting experience
      (2) Observe family members' communication patterns with each other and with newborn
      (3) Instruct parents about newborn behaviors
      (4) Discuss with parents variables that may affect parenting (i.e., expectations about child, expected changes in lifestyle and cultural influences)
      (5) Assess preparations made at home for newborn
      (6) Make home health and public health visit referrals, as indicated
   b. Evaluations
      (1) Parents' caregiving behaviors are safe
      (2) Parents' interactions with infant are appropriate for the normal developmental level of infant
      (3) Parents verbalize appropriate expectations about infant's behaviors
      (4) Parents verbalize acceptance of infant into family unit and describe appropriate preparations at home for infant's arrival
2. Parental knowledge deficit related to cultural differences
   a. Interventions
      (1) Assess parents' cultural beliefs that may influence care and safety of the infant at home
      (2) Instruct parents in safe care of the infant in the home environment
      (3) Provide rationale for newborn care practices (e.g., prevention of aspiration)
      (4) Make home health visit and public health visit referrals, as indicated
   b. Evaluations
      (1) Parents demonstrate safe newborn care practices throughout hospital stay
      (2) Parents verbalize rationale for safe caregiving tasks
      (3) Parents state plan for follow-up care of newborn
3. High risk for alteration in parenting related to unrealistic expectations of infant and lack of attachment behaviors
   a. Interventions
      (1) Assess parental knowledge about infant development and behaviors and past experience with parenting
      (2) Observe parental interactions with infant during feedings, bathing, and comforting
      (3) Instruct parents in newborn behaviors
      (4) Discuss with parents variables that may affect parenting (i.e., expectations about infant, infant's responses to parenting activities, parental feelings about infant)

    b. Evaluations
      (1) Parents' interactions with infant are appropriate to developmental level of infant
      (2) Parents describe what newborn behaviors to expect during the first month of life
      (3) Parents verbalize feelings about infant's arrival and expected changes in parental role and lifestyle
      (4) Parents demonstrate appropriate bonding and attachment behaviors

Health Education

Health education should focus on infant behavior and ways in which parents can engage their infant's attention. The practitioner should also be aware of cultural influences on parenting behaviors in response to infant cues and expectations about the infant's behavior

A. Review of reflexes, sensory capabilities, and common behaviors as outlined in Chapters 22 & 23

B. Changes in behavior that may occur when the infant is ill

C. Ways to attend to the infant's needs when she or he is crying

D. Realistic expectations about infant's behavior, and a description of infant factors that may affect the attachment process (e.g., maternal medications and feeding difficulties)

E. Discussion of feeding behaviors and safety practices with rationale as discussed in Chapter 23

F. Calming and consoling activities include

1. Rocking the infant
2. Bringing the infant's extremities into midline or swaddling the infant to provide security
3. Speaking to the infant in soft, calm, and rhythmic tones

G. Community resources

1. Parent-child interactive programs
2. Babysitting services or day-care organizations
3. Red Cross or other agencies providing cardiopulmonary resuscitation (CPR) and first-aid education
4. Local schools, hospitals, colleges, or recreation departments offering parenting and child development courses and support groups

H. Family dynamics include

1. Reactions to and dealing with stress and fatigue
2. Sibling rivalry
3. Communication patterns, especially communication of needs
4. Extended familiy influences and advice in childrearing

CASE STUDY AND STUDY QUESTIONS

Mrs. White, a first-time mother of a baby girl, calls for her nurse. You enter the room to find both the mother and infant crying. The mother states that the baby refuses to breastfeed, just as she did the evening before. The baby cries each time she attempts to breastfeed and the mother thinks the baby doesn't like her milk.

1. When you find this mother and infant crying, you:

   a. Give the mother a bottle of formula.

   b. Attempt to place the infant on the breast while the infant's mouth is fully open during crying.

   c. Attempt to calm the infant by talking softly, bringing her hands to midline and rocking her to bring her to a quiet state.

   d. Tell the mother not to worry, that the baby will eat when she gets hungry enough.

2. In light of the previous night's events, you know that all of the following are true except

   a. Mothers and babies often work these things out on their own.

   b. Feeding difficulties can affect attachment.

   c. The mother's misperception of the infant's not liking her milk may affect her self-esteem as a parent.

   d. Mrs. White may not know how to breastfeed, especially with a baby who does not take to it easily.

Answers to Study Questions

1. c   2. a

REFERENCES

Axton, S.E. (1989). *Nursing diagnosis pocket guide: Neonatal and pediatric care plans* (2nd ed.). Baltimore: Williams & Wilkins.

Benakappa, D.G., Raju, M., Shivananda, S., & Benakappa, A.D. (1989). Breast-feeding practices in rural Karnataka, India, with special reference to lactation failure. *Acta Paediatrics Japanese Overseas Education, 31*(4), 391–398.

Blackburn, S. (1983). Fostering behavioral development of high-risk infants. *Journal of Obstetric, Gynecologic, and Neonatal Nursing, 12*(3), 76s–86s.

Carpenito, L.J. (1985). *Handbook of nursing diagnosis.* Philadelphia: Lippincott.

Colangelo, C., Bergen, A., & Gottleib, L. (1976). *A normal baby—The sensory-motor process of the first year.* New York: Blythdale Children's Hospital.

Klaus, M.H., & Fanaroff, A.A. (1986). *Care of the high-risk neonate* (3rd ed.). Philadelphia: Saunders.

Hopkins, B., & Westra, T. (1989). Maternal expectations of their infant's development: Some cultural differences. *Developmental Medicine and Child Neurology, 31*(3), 384–390.

Johnson, S.H. (1979). *High-risk parenting: Nursing assessment and strategies for the family at risk.* Philadelphia: Lippincott.

Whaley, L., & Wong, D. (1991). *Nursing care of infants and children* (4th ed.). St. Louis: Mosby.

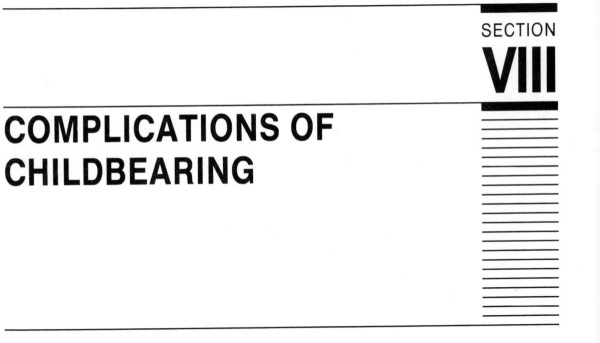

COMPLICATIONS OF CHILDBEARING

Leayn Johnson

Perinatal Loss and Grief

Objectives

1. Define the stages of the grieving process according to Kübler-Ross or Engle

2. Identify ways that effective coping differs from ineffective coping during a crisis

3. Select nursing diagnoses appropriate to specific problems that occur because of perinatal loss

4. State appropriate nursing interventions that facilitate the grieving process

5. Analyze the theoretical basis of grief and loss

6. Discuss strategies that enable the family experiencing perinatal loss to use the bereavement time to learn new coping skills

7. Formulate nursing interventions based on theory and assessment to provide collaborative care to the family experiencing perinatal loss

Introduction

A. Grief is the expected response after a loss, such as death of a loved one, loss of a "perfect" child because of birth defects, loss of the end of the pregnancy because of prematurity, or loss of a fetus from spontaneous abortion

B. Grief can occur with any change since all change involves loss; the loss may be observable or perceived only by the parent, such as the loss of the fantasized perfect child

C. Grief is an alteration in mood and emotions related to an actual or perceived loss

D. Grief is not just sadness; it consists of many emotions and ranges from sadness to anxiety, anger, guilt, fear, or relief

E. The goal for working with parents experiencing perinatal grief and loss is to encourage them to experience emotions and feelings and to work through the various stages of the grieving process to reach resolution

F. There is agreement among theorists on the commonality of the responses to various stages of grief

G. There is also agreement among theorists that one progresses through the grieving process in a highly individual manner within a broad time range; manifestations of grief are highly individual

Clinical Practice

A. Assessment

1. History
   a. Causative factors of the current loss
   b. Past losses
   c. Past coping strategies
   d. Support systems
      (1) Extended family
      (2) Resilience of the marriage
      (3) Religious beliefs and support
   e. Cultural aspects
   f. Developmental stage and tasks of the parents and family members (e.g., Erickson's stages [in Stuart & Sundeen, 1991])
      (1) Parents' ages: adolescence (identity versus identity diffusion)
         (a) The "who am I?" (identity crisis) feeling may be one of confusion: "Do I want to be a parent or am I still a child?"
         (b) Separation anxiety for the adolescent parent may take the form of leaving home for the first time or being without parental guidance and counseling
      (2) Parents' ages: young adult (intimacy versus isolation)
         (a) "I should be able to have healthy children" may be the internal voice of the young woman and the young man
         (b) Feelings may be of punishment or failure when a pregnancy is lost or the baby dies or is born defective
         (c) "I feel so alone" is a typical feeling after perinatal loss
         (d) After a perinatal loss, parents' feelings may be those of never being able to have other children to love, of failure, or of fear that everyone may avoid them because they have failed
      (3) Parents' ages: middle age (generativity versus self-absorption)
         (a) Concerns about the biological clock running out may prevail
         (b) This pregnancy may have represented the last chance to have a child
         (c) Perinatal loss at this age can release intense feelings (e.g., that no one will ever understand how important the loss was); they feel that they cannot share their feelings with anyone who would really under-stand
2. Psychological factors that affect perinatal loss and grief, according to Quirk (Leaphart, 1985) follow
   a. Ambivalence about the pregnancy is normal during early pregnancy; an example of negative ambivalence is that of a woman who wants to be a mother but is not sure that she is ready to be tied down with an infant or can take care of an infant
   b. Motivation for pregnancy and parenthood
      (1) Example of a negative motivation is: "This child will save our marriage"
      (2) Example of a positive motivation is: "I believe we are ready to be won-derful parents"
   c. Expectant parents' relationship with the fetus during pregnancy
      (1) Examples of a negative relationship are a mother's statement: "This has been a terrible pregnancy; I feel so ugly; I hate being pregnant" or a father's statement about how the baby has ruined the mother's figure or their sex life

(2) Examples of a positive relationship are: "I feel the baby enjoys the music I play for her or him" or a father's statement about how strong, energetic, or playful the fetal movements seem to be

d. Pregnancy as a social event or fulfillment of social expectations: examples of a negative event are: "We were expected to have this child—there was so much pressure from the folks" and "We are giving them their grandchild so they will leave us alone"

e. Pregnancy and birth as achievements and indicators of creativity: examples of negative feelings are: "This child proves I am an adult" or "Now, I will finally have someone to love me"

3. Physiological changes that may result from the grief response include
   a. Tachycardia
   b. Shortness of breath
   c. Diaphoresis
   d. Syncope
   e. Confusion
   f. Mental status changes
      (1) Confusion
      (2) Short-term memory impairment
      (3) Decreased comprehension
      (4) Signs of depression
         (a) Appetite changes
         (b) Sleep changes
         (c) Loss of energy and fatigue
         (d) Thoughts of death
   g. Vital sign changes
   h. Respiratory rate increase
   i. Sleep pattern disturbance
   j. Muscular weakness
   k. Tightness of the throat

B. **Theoretical constructs: According to Martocchio (1985), guilt and self-blame are frequently intense after the death of a child; all stages may vary in time and sequence and still be normal**

1. Kübler-Ross's (1969) stages of grieving
   a. Denial: examples of typical statements are
      (1) "When my child improves . . ."
      (2) "Once we get the baby home . . ."
      (3) "Miracles do happen"
   b. Anger: examples of typical statements are
      (1) "Why me?"
      (2) "God is so unfair"
      (3) "This is my husband's fault"
      (4) "The staff at this hospital are responsible"
   c. Bargaining: examples of typical statements are
      (1) "If my baby improves, I will . . ."
      (2) "If God spares my child, I will . . ."
   d. Depression: examples of typical statements are
      (1) "I just want to be alone"
      (2) "I wish I could just die"
      (3) "Just let me sleep"
   e. Acceptance: examples of typical statements are
      (1) "This has been a difficult time but I can cope"
      (2) "We miss our baby very much and she will always be a special part of our lives"

2. Engels's stages (Wilson & Kneisl, 1988)
   a. Acute (approximately 4 to 6 weeks)

(1) Shock and disbelief
  (a) Denial and inability to accept the loss
  (b) Numbness
  (c) Repression of emotional responses
(2) Developing awareness of the loss
  (a) Surfacing of painful feelings
  (b) Crying, anguish, and despair
(3) Resolution
  (a) Formal ritualistic stage defined by society, culture, and religion
b. Long term (approximately 1 to 2 years)
  (1) Sensations of somatic distress
    (a) Shortness of breath
    (b) Exhaustion
    (c) Unreality of life
  (2) Preoccupation with the deceased
    (a) Idealization of the dead infant (or fetus)
    (b) Identification with the dead infant

C. Dysfunctional grieving

1. Prolonged
   a. There is no timetable for grieving
   b. Except for the initial phase, prolonged dysfunctional grieving may involve the following prolonged reactions
     (1) Denial of death
     (2) Intense anger
     (3) Denial of feelings
2. Unresolved
   a. Denial of emotions
   b. Denial of grief
3. Severe depression
   a. Suicidal ideation
   b. Loss of hope
   c. Feelings of helplessness
4. Inability to cry at any time after the loss
5. Prolonged apathetic behavior
6. Continuous and prolonged hallucinations about the dead baby (or fetus): many parents normally experience some type of visual or auditory hallucinations of the dead baby (or fetus) (e.g., they may hear the baby cry); this does not indicate psychosis)

D. Nursing Diagnoses

1. Anticipatory grieving related to premature labor or intrauterine death
2. Dysfunctional grieving related to inability to accept and verbalize the loss or related to denial of the loss
3. Ineffective family coping: disabling, related to infant's anomalies and death
4. Powerlessness related to feelings of despair secondary to perinatal loss

E. Interventions/Evaluations

CASE STUDY

Note: The case study is presented early in this chapter to assist the reader in formulating practical nursing interventions and evaluations on this particular topic.

Mary Jones, a 35-year-old woman, has been diagnosed as being in premature labor at 30 weeks' gestation. Mary and her husband, Tom, have been trying to have a child for 7 years. Mary has had seven spontaneous abortions in 5 years. Mary teaches first grade and Tom is a lawyer. Mary is an only child and her parents live 2000 miles away. Her mother and father have been notified and are planning to

66PD—

join Mary and Tom as soon as possible. Tom has two brothers and his parents also live out of state and are not able to join the couple at this time.

1. Anticipatory grieving related to premature labor or intrauterine death
   a. Interventions
      (1) Promote a trusting relationship with the family
         (a) Encourage verbalization of concerns (example: "Mary, can you talk to me about your fears and concerns?")
         (b) Use nonjudgmental communication
         (c) Answer questions factually
         (d) Describe and explain all procedures
         (e) Assist family members to feel as comfortable as possible within the hospital setting
      (2) Give positive reinforcement for all attempts to verbalize the possible loss
      (3) Support the family's grief reactions
         (a) Use therapeutic communication techniques
            (i) Use reflection, restatement, and clarification to encourage verbalization of the possible loss
            (ii) Encourage the couple to share concerns with the staff
         (b) Use therapeutic communication techniques to encourage verbalization about guilt, previous losses, and coping; examples of statement stems are
            (i) What I am hearing you say is . . .
            (ii) Tell me more about . . .
            (iii) Are you telling me . . .
            (iv) I am not sure I understand; tell me more about . . .
      (4) Provide the couple with the opportunity to talk about anticipatory grieving; an example using the case study is
         (a) Mary: "Why is this happening to me? There is no God"
         (b) Nurse: "The baby coming so early must seem so unfair; can you talk about your concerns?"
      (5) Give Mary and Tom permission to express their anger; examples using the case study are
         (a) Mary: "I hate this hospital; if I had stayed at home, maybe the labor would have stopped"
         (b) Nurse: "You believe that staying at home may have helped?"
         (c) Mary: "Well, no, but I am so frightened"
         (d) Nurse: "Talk to me about your fears; Tom, do you have similar fears?"
      (6) Provide information about the birth, aftercare, and support systems
         (a) Provide factual information
            (i) Inform parents about baby's size, chances for survival, and appearance
            (ii) Neonatal team has been alerted and will be present during the birth
            (iii) Baby will be taken directly to the neonatal intensive care unit and parents may not be able to hold the baby
            (iv) Baby's cry may be weak
         (b) Provide information about religious leaders, social workers, and psychological services available at the facility and in the community, as needed or indicated
         (c) Allow for privacy
            (i) Provide a private room, if possible
            (ii) Pull curtains or provide screen
         (d) Involve the couple in decisions whenever possible (e.g., choice of the neonatologist, if possible)
      (7) Provide consistently familiar personnel for care, whenever possible

(8) Assure the couple and family that everything medically possible is being done
(9) Promote family cohesiveness
   (a) Encourage the family to support and comfort the mother
   (b) Give the father the choice of staying for all procedures
   b. Evaluation: client and family will use anticipatory grieving to express concerns and prepare for a premature birth or stillbirth

---

Mary, after 6 hours of labor, delivered a 1049-g (2 lb, 5 oz) boy who lived for 2 hours. The infant had major anomalies. Mary looked at Tom and said, "What more can we expect? There is no God, no justice. The reason the baby died is because you did not really want this child; we are being punished. I will never cry over this child."

---

2. Dysfunctional grieving related to denial of the loss and inability to accept and verbalize the loss
   a. Interventions
      (1) Develop a trusting relationship
         (a) Touching and hugging can be therapeutic if client and nurse are comfortable with this type of communication
         (b) Allow for privacy
            (i) Private room, if possible; if not, pull the curtains
            (ii) Room at the end of hall away from the nursery
         (c) Encourage the father to express his feelings
      (2) Acknowledge denial as beneficial and part of the grieving process
         (a) Allow the client and family to express feelings; an example using the case study is
            (i) Mary: "This cannot be my perfect baby"
            (ii) Nurse: "This is not the baby you had planned for. Tell me about your expectations"
         (b) Acknowledge that anger is beneficial; an example using the case study is
            (i) Nurse: "Mary, I can see you are angry; you have every right to these feelings; this is a very upsetting time for you and Tom"
            (ii) Mary: "I feel like I just want to throw things against the wall!"
         (c) Encourage expression of feelings using communication techniques
            (i) Observe verbal and nonverbal behavior
               • Facial expressions
               • Clenched fists
               • Blank stare
            (ii) Use reflection and restatement; an example using the case study is
               • "Mary, you said you are being punished; can you tell me more about these thoughts?"
               • "You may feel that you are going crazy because this is the worst thing that has ever happened to you"
            (iii) Use active listening
               • Listen for the words not spoken
               • Make eye contact
               • Realize that listening and caring are more important than advice
            (iv) Use nondefensive communication and remember that the client's anger may be displaced on health care providers; an example using the case study is
               • Mary: "What can you know? You are just a nurse"
               • Nurse: "I can see how upset you are; this has been a very difficult time for you. I want you to know I am here to help you in any way I can"

(v) Use role modeling of effective communication techniques
- Clarify and make sure messages are understood
- Restate and allow the client to hear what she is saying

    (d) Provide information about grieving; an example from the case study is
- (i) Help Mary and Tom come to an intellectual acceptance of the death and start the grieving process
- (ii) "Despite all your wishes to the contrary, this loss has occurred; your baby is dead and you and Tom need to grieve; grieving means allowing yourself to feel the emotion and to talk about the pain"

    (e) Sedation interferes with Mary's experience of the grief process, which she ultimately must face

b. Evaluation: Client and family overcome denial and have the ability to verbalize the loss and show signs of beginning the grief process

3. Ineffective family coping: disabling, related to infant's anomalies and death

a. Interventions

(1) Develop a trusting relationship: realize that emotional bonding has occurred between mother and infant during the past 7 months; examples from the case study are

    (a) Encourage Mary to express her feelings and to verbalize her needs

    (b) "Mary, you have carried this child for 7 long months and now you have lost your child and all your hopes and dreams for this child; can you talk about your feelings?"

(2) Encourage verbalization about the infant's anomalies

(3) Encourage the use of past coping skills that have been successful

(4) Encourage client to verbalize anger

(5) Use therapeutic communication techniques; examples of positive and negative statements are

    (a) "It is okay to cry; tears help with both the sadness and the hurt"

    (b) Do not use statements such as
- (i) "It is for the best"
- (ii) "You can always have another child; you are young"
- (iii) "Just remember, God knows best"
- (iv) "You are lucky this child did not live"

(6) Take a picture of the infant to offer parents (perhaps at a later date)

(7) Ask if the family desires to see or hold the infant

    (a) Respect the parents' wishes

    (b) If the family wishes to see the infant after death, the following preparations are suggested
- (i) Bathe the infant
- (ii) Brush the infant's hair, if possible
- (iii) Dress the infant; use clothes provided by the parents, if possible
- (iv) If the infant is macerated, wrap the torso or body part in a thin, waterproof pad before dressing to minimize wetting of the clothing
- (v) Wrap the baby in a blanket
  - Powder the blanket
  - This often gives the parents a scent by which to remember their baby
- (vi) Offer to take a picture of the infant and parents together
- (vii) Provide the family with time alone with the infant
- (viii) Encourage the family to name the infant
- (ix) Prepare a keepsake package for the family with the following items
  - Identification bracelet
  - Lock of hair, if possible

- Photograph
- Footprints
- Birth and death certificates
- Record of the weight, length, head, and chest measurements
- Receiving blanket
b. Evaluation: Family copes effectively with the infant's death and anomalies
4. Powerlessness related to feelings of despair secondary to perinatal loss
a. Interventions
(1) Explain all procedures, rules, and options to the family about their infant's death
(a) Infant will be placed in the morgue until the mortuary picks up the body
(b) Encourage the couple to make decisions about the following
(i) Funeral arrangements
(ii) Birth and death announcements
(iii) Naming of the infant
(iv) Remaining on the maternity floor or moving to another location
(v) Whether the father will spend the night with the mother in the hospital; make sure that all visiting restrictions are removed for the father
(2) Use active listening to enable the parents to state their feelings
(3) Provide and create opportunities for the parents and family to express feelings
b. Evaluations
(1) The parents verbalize and demonstrate a sense of control and power by using problem-solving skills and making decisions about personal care and the infant's burial
(2) Memories of the newborn are positive (this behavior may not occur until resolution)

Health Education

A. Parents need to be instructed about the normal grieving process

1. Typical feelings to anticipate at various times
2. Normalcy of their feelings and behaviors
3. With the passage of time, the pain lessens
4. Importance of expressing and sharing their grief with one another and with family members

B. Make appropriate referrals for psychological help, spiritual and religious help, and self-help support groups

---

STUDY QUESTIONS

1. Signs of dysfunctional grieving during the first 3 days after the death of the infant include which of the following?

   (1) Anger.

   (2) Denial of emotions.

   (3) Crying.

   (4) Inability to cry.

   a. 1, 2.

   b. 2, 3.

   c. 2, 4.

   d. All of the above.

2. Which of the following appropriate nursing interventions facilitate the grieving process?

   (1) Promotion of a trusting relationship.

   (2) Use of therapeutic communication techniques.

(3) Emotional uninvolvement.

(4) Maintenance of a professional distance.

a. 1, 2.

b. 2, 4.

c. 1, 2, 4.

d. All the above.

3. The client tells the nurse, "I know that this baby may not live." Which of the following is the best reply?

a. Every baby stands a chance of dying.

b. The future cannot be predicted.

c. You seem worried; tell me about your fears.

d. There is a good chance your baby may die.

4. During discharge, the client states, "Nurse, I feel so "low" at times; even before I lost the baby I had these feelings; how will I cope now?" What response is the most therapeutic?

a. "More exercise will help."

b. "You are feeling depressed and low; tell me more."

c. "Most women feel depressed at times."

d. "It must be difficult for you when you feel this sad. How have you coped in the past?"

5. Which of the following interventions is the most beneficial in helping a family start the grieving process?

a. Contacting the hospital social worker.

b. Explaining all procedures in detail.

c. Building of a trusting relationship.

d. Explaining the grieving process.

Answers to Study Questions

1. c	2. a	3. c
4. d	5. c	

REFERENCES

Barranti, C. (1985, March). The grandparent/grandchild relationship in an era of voluntary bonds. *Family Relations*, 343–352.

Bloom-Feshback, J., & Bloom-Feshback, S. (1987). *The psychology of separation and loss.* San Francisco: Jossey-Bass.

Cochran, L., & Claspell, E. (1987). *The meaning of grief: A dramaturgical approach to understanding emotion.* New York: Greenwood.

Collins, S. (1989, November/December). Sudden death counseling protocol. *Dimensions of Critical Care Nursing*, 375–377.

Crosby, J., & Jose, N. (1983). Death: Family adjustment to loss. *Stress in the family: Coping with catastrophe* (Vol. 2). New York: Brunner/Mazel.

Doka, K.J. (1989). *Disenfranchised grief.* Lexington, MA: Heath.

Johnson, S.E. (1987). *After a child dies: Counseling bereaved families.* New York: Springer.

Knapp, R.J. (1986). *Beyond endurance: When a child dies.* New York: Schocken.

Kübler-Ross, E. (1969). *On death and dying.* New York: MacMillan.

Leaphart, E. (1985). Perinatal loss: Strategies to facilitate bereavement. *NAACOG Update Series, Lesson 2,* (Vol. 3). Princeton: Continuing Professional Education Center, Inc.

Levine S. (1984). *Meetings at the edge.* New York: Doubleday Anchor.

Margolis, O.S., Kutscher, A.H., Marcus, E.R., Raether, H.C., Pine, V.R., Sieland, I.B., Cherico, D.J. (Eds.). (1988). *Grief and the loss of an adult child.* New York: Praeger.

Martocchio, B. (1985). Grief and bereavement. *Nursing Clinics of North America, 20*(2), 327–339.

Murphy, S.A. (1990). Preventive intervention following accidental death of a child. *Image: Journal of Nursing Scholarship, 22*(3), 174–179.

Rando, T.A. (1988). *Grieving.* Lexington, MA: Heath.

Shuchter, S., & Zisook, R., (1988, May). Widowhood: The continuing relationship with the dead spouse. *Bulletin of the Menninger Clinic*, 269–272.

Stuart, G., & Sundeen, S. (1991). *Principles and practice of psychiatric nursing.* St. Louis: Mosby.

Toedter, L.J., Lasker, J.N., & Alhadeff, J.M. (1988). The perinatal grief scale: Development and initial validation. *American Journal of Orthopsychiatry, 58*(3), 435–440.

Valeriote, S., & Fine, M. (1987, Fall). Bereavement following the death of a child: Implications for family therapy. *Contemporary Family Therapy*, 202–217.

Varcarolis, E.M. (1990). *Foundations of psychiatric mental health nursing.* Philadelphia: Saunders.

Wilson, H.S., & Kneisl, C.R. (1988). *Psychiatric nursing.* Menlo Park, CA: Addison-Wesley.

CHAPTER 26

Barbara Petree
Susan Mattson

Hypertensive States in Pregnancy

Objectives

1. Define the types of hypertensive states in pregnancy

2. Identify the signs and symptoms of the HELLP syndrome

3. Describe the treatment modalities of pre-eclampsia, chronic hypertension, transient hypertension, and the HELLP syndrome

4. Discuss the drugs used in treatment

5. Analyze data obtained to determine overt and covert risk factors to mother and fetus

6. Correlate subtle history and physical findings (of mother at risk) with early indicators of hypertension

7. Predict maternal and fetal complications based on the data base

8. Formulate nursing interventions to alleviate or prevent anticipated problems from nursing assessment

9. Analyze the drug regimen to be used and its maternal and fetal effects

Introduction

A. Hypertensive disorders include a variety of vascular disturbances that may predate the pregnancy or occur during the gestational or postpartum periods

B. The term pregnancy-induced hypertension (PIH) covers those specific conditions developing during pregnancy and the puerperium

1. Pre-eclampsia and eclampsia are two categories of PIH that represent the same process, but eclampsia is reserved for describing the occurrence of generalized convulsions

2. PIH may be superimposed on chronic hypertension, or a woman may develop transient hypertension during the pregnancy or puerperium

3. The HELLP syndrome is a severe sequela of PIH (see further discussion later in this chapter)

C. Incidence of PIH is 5 to 7% of all pregnancies

1. PIH is among the three leading causes of maternal death in the United States, and it is the leading cause in Great Britain
2. If a woman has chronic hypertension, she has a 25 to 35% risk of developing PIH
3. PIH does not necessarily predispose a woman to developing essential hypertension at a later date
4. A sign of latent essential hypertension may be a recurring hypertension with a subsequent pregnancy

D. Although the cause of PIH generally remains unknown, several theories have been proposed

1. A hormonal cause has been suggested, but no single hormone or combination of particular hormones has been proved to cause PIH
2. A second hypothesis is that there is an imbalance between prostaglandin dilators and vasoconstrictors
3. Uteroplacental ischemia is the third postulation (Brinkman, 1986)

E. Although the pathophysiology of the disease is not well defined, the primary underlying mechanism appears to be vasospasm

1. Therapy is aimed at controlling hypertension and convulsions
2. Because development of the disease depends on the presence of trophoblastic tissue, the only true cure is delivery of the infant (Doan-Wiggins, 1987)

F. Although the cause remains unknown, the accepted underlying pathology of generalized arteriolar constriction results in many system responses

1. Rise in blood pressure results, probably as a result of the elevated systemic vascular resistance
2. Renal blood flow and glomerular filtration rate (GFR) are lower than in normal pregnancies; glomerular membranes are also damaged from the vasoconstriction, increasing their permeability to proteins
3. Studies done on cerebral and uteroplacental circulation have shown a decreased blood flow and increased vascular resistance in these organs as well
4. In effect, major maternal systems are affected
   a. Renal
   b. Pulmonary
   c. Hepatic
   d. Hematological
   e. Uteroplacental and fetal
   f. Central nervous
5. Fetal complications are due to reduced uterine blood flow and vasospasm, causing
   a. Intrauterine growth–retarded (IUGR) fetus
   b. Hypoxia
   c. Possibly death

G. Prenatal factors increasing the risk of PIH include

1. Primigravida
2. Essential hypertension (especially in Afro-American women)
3. Low socioeconomic status
4. Age extremes (under 17 or over 35 years old)
5. Underweight or overweight
6. Family history of hypertension or vascular disease
7. Diagnosis of PIH in previous pregnancy
8. Diabetes mellitus
9. Pre-existing hypertensive, vascular, or renal disease

H. Factors that develop during pregnancy and increase the risk of developing PIH include

1. Diabetes mellitus
2. Multiple gestation
3. Gestational trophoblastic disease
4. Fetal hydrops
5. Hydramnios
6. Renal infections

I. Sequelae of PIH represent serious threats to maternal and fetal well-being; they include

1. Abruptio placentae
2. Retinal detachment
3. Acute renal failure
4. Cardiac failure
5. Cerebral hemorrhage
6. Maternal death
7. Fetal growth retardation, hypoxia, and death

J. Definitions

1. PIH
   a. Pre-eclampsia
      (1) Hypertension
         (a) Systolic pressure of 140 mm Hg or a rise of 30 mm Hg over baseline (before pregnancy or at first prenatal visit)
         (b) Diastolic pressure of 90 mm Hg or a rise of 15 mm Hg over baseline
         (c) Rise in blood pressures manifested when taken at least twice 6 or more hours apart
      (2) Proteinuria
         (a) 300 mg or more protein in 24-hour urine collection
         (b) Protein concentration of 1 g or more per liter in two random urine samples collected at 6 hours or more apart (1+ to 2+ on dipstick)
      (3) Edema
         (a) Greater than 1+ pitting edema after 12 hours of bed rest
         (b) Weight gain of 2.3 kg (5 lb) or more in 1 week
         (c) Both after the 20th week of pregnancy
      (4) Classic triad

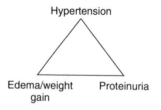

Hypertension

Edema/weight gain   Proteinuria

      (5) Rarely, pre-eclamptic findings may be seen in the presence of lupus anticoagulant
   b. Severe pre-eclampsia is defined in the presence of one or more of the following
      (1) Blood pressure
         (a) Systolic pressure of 160 mm Hg (with client on bed rest in left lateral position)
         (b) Diastolic pressure of 110 mm Hg (with client on bed rest in left lateral position) on two occasions 6 hours apart
      (2) Proteinuria: 5 g in 24-hour urine collection or 3+ to 4+ on random dipstick

(3) Oliguria: 24-hour urinary output of less than 700 to 800 ml in 24 hours or 30 ml/hr
(4) Hyperreflexia of 4+, possibly with clonus
(5) Cerebral and visual disturbances: altered consciousness, headache, blurred vision, scotomata
(6) Pulmonary edema or cyanosis
(7) Epigastric pain or right upper quadrant pain related to stretching of the liver capsule (Glisson's capsule), which could precede hepatic rupture (a rare but catastrophic complication)
(8) Impaired liver function of unclear cause
(9) Thrombocytopenia: platelet adherence to disrupted vascular endothelium

c. Eclampsia
  (1) Presence of seizures: clonic/tonic
    (a) Seizures are not attributed to other causes
    (b) Periods of hypoxia occur in mother and fetus
    (c) Risk of aspiration is great
    (d) Cardiovascular, hematological, renal, hepatic, central nervous and other organ systems are damaged secondary to hypertension and impaired tissue perfusion

2. Chronic hypertension: presence of hypertension before 20th week of pregnancy; morbidity is higher if diastolic pressure is over 105 mm Hg
3. Chronic hypertension with superimposed pre-eclampsia/eclampsia
   a. Morbidity is 25 to 35% higher than with pre-eclampsia alone
   b. Increased incidence or possibility of intracranial bleed
   c. May be related to renal or vascular disease
   d. May see the presence of hypertension before 20 weeks, edema, and proteinuria
4. Transient hypertension
   a. Development of elevated blood pressure during pregnancy or in the first 24 hours postpartum without pre-existing signs of pre-eclampsia or hypertension
   b. Blood pressure spontaneously returns to normal within 10 days
5. HELLP syndrome
   a. Is a severe sequela of PIH; occurs in 2 to 12% of cases
   b. Is seen most often in older white women (Poole, 1988)
   c. Is an acronym of
     (1) H: hemolysis: red blood cell (RBC) breakdown in vessels in vasospasm
       (a) Reduced oxygen-carrying capacity
       (b) Abnormal peripheral blood smear, with burr cells and schistocytes present
       (c) Increased bilirubin level of 1.2 mg/dl
       (d) Increased lactic dehydrogenase over 600 IU/L
     (2) EL: elevated liver enzymes
       (a) Increased serum glutamic oxalacetic transaminase (SGOT) of over 72 IU/L
       (b) Increased lactic dehydrogenase of over 600 IU/l
     (3) LP: low platelets—platelets aggregated in damaged vascular endothelium
   d. Pathophysiology (Fig. 26–1)
     (1) Arteriolar vasospasms damage the endothelial layer of small vessels, causing lesions
       (a) These lesions allow formation of platelet aggregations and, in turn, of a fibrin network
       (b) As RBCs are forced through the network under high pressure, the cells are hemolyzed

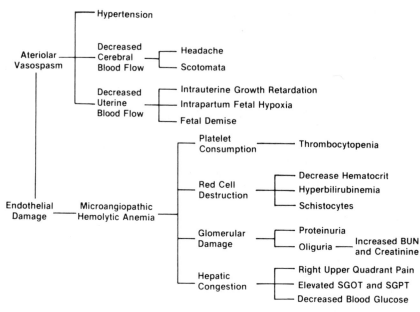

Figure 26–1
Physiological alterations that occur in the HELLP syndrome. SGPT, serum glutamic pyruvic transaminase. (From Whittaker, A.A., et al. [1986]. Hemolysis, elevated liver enzymes, and low platelet count syndrome. Nursing care of the critically ill obstetrical patient. *Heart & Lung, 15,* 402–408.)

          (c) The cells assume characteristic shapes (burr cells and schistocytes) as further evidence of damage

          (d) As hemolysis progresses, maternal hyperbilirubinemia is seen

      (2) Maternal hepatic failure results from microemboli in the liver

          (a) Ischemia and tissue damage result from the emboli

          (b) Obstruction to the hepatic blood flow and fibrin deposits cause hepatic distension

          (c) The increasing intrahepatic pressure potentiates liver rupture (the most common cause of maternal death)

      (3) The circulating volume of platelets decrease as a result of an increase in consumption

          (a) Circulating platelets adhere to damaged endothelium sites

          (b) As the platelets are consumed, thrombocytopenia results (Poole, 1988)

Clinical Practice

A. Assessment

Pregnancy-Induced Hypertension

1. History
   a. Estimated date of confinement (EDC)
   b. Major risk factors
      (1) Primigravida
      (2) Low socioeconomic status
      (3) Race or ethnic group: Afro-American or hispanic
      (4) Age under 17 or over 35 years old
      (5) Weight: under 90 lb (40.9 kg) or over 250 lb (113.6 kg)
      (6) Family history of hypertension or vascular or renal disease

      (7) Family history of PIH (especially mother or sister)

      (8) Diagnosis of PIH in previous pregnancy

      (9) Diabetes mellitus

      (10) Pre-existing hypertension or vascular or renal disease

      (11) Psychosocial history of drug, tobacco, alcohol (more than 3 drinks per day) use

  c. Dietary findings

      (1) Exercise (amount, frequency)

      (2) Intake: protein and general calories

         (a) A link has been seen between decreased protein intake and development of PIH

         (b) Abrams and Parker (1988) reported that moderately and severely overweight women demonstrated an increased incidence of PIH

         (c) Preliminary observations support the hypothesis that calcium supplementation reduces the occurrence of PIH (Belizan, Villar, & Repke, 1988)

2. Physical findings

  a. EDC established

      (1) Fundal height is measured with tape measure

      (2) Ultrasonography is used to assess gestational age, fetal growth, and placental aging (see Chapter 11 for further discussion of antepartum testing)

  b. Fetus assessed

      (1) Heart rate is taken with stethoscope or electronic fetal monitor

      (2) Ultrasound test is done for possible growth retardation

  c. Maternal subjective reports

      (1) Decreased fetal movements

      (2) Heartburn or stomachache

      (3) Headache

      (4) Visual disturbances

      (5) Numbness in hands and feet

  d. Blood pressure values

      (1) Correct for variables that affect accuracy

         (a) Correct size cuff is used

         (b) Client is in left lateral recumbent position

         (c) Blood pressure is taken on left (inferior) arm (hydrostatic pressure research has demonstrated that in left lateral recumbent position, blood pressure is lower in upper arm above heart and higher in left arm below heart)

         (d) Blood pressure is taken with client in same position on same arm each visit

      (2) Rollover test

         (a) First described in 1974

            (i) At 28 to 32 weeks, the client is placed in left lateral position for 20 minutes, then rolled onto her back

            (ii) Blood pressure is taken immediately and 5 minutes later

            (iii) A 20 mm Hg diastolic rise is a response that predicts the development of PIH

         (b) Unfortunately, too many false-negative and false-positive results have been reported and test is considered too imprecise for general use

      (3) Mean arterial pressure (MAP) may also be useful

         (a) It reflects the resistance against which heart works

         (b) Calculating MAP

            (i) Add systolic pressure to twice diastolic pressure

            (ii) Divide the product by 3

         (c) An increase of 20 mm Hg in MAP is considered ominous (Reeder & Martin, 1987)

(d) A MAP of 100 is abnormal, and a MAP of 105 indicates hypertension (Sherwen, Scoloveno, & Weingarten, 1991)

e. Urine

(1) Clean-catch specimen is assessed for protein with dipstick (1+ to 2+ with mild PIH, 3+ to 4+ with severe PIH)

(2) 24-hour collection is more accurate (300 mg or more in mild PIH and 5 g in severe PIH)

(3) Reduced urinary output (below 30 ml/hr) may be present

f. Deep tendon reflexes

(1) Reflexes graded from 0 to 4+

(a) 0: no response

(b) 1+: low normal

(c) 2+: average, normal

(d) 3+: brisker than average

(e) 4+: hyperactive; may be associated with clonus

(2) Clonus

(a) Briskly dorsiflex the foot while slightly flexing the knee

(b) Involuntary oscillations may be seen between flexion and extension when continuous pressure is applied to the sole of the foot

(c) Clonus is a sign of extreme hyperreflexia

g. Weight gain: note gain of more than 2 lb (907 g) per week

h. Edema

(1) Weight gain can be an indicator of edema, which reduces tissue perfusion

(2) Nonpitting edema of hands and face may be seen

(3) Pitting edema may also be seen

(a) 1+: edema is minimal at pedal and pretibial sites

(b) 2+: edema of lower extremities is marked

(c) 3+: edema is evident in face, hands, lower abdominal wall, and sacrum

(d) 4+: generalized massive edema is evident, including ascites from the accumulation of fluid in the peritoneal cavity (Scherwen, Scoloveno, & Weingarten, 1991)

i. System changes

(1) Respiratory

(a) Generalized arteriolar vasospasm produces reduced oxygen use in every organ

(b) Abnormal breath sounds are rales and wheezing

(c) Lungs are dull to percussion, denoting fluid overload (pulmonary edema)

(d) Dyspnea occurs

(2) Cardiovascular

(a) There is an increase in total peripheral vascular resistance

(i) Vascular sensitivity to substances such as angiotension II and catecholamines leads to vasospasm

• Cold or warm extremities

• Reduced capillary filling time

• Tachycardia

(ii) Left ventricular work is increased because of vasospasm

• Increased neck vein distension

• Gallop rhythm with impending congestive heart failure

(b) Coagulation factors are altered as a result of microcoagulation resulting from vasospasm

(c) Poor correlation exists between pulmonary capillary wedge pressure (PCWP) and central venous pressure (CVP)

(i) CVP does not give accurate information about left side pressure; PCWP is required

(ii) CVP is often low (0 to 5 cm H_2O)

(iii) PCWP is low to normal (0 to 7 mm Hg)

(d) Clients with severe pre-eclampsia experience hypovolemia and hemoconcentration

   (i) Probably caused by the contracted vascular bed and increased vascular permeability that lead to extravasation of fluid into the extravascular compartment (Scherwen, Scoloveno, & Weingarten, 1991)

   (ii) May have a rapid rise in hematocrit from 36 to 44% in a week

(3) Cerebral

(a) Loss of autoregulation of cerebral blood flow with acute hypertension leads to abnormally high cerebral perfusion

   (i) Causes constriction and dilation of arterioles

   (ii) Dilated ischemic segments lead to extravasation of fluid and edema formation, causing reduced blood flow

   (iii) Petechial hemorrhages

   (iv) Vessel wall necrosis

(b) Cerebral edema with transient neurological deficits

   (i) Drowsiness

   (ii) Dizziness

   (iii) Tinnitis

   (iv) Visual disturbances
   - Diplopia
   - Blurred vision
   - Scotomata

(c) Severe, continuous headaches or pressure in the head, often frontal or occipital

(d) vomiting

(4) Renal

(a) Glomerular function is altered

   (i) Decreased GFR is partially explained by decreased renal plasma flow (RPF)

   (ii) Glomeruloendotheliosis causes many glomeruli to be nonfunctional (as a result of an occlusion of glomerular capillaries by swollen endothelial cells)

(b) Protein leakage into the urine occurs

   (i) Normally, there is no leakage because of the impermeability of glomeruli to large protein molecules and tubular reabsorption of smaller proteins

   (ii) In PIH, glomerular damage occurs and permeability to proteins increases

   (iii) As damage increases, both large and small protein molecules cross the glomerular membrane

(c) Renal tubular function is altered

   (i) Uric acid clearance
   - Urate clearance is about 10% of creatinine clearance
   - Abnormal uric acid clearance is present in PIH as a function of decreased GFR and suggests tubular dysfunction
     □ Normal values of uric acid are 4.03 to 5.38 mg/dl
     □ Values above 5 mg/dl are associated with poor outcome
   - Renal ischemia increases renal medullary lactic acid

   (ii) Urine-concentrating capacity
   - Urine-concentrating ability is decreased in hypertensive women; specific gravity is normally 1.005 to 1.030.
   - Specific gravity is considered by some to be an unreliable measure of osmolality, and a urine osmolality test is recommended (normal urine osmolality is 25 to 88 mOsm/kg)

(iii) Renin–angiotensin–aldosterone system
- In a normal pregnancy, an important factor in pressure/volume regulation is the renin–angiotensin–aldosterone system
- Studies of this system in pregnancy are inconclusive; it appears to be altered in PIH

(iv) Sodium excretion
- Little sodium and chloride are found in the urine of women with PIH
- With a small amount of urine produced, sodium is retained by tubular reabsorption
- Known anomalies of renal function cause sodium retention; many factors affect GFR and tubular reabsorption
- Reduction of sodium in diet or increasing sodium excretion (with diuretics) has no effect on occurrence of PIH, and it even aggravates the hypovolemia of the disease

(5) Hepatic system
- (a) Ten percent of women with severe PIH have hepatic involvement
- (b) With hepatic involvement, mild SGOT elevation is seen
- (c) Bilirubin level usually remains normal
- (d) HELLP syndrome may occur
- (e) Hemorrhagic changes in the liver are present in 66% and necrotic changes in 40% of eclamptic women, and in 50% of pre-eclamptic women
- (f) Thrombosis of hepatic vessels, and disseminated intravascular coagulopathy (DIC) are seen
- (g) Stretching of the liver capsule (Glisson's capsule) occurs from edema
- (h) Hepatic rupture is a dramatic complication, with a maternal mortality rate of 70%; hepatic rupture is biphasic
  - (i) Phase 1: necrosis, intrahepatic hemorrhage, subcapsular hemorrhage—conservative management is possible
  - (ii) Phase 2: rupture of Glisson's capsule—surgery is mandated for lives of mother and fetus
- (i) Hepatic hematomas have been noted on ultrasound scans, computerized tomographic scans and at time of laparotomy; no rupture occurred

3. Psychosocial responses
   a. The additional crisis of high-risk pregnancy exacerbates the normal crisis situation, with client concerns for herself, her fetus, and her family
   b. Concerns
      (1) Need for long-term bed rest or hospitalization
          (a) Boredom
          (b) Need to be off from work
          (c) Family's need for "substitute" for household and family activities
      (2) Separation from family, friends, and other children when hospitalized
          (a) Need for satisfactory child care
          (b) Need for substitute interaction (e.g., phone calls, letters)
   c. Behaviors
      (1) Expressed feelings of ambivalence
      (2) Crying or withdrawal; grief over loss of "perfect" pregnancy
   d. Stress responses
      (1) Crying, withdrawal, or silence
      (2) Fear
      (3) Anxiety

(4) Hospital psychosis: aberrant behavior that occurs when hospitalized for long periods, especially when deprived of sunlight and time orientation

4. Diagnostic procedures
   a. Blood pressure as determined in lateral position
   b. Laboratory tests (Table 26–1)
      (1) Complete blood count with platelets
      (2) Type and screen or crossmatch for two units of packed blood cells
      (3) Urine for protein and specific gravity
      (4) Additional tests for women with severe pre-eclampsia
         (a) Electrolytes
         (b) Fibrinogen
         (c) Clot observation: a tube of blood is drawn to observe for clot formation and potential clot degradation
         (d) Serum creatinine
         (e) Liver function tests
   c. Fetal assessment
      (1) Non stress test (NST)/contraction stress test (CST)
      (2) Ultrasound test for growth pattern
      (3) Amniocentesis for pulmonary maturity if need for delivery is imminent
      (4) Biophysical profile
      (5) Doppler flow studies (see Chapter 11 for complete discussion)

Table 26–1.
LABORATORY TESTS AFFECTED BY PIH AND HELLP

	Pregnancy	PIH
Hemoglobin	10–12 g/dl	Decreased in HELLP
Hematocrit	32–40%	Increased Decreased in HELLP
Platelets	150,000–400,000	Decreased
Fibrinogen	300–600 mg/dl	Decreased
Fibrin split products	Absent or minimal	Increased
Prothrombin	12–16 sec	Unchanged
PT	75–125% in 1 hour	Unchanged
PTT	12–14 sec	Unchanged
Bleeding time	1–3 min (Duke)	Unchanged
	2–4 min (Ivy)	Decreased
	2–8 min (Template)	Increased
Respiratory		
Oxygen consumption	180–270 ml/min	Increased
Functional residual capacity (FRC)	1.41 L	Decreased
Carbon dioxide content	18–26 mmol/L	Increased
Factors VII, VIII, IX, X	Increased	Increased
Factors XI, XIII	Decreased	Decreased
Renal		
Creatinine	0.4–1.0 mg/dl	Increased
BUN	5–10 g/dl	Increased
Uric acid	<6 mg/dl	Increased in HELLP
Creatinine clearance	130–180 ml/min	Decreased in HELLP
Uric acid clearance	10% of creatinine clearance	
Hepatic		
Alkaline phosphatase	60–480 U/ml	Increased in HELLP
Albumin	2.8–3.7 g/dl	Decreased
Bilirubin	Slight elevation from 0.2–0.9 mg/dl	Increased in HELLP
SGOT	5–40 IU	Increased in HELLP
SGPT	3–21 IU	Increased in HELLP
LDH	90–200 IU	Increased in HELLP

Chronic Hypertension

1. History
   a. Risks dependent on
      (1) Maternal age
      (2) Duration of hypertension
      (3) Presence of medical complications
      (4) Severity of hypertension early in pregnancy
   b. Maternal mortality is usually caused by a malignant rise in blood pressure with subsequent congestive heart failure or cerebrovascular accidents
2. Physical findings
   a. Hypertension diagnosed before the 20th week of pregnancy
   b. Increased morbidity and mortality
   c. Increased incidence of superimposed pre-eclampsia
   d. Increased incidence of abruptio placentae
   e. Clients with labile or borderline hypertension have pathophysiologic alterations with
      (1) Elevated cardiac output
      (2) Central redistribution of blood volume
      (3) Enhanced activity of autonomic nervous system
      (4) Increased left ventricular ejection rate
      (5) Normal total vascular resistance
   f. Vascular resistance and arterial pressure are elevated, with increased ventricular workload
   g. Heart rate is increased but stroke volume and left ventricular ejection rate are normal
   h. Danger of pulmonary edema
   i. Primary essential hypertension: cardiac strain is evident with moderate essential hypertension
      (1) Stroke volume remains normal or starts to fall
      (2) Myocardial contractility is normal
3. Diagnostic procedures
   a. Electrocardiographic (ECG) studies show increased thickness in left ventricular wall
4. Treatment: see Table 26–2.

Secondary Hypertension

1. History
   a. It is important to know the duration of hypertension
   b. The client may have
      (1) Essential hypertension
      (2) Acute or chronic glomerulonephritis
      (3) Chronic pyelonephritis
      (4) Collagen vascular disease
      (5) Systemic lupus erythematosus
   c. Renal disorder is usually the main cause of other origins
2. Physical findings
   a. Diastolic blood pressure above 105 mm Hg
   b. Involvement of systems
      (1) Renal conditions
         (a) Acute glomerulonephritis
         (b) Chronic nephritis
         (c) Lupus nephritis
         (d) Diabetic nephropathy
      (2) Endocrinological conditions
         (a) Cushing's syndrome

(b) Primary aldosteronism
(c) Pheochromocytoma
(d) Thyrotoxicosis
(3) Neurological conditions
(a) Cerebrovascular accident
(b) Quadriplegia
(c) Blindness
c. Mortality increases twofold with blood pressure above 160/90 mm Hg, versus blood pressure below 140/90 mm Hg
3. Treatment
a. Morbidity is lower in treated women
b. Thiazide diuretics are not used during pregnancy
c. See drugs in Table 26–2

Transient (Gestational) Hypertension

1. History
a. Transient hypertension in the second half of pregnancy, during labor, or within 48 hours after delivery
b. It is difficult to differentiate from pre-eclampsia
2. Physical findings
a. Proteinuria of less than 300 mg/L
b. Renal disease must be ruled out
3. Treatment: although no treatment is required, the client is often placed on antihypertensive drugs (see Table 26–2)

Chronic Hypertension With Superimposed Pre-Eclampsia

1. The client demonstrates significant proteinuria as well as edema, as assessed by weight gain
2. Treatment is the same as for PIH (see Table 26–2)

B. Nursing Diagnosis

1. High risk for central nervous system (CNS) injury related to hypertension and excessive fluid volume
2. Altered tissue perfusion related to renal disturbances
3. Altered tissue perfusion related to cardiovascular disturbances
4. High risk for altered respiratory function: decreased related to excessive fluid volume
5. High risk for hepatic injury related to hypertension
6. High risk for impaired fetal well-being, related to altered uteroplacental perfusion
7. Anxiety and fear related to risk of harm to self and fetus

C. Interventions/Evaluations

1. High risk for CNS injury related to hypertension and excessive fluid volume
a. Interventions
(1) Monitor blood pressure every 15 minutes or more frequently
(2) Maintain fluid balance and document intake and output (I&O)
(a) May restrict fluids to 125 ml/hr of combined IV and oral fluids if so ordered
(b) Monitor urinary output
(c) Measure and document any emesis
(d) Central monitoring lines may be ordered with severe pre-eclampsia
(3) Assess deep tendon reflexes (DTR) and clonus
(4) Assess for subjective symptoms
(a) Headaches or pressure

Table 26–2.
DRUGS USED IN TREATMENT OF HYPERTENSION IN PREGNANCY

Drugs	Dosage and Route of Administration	Nursing Interventions	Side Effects	Fetal Implications
Magnesium sulfate Decreases the amount of acetylcholine released by motor nerve impulse; thereby depresses CNS and provides anticonvulsant effects; also acts peripherally as vasodilator, thus reducing blood pressure *Effect* *Serum Magnesium Levels* Anticonvulsant 4–6 mEq/L prophylaxis ECG changes 5–10 mEq/L Loss of DTRs 10 mEq/L Respiratory paralysis 15 mEq/L General anesthesia Over 15 mEq/L Cardiac arrest Over 25 mEq/L Use with caution in clients with impaired renal function; contraindicated in clients with heart block or myocardial damage	IV: 4-g loading dose (50% solution diluted to make a 10% solution—not to exceed 200 mg/ml) followed by 1 to 2-g/hr infusion, monitored by infusion pump or controller IM: 10 g of 50% solution (5 g in each buttock by Z-track technique); this route is rarely used and should be used only to maintain adequate plasma levels when nursing staff is unavailable to adequately monitor client	1. Respiratory status: at least 12/min 2. Reflexes: DTR, patellar, biceps, triceps—should be at least 1+ (absence is early sign of magnesium toxicity) 3. Blood pressure and pulse: 5–15 minutes initially, then every 15 minutes 4. Urinary output at least 30 ml/hr; use urimeter with severe pre-eclamptics (magnesium is excreted by the kidney) 5. Place resuscitation and seizure supplies in room 6. Monitor fetal status 7. Monitor serum magnesium levels every 4 hours 8. Place magnesium antidote at bedside: calcium gluconate or gluceptate, 1 g pushed over 3 minutes for magnesium toxicity	Respiratory depression Decreased urinary output Hypotonia Magnesium toxicity	Hypotonia Temperature control Respiratory depression
Hydralazine (Apresoline) Antihypertensive: reduces blood pressure by direct relaxation of vascular smooth	IV: 5–10 mg slowly; takes effect in 10 to 80 minutes; if no response,	1. Monitor blood pressure every 2–3 minutes after dosing for 30	Headache Palpitations Lupuslike syndrome	Improvement of uteroplacental blood flow

Drug/Action	Dosage	Nursing considerations	Side effects	Fetal/other effects
muscle: resultant vasodilation reduces peripheral vascular resistance, increases cerebral and renal blood flow and uterine perfusion	repeat dose in 20 minutes IM: 10–50 mg; takes effect over 15 minutes and lasts 3–4 hours; this route is not usually recommended because of generalized edema and inconsistent absorption	minutes 2. Assess urinary output 3. Monitor fetus	Hypotension	Reduction of blood flow to fetus decreases oxygenation Fetal distress
Sodium nitroprusside Direct dilatation of arterioles and veins	IV: IV solution 0.01 g/L infused at a rate of 0.2–0.8 mg/min; takes effect in 1/2–2 minutes and lasts 3–5 minutes	1. Blood pressure monitoring 2. ICU nurse in attendance 3. Useful only for short-term control	Hypotension	Cyanide toxicity in fetus
Other drugs for hypertension Methyldopa (Aldomet)	Oral agents 1 g initially oral route and maintainance 1 to 2 g/day in four divided doses	1. Assist client when ambulating 2. Monitor fetal heart rate	Postural hypotension, drowsiness, fluid retention	To improve blood flow and promote fetal growth; however, beta-blockers can cross the placenta: a question is raised regarding IUGR Safety and efficacy unknown during pregnancy
Clonidine	IV: 150 µg in 10 cc saline given over 5 minutes	Take blood pressure every 2–3 minutes for 30–45 minutes	Rebound hypertension abrupt discontinuation	
Prazosin (Minipress)	1 mg twice daily, used in doses as high as 20 mg/day orally	Observe client or give instructions to client and family	Hypotension (especially with first dose) Drowsiness	Improves blood flow by lowering systolic and diastolic pressures Experience is limited
Atenolol (Tenormin)	100–200 mg orally	Give instructions to client and family	Weariness, exhaustion	
Propranolol	40–240 mg orally			Associated with neonatal bradycardia, hypoglycemia, IUGR, and neonatal respiratory depression
Thiazide diuretics	Not recommended		Adverse maternal effects: Hypokalemia Hyponatremia Elevated uric acid Hemorrhagic pancreatitis and even death	Electrolyte imbalance Thrombocytopenia Small for gestational age
Nifedipine (Procardia)	10 mg orally every 30 minutes × 3 doses, then every 4–8 hours	Assess blood pressure every 2–3 minutes for 1 hour	Rapid lowering of blood pressure Hypotension	Maximizes blood flow

(b) Visual changes and disturbances

(c) Level of consciousness

(5) Maintain client on bed rest in the left lateral position (Fig. 26–2)

(6) Administer drugs to dilate vasculature (see Table 26–2 for drug information)

(7) As preventive measure for PIH in general, low-dose aspirin, 60 to 150 mg/day may be prescribed (Benigni, Gregorini, Frusca, Chiabrando, Ballerini, Valcomonico, Orisio, Piccinelli, Pinciroli, Fanelli, Gastaldi, & Remuzzi, 1986; Lubbe, 1987; Schiff, Peleg, Goldenberg, Rosenthal, Ruppin, Tamarkin, Barkai, Ben-Baruch, Yahat, Blanstein, Goldman, & Mashiach, 1989; Wallenburg, Dekker, Makovitz, & Rotmans, 1986); assess bleeding at any site

(a) Urine (hematuria)

(b) Gums

(c) IV site

(d) Skin (petechiae)

b. Evaluations

(1) Blood pressure remains within acceptable limits

(2) Fluid balance is maintained, with urinary output greater than 30 ml/hr

(3) Deep tendon reflexes are within normal limits, with no clonus observed

(4) There are no reported symptoms of headaches or visual disturbances

(5) Level of consciousness is appropriate

(6) No seizures or other CNS damage is seen

2. Altered tissue perfusion related to renal disturbances

a. Interventions

(1) Assess for edema of face and hands and pitting edema of feet and ankles

(2) Document I & O

(a) Use urimeter for hourly output measurement with severely preeclamptic clients

(b) Monitor urinary protein status

(3) Weigh the client daily

(4) Administer drugs to dilate vasculature (see Table 26–2 for complete drug information)

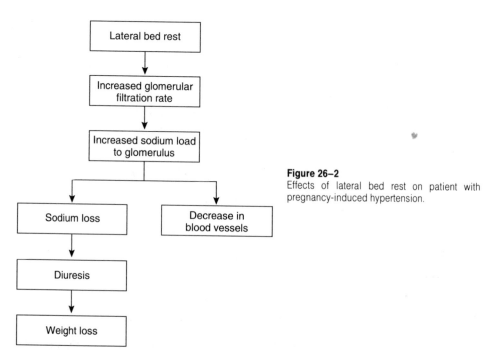

Figure 26–2
Effects of lateral bed rest on patient with pregnancy-induced hypertension.

b. Evaluations
    (1) No excessive edema is observed
    (2) I & O balance is maintained with urinary output greater than 30 ml/hr
    (3) Weight gain is within normal limits
3. Altered tissue perfusion related to cardiovascular disturbances
  a. Interventions
    (1) Take vital signs every 15 to 30 minutes
    (2) Observe for and report any cardiac irregularities, tachycardia, or chest pain
    (3) Observe for neck vein distension
    (4) Assess for generalized edema
    (5) Assess capillary refill time (may be decreased)
    (6) Assess temperature of extremities
  b. Evaluations
    (1) Vital signs remain within normal limits
    (2) No cardiac disturbances are observed
    (3) No neck vein distension is observed
    (4) No signs of congestive heart failure (CHF) are noted
    (5) Capillary refill is within normal limits
    (6) Extremities are neither cold nor excessively warm
4. High risk for altered respiratory function: decreased related to excessive fluid volume
  a. Interventions
    (1) Take vital signs, especially respiratory rate, every 15 to 30 minutes
    (2) Assess breath sounds and listen for rales
    (3) Observe pulmonary status
      (a) Dyspnea
      (b) Shortness of breath
      (c) Tachypnea
    (4) Listen for dry, hacking cough
    (5) Administer oxygen at 10 to 12 L/min as needed
    (6) Interpret blood gases
  b. Evaluations
    (1) Vital signs are within normal limits
    (2) No pulmonary edema is documented
    (3) No signs of respiratory distress are noted
    (4) Blood gases remain within normal limits
5. High risk for hepatic injury related to hypertension
  a. Interventions
    (1) Assess epigastric pain
    (2) Observe for and assess degree of jaundice, if present
    (3) Observe for signs of shock and be prepared for immediate intervention
    (4) Avoid fundal pressure at time of delivery
  b. Evaluations
    (1) No signs of hepatic injury or rupture are observed
    (2) Jaundice is documented
6. High risk for impaired fetal well-being related to altered uteroplacental perfusion
  a. Interventions
    (1) Maintain client on bed rest in the lateral position
    (2) Treat mother for altered tissue perfusion
    (3) Provide for prenatal care
      (a) Provide for antepartum testing as ordered
        (i) NST, CST
        (ii) Biophysical profile, with amniotic fluid index
        (iii) Ultrasound for possible IUGR
        (iv) Doppler flow studies for impaired uterine artery perfusion

(b) Instruct mother in technique for daily fetal movement counts (see Chapter 11 for complete discussion of antepartum tests)
(4) Continuous electronic fetal monitoring (EFM) while in labor
  (a) Observe for signs indicative of fetal distress (see Chapter 16 for complete discussion of fetal assessment during labor)
    (i) Tachycardia or bradycardia
    (ii) Severe variable decelerations, especially with documented oligo-hydramnios
    (iii) Late decelerations
    (iv) Decreased variability
  (b) Report any nonreassuring signs to physician or certified nurse midwife (CNM)
b. Evaluations
  (1) Bed rest in the lateral position is maintained
  (2) Mother is treated for altered tissue perfusion
  (3) Antepartum tests are within normal limits
  (4) Reassuring heart rate and variability are seen during labor
6. Anxiety and fear related to risk of harm to self and fetus
  a. Interventions
    (1) Explain disease process appropriately for client's and family's level of understanding
    (2) Explain rationale for interventions and anticipate possible actions
    (3) Clarify and interpret results of antepartum tests
    (4) Reassure the client as to fetal status
    (5) Involve the family in care
      (a) Explain the need for the client to remain on bed rest
      (b) Assist in mobilizing resources to take over the client's usual functions
      (c) Refer to social services if necessary for community and financial support
  b. Evaluations
    (1) Mother reports a decrease in anxiety
    (2) Family members act as support system
    (3) Assistance is obtained from other resources as needed

Health Education

A. Provide the client and her family with the following information

1. The effect of hypertension on all organ systems and the potential for harm resulting from altered tissue perfusion and edema
2. The effect of hypertension on the fetus: with reduction of blood flow to the uterus, and resultant decrease in nutrients and oxygen, the fetus may be growth retarded and experience hypoxia
3. The importance of activity restriction and rest, especially in the left lateral position
4. The signs and symptoms of worsening of condition and when to report them to the health care provider
5. The prenatal monitoring that will be done
   a. Antepartum tests for fetal well-being
   b. Laboratory work
   c. Frequent visits to health care provider

B. Methods of teaching

1. Participate in one-to-one teaching with diagrams of blood vessels, heart, and kidneys if the client has mild PIH
2. Meet with the family to discuss the requirements of care

3. Arrange a meeting with the social worker to assess financial needs, emotional needs, and plan solutions
4. Use interpreters (or other teaching aids) if the client or family cannot speak English
5. Use videotapes or books
6. Review teaching in 1 to 2 weeks, because the client's perception is clouded owing to her state of denial, anxiety, lack of comprehension, general knowledge base
7. Help the family to recognize the life-threatening potential of this condition
8. Assist the client with developing her support systems to assist with her care (including special preparation of food, if necessary) and with child care if needed

CASE STUDIES AND STUDY QUESTIONS

Christine, a 22-year-old, G1,P0 Afro-American woman, is admitted with blood pressure of 148/96, which at her last two prenatal visits had been 130/80 and 140/90. Her prenatal blood pressure was 90 to 100/60 to 70. She has been on lateral bed rest for 1 week. Her weight gain in the past 2 weeks has been 3.2 kg (7 lb) and 3.6 kg (8 lb) each week. She has pedal edema and is spilling 3+ protein in her urine. Christine is given a 4-g loading dose of magnesium sulfate followed by a 2-g/hr maintenance dose. Her laboratory reports remain within normal limits, with the exception of the elevated urine protein. The decision is made to continue with lateral bed rest. Orders are written for blood pressure checks every 30 minutes, I & O, daily weight, deep tendon reflexes checks, and a protein check with every voiding. Serial fetal surveillance with ultrasound scans and NST is instituted.

1. Which of the following is the most common warning sign of pre-eclampsia?

   a. Proteinuria.

   b. Headache.

   c. Edema.

   d. Increased blood pressure.

   e. Epigastric pain.

2. The nurse would suspect the diagnosis of PIH if she found which of the following in her assessment?

   a. Ankle edema and glucosuria.

   b. Glucosuria and proteinuria.

   c. Proteinuria and hypertension.

   d. Hypertension and hyporeflexia.

3. All of the following physiological changes may be present in Christine except:

   a. Increased arterial blood pressure.

   b. Decreased peripheral vascular resistance.

   c. Decreased plasma renin activity.

   d. Increased pressor responsiveness to angiotensin II.

4. Christine has the signs and symptoms of severe pre-eclampsia. Her conditon is worsening. What signs might you expect?

   a. Blood pressure of 160/110.

   b. Proteinuria 3+ to 4+, 5 g in 24-hour urine testing.

   c. Hematuria.

   d. Diminished reflexes.

The client has a clonic/tonic seizure. She is turned to a lateral position. After the seizure, reflexes are hyperactive and clonus is present. The fetus experienced a bradycardic episode from the maternal apnea. Oxygen is administered at 10 L/min via a face mask to assist the fetus with intrauterine resuscitation. Delivery is not attempted at this time, so the patient can be stabilized. Diazepam was used at the time of the seizure.

5. Which of the following is the major complication from a seizure?

   a. Aspiration

   b. CHF

   c. Uremia

   d. Infection

6. In eclampsia, where are lesions found?

    a. The brain.

    b. The kidney.

    c. The heart.

    d. The lungs.

    e. All organs.

7. What renal lesion is most associated with eclampsia?

    a. Glomerular endothelial swelling.

    b. Pyelonephritis.

    c. Hydroureter.

    d. Cortical necrosis.

    e. Acute tubular necrosis.

8. If a client is eclamptic in more than one pregnancy, she is more likely to develop which of the following?

    a. Epilepsy.

    b. Diabetes.

    c. Hypertension.

    d. Arthritis.

    e. Amniotic fluid embolus.

Celia, a 29-year-old, G2,P1 woman with chronic hypertension of 2 years' duration and superimposed pre-eclampsia is at 34 weeks' gestation. Her baseline blood pressure had been 130/90; 1 week ago her blood pressure was 160/105, 2 days ago it was 165/110, and today it is 170/110. Celia has had a 2.3-kg (5-lb) weight gain in one week, 3+ pitting edema, and 4+ proteinuria. Her usual hypertension medications are methyldopa (Aldomet) and hydralazine. Celia is managed with one-to-one nursing care, with precautions taken to prevent seizures, administration of IV magnesium sulfate, an indwelling catheter with a urimeter, blood pressure checks every 15 minutes, reflexes and clonus checks, IV fluid balance monitoring, hypertensive medications, and EFM. Laboratory work was drawn for CBC, liver enzymes tests, and renal function studies. Induction of labor will be initiated once the client is stabilized.

9. What laboratory values would you expect with Celia?

a. Creatinine of 0.9 mg/dl.

b. Uric acid of over 10 mg/dl.

c. Urine protein of 4 g.

d. SGOT of 40 IU/L.

10. Clients with hypertension are at risk for damage to many organs during pregnancy. What change increases that risk?

    a. Poor renal function.

    b. Cardiac enlargement.

    c. Advanced retinal changes.

    d. Poor pulmonary function.

    e. History of pre-eclampsia superimposed on the hypertension.

11. Magnesium sulfate should not be administered if which of the following is true?

    a. Respirations are 16/min.

    b. Reflexes are 2+.

    c. Irritability and nervousness are evident.

    d. Urinary output is below 20 ml/hr.

Estelle, a 37-year-old, G4,P3 woman, gave birth 1 hour ago. She had a normal spontaneous vaginal delivery of a female infant weighing 8 lb 10 oz. (3912 g) with Apgar scores of 9 and 9. During recovery, Estelle's blood pressure was 147/90, 152/97, 160/96, 160/90. No edema is evident, and her urine is negative for protein. All laboratory values were normal. The following day, Estelle's blood pressure remained elevated. The client and infant were discharged with office follow-up. Her blood pressure remained elevated for 10 days.

12. When all laboratory values are returned normal, and the patient has only hypertension, one must suspect _____ _____ hypertension.

Debbie, a 32-year-old woman, G1,P0 at 33 weeks' gestation, has had an elevated blood pressure of 140/90 for 2 weeks, with proteinuria and generalized edema, and has stayed at home on bed rest. She was hospitalized with severe epigastric pain. Laboratory values demonstrated hemolysis with an abnormal peripheral blood smear, an increased bilirubin of over 1.2 mg/dl, elevated liver enzymes (SGOT of over 72 IU/L and lactate dehydrogenase (LDH) increased above 600 IU/L) and a platelet count of less than 100,000.

13. The HELLP syndrome has potential maternal and fetal mortality and morbidity. Which of the following factors are involved?

    (1) Low platelets.

    (2) Hemolysis.

    (3) Hyperbilirubinemia.

    (4) Proteinuria.

    (5) Elevated liver enzymes.

    a. 1, 2, 3.

    b. 2, 4, 5.

    c. 1, 2, 5.

    d. 5 only.

14. Josie is a 16-year-old woman at 37 weeks' gestation with a blood pressure of 155/105, 3+ proteinuria, 4+ pitting edema of the feet and ankles, nonpitting edema of face and neck, and no seizure activity. She probably has which of the following?

    a. Mild pre-eclampsia.

    b. Severe pre-eclampsia.

    c. Gestational hypertension.

    d. Eclampsia.

    e. None of the above.

15. Which of the following is found in severely pre-eclamptic patients?

    a. Decreased response to angiotensin II.

    b. Reduced plasma volume and increased hematocrit.

    c. Decrease in total body sodium.

    d. Increase in uric acid.

    e. Reduced potassium.

16. Which of the following are warning signals of PIH that should be watched for during the course of prenatal care?

    (1) Sudden excessive weight gain (greater than 2 or 3 lb/wk.) (0.9-1.4 kg)

    (2) Generalized skin rash.

    (3) An elevation of blood pressure greater than 15 mm Hg in diastolic pressure over previously recorded levels.

    (4) An elevation of more than 30 mm Hg in systolic pressure over previously recorded levels.

    a. 1, 2, 3.

    b. 1, 2.

    c. 3, 4.

    d. 1, 3, 4.

17. A 40-year-old, G5, P4 hypertensive woman at 32 weeks' gestation who has a blood pressure of 180/120 (which has not changed during her pregnancy) and no edema or proteinuria—but who has retinal changes—has which of the following?

    a. Pre-eclampsia.

    b. Severe pre-eclampsia.

    c. Chronic hypertension.

    d. Superimposed pre-eclampsia.

    e. Renal disease.

18. Which of the following is not characteristic of magnesium sulfate used in treatment of pre-eclampsia.

    a. It has no effect on the fetus.

    b. It is a smooth muscle relaxant.

    c. It has a large margin of safety.

    d. It is a CNS depressant.

    e. It improves uterine blood flow.

19. A 30-year-old woman at 16 weeks' gestation with a blood pressure of 144/95, no edema, and no proteinuria (once hydatidiform mole is ruled out) probably has which of the following?

    a. Pre-eclampsia.

    b. Pre-existing hypertension.

    c. Renal disease.

    d. Diabetes.

Answers to Study Questions

1. d	2. c	3. b	13. c	14. b	15. b
4. a, b	5. a	6. e	16. d	17. c	18. a
7. a	8. c	9. b	19. b		
10. e	11. d	12. transient			

REFERENCES

Abrams, B., & Parker, J. (1988). Overweight and pregnancy complications. *International Journal of Obesity, 12*(4), 293–303.

ACOG Technical Bulletin (1986). *Management of preeclampsia. 19.* Washington, DC: ACOG.

Anderson, G.D., & Sibai, B.M. (1986). *Obstetrics: Normal and problem pregnancies.* New York: Churchill Livingstone.

Belizan, J., Villar, J., & Repke, J. (1988). The relationship between calcium intake and pregnancy-induced hypertension: Up-to-date evidence. *American Journal of Obstetrics and Gynecology, 158*(4), 898–902.

Benigni, A., Gregorini, G., Frusca, T., Chiabrando, C., Ballerini, S., Valcamonico, A., Orisio, S., Piccinelli, A., Pinciroli, V., Fannelli, R., Gastaldi, A., & Remuzzi, G. (1986). Blood supply to the uterus in preeclampsia: Effect of low-dose aspirin on fetal and maternal generation of thromboxane by platelets in women at risk for pregnancy-induced hypertension. *New England Journal of Medicine, 321,* 357–362.

Brinkman, C.R., III (1986). *Essentials of obstetrics and gynecology.* Philadelphia: Saunders.

Campbell, S., Bewley, S., & Cohen-Overbeek, T. (1987). Investigation of the uteroplacental circulation by Doppler ultrasound. *Seminars in Perinatology, 11*(4), 362–368.

Chesley, L. (1978). *Hypertension and renal diseases, hypertensive disorders in pregnancy* (2nd ed.). New York: Appleton-Century-Crofts.

Chesley, L. (1985). Hypertensive disorders in pregnancy. In N. Gleicher (Ed.), *Principles of medical therapy in pregnancy* (p. 751). New York: Plenum.

Doan-Wiggins, L. (1987). Hypertensive disorders of pregnancy. *Emergency Medicine Clinics of North America, 5*(3), 495–508.

Gant, N., Whalley, P., Everett, R., Worley, R., & MacDonald, P. (1987). Control of vascular reactivity in pregnancy. *American Journal of Kidney Disease, 9*(4) 303–307.

Gant, N., & Worley, R. (1980). *Hypertensions in pregnancy: Concepts and management.* New York: Appleton-Century-Crofts.

Gavette, L., & Roberts, J. (1987). Use of mean arterial pressure (MAP-2) to predict pregnancy-induced hypertension in adolescents. *Journal of Nurse-Midwifery, 32*(6), 357–364.

Hacker, N., & Moore, J. (1986). *Essentials of obstetrics and gynecology.* Philadelphia: Saunders.

Jensen, M., Bobak, I. (1985). *Maternity and gynecologic care* (3rd ed., pp. 14–25). St. Louis: Mosby.

Koniak-Griffin, D., & Dodgson, J. (1987). Severe pregnancy-induced hypertension: Postpartum care of the critically ill patient. *Heart & Lung, 16*(6), 661–669.

Lubbe, W. (1987). Hypertension in pregnancy: Whom and how to treat. *British Journal of Clinical Pharmacology, 24*(Suppl. 1), 15S–20S.

Metcalfe, J., McAnulty, J., & Ueland, K. (1986). *Heart disease and pregnancy* (pp. 279–289). Boston: Little, Brown.

Poole, J. (1988, November/December). Getting perspective on HELLP syndrome. *Maternal Child Nursing, 13,* 432–437.

Pritchard, J., Cunningham, F., & Mason, R. (1976). Coagulation changes in eclampsia: Their frequency and pathogenesis. *American Journal of Obstetrics and Gynecology, 124*(8), 855–864.

Pritchard, J., MacDonald, P., & Gant, N. (Eds.). (1985). *Williams' obstetrics* (17th ed.) Norwalk, CT: Appleton-Century-Crofts.

Reeder, S., & Martin, L. (1987). *Maternity nursing: Family, newborn, and women's health care* (16th ed.). Philadelphia: Lippincott.

Rubin, P. (1987). Hypertension in pregnancy. *Journal of Hypertension Supplement, 5*(3), 557–560.

Schiff, E., Peleg, E., Goldenberg, M., Rosenthal, T., Ruppin, E., Tamarkin, M., Barkai, G., Ben-Baruch, G., Yahat, I., Blanstein, J., Goldman, B., & Maschiach, S. (1989). The use of aspirin to prevent pregnancy-induced hypertension and lower the ratio of thromboxane A2 to prostacyclin in relatively high-risk pregnancies. *New England Journal of Medicine, 321,* 351–356.

Shannon, D. (1987). HELLP syndrome: A severe consequence of pregnancy-induced hypertension, hemolysis, elevated liver enzymes and low platelets. *Journal of Obstetric, Gynecologic, and Neonatal Nursing, 16*(6), 395–402.

Sherwen, L., Scoloveno, M., & Weingarten, C. (1991). *Nursing care of the childbearing family.* Norwalk, CT: Appleton & Lange.

Talledo, O., Chesley, L., & Zuspan, F. (1968). Renin-angiotensin system in normal and toxemic pregnancies. III. Differential sensitivity to angiotensin II and norephinephrine in toxemia of pregnancy. *American Journal of Obstetrics and Gynecology, 100*(2), 213–221.

Van Assche, F., Spitz, B., & Vansteelant, L. (1989). Severe systemic hypertension during pregnancy. *American Journal of Cardiology, 63*(6), 22C–25C.

Wallenburg, H., Dekker, G., Makovitz, J., & Rotmans, P. (1986). Low-dose aspirin prevents pregnancy-induced hypertension and pre-eclampsia in angiotensin-sensitive primigravidae. *Lancet, 1,* 1–3.

Wasserstrum, N., & Cotton, D. (1986). Hemodynamic monitoring in severe pregnancy-induced hypertension. *Clinics in Perinatology, 13*(4), 781–799.

Barbara A. Moran

Maternal Infections

Objectives

1. Define TORCH

2. List one symptom related to each infection that TORCH comprises

3. Identify causative pathogens in perinatal infections

4. Identify risk groups for AIDS and other STDs

5. Define health education strategies to prevent maternal infections

6. Recognize clinical signs and symptoms of perinatal infections

7. Correlate history and physical findings with early indicators of maternal infection

8. Formulate nursing interventions from information obtained in the history

9. Discuss potential fetal complications associated with maternal infections

TORCH

Introduction: TORCH

A. **TORCH is an acronym for a group of five infectious diseases**

1. Toxoplasmosis
2. Other (hepatitis B)
3. Rubella
4. Cytomegalovirus (CMV)
5. Herpes simplex virus (HSV)

B. **Each disease is teratogenic**

1. Each crosses the placenta
2. Each may adversely affect the developing fetus
3. The effect of each varies, depending on developmental stage at time of exposure

C. Statistics: Active maternal infection is present in approximately 15% of all pregnancies

D. Nursing interventions
1. Health education
2. Prevention

Clinical Practice: TORCH

See Table 27–1 for complete discussion of each component of TORCH, maternal and fetal effects, and treatment.

A. Assessment
1. History
   a. Flulike illness
   b. Fever of unknown origin
   c. Exposure to sick children
   d. Rash
   e. Painful genital lesions
   f. Close contact with possibly infected cats (outside-dwelling cats)
   g. Chronic fatigue
   h. Blood or secretion exposure
   i. Raw meat ingestion
2. Physical findings
   a. Lymphadenopathy: suboccipital, postauricular, cervical
   b. Rash: pink or red maculopapules
   c. Ulcerated, painful lesions on the cervix, vagina, and genital area
   d. Low-grade temperature
   e. Headache
   f. Malaise
   g. Anorexia
   h. Jaundice
   i. Hepatomegaly
   j. Arthralgias or arthritis
   k. Nausea and vomiting
   l. Clay-colored stool
3. Psychosocial findings
   a. Anxiety
   b. Fear
   c. Apprehension
4. Diagnostic findings
   a. Complete blood count (CBC) (WBC count increased to over 12,000)
   b. TORCH screen
   c. IgG-specific antibody (i.e., rubella-specific IgG to document prior infection)
   d. IgM-specific antibody (i.e., rubella-specific IgM to confirm recent infection; it becomes detectable about 1 week after onset of illness and persists for about 1 month)
   e. Papanicolaou's (PAP) smear for herpetic morphologic changes
   f. Culturing of lesions for CMV and HSV
   g. Hepatitis B surface antigen (HBsAg) is present in blood 30 to 50 days after exposure and 7 to 21 days before the onset of jaundice
   h. Alanine amino transferase (ALT) levels rise about 50 days after exposure and persist for 30 to 60 or more days
   i. Hepatitis B e antigen (HBeAg): the presence of e antigen denotes a high degree of infectivity

    j. Enzyme-linked immunosorbent assay (ELISA)
    k. Liver function
       (1) Elevated bilirubin levels
       (2) Elevated transaminase enzyme levels
    l. Serial sonography (to detect intrauterine growth retardation [IUGR])

B. Nursing Diagnoses

1. Knowledge deficit related to infection and its treatment
2. Anxiety and fear related to possible sequelae
3. High risk for injury related to infection

C. Interventions/Evaluations

1. Knowledge deficit related to infection and its treatment
    a. Interventions
       (1) Give factual information on the infection: mode of transmission and possible sequelae
       (2) Give directions on any medication the client needs to take
       (3) Provide written material that contains the same information at the client's level of understanding
       (4) Review options in cases of known teratogenic effects
    b. Evaluations
       (1) Client is able to verbalize knowledge about the infection and treatment needed
       (2) Client is able to verbalize signs and symptoms that would indicate a need to seek further care
       (3) Client is able to use self-care measures and to comply with recommended regimen
2. Anxiety and fear related to possible sequelae
    a. Interventions
       (1) Provide information as described above to increase the client's sense of control and decrease anxiety by minimizing fear of unknown
       (2) Develop trust and rapport by being nonjudgmental
       (3) Give information in a calm and consistent manner
       (4) Have client's significant other involved in counseling if the client desires
       (5) Encourage questions and verbalizations of fears
    b. Evaluation: client is able to verbalize decreased anxiety related to infection
3. High risk for injury related to infection
    a. Interventions
       (1) Teach importance of follow-up care
       (2) Teach mode of transmission
       (3) Breastfeeding is usually not discouraged
    b. Evaluation: client is able to minimize and prevent further risk factors

Health Education

A. Stress the need to vaccinate susceptible women before conception or immediately postpartum

B. Instruct the client on good handwashing, especially after handling raw meat

C. Wash all kitchen surfaces that come into contact with uncooked meat

D. Instruct the client to avoid eating insufficiently cooked meat

E. Instruct the client to avoid contact with cat feces in litter boxes during pregnancy and avoid gardening in soil contaminated with cat feces

Table 27–1
TORCH DISEASE

Infection	Agent	Mode of Transmission	Detection	Maternal Effects
Toxoplasmosis	• Protozoa • *Toxoplasma gondii*	• Eating raw meat containing *T. gondii* • Ingesting *T. gondii* cysts secreted in feces of infected cats • Transplacentally • Impossible to transmit to others since the infecting organisms are tissue bound and are not excreted	• Serological antibody testing • ELISA	• 90% of women are asymptomatic • Posterior cervical lymphadenopathy • Malaise • Premature labor and delivery
Hepatitis B	• Hepatitis B virus (HBV) • Incubation: usually 50–180 days	• Sexually • Perinatally • Transplacentally • Contact with maternal blood • Close personal contact • Blood, stool, and saliva transmission • Shared razors, toothbrushes, towels, and other personal items	• HbsAg • HbeAg • Alanine amino transferase (ALT) increased 50 days after exposure • Anti-HBsA: individual is immune and noninfectious • Anti-HBeAg: individual is less likely to be infectious	• Fever • Jaundice • Hepatomegaly • Malaise • Premature labor
Rubella	• Rubella virus • Incubation: 2–3 weeks	• Nasopharyngeal secretions • Transplacentally	• Serological antibody titer testing (IgG-specific rubella antibody) • Virus isolation from throat	• Pink, maculopapular rash on face, neck, arms, and legs lasting 3 days • Lymph node enlargement • Slight fever • Malaise, • Headache • History of exposure 3 weeks earlier
Cytomegalovirus (CMV)	• Virus • Incubation: unknown	• Intimate contact with infected secretions (breast milk, cervical mucus, semen, saliva, and urine) • Transplacentally • Organ transplantation	• ELISA • IgM-specific • Isolation of virus from urine or endocervical secretions	• Clinically "silent"—only 1–5% develop symptoms: Low-grade fever Malaise Arthralgia Hepatomegaly

Neonatal Effects	Treatment	Incidence and Prevention	High-Risk Potential
• Severity varies with gestational age (usually, earlier infection results in more severe effects) • Neurological, opthalmological, and cognitive sequelae are variable • IUGR • Hydrocephaly • Microcephaly	• Pyrimethamine and sulfadiazine during second and third trimesters can reduce incidence of congenital toxoplasmosis by about 50%	• Incidence varies throughout world (1–4 infants per 1000 live births) • 20–30% of U.S. women have been exposed • Incidence of congenital toxoplasmosis infection in U.S. is 1 in 1000–8000	• Populations that consume raw or poorly cooked meat • High-risk gestational age is 10–24 weeks
• Increased risk of transmission to infant if mother is HBeAg-positive (indicating acute infection) • Stillbirth • Clinical illness is relatively infrequent • Most (90–95%) of those infected are asymptomatic and become chronic hepatitis B carriers	• Mother: rest • Infant: vaccine • Heptavax-B • Recombivax-Hb • If mother is carrier, infant receives hepatitis B immunoglobulin	• Acute infection occurs in 1–2 per 1000 pregnancies • 4–13% of population of Southeast Asia • 1500 reported cases in Canada in 1988 • Minimize exposure of close physical contact • Heptavax-B (pregnancy does not contraindicate vaccination)	• Southeast Asians • Eskimos • Africans • Prostitutes • Homosexuals • IV drug users • Hemophiliacs • Transfusion recipients

• Significant damage occurs in approximately
   50% of fetuses in first month
   20–25% of fetus in second month
   6–10% of fetus in third month
• Spectrum anomalies:
   Deafness: 60–70%
   Eye defects: 10–30%
   CNS defects: 10–25%
   Heart defects: 10–20%
• Virus sheds for 6–12 months ("cloud baby")
	• Women with rubella require no special therapy other than mild analgesics and rest
	• Neonates must be recognized as potential sources of rubella infection and should be isolated
		• Last epidemic in 1964; since introduction of vaccine in late 1960s, rubella is rare
		• Occurs more commonly in springtime
		• Vaccine is contraindicated during pregnancy
			• Occurs primarily in young children and adolescents
			• Unimmunized populations (10–20)% of U.S. population is not immune)

• Most (90–95%) of those infected are asymptomatic
• Infection is most likely to occur with primary maternal infection
• Cytomegalic inclusion disease (CID) is rare (1/10,000–20,000 newborns):
   IUGR
   Microcephaly
   Periventricular calcification
   Sensorineural deafness
   Blindness with chorioretinitis
   Mental retardation
   Hepatosplenomegaly
	• Mother: treat symptoms
	• Infant: no satisfactory treatment is available
	• Isolate infant
		• Most common viral perinatal infectious agent
		• Occurs in 1–2% of pregnant women
		• Most people in U.S. have been infected
		• Prevalence depends on age, race, sex, class, sexual behavior, and occupational or institutional exposure
		• Rigorous personal hygiene throughout pregnancy
		• Vaccine is experimental
			• Workers in daycare centers
			• Persons undergoing renal dialysis
			• Immunocompromised persons

Table continued on following pages

Table 27–1 *Continued*

Infection	Agent	Mode of Transmission	Detection	Maternal Effects
Herpes simplex virus (HSV)	• Herpesvirus • Incubation 2–10 days	• Intimate mucocutaneous exposure • Passage through an infected birth canal • Ascending infection especially with rupture of membranes (ROM) • Transplacentally (although rare) if initial infection occurs during pregnancy	• Tissue culture (swab specimen from vesicles) • Vesicles on cervix, vagina, or external genital area • Swelling, redness, and painful lesions • Papanicolaou smear	• Painful genital lesions • Primary infection is commonly associated with fever, malaise, myalgias • Numbness, tingling, burning, itching, and pain with lesions • Lymphadenopathy • Urinary retention

Acquired Immunodeficiency Syndrome

Introduction: Acquired Immunodeficiency Syndrome

A. Major public health issue: first recognized in 1981

B. Human immunodeficiency virus (HIV)

1. Agent: retrovirus (RNA virus)
2. Transmitted by exposure to blood and blood products
   a. Transfusions
   b. Needle sharing among addicts
   c. Accidental inoculation in health care workers
3. Perinatal exposure
   a. Intrauterine
   b. Peripartum
   c. Breastfeeding
4. Sexual contact
5. Not transmitted through casual contact (e.g., water, food, and environmental services)

C. High-risk groups

1. Male homosexuals
2. Male bisexuals
3. Prostitutes
4. Hemophiliacs
5. Drug abusers
6. Sexual partners of these groups

D. Women and the acquired immunodeficiency syndrome (AIDS)

1. Total number of AIDS cases reported in the United States through November 1991 was 202,843
2. Total number of female AIDS cases reported in the United States was 20,739 (10.9% of all reported cases) See Figs. 27–1 and 27–2

Table 27–1 *Continued*

Neonatal Effects	Treatment	Incidence and Prevention	High-Risk Potential
• Rare transplacental transmissions have resulted in miscarriages • Mortality of 50–60% if neonatal exposure is with active primary infection • Neurological or ophthalmic sequelae • Disseminated infection in 70% of cases, with jaundice, respiratory distress, and CNS involvement	• Acyclovir is not used during pregnancy • Protect neonate from exposure at time of delivery • Cultures are done when mother has active lesions • Avoid routine use of scalp electrodes • If lesions are visible, delivery should be by cesarean section	• Not reported to CDC • Estimated 300,000 new cases per year • 1 in 5000–7500 live births with perinatal transmission • Up to 70% of women delivering infected infants have no history of genital herpes • Avoid genital contact when male partner has penile lesions • Use condoms	• Multiple sex partners

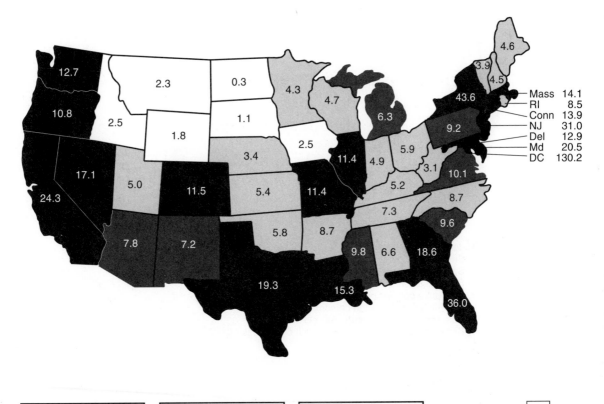

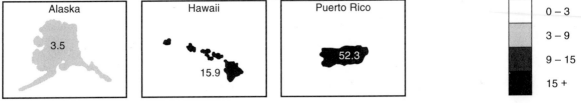

Figure 27–1
AIDS annual rates per 100,000 population for cases reported March 1990 through February 1991 in the United States. (HIV/AIDS Surveillance Report. [March, 1991]. Atlanta, GA: Centers for Disease Control.)

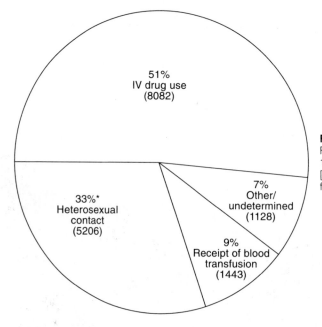

Figure 27–2
Female exposure category, January 1991 (HIV/AIDS Surveillance Report [February 1991]. Atlanta, GA: Centers for Disease Control)

*Heterosexual contact
   Sex with an IV drug abuser: 3257 (63%)
   Sex with a bisexual woman: 510 (10%)
   Sex with a person with hemophilia: 76 (.01%)
   Sex with a transfusion recipient with HIV infection: 110 (22%)
   Sex with an HIV-infected person: 634 (12%)
   Born in a Pattern II country: 563 (11%)
   Sex with a person born in a Pattern II country: 56 (.01%)

3. 100,000 women are infected with the virus
4. 11.4 million women are at risk
5. Percentage of infected women is increasing
    a. 1981: women were 3% of total cases
    b. 1985: women were 6.6% of total cases
    c. 1989: women were 10.9% of total cases
6. 30% of women with AIDS are infected through heterosexual contact with infected partner
7. Perinatal transmission is estimated to be 25 to 50%

E. Azidothymidine (AZT)

1. AZT is used for symptomatic clients
2. No data on safety in pregnancy are available
3. It is not known whether AZT alters perinatal transmission

F. Opportunistic infections associated with AIDS

1. *Pneumocystis carinii* pneumonia (most common)
2. Toxoplasmosis
3. Candidiasis (thrush)
4. Mycobacterial infections
5. CMV
6. HSV
7. Syphilis
8. Tuberculosis

Clinical Practice: Acquired Immunodeficiency Syndrome

A. Assessment

1. History
    a. Fatigue
    b. Malaise
    c. Fever
    d. Night sweats
    e. Diarrhea
    f. Weight loss
    g. Anorexia
    h. Cognitive changes
    i. Neurological disorders
    j. History of blood transfusion before 1985
    k. Oral or gingival lesions
    l. Nasal congestion
    m. Cough and shortness of breath
    n. Lymphadenopathy
    o. Tuberculosis (TB)
    p. IV drug abuse
    q. Prostitution
    r. Multiple sex partners
    s. Partner who is an IV drug user or bisexual
2. Physical findings
    a. Lymphadenopathy
    b. Oral or gingival lesions
    c. Presence of opportunistic infection
        (1) *Pneumocystis carinii* pneumonia
        (2) Kaposi's sarcoma
        (3) Candidiasis (thrush)

(4) Disseminated mycobacterial infections
(5) Ulcerative herpes simplex
(6) *Salmonella*
(7) Hepatitis
(8) CMV
(9) Toxoplasmosis
(10) HSV
(11) Syphilis
3. Psychosocial findings
   a. Anxiety
   b. Fear
   c. Lack of social support and social isolation
   d. Stress
   e. Depression
   f. Emotional liability
   g. Denial
   h. Financial problem
4. Diagnostic
   a. CBC with differential, platelet count (to monitor anemia, leukocytopenia and thrombocytopenia)
   b. Type, Rh factor, antibody screen
   c. Rubella titer
   d. HbsAg
   e. Purified Protein Derivative (PPD)/x-ray (incidence of active TB markedly elevated among HIV-infected patients)
   f. T-cell count (absolute T4 or helper T cells or CD4)
      (1) Lymphocyte count is markedly decreased
      (2) T lymphocytes are decreased, misshapen, and qualitatively deficient
      (3) Ratio of helper T cells (CD4 or T4) to suppressor T cells (CD8 or T8) is normally 2:1; it is 1:2 in persons with AIDS
      (4) Immunoglobulin levels are elevated
   g. Pap smear
   h. Gonorrhea, chlamydia cultures, and TORCH screen
   i. Serial ultrasonography to detect IUGR
   j. Venereal Disease Research Laboratory testing (VDRL)
   k. Urinalysis: may reveal proteinuria due to AIDS nephropathy
   l. Blood chemistries
      (1) Elevated BUN and creatinine levels may indicate presence of AIDS-related renal disease
      (2) Abnormal liver enzymes may indicate liver infiltration by opportunistic infection
      (3) Elevated total protein may indicate hypergammaglobulinemia
      (4) Decreased albumin may indicate poor nutrition
   m. Antigen capture assay
   n. Viral culture
   o. Detection of antibody to HIV (Fig. 27–3)
      (1) Enzyme-linked immunosorbent assay (ELISA)
      (2) Western blot

B. Nursing Diagnoses

1. Knowledge deficit related to infection, its treatment, and sequelae
2. Fear related to potential for infection and deterioration of maternal condition
3. Anticipatory grief related to decreased quality of life for self and fetus
4. Altered family processes
5. Altered nutrition related to infection
6. Ineffective individual coping related to infection

C. Interventions/Evaluations

1. Knowledge deficit related to infection, its treatment, and sequelae
   a. Interventions
      (1) Provide information about HIV antibody testing and its significance
      (2) Provide information about the infection and how it is transmitted in an open and nonjudgmental manner; AIDS is transmitted through blood, semen, vaginal secretions and breast milk
      (3) Discuss safer sex
      (4) Provide information on implications of HIV infection versus the disease of AIDS; 8-year median interval between acute infection and immunodeficiency
      (5) Counsel the client about the risk to sexual partners and lack of risk to casual contacts at home and work. Explain precautions regarding blood and body fluids
      (6) Give written information on above at level that client can understand
      (7) Assure the client of confidentiality
      (8) Explain all procedures and treatments
   b. Evaluations
      (1) Client verbalizes meaning of HIV antibody testing
      (2) Client understands implications of a positive result
      (3) Client expresses understanding of procedures
      (4) Client will use condoms correctly
      (5) Client understands rights related to confidentiality

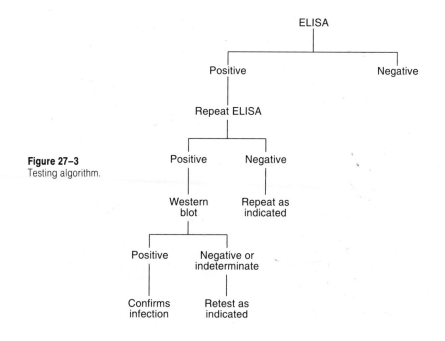

Figure 27–3
Testing algorithm.

2. Fear related to potential for infection and deterioration of maternal condition
   a. Interventions
      (1) Acknowledge client's fears
      (2) Encourage ventilation of feelings of anger and guilt in an emotionally supportive environment
      (3) Provide appropriate information to enable the client to make informed decisions
      (4) Assess coping mechanism in prior crises and history with illness
      (5) Encourage the client to use family and significant others for support if available
      (6) Assess available support (family, friends, church)
      (7) Provide factual information and correct misconceptions
      (8) Assist significant others to provide needed support
      (9) Provide information on support groups
      (10) Give as many options as possible to maintain feeling of control
   b. Evaluations
      (1) Client is able to express her concerns openly
      (2) Client identifies source of fear and concern
      (3) Client exercises control in decision making
      (4) Client is able to accept support
3. Anticipatory grief related to decreased quality of life for self and fetus
   a. Interventions
      (1) Acknowledge the client's grief and anger
      (2) Assist in understanding grief process
      (3) Encourage expression of feelings of potential loss
      (4) Assist support people to adjust to situation
      (5) Assess support systems within the client's life
      (6) Help the client to identify the potential loss
      (7) Encourage the client to identify strengths and positively reinforce them
   b. Evaluations
      (1) Client is able to move through the grieving process
      (2) Client identifies potential loss
      (3) Client communicates understanding of grief process
      (4) Client seeks support groups
4. Altered family processes
   a. Interventions
      (1) Assess client's perception of pregnancy and her role as mother
      (2) Assess significant others' support of client and self
      (3) Refer the client for stress management techniques
   b. Evaluations
      (1) Client is able to communicate with her family and significant others about her pregnancy and the potential of the disease process
      (2) Family is willing to meet emotional and physical needs of the client
5. Altered nutrition related to infection
   a. Interventions
      (1) Supplemental vitamins
      (2) Ferrous sulfate
      (3) Folic acid (if low folate levels)
      (4) Provide nutritional information, emphasizing increased protein intake
      (5) Refer the client to a nutritionist
   b. Evaluations
      (1) Client prevents further nutritional decline
      (2) Client has appropriate uterine growth for gestational age
6. Ineffective individual coping related to infection
   a. Interventions
      (1) Assist the client in objectively viewing illness

(2) Provide accurate information of potential procedures

(3) Assist the client in developing appropriate coping skills

(4) Assist the client in identifying feelings such as anger and guilt

(5) Refer the client to health care workers who focus on AIDS

(6) Refer the client to mental health worker or support group

   b. Evaluations

(1) Client verbalizes the threat of disease accurately

(2) Client appropriately expresses her feelings, including anger and guilt

(3) Client has the ability to solve problems and make decisions

Health Education: Acquired Immunodeficiency Syndrome

A. **Testing:** strongly encourage the following to have HIV testing—intravenous drug users; homosexual or bisexual males; hemophiliacs; clients being evaluated for sexually transmitted diseases (STDs), victims of sexual abuse; clients who have had transfusions, tattoos, or acupuncture since 1977; and clients who are uncertain about the risk factors of their partners

B. **Prevention**

1. Mutually monogamous sexual relationships minimize sexual transmission
2. Avoid sex with multiple partners, partners with multiple partners, or prostitutes
3. Avoid sexual contact with people with discharge, genital warts, or herpes lesions
4. Use latex condoms in combination with spermicide (Nonoxynol 9) to avoid transmission of semen or vaginal secretions
5. Never share needles or syringes
6. Avoid breastfeeding because it is associated with transmission

C. **Resources**

1. Foundation for Children With AIDS: (617) 783–7300
2. National Self-Help Clearinghouse: (212) 840–1258
3. AIDS hotline: 1–800–342–AIDS; 1–800–344–7432 (Spanish); 1–800–243–7889; (1-800–AIDS-TTY) (hearing impaired)

D. **Provide information about self-help groups**

E. **Provide information about effective birth control after pregnancy**

Sexually Transmitted Diseases

Introduction: Sexually Transmitted Diseases

A. **Other sexually transmitted diseases (STDs) include the following**

1. Gonorrhea
2. Syphilis
3. Human papillomavirus (HPV)
4. Chlamydia
5. Trichomonas
6. Candida

B. **Definition**

1. Diseases are transmitted from one person to another during sexual intercourse
2. Transmission occurs through contact with the genitalia, mouth, or rectal area of an infected person

C. High-risk population

1. Adolescents
2. Women with multiple sex partners
3. Indigent women with no prenatal care

D. Statistics

1. Twelve million cases of STDs occur per year
2. Most cases occur among persons under 25 years of age

Clinical Practice: Sexually Transmitted Diseases

See Table 27–2 for complete discussion of HIV and STDs: mode of transmission, maternal and fetal effects, and treatment

A. Assessment

1. History
   a. Previous STD infection for self or partner
   b. Multiple sexual partners
   c. Sex with a new partner in the preceding 2 months
   d. Sexual partners with penile discharge, condyloma, or ulcer
   e. Dysuria
   f. Fever
   g. Dyspareunia
   h. Vaginal discharge, itching, or odor
   i. Exposure to infected sexual partner
   j. Recent use of antibiotics or other medications
   k. Allergy history (allergic reactions to soap or medications often mimic STD lesions)
2. Physical findings
   a. Purulent urethral or cervical discharge
   b. Friable cervix
   c. Genital lesion that may or may not be painful
   d. Tender uterus, adnexal structures, or both
   e. Pain on motion of cervix
   f. Inguinal adenopathy
   g. Low-grade temperature
   h. Disseminated lymphadenopathy
   i. Rash on palms and soles of feet in secondary syphilis
   j. Papillomatous excrescences (genital warts)
   k. Poor personal hygiene
3. Psychosocial findings
   a. Anxiety
   b. Fear
   c. Confusion
   d. Difficulty in communicating
   e. Guilt
4. Diagnostic findings
   a. Positive cervical, oral, or rectal culture for gonorrhea
   b. Positive cervical culture for *Chlamydia* and *Streptococcus*
   c. Gram stain showing gram-negative diplococci
   d. VDRL or rapid plasma reagin test (RPR) for general screening
   e. Fluorescent treponemal antibody absorption test (FTA-Abs) for specific testing
   f. Tissue cultures

   g. Potassium hydroxide (KOH) smear and wet prep (to identify *Trichomonas*, monilia, and "clue cells")
   h. Biopsy of lesions
   i. Culture of herpes lesions
   j. Microscopic darkfield examination for motile spirochetes

B. Nursing Diagnoses

1. Knowledge deficit related to infection, its treatment, and sequelae
2. Alteration in comfort related to infection
3. Anxiety and fear related to infection and its possible sequelae

C. Interventions/Evaluations

1. Knowledge deficit related to infection and its treatment
   a. Interventions
     (1) Provide factual information about cause, mode of transmission, and rationale for treatment of the related STD
     (2) Explain importance of taking prescribed medication and completion of entire course even if symptoms subside
     (3) Provide written material for the client to take home
     (4) Instruct the client in warning signs of complications (e.g., fever, increased pain, bleeding)
     (5) Advise the client to abstain from intercourse until she is free of infection
     (6) Advise the client of possible side effects of medications
     (7) Instruct the client in good hygiene to prevent secondary infection
     (8) Advise the client of importance of having her sexual partners evaluated and treated
   b. Evaluations
     (1) Client is able to verbalize understanding of the infection and its treatment
     (2) Client is able to use self-care measures
     (3) Client complies with medication treatment and returns for follow-up appointments
     (4) Client has her partner examined and treated
     (5) Client states the warning signs of complications and side effects of medications and ways to prevent re-infection
2. Alteration in comfort related to infection
   a. Interventions
     (1) Assess level of discomfort
     (2) Administer analgesics as ordered (acetaminophen or aspirin)
     (3) Aid the client in taking warm sitz baths
     (4) Advise the client to use a hair dryer to dry the genital area
     (5) Advise the client to expose lesions to air
   b. Evaluations
     (1) Client appears comfortable
     (2) Client has fewer complaints of pain
     (3) Client returns to an infection-free state
3. Anxiety and fear related to infection and its possible sequelae
   a. Interventions
     (1) Provide information in a nonjudgmental, nonthreatening manner
     (2) Offer to include family member or significant other in discussion
     (3) Encourage the client to verbalize feelings about having infection and its impact on her life and her fetus
   b. Evaluations
     (1) Client is able to verbalize decreased anxiety related to infection

Table 27–2
SEXUALLY TRANSMITTED DISEASES

Infection	Agent	Detection	Maternal Effects
Acquired immuno-deficiency syndrome (AIDS)	• Retrovirus HTLV III (human T-cell lymphotrophic virus) • Human immune deficiency virus (HIV)	• ELISA for general screening • Western blot • Virus isolation from blood, semen, vaginal secretions, breast milk, spinal fluid, saliva, or tears	• Some studies suggest infected pregnant women progress more rapidly than nonpregnant women • 20% of HIV-infected adults develop AIDS • 70% of patients with AIDS die within 2 years
Human papillomavirus	• Human papillomavirus (HPV) • Incubation: 3–9 months or longer	• Single or multiple irregular painless papules in the genital or perianal area • Colposcopy used as adjunct in equivocal situations • Cervical cytological testing	• A significant number of lesions enlarge during pregnancy • Usually multicentric in pregnancy

Chlamydia	• Bacteria: *Chlamydia trachomatis*	• Endocervical and urethral culture
		• ELISA (less sensitive and less specific)
			• Most of those infected are asymptomatic
			• Mucopurulent cervicitis
			• May be associated with other sexually transmitted diseases
			• Occasionally
			  Premature rupture of membranes (PROM)
			  Preterm labor
			  IUGR
			  Infertility
			  Chorioamnionitis

Gonorrhea	• Bacteria: *Neisseria gonorrhoeae*, gram-negative diplococcus • Incubation 10 days	• Endocervical, oral, or rectal cultures • Genital or blood cultures • Gram stain	• 60–80% of those infected are asymptomatic • Occasionally pelvic peritonitis • Premature rupture of membranes (PROM) • Postpartum endometritis • Chorioamnionitis • Increased infertility and ectopic pregnancies
Syphilis	• Spirochete: *Treponema pallidum* • Incubation: 10–90 days (average, 21 days)	• Venereal Disease Research Laboratory (VDRL) • Rapid plasma reagin (RPR) • Fluorescent treponemal antibody absorption test (FTA-Abs) • Secondary syphilis: increased liver enzymes	• Primary chancre: painless ulcerative lesion • Secondary syphilis: fever and malaise, red macules on palms or soles of feet • Generalized lymphadenopathy • Early latent positive serology <1 year duration • Latent cardiovascular syphilis • Neurosyphilis
Trichomonas	• Protozoan: *Trichomonas vaginalis*	• "Wet prep" saline examination • Papanicolaou's smear • Urinalysis	• Malodorous, discolored vaginal discharge • Dysuria

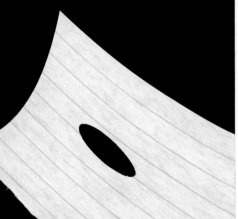

Neonatal Effects	Treatment	Incidence
• 30–50% chance of transmission from infected mother • 65% of infected infants may develop AIDS within a few months after birth	• If HIV-positive as a newborn, repeat antibody testing at 6 and 12–15 months	• First recognized in 1981 and appears to have originated in Africa • 1991; estimated 200,000 cases in U.S.

• Potential transmission of laryngeal papillomata
• Very rare (less than 1 as per 1000–1500 pregnancies in which mothers have genital condyloma)
	• Trichloroacetic acid (TCA) or bichloroacetic acid (BCA)
	• Small lesions:
	   Cryotherapy
	   CO_2 laser therapy
	   Electrocautery
	• Large lesions
	   Surgical excision (but increased morbidity due to increased vascularity)
	   CO_2 laser vaporization
	• Podophyllin or 5-fluorouracil (5-FU) *contraindicated* in pregnancy
		• Estimated 40–60 million persons infected
		• Although exact prevalence is not known, HPV is probably more frequent in pregnant women because of increased vascularity and increased hormones
		• Increasing incidence noted in STD clinics and private offices
		• Peak occurrence at age 15–35
		• Associated with other STDs

• 25% of exposed infants develop Conjunctivitis • 10% of exposed infants develop pneumonia	• Erythromycin, 500 mg PO qid for 7 days (when pregnant) • Erythromycin ophthalmic ointment for newborns • Doxicycline (postpartum) 100 mg bid for 7 days • Tetracycline (for nonpregnant women) • Simultaneous treatment of partner	• Most common sexually transmitted disease • An estimated 4 million cases occur annually in U.S. • 5%–35% of pregnant women are infected (depending on population)
• Purulent conjunctivitis • Sepsis or meningitis	• Aqueous procaine penicillin • Amoxicillin • Probenecid	• Over 1 million cases are reported in U.S. each year • Over 20,000 cases were reported in Canada in 1988, over 9000 in women of childbearing age • Frequency in pregnancy ranges from 0.5–7, depending on population • Incidence has declined during the past 5 years because of increased use of condoms
• Vary depending on gestation • Stillbirth • IUGR • Nonimmune hydrops • Premature labor	• Penicillin G • Erythromycin (if penicillin allergy) • Tetracycline (not used during pregnancy)	• 100,000 cases are reported in U.S. each year; 80% of these women are of reproductive age • 1500 cases were reported in Canada in 1988 • Some 160 cases of congenital syphilis are reported in U.S. each year
• Infant contact through infected vagina • Usually asymptomatic	• Metronidazole for mother and sex partner (avoid during first trimester) • Local therapy	• Not reported to CDC but estimated in as many as 20% of pregnancies • Estimates of 10–15% of all cases of vaginitis

Health Education: Sexually Transmitted Diseases

A. Provide information on prevention of STDs

1. Limit number of sexual partners
2. Use condoms or diaphragms with spermicide Nonoxynol 9
3. Use cotton underwear and cotton base clothing

B. Instruct the client on self-care measures

1. Burrow's solution
2. Warm sitz baths
3. Dry heat from hair dryer

C. Provide information about hygiene measures, including wiping vulva from front to back after urination

D. Encourage handwashing

E. Educate the client about the importance of reporting symptoms to health care provider, especially in last trimester

F. Educate the client on the need to take all of medication prescribed for self and partners

Urinary Tract Infection and Pyelonephritis

Introduction: Urinary Tract Infection and Pyelonephritis

A. Anatomical and physiological changes

1. A change in urine composition occurs that supports bacterial growth
2. Dilation of the upper part of the ureter occurs
3. Enlarging uterus compresses ureters
4. Smooth muscle relaxation effect of progesterone leads to stasis of urine

B. Predisposing history

1. History of urinary tract infection (UTI) before pregnancy
2. History of childhood UTI
3. Advanced maternal age
4. Low socioeconomic status
5. Underlying chronic diseases
6. Hypertension

C. Statistics

1. Asymptomatic bacteriuria is found in 2 to 15% of pregnancies
2. Pyelonephritis develops in 20 to 40% of cases if untreated
3. Acute pyelonephritis may cause premature labor and delivery

Clinical Practice: Urinary Tract Infection and Pyelonephritis

A. Assessment

1. History

   d. Hematuria
   e. Fever or chills
   f. Urgency
   g. Nocturia
   h. Malodorous urine
   i. Back pain
   j. Recent catheterization
   k. Frequent intercourse
   l. Low abdominal pain and tenderness
   m. Nausea, vomiting, or diarrhea
   n. Presence of predisposing diseases such as hypertension, diabetes, sickle cell trait, or kidney disease
   o. Abdominal or pelvic surgery or trauma to the pelvis
2. Physical findings
   a. Tender urethra
   b. Tender trigone (bladder neck)
   c. Elevated temperature 37.2° to 38.9°C (99° to 102°F) (with pyelonephritis may be above 38.9°C [102°F])
   d. Costovertebral angle (CVA) tenderness
   e. Decreased bowel sounds (with pyelonephritis)
3. Psychosocial findings: anxiety
4. Diagnostic findings
   a. Urine
     (1) Pyuria (more than five WBCs per high-power field)
     (2) Hematuria
     (3) Bacteria (10^5 or more organisms/ml)
       (a) *Escherichia coli* can account for 90% of UTIs
       (b) A mixed culture suggests a specimen contamination
       (c) Other organisms may include the following
         (i) *Proteus*
         (ii) *Klebsiella*
         (iii) *Enterobacteria*
         (iv) *Pseudomonas*
   b. CBC with differential
     (1) Elevated WBC count (12,000 to 20,000 WBCs) and 80% polymorphonuclear leukocytes (PMNs)
     (2) Anemia (from chronic bacteriuria)
   c. Fever and anatomical location of the pain and tenderness are the findings most commonly used to tentatively distinguish cystitis from pyelonephritis

B. Nursing Diagnoses

1. Knowledge deficit related to infection, its treatment, and possible sequelae
2. High risk for injury related to infection
3. Anxiety and fear related to possible sequelae

C. Interventions/Evaluations

1. Knowledge deficit related to infection, its treatment, and possible sequelae
   a. Interventions: provide information related to the following
     (1) The signs and symptoms of a UTI (pain with urination, urgency, frequency) and importance of reporting them to health care provider
     (2) The importance of adequate hydration
     (3) The correct method of wiping perineal area
     (4) Possible effects of UTI on pregnancy
   b. Evaluation: Client is able to state the signs and symptoms of a UTI and the importance of seeking treatment quickly

2. High risk for injury related to infection
   a. Interventions
      (1) The importance of completing treatment with antibiotics must be explained so the client will take all of her medications
      (2) Obtain a follow-up urine culture 48 hours after therapy, 2 weeks after the client finishes her antibiotics regimen, and every 4 to 6 weeks until delivery
      (3) Instruct the client on the signs and symptoms of early labor, and tell her to report them promptly
   b. Evaluation: The client returns to an infection-free state and remains free of infection throughout pregnancy
3. Anxiety and fear related to possible sequelae
   a. Interventions
      (1) Providing information as above increases the client's sense of control
      (2) Give information in a calm, consistent manner
   b. Evaluation: Client verbalizes a decrease in her anxiety level

Health Education: Urinary Tract Infection and Pyelonephritis

A. Provide information about hygiene measures, including wiping from front to back after urinating and washing hands frequently

B. Instruct the client to void before and after intercourse

C. Instruct the client on the need to drink 8 to 10 glasses of water daily; include cranberry juice to lower the pH of the urinary tract

D. Instruct the client to void frequently as the need arises; holding urine increases time bacteria are in bladder

E. Suggest the use of lubrication such as K-Y jelly during intercourse as needed

F. Instruct the client in the importance of completing antibiotic therapy, even if she no longer has symptoms

Introduction: Other Communicable Diseases

A. Other communicable diseases include the following

1. Measles
2. Mumps
3. Chickenpox
4. Influenza
5. Mononucleosis
6. Upper respiratory infection (URI)
7. Parvovirus

B. Effects

1. Pregnant women are exposed to the same communicable diseases as the general population
2. Both mother and fetus must be considered
3. Effect of infection varies depending on disease and stage of pregnancy during which infection occurs

ble Diseases

of the above-named communicable

A. Assessment

1. History
   a. Previous exposure
   b. Lack of immunization
   c. Stuffy nose
   d. Watery eyes
   e. Fever or chills
   f. Adenopathy
   g. Fatigue
   h. Myalgia (muscle aches)
   i. Rash
   j. Sore throat and cough
   k. Malaise
2. Physical findings
   a. Fever
   b. Rash: macule, papule, or vesicle
   c. Adenopathy
   d. Pharyngitis
   e. Parotitis (swollen salivary glands)
   f. Low-grade temperature
3. Psychosocial findings
   a. Anxiety
   b. Fear
   c. Apprehension
4. Diagnostic findings
   a. CBC (increased WBC count)
   b. Throat culture
   c. Mononucleosis spot test and heterophile test
   d. Disease-specific serology antibody tests of IgG and IgM
   e. Virus isolation
   f. Serological testing: ELISA or fluorescent antibody membrane antigen (FAMA)

B. Nursing Diagnoses

1. Knowledge deficit related to infection, its treatment, and possible sequelae
2. Anxiety and fear related to infection, its treatment, and possible sequelae

C. Interventions/Evaluations

1. Knowledge deficit related to infection, its treatment, and possible sequelae
   a. Interventions
      (1) Provide information on the signs and symptoms of the communicable disease, its mode of transmission and prevention, and the importance of reporting exposure to health care provider
      (2) Provide written material containing information at appropriate level for the client
      (3) Reinforce need for the client to take all of medication
      (4) Provide information about the safety of vaccines during pregnancy
   b. Evaluations
      (1) Client understands disease process
      (2) Client is able to prevent or decrease occurrence of the disease
      (3) Client will report any signs or symptoms
2. Anxiety and fear related to infection, its treatment, and possible sequelae

Table 27–3
COMMUNICABLE DISEASES

Infection	Agent	Mode of Transmission
Varicella (chickenpox) zoster (shingles)	• Varicella zoster virus • Incubation: 11–20 days	• Probably by aerosolized respiratory droplets • Portal of entry is respiratory tract • Transplacentally
Mumps	• Paramyxovirus • Incubation: 16–18 days	• Respiratory secretions
Influenza	• Virus • Incubation: 24–72 hours	• Respiratory secretions
Measles (rubella)	• Ribonucleic acid (RNA) virus • Incubation: 10–14 days	• Respiratory secretions • Airborne
Parvovirus B19 (Fifth disease)	• DNA virus • DNA-deoxyribonucleic acid	• Respiratory secretions

a. Interventions
   (1) Provide information as above to increase the client's sense of control and to decrease her uncertainty
   (2) Give information in a calm, consistent manner
b. Evaluations
   (1) Client expresses her concerns about communicable disease
   (2) Client's anxiety about the effect of the disease process on her pregnancy is decreased

Health Education: Other Communicable Diseases

A. Prevention: educate the client on the need for immunizations

Maternal Effects	Neonatal Effects	Incidence and Prevention
• Varicella is severe in adults • Death/case ratio: 50 in 100,000 in adults compared with 2 in 100,000 in children • Risk of premature labor due to high temperature • Risk of varicella pneumonia appears to be increased during pregnancy	• Affects 30–40% of fetuses born to mothers with active disease • Congenital varicella syndrome Limb-reduction anomalies IUGR Cataracts Microphthalmos Chorioretinitis Microcephaly • If mother contracts infection 4 days or less before delivery, administer zoster immune globulin	• Most commonly reported infectious disease • 1.8% of cases occur after age 20 • Occurs in 5–15% women of childbearing age • 100% of population is seropositive by age 60 • Generally occurs during late winter or early spring • Occurs in 1 in 7500 pregnancies
• Spontaneous abortion rate is increased 2-fold	• Tetratogenicity is unknown; probably rare or nonexistent	• 600 cases were reported in Canada in 1988 (50 in women of childbearing age) • Mumps vaccine is contraindicated during pregnancy
• Usually brief but incapacitating disease • Deaths occur from secondary bacterial pneumonia	• Any risk of malformation has been confined to first trimester • Most studies fail to support tetratogenicity	• Killed virus vaccine • Vaccine during pregnancy is indicated if mother is at medical risk because of other diseases
• Serious morbidity is rare • Possible increased rate of miscarriage or preterm birth	• Tetratogenicity is unknown; probably rare or nonexistent	• Greatest incidence with adolescents and young adults • 600 cases were reported in Canada in 1988 (33 in women of childbearing age) • Measles vaccine is contraindicated during pregnancy
• Erythema • Elevated temperature • Arthralgia	• Spontaneous abortions	• Risk of women with primary infection during first 20 weeks of pregnancy is 15–17%

Introduction: Chorioamnionitis

A. Definition

1. Inflammation of the chorion and amnion occurs
2. Mononuclear leukocytes and PMNs infiltrate the membranes
3. Organisms are usually present in vagina (most commonly Streptococcus)

B. Chorioamnionitis is associated with the following

1. Premature rupture of membranes
2. Prolonged rupture of membranes

C. Management

1. Identification of the infecting organism
2. Parenteral antibiotic therapy
3. Delivery of the infant

4. Vaginal delivery is preferred, but cesarean section may be done in presence of severe infection

Clinical Practice: Chorioamnionitis

A. Assessment

1. History
   a. Premature rupture of membranes before the onset of labor
   b. Prolonged rupture of membranes during or before the onset of labor
   c. Uterine tenderness
   d. Prenatal infection
   e. Poor prenatal care
2. Physical findings
   a. Maternal fever (39°C [102.2°F] in mild infection and 40°C [104°F] in severe infection)
   b. Fetal tachycardia (usually over 180 beats/min)
   c. Fetal monitoring tracing consistent with hypoxia
   d. Chills
   e. Uterine pain and tenderness
   f. Foul-smelling vaginal discharge
   g. Hypotension
   h. Tachycardia
3. Psychosocial findings
   a. Fear
   b. Anxiety
4. Diagnostic findings
   a. Unspun smear of amniotic fluid (bacteria and neutrophils seen)
   b. Culture of amniotic fluid and cervix: possible pathogens include the following
      (1) Group A and B streptococci
      (2) *Neisseria gonorrhoeae*
      (3) *Chlamydia*
      (4) *Staphylococcus aureus*
      (5) *Haemophilus influenzae*
      (6) *Escherichia coli*
      (7) Anaerobic gram-positive cocci
   c. CBC: increased WBC count (over 15,000 to 20,000/mm^3 with over 90% PMNs and bands)
   d. Urinalysis to rule out urinary tract infection

B. Nursing Diagnoses

1. Knowledge deficit related to infection, its treatment, and sequelae
2. Anxiety related to well-being of self and baby
3. Ineffective individual coping related to stress of increased discomfort and illness

C. Interventions/Evaluations

1. Knowledge deficit related to infection, its treatment, and sequelae
   a. Interventions
      (1) Provide information on antibiotic treatment in a calm, reassuring manner

(2) Involve the client and her family or significant other in the learning process

(3) Reinforce information provided by the physician on the possible course of labor, including possibility of cesarean section (C/S)

b. Evaluation: client accurately verbalizes what chorioamnionitis is and how it is treated

2. Anxiety related to well being of self and baby

a. Interventions

(1) Develop trust and rapport by being nonjudgmental and interested in the client

(2) Facilitate client communication with the physician

(3) Provide information that will increase the client's sense of control and decrease her uncertainty

(4) Suggest to the client coping strategies that are distracting or relaxing or that change how the client perceives her situation

b. Evaluations

(1) Client verbalizes sources of anxiety, concerns, and issues in a supportive environment

(2) Client verbalizes a decrease in anxiety

(3) Client uses coping skills effectively as evidence by following instructions, problem solving, and using relaxation techniques

(4) Client appropriately expresses her feelings

(5) Client maintains communication with health care providers and her family or significant other

Health Education: Chorioamnionitis

A. Prevention

1. Adequate prenatal care
2. Treatment of prenatal vaginal infection
3. Notify health care provider of premature rupture of membranes (PROM)

CASE STUDIES AND STUDY QUESTIONS

TORCH

Sally Green, a health care worker in a daycare setting, is a 27-year-old multigravida with her last menstrual period 11 weeks ago. Her 3-year-old daughter developed a fever and rash 5 days earlier. Two days later, the pediatrician established a diagnosis of rubella. On examination, Sally is found to be healthy and her uterus is 10 to 11 weeks in size. She does not remember having had rubella. Her friend told her to be tested for TORCH. She wants to know what it is.

1. What does TORCH stand for?

2. What laboratory test could determine her susceptibility?

a. CBC.

b. Rubella titer.

c. Nasopharyngeal swab.

3. If Sally develops rubella, what is the likelihood of fetal involvement?

a. 6 to 10% of fetuses are affected if exposed in third month of pregnancy.

b. There is no chance of this fetus being affected.

c. 25% of fetuses are affected if exposed in the third month of pregnancy.

d. There is a good chance of the fetus being affected if exposed any time during the pregnancy.

4. Sally could be at risk for what other TORCH disease?

   a. AIDS

   b. Cytomegalovirus

   c. Toxoplasmosis

   d. Rubeola

5. Which of the following will reduce her chances of exposure?

   a. Cooking chicken until it is well done.

   b. Using a mask to protect her from airborne diseases.

   c. Rigorous personal hygiene while at work and home.

   d. Taking Acyclovir

   e. Having serial cervical cultures

   (1) a,c,d

   (2) b,d

   (3) a,b,c

   (4) none of the above

Acquired Immunodeficiency Syndrome

Mildred Purcell is a 21-year-old primigravida (G1) woman with her last menstrual period 12 weeks ago. She is in for her initial prenatal visit. Her uterus is approximately 12 weeks in size and her blood pressure is 110/72. During your discussion with Mildred, she expresses some concern over the possibility of being exposed to AIDS. She states she has had only one sexual partner and they have been in a monogamous relationship for 2 years. When questioned, her concern stems from the fact that a colleague at work recently tested positive for HIV.

6. As part of your assessment, what other information do you need to know?

   a. Does she live with other people?

   b. Has she eaten at her colleague's home?

   c. Sexual history of her partner.

7. In your discussion with Mildred about AIDS, you may tell her (answer the following true or false):

   a. AIDS is spread only through sexual contact.

   b. The occurrence of AIDS in women has not been increasing.

   c. She may take AZT prophylactically.

   d. Symptoms of AIDS include fatigue, night sweats, and lymphadenopathy.

8. If it is established that Mildred's partner had previous partners, which of the following would you recommend for general screening?

   a. ELISA.

   b. Western blot.

   c. T-cell count.

9. If this test were positive, what test would confirm HIV infection?

   a. ELISA.

   b. Western blot.

   c. T-cell count.

10. The HIV virus has been found in all except which of the following?

   a. Saliva.

   b. Tears.

   c. Sweat.

   d. Semen.

Sexually Transmitted Diseases

Gail Andress is a 17-year-old single primigravida (G1) woman who is seen for her first prenatal visit at 20 weeks' gestation. Her history is unremarkable with the exception of treatment for gonorrhea 1 year previously. Examination of the skin, head, ears, nose, and throat is normal. Gail is afebrile, her pulse is 88, and her blood pressure is 118/72. The size of her uterus corresponds with gestational age by dates. There is a small amount of yellow discharge at the cervix. The vulva appears red and inflamed.

11. What is the causative agent of gonorrhea?

   a. Gram-negative diplococcus.

b. Gram-positive diplococcus.

c. Protozoa.

d. Spirochete

12. Match the disease with the type of infectious organism that causes it.

Gonorrhea	1. Protozoa
Syphilis	2. Bacteria
Trichomonas	3. Virus
HIV	4. Spirochete
Human papillomavirus	
Chlamydia	

13. Answer the following true or false.

a. Because Gail does not appear to have symptoms, you need not worry about gonorrhea or chlamydia.

b. Untreated gonorrhea may cause PROM.

c. Gonorrhea has been on the decline for the past 5 years because of better hygiene.

d. An allergic reaction to soap or medications can mimic STD symptoms.

Urinary Tract Infection and Pyelonephritis

Ann Nelson is a 23-year-old gravida 2, para 1 (G2,P1) woman whose last menstrual period began 24 weeks ago. She has had one prenatal visit. She now complains of increasing urinary frequency for 5 days and of burning on urination for 2 days. For the past 24 hours, she has had a constant aching pain in her back and right side, along with chills and fever. Her temperature is 38.9°C (102°F), her pulse is 110, and her blood pressure is 110/70. There is marked costovertebral angle tenderness on the right. Her uterus measures 23 cm; the fetal heart rate is 146; and her cervix is long and closed. Based on urine laboratory values, Ann is diagnosed as having acute pyelonephritis.

14. Name three physiological changes that occur during pregnancy and predispose women to UTI.

a. Changes in urine composition

b. Dilatation of the upper third of ureters

c. Decreased frequency of urination

d. Compression of ureters by enlarging uterus

e. Increased intake of liquids

(1) a,b,c

(2) b,c,e

(3) a,b,d

(4) b,c,d

15. A history of which of the following places a pregnant woman at an increase risk for UTI?

a. History of childhood UTIs.

b. Chronic disease and hypertension.

c. Prior UTIs.

d. a,c.

e. a,b,c.

16. Answer the following as true or false.

a. Pyuria is defined as more than five WBCs per high-power field.

b. *Proteus* is the most common cause of UTI.

c. The client should be instructed to take prescribed medication until symptoms are gone.

d. Drinking 8 to 10 glasses of water daily helps prevent UTIs.

Vicki Howett is a 24-year-old school teacher approximately 14 weeks pregnant with her first pregnancy. She is concerned about many of the diseases she may be exposed to and asks many questions.

17. How is chickenpox transmitted?

a. Aerosolized droplets.

b. Blood and mucus.

c. Skin to skin contact.

18. Mumps is caused by what agent?

a. Paramyxovirus.

b. Protozoa.

c. RNA virus.

19. What is the incubation period for measles?

a. 5 to 9 days.

b. 10 to 14 days.

c. 15 to 20 days.

20. Answer the following questions true or false.

a. Immunizations are not indicated during pregnancy.

b. Varicella is another name for chickenpox.

c. Teratogencity of chlamydia is rare or nonexistent.

Sarah Carr is a 16-year-old unwed primigravida (G1) woman who is admitted at 36 weeks' gestation with a temperature of 39.4°C (103°F), uterine tenderness, chills, and a blood pressure of 102/72. Fetal heart rate is 180. Fetal monitoring tracing shows absent short-term variability but no decelerations. Catherized urinalysis is unremarkable. CBC shows hemoglobin values of 10.5 g/dl, hematocrit of 36%, and WBC count 22,000/mm³ with 85% PMNs, 10% bands, and 5% lymphocytes.

21. All of the following are possible pathogens associated with chorioamnionitis except which?

a. *Escherichia coli.*

b. Group A and B streptococci.

c. *Toxoplasma gondii.*

22. All of the following are diagnostic for chorioamnionitis except which?

a. Culture of cervix.

b. Amniotic fluid smear.

c. Vaginal smear.

23. Chorioamnionitis is associated with premature rupture of membranes and what other factor?

a. Cerclage use.

b. Prolonged rupture of membranes.

c. Inadequate hydration.

24. Answer the following true or false.

a. Mononuclear leukocytes and PMNs infiltrate the chorion.

b. Teenage unwed pregnancy and poor nutrition are factors that predispose to chorioamnionitis.

c. A cesarean section is the preferred method of delivery in a client with chorioamnionitis.

Answers to Study Questions

1. Toxoplasmosis, other (hepatitis B), rubella, cytomegalovirus, herpes simplex.
2. b
3. a
4. b
5. 3

6. c
7. a. False b. False c. False d. True.
8. a
9. b
10. c

11. a
12. Gonorrhea—bacteria (2.)
    Syphilis—spirochete (4.)
    Trichomonas—protozoa (1.)
    HIV—virus (3.)
    Human papillomavirus—virus (3.)
    Chlamydia—bacteria (2.)
13. a. False b. True c. False d. True.

14. 3

15. e
16. a. True b. False c. False d. True.

17. a
18. a
19. b
20. a. False b. True c. True.

21. c
22. c
23. b
24. a. True b. True c. False.

REFERENCES

Abrams, R.S. (1989). *Medical problems during pregnancy*. Norwalk, CT: Appleton & Lange.

American Academy of Pediatrics Committee on Infectious Disease. (1990). Parvovirus, erythema infectiosum, and pregnancy. *Pediatrics, 85*(1), 131–3.

Barton, J.J., O'Connor, T.M., Cannon, M.J., & Linne, C.M. (1988). Prevalence of human immunodeficiency virus in a general prenatal population. *American Journal of Obstetrics and Gynecology, 160*(6), 1316–1320.

Blanche, S., Rouzioux, C., Moscato, M.G., Verber, F., Mayaux, M.J., Jacomet, C., et al. (1989). Prospective study of infants born to women seropositive for human immunodeficiency virus type 1. *New England Journal of Medicine, 320*(25), 1643.

Bobak, I., Jenson, M., & Zalar, M. (Eds.) (1989). *Maternity and gynecologic care: The nurse and the family*. St. Louis: Mosby.

Cohn, J.A. (1989). VIrology immunology, and natural history of HIV infection. *Journal of Nurse-Midwifery, 34*(5), 242–252.

Dowen, R.H., & Dillon, M. (1985). Herpes infection of pregnancy. *NAACOG Update Series, 3*(4), 1–6.

Fears, J. (1987). A review of immune defects in AIDS. *Topics in Emergency Medicine, 9*(2), 13.

Feinkind, L., & Minkoff, J.L. (1988). HIV in pregnancy. *Clinics in Perinatology, 15*(2), 189–202.

Fekety, S.E. (1988). Managing the HIV-positive patient and her newborn in a CNM service. *Journal of Nurse-Midwifery, 34*(5), 253–258.

Felberbaum, M., & Salzberg, M. (1987). Epidemiology and risk factors associated with AIDS. *Topics in Emergency Medicine, 9*(2), 1.

Frigoletto, F., & Little, G. (1988). *Guidelines for perinatal care* (2nd ed.). Washington, DC: American Academy of Pediatrics and American College of Obstetricians and Gynecologists.

Gabbe, S., Niebyl, J., & Simpson, J.L. (Eds.) (1986). *Obstetrics: Normal and problem pregnancies*. New York: Churchill Livingstone.

Gloeb, J., O'Sullivan, M.J., & Efantis, J. (1988). Human immunodeficiency virus infection in women. *American Journal of Obstetrics and Gynecology, 159*(3), 756–761.

Haggerty, L. (1985). TORCH: A literature review and implications for practice. *Journal of Obstetric, Gynecologic, and Neonatal Nursing, 14*(2), 124–129.

Hayes, C.E., Sharp, E.S., & Miner, K.R. (1989). Knowledge, attitudes, and beliefs of HIV-seronegative women about AIDS. *Journal of Nurse-Midwifery, 34*(5), 291–295.

Hanson-Smith, B. (Ed.). (1989). *Nursing care planning guides for childbearing families*. Baltimore: Williams & Wilkins.

Holman, S. (1989). Epidemiology and transmission of HIV infection in women: Considerations for nurse-midwives. *Journal of Nurse-Midwifery, 34*(5), 233–241.

Holman, S., Berthaud, M., Sunderland, A., Moroso, G., Cancellieri, F., Mendez, H., et al. (1989). Women infected with HIV: Counseling and testing during pregnancy. *Seminars in Perinatology, 13*(1), 7–15.

Katz, B.Z. (1989). Natural history and clinical management of the infant born to a mother infected with HIV. *Seminars in Perinatology, 13*(1), 27–34.

Kneisl, C., & Wilson, H. (1984). *Handbook of psychosocial nursing care*. Menlo Park, CA: Addison-Wesley.

Krutsky, C., & Weiner, J. (1989). Integrating HIV/AIDS risk assessment into a nurse-midwifery practice. *Journal of Nurse-Midwifery, 34*(5), 275–276.

Kurth, A., & Hutchison, M. (1989). A context for HIV testing in pregnancy. *Journal of Nurse-Midwifery, 34*(5), 259–266.

Landers, D., & Sweet, R. (1990). Perinatal infections. *Danforth's obstetrics and gynecology* (6th ed.). Philadelphia: Lippincott.

Loucks, A. (1987)., Chlamydia: An unheralded epidemic. *American Journal of Nursing, 87*(7), 920–922.

Loveman, A., Colburn, V., & Dobin, A. (1986). AIDS in pregnancy. *Journal of Obstetric, Gynecologic, and Neonatal Nursing, 15*(2), 91.

Marecki, M. (1988). Chlamydia trachomatis: A developing perinatal problem. *Journal of Perinatal and Neonatal Nursing, 1*(4), 1.

Marvin, C., & Slevin, A. (1987). Chlamydia: Cause, prevention and cure. *MCN: American Journal of Maternal Child Nursing, 12*(5), 318–321.

McFarland, G., & McFarlane, E. (1989). *Nursing diagnosis and intervention*. St. Louis: Mosby.

Minkoff, H. (1986). Acquired immunodeficiency syndrome. *Journal of Nurse-Midwifery, 31*(4), 189–193.

Nettina, S., & Kauffman, F. (1990). Diagnosis and management of sexually transmitted genital lesions. *Nurse Practitioner, 15*(1), 20–39.

Nicholas, S.W., Sondheimer, D.L., Willoughby, A.D., Yaffe, S.S., & Katz, S.L. (1989). Human immunodeficiency virus infection on childhood, adolescence and pregnancy: A status report and national research agenda. *Pediatrics, 83*(2), 293.

Niebyl, J. (1990). Teratology and drugs in pregnancy and lactation. *Danforth's obstetrics and gynecology* (6th ed.). Philadelphia: Lippincott.

Pernoll, M., & Benson, R. (Eds.). (1987). *Obstetric and gynecologic diagnosis and treatment*. Los Altos, CA: Appleton & Lange.

Pritchard, J., MacDonald, P., & Gant, N. (1985). *Williams obstetrics* (17th ed.). Norwalk, CT: Appleton-Century-Crofts.

Reed, G.B., Claireaux, A.E., & Bain, A.D. (1989). *Diseases of the fetus and newborn*. St. Louis: Mosby.

Rich, K.C. (1989). Maternal AIDS: Effects on mother and infant. *Annals of the New York Academy of Sciences, 562*, 241–247.

Ritter, S., & Vermund, S. (1985). Congenital toxoplasmosis. *Journal of Obstetric, Gynecologic, and Neonatal Nursing, 14*(6), 435–439.

Ryder, R.W., Nsa, W., Hassig, S.E., Behets, F., Rayfield, M., Ekungola, B., et al. (1989). Perinatal transmission of the HIV type 1 to infants of seropositive women in Zaire. *New England Journal of Medicine, 320*(25), 1637–1642.

Selwyn, P., Schoenbaum, E.E., Davenny, K., Robertson, V.J., Feingold, A., Shulman, J., et al. (1989). Prospective study of human immunodeficiency virus: Infection and pregnancy outcomes in intravenous drug users. *Journal of the American Medical Association, 261*(9), 1289–1294.

Sever, J., Larsen, J., & Grossman, J. (1989). *Handbook of perinatal infections*. Boston: Little, Brown.

Stear, L.A., & Elinger, S.S. (1988). Understanding AIDS: Implications for pregnancy. *Journal of Perinatal and Neonatal Nursing, 1*(4), 33–46.

Sutton-DeBarros, C. (1989, April). How to clinically evaluate the pregnant substance abuser for HIV infection. *AIDS Patient Care*, 29–32.

Swiet, M. (1989). *Medical disorders in obstetric practice*. Oxford, UK: Blackwell Scientific.

Taylor, P.K. (1989). The impact of AIDS on women's lives and implications for nurse-midwifery practice. *Journal of Nurse-Midwifery, 34*(5), 272–274.

Traux, B. (1987). Psychosocial aspects of AIDS. *Topics in Emergency Medicine, 9*(2), 61.

Weiner, J. (1989). Integrating HIV/AIDS risk assessment into a nurse-midwifery practice. *Journal of Nurse-Midwifery, 34*(5), 275–276.

Wilson, D. (1988). An overview of sexually transmissible diseases on the perinatal period. *Journal of Nurse-Midwifery, 33*(3), 115–128.

Judy Schmidt

Hemorrhagic Disorders

Objectives

1. Define the hemorrhagic complications of placenta previa, abruptio placentae, disseminated intravascular coagulation (DIC), and gestational trophoblastic disease

2. Recognize the common signs and symptoms of placenta previa, abruptio placentae, DIC, and trophoblastic disease

3. State the appropriate initial nursing interventions

4. Record client response to nursing treatment

5. Associate less common signs and symptoms of placenta previa, abruptio placentae, and DIC with their respective conditions

6. Correlate client response with desired response to treatment to anticipate subsequent care

7. Assemble the appropriate health care provider team and coordinate the health care team as long as is necessary

Placenta Previa

INTRODUCTION

Placenta previa is an implantation of the placenta near or over the cervical os.

A. The extent to which the placenta is in contact with the os is described as total (complete or central), partial, marginal, or low lying.

B. Approximately 3.5 to 8 pregnancies/1000 will have placenta previa after 20 weeks' gestation, with a range of 1/1500 nulliparas to 1/20 grand multiparas

CLINICAL PRACTICE

A. Assessment

1. History
   a. Presents with confirmed placenta previa or vaginal bleeding
      (1) Previously diagnosed by ultrasonogram

(a) Many women (4 to 45%) may be diagnosed with placenta previa in the second trimester; however, 1/150 to 250 have placenta previa in the third trimester

(b) Second-trimester placenta previa usually resolves (88 to 98%) unless the placenta previa is total

(2) Is documented on medical record

(3) Is common to have a history of one or more prior bleeding episodes

(4) Risk factors include

(a) Prior placenta previa

(b) Short interval between pregnancies

(c) Uterine scars

   (i) Previous abortions

   (ii) Previous cesarean sections

   (iii) Previous endometritis

   (iv) Previous molar pregnancy

(d) Smoking

(e) Living at high altitude

(f) Multiple gestation

(g) Male fetus

(5) Most risk factors involve need for increased uteroplacental surface area

b. Presents with initial bleeding episode

(1) Usually is painless but may be painful if combined with abruptio placentae

(2) First bleeding is usually self-limiting

(a) Before admission: second-trimester placenta previa may resolve

(b) After admission: second-trimester placenta previa may be stabilized and the client discharged

(c) First bleeding may be combined with abruptio placentae and continuous bleeding

(d) At presentation with placenta previa, 30 weeks is average gestational age

   (i) One-third present before 31 weeks

   (ii) One-third present between 31 to 36 weeks

   (iii) One-third present after 36 weeks

2. Physical findings

a. Bleeding

(1) Blood is bright red (10 to 20% of women with placenta previa), with or without uterine contractions

(2) Presence of clots usually indicates normal coagulation process is occurring

(3) Absence of clots may indicate coagulopathy

(4) Painless bleeding is common in placenta previa (70 to 80%)

(5) Painless bleeding or referred pain is common if abruptio placentae has occurred, with or without placenta previa

b. Shock with significant blood loss

(1) Rising, thready pulse rate

(2) Pallor and clammy skin

(3) Falling blood pressure

(4) Air hunger

c. Fetal heart rate (FHR) response to maternal shock

(1) Increased or absent FHR

(2) Loss of variability of FHR

(3) Abnormal FHR and loss of variability

(a) Initial compensatory tachycardia

(b) Subsequent bradycardia

d. Complications associated with placenta previa

(1) Coagulopathy

(2) Placental abnormalities
  (a) Placenta accreta : implants to the myometrium
  (b) Placenta increta: implants into the myometrium
  (c) Placenta percreta : implants through the myometrium
(3) Postpartum hemorrhage from implantation in less muscular, lower uterine segment
(4) Uterine rupture
(5) Vasa previa consists of the following
  (a) Exposed velamentous cord insertion with vessels running unsupported through the membranes before entering the placental surface
  (b) Rupture of the vessels when rupture of membranes (ROM) occurs
  (c) A 60 to 90% fetal mortality rate
  (d) Greater risk of compression, rupture, or both when vessels are close to cervix and experience more trauma
e. Fetal malpresentation
(1) Nonpolar fetal lie is common
(2) Occurs in 30% of cases of placenta previa
(3) Includes transverse lie, breech, and unengaged vertex
3. Psychosocial findings
a. Maternal stress factors
(1) Anxiety
(2) Fear of pregnancy loss
(3) Fear for self
(4) Confusion and panic
b. Maternal behavioral factors
(1) Difficulty in making decisions
(2) Loss of pregnancy and loss of own life and health questioned
(3) Tense body posture and expression
4. Diagnostic procedures
a. Ultrasonography
(1) Need more than one view to locate placenta, including lateral uterine walls to diagnose placenta previa
(2) Differentiate placenta previa from abruptio placentae or other causes of bleeding
(3) Determine if placenta previa and abruptio placentae coexist
(4) Approximately 7 to 10% of women are asymptomatic and placenta previa is found on routine ultrasonogram
(5) Magnetic resonance imaging (MRI) may be used to diagnose placenta previa; especially useful for posterior uterine wall placenta (fetal risk of magnetic resonance imaging is unknown)
(6) Doppler color flow aids diagnosis of placental vessel abnormalities associated with placenta previa, such as velamentous insertion of cord
b. Avoid speculum and digital vaginal examinations to diagnose placenta previa
(1) Speculum examination may be done after placenta previa has been ruled out by ultrasonography
(2) Digital examination risks perforation or abruption of placenta previa
c. If there is significant blood loss, clotting problems develop: evaluate baseline values
d. Clotting studies (e.g., prothrombin time [PT], partial thromboplastin time [PTT], platelets, complete blood count [CBC], fibrinogen, fibrin split products [FSP], or fibrin degradation products)
e. Type and crossmatch at least 2 units of blood products
f. Kleihauer-Betke stain or APT test for presence of fetal red blood cells (RBC) in maternal blood sampling or vaginal blood
g. If ultrasound test inconclusive for low-lying position, a double set-up is prepared for either delivery by cesarean section or vaginal examination

B. Nursing Diagnoses

1. Alteration in tissue perfusion related to blood loss
2. Alteration in fetal perfusion and oxygenation related to maternal blood loss
3. Maternal anxiety related to threat to self and fetus

C. Interventions/Evaluations

1. Alteration in tissue perfusion related to blood loss
   a. Interventions
      (1) Draw blood and send for clotting studies, as ordered
      (2) Establish IV line with large bore intracatheter (16 gauge preferable, or 18 gauge)
      (3) Rapidly administer nondextrose crystalloids, such as Ringer's lactate or normal saline to increase blood volume
         (a) Measure urine output
         (b) Measure urine specific gravity
         (c) Obtain electrolyte values periodically, as ordered
         (d) Obtain hematocrit as ordered
      (4) Avoid vaginal examinations
      (5) Administer oxygen at 8 l per mask (10 to 12 l if rebreather bag used)
      (6) Monitor maternal pulse and blood pressure
         (a) Use automated cuff, if available
         (b) Use electrocardiogram (ECG) monitor or maternal rate mode on electronic fetal monitor (EFM), as needed
         (c) Monitor central venous pressure (CVP) or Swan-Ganz catheter, if used
      (7) Observe for clotting of blood
      (8) Measure or estimate blood loss
         (a) Metric scale: 1 g = 1 ml
         (b) Nonmetric scale: 1 oz = 29 ml
      (9) Tocolysis indicated if client is not in active labor with bleeding
   b. Evaluations: improved tissue perfusion shown by the following
      (1) Clotting of blood
      (2) Improved vital signs
      (3) Decreased blood loss
      (4) Improved or stable color and warmth of skin
      (5) Improved or stable clotting studies
      (6) Respiratory rate normal and breathing unlabored
      (7) Few or no uterine contractions
2. Alteration in fetal perfusion and oxygenation related to maternal blood loss
   a. Interventions
      (1) Continuously monitor FHR, preferably with EFM, to evaluate variability
      (2) Observe for abnormal FHR patterns (see Chapter 16 for further discussion of FHR patterns)
         (a) Loss of variability
         (b) Sinusoidal pattern
         (c) Tachycardia
         (d) Persistent late decelerations
      (3) Place client in lateral position or wedge to left
      (4) Treat client for alteration in tissue perfusion (as needed)
         (a) Oxygen therapy
         (b) Fluids
         (c) Position change
         (d) Tocolysis
   b. Evaluations
      (1) Normal or improved FHR patterns seen
      (2) Normal or improved FHR variability seen

3. Maternal anxiety related to threat to self and fetus
    a. Interventions
        (1) Speak calmly to client and support persons
        (2) Explain interventions and why they are being performed
        (3) Reassure client about fetal status
    b. Evaluations
        (1) Client reports less anxiety
        (2) Client's body posture and expressions are less tense

Abruptio Placentae

INTRODUCTION

When the placenta separates from the uterine wall before delivery of the fetus, it is an abruption of the placenta.

A. **This condition can be either a partial or a total abruptio placentae**

B. **The resultant loss of blood may be either revealed (external) or concealed (internal)**

CLINICAL PRACTICE

A. Assessment

1. History
    a. Presents with signs and symptoms of blood loss
    b. Presents with external bleeding or enlarging uterus (without external bleeding)
    c. May present with painful abdomen or firm, tender uterus, and uterine contractions
    d. Occurs in 1/120 deliveries and extent of abruption varies
        (1) Recurrence rate is 5.5 to 16% or 30 times higher in repeat pregnancies
        (2) Poor future reproduction potential is indicated
    e. Possible etiological factors
        (1) Maternal hypertension
            (a) Vascular pathology involved
            (b) Abruption risk five times higher
        (2) Cigarette smoking
            (a) Decidual necrosis found
            (b) Preventable
        (3) Multigravida
            (a) Grand multipara's risk is 2½ times higher
            (b) Factors include endometrial damage and poor nutrition
        (4) Cocaine use
        (5) Methamphetamine use
        (6) Short umbilical cord
        (7) Abdominal trauma
        (8) Controversial etiology
            (a) Folic acid deficiency
            (b) Vena caval compression
2. Physical findings: common, not absolute
    a. Blood loss, painful abdomen, or both, and firm, tender uterus
        (1) Prediction of an abruptio placentae is difficult
        (2) Antepartum testing results are normal until placenta abrupts
        (3) Continuous dull back pain and abdominal pain may occur
        (4) Intermittent abdominal cramping may occur

      b. Uterine contractions: frequent and mild; tonus may be elevated

      c. Symptoms of significant bleeding from abruptio placentae

         (1) Rising pulse rate with falling blood pressure

            (a) Blood pressure in normal range with hypertensive clients

            (b) True blood pressure returns after intravascular volume replaced

         (2) Pale, clammy skin

         (3) Increasing uterine distension

            (a) Abdominal girth and fundal height measurements useful

            (b) Measurement of abdominal girth and fundal height is not conclusive of benign course

         (4) Concealed (internal) bleeding in 10% of clients

         (5) Syncope

         (6) Nausea and vomiting

      d. FHR in the presence of maternal shock

         (1) Increased or absent

         (2) Decreased variability

  3. Psychosocial findings

      a. Maternal stress factors

         (1) Anxiety

         (2) Fear of loss of pregnancy

         (3) Fear for self

         (4) Confusion

      b. Maternal behavioral factors

         (1) Client has difficulty in communicating facts and concerns

         (2) Client expresses pain verbally, by body posture, or both

         (3) Client expresses fear of events and situation

  4. Diagnostic procedures

      a. Observe for coagulation abnormalities with clotting studies (PT, PTT, platelet count, fibrinogen, FSP)

      b. Type and crossmatch at least 2 units of blood products

      c. Consider ultrasonography for placental condition, if possible, and to differentiate from placenta previa

         (1) Abruptio placentae viewed on ultrasonography may be unreliable

         (2) Ultrasonography may not differentiate uterine rupture, amnionitis, pyelonephritis, and preterm labor

      d. Palpation of abdomen

         (1) Tenderness

         (2) Rigidity

         (3) Elevated tonus

         (4) Frequent uterine contractions

  5. Complications

      a. Couvelaire uterus

         (1) Bleeds into and through the myometrium

         (2) Abrupts in center of placenta; blood is trapped

         (3) Immediate blood loss is concealed

         (4) Bleeds unclotted into amniotic sac; color of amniotic fluid is that of port wine

         (5) Actual and observed blood losses are disproportionate and inaccurate

      b. Intrauterine growth retardation

      c. Fetal anoxia

      d. Fetal exsanguination

      e. Prematurity

      f. Maternal shock

      g. Maternal or neonatal coagulopathy, or both

      h. Renal failure

      i. Hypoxic damage to liver, adrenal glands, and anterior pituitary

B. **Nursing Diagnoses**

1. Alteration in maternal tissue perfusion

2. Alteration in fetal oxygenation and tissue perfusion
3. Anxiety related to fear for self and fetus
4. Alteration in comfort: abdominal pain

C. Interventions/Evaluations

1. Alteration in maternal tissue perfusion
    a. Intervention
       (1) Ensure laboratory studies are performed
          (a) CBC
          (b) Electrolyte values
          (c) Urinalysis
          (d) Type and crossmatch for blood products
          (e) Clotting studies
       (2) Establish one or more IV lines with 18-gauge or larger intracatheter
       (3) Rapidly administer IV normal saline, Ringer's lactate, or Plasmanate, as ordered
       (4) Avoid vaginal examinations
       (5) Administer oxygen via face mask at 8 to 10 l/min
       (6) Assist with CVP or insertion of Swan-Ganz catheter as needed; recommended ranges vary
          (a) CVP 5 to 12 torr
          (b) Pulmonary arterial pressure (PA) 10 to 20 torr
          (c) Pulmonary wedge pressure (PWP) <6 to 8 torr
       (7) Insert Foley catheter: 30 to 60 ml/hour output desired
       (8) Prepare for immediate cesarean delivery based on the following
          (a) Gestational age and viability of fetus
          (b) Maternal condition
       (9) Administer blood transfusion, if necessary
          (a) >10 U is considered a massive transfusion
          (b) After administration of 4 to 6 U, reevaluate clotting studies and potassium level
       (10) Monitor maternal pulse and blood pressure
       (11) Measure and estimate blood loss
          (a) Weigh blood loss on metric scale (1 g = 1 ml) or on nonmetric scale (1 oz = 29 ml)
          (b) Measure and mark on abdomen height of fundus, especially if bleeding is concealed
          (c) Measure and record abdominal girth
       (12) Position for comfort (analgesics may be contraindicated if maternal or fetal compromise indicated)
    b. Evaluations: improved tissue perfusion shown by the following
       (1) Improved vital signs
       (2) Improved or stable clotting studies
       (3) Improved or stable color and warmth of skin
       (4) Decreased blood loss
       (5) Normal respiratory rate and unlabored breathing
       (6) Improved comfort level
2. Alteration in fetal oxygenation and tissue perfusion
    a. Interventions
       (1) Continuously monitor fetal heart for the following
          (a) Baseline rate changes
          (b) Variability
          (c) Sinusoidal pattern
       (2) Avoid supine hypotension by positioning client laterally or wedged to left
       (3) Treat client for alteration in tissue perfusion
    b. Evaluation: normal or improved FHR and variability seen
3. Anxiety related to fear for self and fetus

a. Interventions
   (1) Speak calmly to client and support persons
   (2) Reassure with information about events and efforts of team
   (3) Explain status of problem and plan
      (a) Imminent delivery
      (b) Observation
   (4) Answer questions straightforwardly
b. Evaluations
   (1) Client expresses fewer concerns and fears
   (2) Client's body posture and facial expression are less tense
4. Alteration in comfort: abdominal pain
   a. Interventions
      (1) Position for comfort (except not supine)
      (2) Medicate or assist with regional anesthesia, as ordered
      (3) Assist with supportive strategies used in labor if unable to medicate client
      (4) Explain rationale of avoiding medication
   b. Evaluations
      (1) Client reports increased comfort
      (2) No side effects seen from analgesia or regional anesthesia in mother or fetus

Disseminated Intravascular Coagulation

INTRODUCTION

A. DIC indicates the acceleration of the coagulation system and activation of the fibrinolytic system

B. The lysis, or breakdown, of fibrinogen creates low fibrinogen levels and elevated FSP (fibrin split products or fibrin degradation products)

C. Platelets are also depleted in the accelerated coagulation process

CLINICAL PRACTICE

A. Assessment

1. History
   a. Client presents with previous obstetrical complications such as the following
      (1) Abruptio placentae
      (2) Intrauterine fetal death
      (3) Pregnancy-induced hypertension (PIH), and HELLP (hemolysis, elevated liver [enzymes], low platelets) syndrome
      (4) Sepsis of pregnancy
      (5) Amniotic fluid embolus
      (6) Gestational trophoblastic disease
      (7) Placenta accreta
      (8) Couvelaire uterus with concealed (internal) abruptio placentae
   b. Client presents with medical complication during pregnancy such as the following
      (1) Thrombocytopenia
      (2) Vascular disorders
      (3) Acid-base imbalance
      (4) Malignancy
      (5) Hypovolemic shock after hemorrhage
      (6) Massive transfusion therapy
2. Physical findings

   a. Bleeding
      (1) May occur from gums, puncture sites, bladder, uterus, and nose
      (2) Is usually without clots
      (3) May distend abdomen after cesarean section
      (4) Low-grade DIC increases the risks of thrombosis or hemorrhage
   b. Signs and symptoms of shock
      (1) Pale, clammy skin
      (2) Rising thready pulse rate and falling blood pressure
      (3) Altered level of response and consciousness
      (4) Respiratory distress
      (5) Renal failure
   c. Abnormal clotting studies (some but not all may be abnormal)
      (1) Fibrinogen levels less than 100 mg/dl; normal is 300 to 600 mg/dl during pregnancy
      (2) Platelet count less than 50,000 (normal is 150,000 to 400,000 mm^3); symptomatic is less than 100,000 mm^3
      (3) FSP present, elevated, or both; normal is 10 μg/ml
      (4) Plasma antithrombin III (AT III) consumption
      (5) Elevated fibrinopeptide A
         (a) Values depend upon methodology
         (b) Is rarely used and availability is limited
         (c) May rule out thrombotic episode when other methods fail
      (6) Abnormal PT and PTT values may vary with methodology
         (a) Thrombin time (TT) is 15 seconds
         (b) PT is 11 seconds, at least 60%
         (c) Whole blood clotting time (WBCT) is 4 to 12 minutes
         (d) Activated coagulation time (ACT) by hand is 75 to 90 seconds
         (e) Activated partial thromboplastin time (aPTT) is 26 to 39 seconds
      (7) Schistocytosis
         (a) Arteriolar vasospasms damage the endothelial layer of small blood vessels, forming lesions that allow platelet aggregation and formation of a fibrin network
         (b) The RBCs that are forced through the fibrin network under high pressure are hemolyzed
         (c) The same process results in the formation of schistocytes, which are abnormally shaped RBCs that are further evidence of erythrocyte damage (Poole, 1988)
      (8) Leukocytosis
      (9) Positive protamine sulfate test
      (10) Abnormal clot retraction
   d. FHR patterns indicative of fetal distress
      (1) Loss of variability
      (2) Tachycardia or bradycardia
      (3) Occasional sinusoidal pattern
3. Psychosocial findings
   a. Maternal anxiety
      (1) Related to self
      (2) Related to baby
   b. Maternal sense of impending doom
   c. Maternal altered consciousness and response
4. Diagnostic procedures
   a. Complete clotting studies
   b. Liver studies
   c. Arterial blood gas studies
   d. Type and crossmatch for blood products
   e. Measurement of abdominal height and girth as appropriate (see physical findings)
   f. Palpate for uterine tone and contractions

B. Nursing Diagnoses

1. Alteration in maternal tissue perfusion
2. Alteration in fetal tissue perfusion (if undelivered)
3. Alteration in respiratory function, decreased
4. Maternal anxiety related to threat to self and fetus
5. High risk for altered consciousness, related to altered respiratory function

C. Interventions/Evaluations

1. Alteration in maternal tissue perfusion
   a. Interventions
      (1) Draw blood for clotting studies and send to laboratory
         (a) Serial levels may be helpful in diagnosis
         (b) Some studies may be repeated
      (2) Establish IV line with large-bore intracatheter (16 gauge or 18 gauge)
      (3) Administer fluids and blood products, as ordered
         (a) Anticipate aggressive fluid therapy
         (b) Crystalloids, colloids, fresh frozen plasma, cryoprecipitate, platelets, fresh whole blood, and packed RBCs may be used
      (4) Administer oxygen via face mask at 8 l/min
      (5) Monitor vital signs, including quality of respiration rate and baseline characteristics
      (6) Position client for comfort
      (7) Administer medications ordered (e.g., heparin, which is used to normalize PTT and prevent thrombosis)
         (a) Variable results
         (b) More therapeutic if AT III is over 70%
         (c) Usual dose: 2500 to 5000 U subcutaneously every 8 to 12 hours
         (d) Other medications: AT III concentrates and antiplatelet drugs
   b. Evaluations: improved tissue perfusion shown by the following
      (1) Decreased blood loss
      (2) Improved results in clotting studies
      (3) Improved vital signs
      (4) Normal or improved respirations
      (5) Improved color and warmth of skin
2. Alteration in fetal perfusion (if undelivered)
   a. Interventions
      (1) Continuously monitor fetal heart for rate, variability, and sinusoidal pattern
      (2) Avoid supine position when positioning client for comfort
      (3) Treat mother for alteration in tissue perfusion
   b. Evaluations: normal or improved FHR and variability
3. Alteration in respiratory function; decreased
   a. Interventions
      (1) Administer oxygen as needed via face mask, tracheostomy, or endotracheal tube
      (2) Position for improvement in respiration
      (3) Observe rate and quality of respirations
   b. Evaluations: stable or improved respiratory status as evidenced by the following
      (1) Adequate oxygenation maintained as confirmed by blood gas studies
      (2) Respiration within normal limits
4. Maternal anxiety related to threat to self and fetus
   a. Interventions
      (1) Speak calmly to client and support persons
      (2) Reassure about fetal status
      (3) Explain interventions and their rationale

b. Evaluation: client reports less anxiety
5. High risk for altered consciousness related to altered respiratory function
   a. Interventions
      (1) Assess level of consciousness in client
         (a) Is oriented to place, person, and time
         (b) Answers questions appropriately
         (c) Responds to stimuli
         (d) Follows commands
      (2) Explain and provide information
   b. Evaluation: level of consciousness remains within normal limits

Gestational Trophoblastic Disease

Introduction

A. Gestational trophoblastic disease describes a spectrum of trophoblastic diseases that have common clinical findings such as abnormal, proliferative tissues and abnormally high chorionic gonadotropin (HCG) levels.

B. Classifications have varied over the years, but the symptoms are unchanged for the hydatidiform mole and neoplasia.

C. Molar pregnancy is characterized by chronic or acute bleeding and a uterus that is large for gestational age after all other causes have been ruled out such as

1. Myoma
2. Hydramnios
3. Multiple fetuses
4. Inaccurate gestational dating

Clinical Practice

A. Assessment

1. History
   a. Hydatidiform mole (molar pregnancy)
      (1) Complete (classic)
         (a) Maternal genetic tissues lost: no nucleus in fertilized egg
         (b) No fetal tissue
         (c) Neoplasia rate of 20% occurs
         (d) Other microscopic differences from incomplete type occur
      (2) Incomplete (atypical)
         (a) Fetal tissue noted: amniotic sac, fetus, or both
         (b) Triploid karyotype: 69 chromosomes often present
         (c) Neoplasia rate of 5% occurs
      (3) Incidence
         (a) In 1/1500 to 2000 pregnancies in United States and Europe
         (b) Is higher in countries outside United States and Europe
         (c) Is 10 times higher if mother is older than 45 years
         (d) Has four to five times increased risk of recurrence
   b. Invasive mole (chorioadenoma destruens)
      (1) Severity is intermediate between mole and choriocarcinoma: usually a locally invasive lesion
      (2) Occurs when trophoblastic tissue continues to grow
      (3) Trophoblastic tissue locally invades
         (a) Uterine myometrium
         (b) Pelvic blood vessels
         (c) Vagina, occasionally

        (4) Occurrence rate is 15% after hyatidiform mole

   c. Choriocarcinoma

       (1) Is highly malignant, with wide spread metastasis

       (2) Spreads to

          (a) Lungs

          (b) Brain

          (c) Liver

          (d) Kidneys

          (e) Intestines

          (f) Spleen

          (g) Vagina

       (3) Is not always preceded by mole

          (a) About 25% of diagnosed choriocarcinoma is preceded by spontaneous abortion

          (b) 20% of cases of diagnosed choriocarcinoma occur after normal pregnancy with abnormal tissue proliferation

       (4) Five percent of molar pregnancies turn into choriocarcinoma

       (5) High levels of HCG persist after delivery

  2. Physical findings

   a. Hydatidiform mole (molar pregnancy)

       (1) Trophoblast proliferates

          (a) Villi become edematous because of lack of fetal circulation

          (b) In classic type, villi become mass of clear vesicles hanging in clusters

          (c) Can be located in uterus, oviduct, or ovary

       (2) Chronic or acute bleeding seen by 12 weeks' gestation

          (a) Overt or concealed

          (b) Brown or bright red blood

       (3) Signs and symptoms may include anemia, hypervolemia, nausea, vomiting, abdominal cramping, and expulsion of vesicles

       (4) Uterus rapidly enlarges

          (a) Palpation is difficult because of soft tissue

          (b) Ovaries may be enlarged and tender

       (5) Fetal heart tones are absent or have one heartbeat only in a twin molar pregnancy

       (6) Pregnancy-induced hypertension occurs at less than 24 weeks' gestation

       (7) Emboli are more frequent, especially pulmonary emboli

       (8) Ultrasonography shows molar pregnancy

   b. Neoplasia: chorioadenoma destruens or choriocarcinoma

       (1) Prognosis can be good or poor, depending on extent of disease

       (2) Condition often develops early as blood-borne trophoblast

       (3) Lungs are commonly invaded (75% of metastases)

          (a) Cough and bloody sputum are present

          (b) Original lesion may disappear

       (4) Also invades vagina (50%), vulva, kidney, liver, brain, ovaries, and bowel

       (5) Good prognosis

          (a) Detected and therapy started within 4 months of onset

          (b) HCG levels of less than 40,000 l IU/ml

          (c) No prior chemotherapy

          (d) Cure rate of 90 to 100%

       (6) Poor prognosis

          (a) Detected at more than 4 months' duration

          (b) HCG levels of greater than 40,000 l IU/ml or rising indicate extensive disease

          (c) Prior chemotherapy failure

          (d) Metastasis to brain and liver (irradiation may be useful)

          (e) Occurs after a term pregnancy

(f) Remission rate of 45 to 65%
(g) Death usually a result of hemorrhage
c. Other placental trophoblastic tumors
(1) Chorioangioma or hemangioma
(a) Small tumors: asymptomatic
(b) Large tumors: may lead to antepartum hemorrhage, hydramnios, fetal anemia, or fetal death
(2) Metastatic placental tumors
(a) Any blood-borne metastasis may involve placenta
(b) Leukemias and lymphoma make up 30%
(c) Malignant melanoma makes up 30%

B. Nursing Diagnoses

1. High risk for fluid volume deficit related to evacuation of hydatidiform mole
2. Grief related to loss of pregnancy
3. High risk for altered health maintenance related to insufficient knowledge of trophoblastic disease
4. Anxiety related to fear of carcinoma secondary to trophoblastic disease

C. Interventions/Evaluations

1. High risk for fluid volume deficit related to evacuation of hydatidiform mole
   a. Interventions
      (1) Monitor vital signs and blood pressure
      (2) Monitor amount of bleeding by menstrual pad count
      (3) Order preoperative laboratory work
         (a) CBC
         (b) Clotting studies
         (c) Type and crossmatch for blood products
         (d) Urinalysis
      (4) Begin or maintain IV line with 18-gauge or larger intracatheter
      (5) Administer ordered IV fluids for volume expansion
   b. Evaluations
      (1) Vital signs are within normal limits
      (2) Vaginal bleeding is absent or minimal
2. Grief related to loss of pregnancy (see Chapter 25 for complete discussion of perinatal grief)
3. High risk for altered health maintenance related to insufficient knowledge of trophoblastic disease
   a. Interventions
      (1) Encourage compliance with follow-up regimen (see health education section for specifics of follow-up)
      (2) Discuss contraceptive options to prevent pregnancy for 1 year (see Chapter 20 for complete discussion of contraception)
   b. Evaluations
      (1) Client agrees to comply with follow-up plan
      (2) Client has made plans for contraception
4. Anxiety related to fear of carcinoma secondary to trophoblastic disease
   a. Interventions
      (1) Encourage client to verbalize concerns
      (2) Clarify the relatively low risk of conversion to carcinoma
      (3) Reiterate the importance of follow-up care
   b. Evaluations
      (1) Client's anxiety is decreased
      (2) Client verbalizes concerns, fear, and frustrations related to trophoblastic disease

Health Education

A. Second-trimester placenta previa

1. Client may be prepared for discharge
    a. If transportation is immediately available
    b. If located within 20 minutes of hospital
2. Explain diagnosis, using pictures
3. Review symptoms necessitating return to hospital
    a. Bleeding
        (1) Describe amounts in metric or nonmetric units
        (2) Describe appearance of clots
    b. Uterine and abdominal pain
    c. Uterine contractions
    d. Rupture of membranes
4. Review risk of intrauterine growth retardation
    a. Importance of good nutrition
    b. Avoidance of smoking
    c. Importance of rest and side-lying position
    d. Avoidance of supine hypotension
        (1) Tilt to side, even with semi-fowler's position
        (2) Side-lying position
5. Explain importance of follow-up
    a. Serial ultrasound tests at 2 to 4 week intervals
        (1) Placental status and position
        (2) Fetal growth
    b. Other antepartum testing
    c. Maternal status
        (1) Hypovolemia
        (2) Anemia
        (3) Coagulopathy
        (4) Fatigue
        (5) Signs of labor
        (6) Avoidance of coitus

B. Late third-trimester placenta previa

1. Explain reasons for hospitalization
    a. Cervical changes occurring near delivery
    b. Bleeding risk
        (1) Need for transfusion
        (2) Need for observation and blood testing
    c. Viability of fetus
        (1) Neonatal resuscitation anticipated
        (2) Immediate neonatal care needed, especially if preterm
    d. Need to observe labor status
        (1) Tocolytics, as needed
        (2) Likelihood of cesarean section
    e. Need for fetal observation and testing
        (1) FHR monitoring
        (2) Fetal lung maturity
        (3) Ultrasound testing
    f. Provide educational videotapes and reading materials (as available), such as information about the following
        (1) Labor and delivery
        (2) Baby care
        (3) Nutrition

C. Abruptio placentae

1. Explain problem of placental separation before delivery
   a. Risk to fetus
   b. Risk to mother
   c. Symptoms to report to nurse and physician
      (1) Feeling of increased blood loss
      (2) Increased pain and contractions
      (3) Difficulty in breathing and dizziness
2. Explain plan of care
   a. Fluid replacement
   b. Blood replacement, as needed
   c. Need to monitor FHR and maternal vital signs
   d. Need for possible ultrasound test
   e. Preoperative preparation for possible cesarean section
   f. Close observation of both mother and baby

D. Chronic DIC

1. Explain that blood is not clotting properly
2. Explain necessity for observation and tests
   a. Fetal monitoring
   b. Coagulation factors
   c. Signs of increased bleeding
   d. Signs of other complications
3. Prepare for events of care
   a. Explain present orders
   b. Explain plans if condition worsens

E. Acute DIC

1. Explain that blood is not clotting properly
2. Explain immediate actions in progress
   a. Fluid replacement
   b. Use of blood products
   c. Use of Foley catheter
   d. Measurement of CVP or use of Swan-Ganz catheter
3. Reassure client of procedures and activity in progress
4. Prepare client for imminent events, such as
   a. Possible cesarean section
   b. Measurement of CVP or use of Swan-Ganz catheter

F. Gestational trophoblastic disease

1. Provide information on condition, symptoms, and cause; explain the following
   a. Abnormal pregnancy
   b. Cause or control unknown
   c. What is in uterus
   d. Symptoms of nausea, vomiting, cramping, and bleeding
2. Describe events to expect during evacuation procedures
   a. Vacuum curettage is usually the preferred procedure
      (1) Medication for pain
      (2) Cramping and bleeding
      (3) Environment and equipment
   b. Hysterectomy procedure performed
      (1) If excessive bleeding is present
      (2) If mother over 40 to 45 years of age
3. Provide information regarding need for follow-up of 1 year, which may consist of the following
   a. HCG levels

(1) Weekly for 3 weeks
(2) Monthly for 6 months
(3) Every 2 months for 6 months
   b. No pregnancy for 1 year
   c. Chest x-ray film
4. Acknowledge family concerns and provide information about resources for support and additional understanding

CASE STUDIES AND STUDY QUESTIONS

W.A., a 29-year-old gravida 6, para 1 (G6, P1), has been admitted to a local level I hospital at 26 or 27 weeks' gestation complaining of bleeding without pain. Vital signs are stable, her hematocrit is 30.5%, and an ultrasound scan reveals a complete placenta previa. She is given IV magnesium sulfate and oral terbutaline for mild uterine contractions and transferred to a level III (tertiary) regional hospital. After 12 days' hospitalization, no further bleeding is noted and W.A. is discharged on bed rest. She lives within 15 minutes of the hospital.

Upon readmission for bleeding at 29 weeks, about 200 ml of vaginal blood is noted. W.A. is started on a graduated dose regimen of magnesium sulfate, 5 g the first hour, 4 g the second hour, 3 g the next hour, and then a maintenance dose. At this time, an ultrasound scan reveals a complete previa, grade II placenta, and transverse fetal lie.

On the 10th day of admission, uterine contractions and increased amounts of bleeding begin. Her hematocrit is 25.9%, hemoglobin value is 8.5 g/dl, vital signs are stable, and a nonstress test (NST) is reactive. On day 14, W.A. experiences spontaneous rupture of membranes (SROM) with clear amniotic fluid, increasing uterine contractions, persistent bloody drainage; an ultrasonography shows an oblique lie. A cesarean section is performed and the placenta previa is noted to have abrupted free of the internal os. The combined blood loss before and during surgery is estimated at 2000 ml.

In the recovery room, lochia rubra is light to moderate, the fundus is firm at the umbilicus, and oxygen saturation in arterial blood (SaO_2) is 98 to 99%. W.A. receives a continuous IV infusion of Ringer's lactate with 20 U of oxytocin (Pitocin), morphine sulfate for pain, an additional 2 U of packed RBCs, and prophylactic ampicillin.

1. As W.A.'s nurse you should know that a transverse lie

   a. Is an isolated condition.

   b. Indicates an occiput presentation of either left occipitotransverse (LOT) or right occipitotransverse (ROT).

   c. Is more common with a placenta previa.

   d. Will be rotated by her physician to a normal presentation.

2. Measuring W.A.'s hematocrit periodically

   (1) Is referred to as serial hematocrit.

   (2) Reflects the normal hemodilution of W.A.'s pregnancy.

   (3) Reflects the need for transfusion.

   (4) Reflects the blood loss from her previa.

   a. 1, 3.

   b. 2.

   c. 3, 4.

   d. 1, 3, 4.

3. In providing intrapartum and recovery care to W.A., your observations and care are influenced by the knowledge that with a placenta previa

   a. The risk of postpartum hemorrhage is the same as that for any cesarean delivery.

   b. The risk of an accreta placenta is greater and postpartum hemorrhage is greater.

   c. The risk of accreta placenta is less and postpartum hemorrhage is greater.

   d. Coagulopathy is an unlikely occurrence.

4. As the high-risk antepartum nurse for W.A., which of the following actions would you try to initiate?

a. Acquisition of an eggcrate mattress or similar mattress.

b. Instruction before her first hospital discharge about the danger signs of bleeding and cramping.

c. Refusal to discharge her to her home.

d. Both a and b.

V.P. is a 21-year-old Laotian Hmong, gravida 4 para 3 (G4, P3), with a history of one cesarean section followed by two vaginal births after cesarean (VBAC) who appears at the hospital complaining of vaginal bleeding. She is uncertain of her estimated date of confinement, and an ultrasound scan places her at 27 to 28 weeks' gestation with an anterior fundal placenta and breech presentation. Her vital signs are stable, hematocrit level is 34.1%, hemoglobin value is 11.5 g/dl, and during the next 2 weeks, V.P. has small amounts of dark, bloody discharge with occasional scant, bright red, mucouslike bleeding.

V.P. remains hospitalized and receives a tapering magnesium sulfate regimen; oral terbutaline, 2.5 mg every 3 hours; oral indomethacin, 25 mg every 6 hours; and steroids for stimulating fetal lung maturity.

On day 14, V.P. has increased mucous and bloody discharge, low back pain, cramps, and seems tense. She refuses lunch and now the uterine tone is palpable, and cervical changes are noted; the FHR is 160 beats/min with decreased long-term variability, and variable decelerations occur with uterine contractions.

A decision is made to perform a cesarean section at 29 to 30 week's gestation during which a 20 to 25% abruption is noted with a 200-g retroplacental clot; estimated blood loss at delivery is 800 ml. A 1360-g (3 lb) girl with Apgar scores of 5 and 6 is delivered and no immediate fetal respiratory distress is noted.

Although V.P. recovers well, her second-day hematocrit is 22% and her hemoglobin value is 7.3 g/dl; 2 U of packed RBCs are administered. On postpartum day 3 she is discharged in stable condition with a hematocrit of 30%, and a hemoglobin value of 9.7 g/dl.

5. A breech presentation in this situation

a. Is common with abruptio placentae.

b. Is an isolated event.

c. Adds danger of uterine bleeding.

d. Adds danger of uterine rupture.

6. At delivery, a retroplacental clot was noted near the center of the placenta. If V.P. continued to bleed from the clot site, she would have been likely to develop which of the following?

(1) Concealed bleeding.

(2) Revealed bleeding.

(3) Couvelaire uterus.

(4) Uterine rupture.

a. 2.

b. 2, 4.

c. 1, 3.

d. 1.

7. At 9 cm, V.P. suddenly loses consciousness; becomes cyanotic; has shallow, irregular respirations and a rapid, thready pulse; and the FHR decreased to 50 beats/min. These are symptoms of which of the following?

a. Precipitous delivery.

b. Abruptio placentae.

c. Impending cardiac arrest.

d. Supine hypotension.

8. The above situation

a. Is unrelated to abruptio placentae.

b. Is associated with abruptio placentae.

c. Occurs frequently with abruptio placentae.

d. Is an unrealistic description.

P.R. is a 23-year-old gravida 4, para 1 (G4, P1), 167.6-cm, 73.5-kg (5 ft 6 in, 162-lb) woman who is at 27 to 28 weeks' gestation by ultrasonography and at 30.5 weeks' gestation by dates. She presents to her local level I hospital when she notes vaginal spotting of bright red blood and is transferred to a level III tertiary hospital for preterm labor and partial separation of the placenta. Her total blood loss is 400 to 500 ml and 4 days later, her hematocrit is 32.7%. P.R. tests positive for amphetamine and methamphetamine and negative for cocaine. She smokes 1½ pack of cigarettes daily and drinks five to eight cups of coffee per day. P.R. begins a regimen of magnesium sulfate, oral indomethacin, prophylactic ampicillin, and steroids. She remains stable on bed rest for 5 days, is weaned from her tocolytics, and is discharged to return to her local obstetrical care.

9. It is possible that the bleeding P.R. experienced was caused by which of the following?

    a. Amphetamine sulfate.

    b. Intrauterine growth retardation.

    c. Increased activity.

    d. Cocaine use.

10. In P.R.'s situation, it is important that a nurse or an appropriate professional evaluate which of the following?

    (1) Her nutritional history.

    (2) Her source of amphetamines.

    (3) Her preparation for an unmedicated childbirth.

    (4) Her awareness of prenatal substance use on the fetus.

    a. 1, 2.

    b. 1, 3, 4.

    c. 1, 4.

    d. 2, 3.

11. The health of P.R.'s fetus may be influenced by which of the following?

    (1) Past use of amphetamines, nicotine, and caffeine.

    (2) Past nutritional intake.

    (3) Future nutritional and substance use.

    (4) Prepregnant use of nicotine and caffeine.

    a. 1, 2.

    b. 1, 2, 3.

    c. 2, 4.

    d. 3, 4.

12. P.R. is returned to her local level I hospital because of which of the following?

    a. She has no insurance.

    b. She uses drugs.

    c. There is no further medical problem.

    d. a, b, c.

Answers to Study Questions

1. c	2. d	3. b
4. d	5. b	6. c
7. c	8. b	9. a
10. c	11. b	12. c

REFERENCES

Abdella T., Sibai, B., Hays, J., & Anderson, G. (1984). Relationship of hypertensive disease to abruptio placentae. *Obstetrics and Gynecology 63*, 365–370.

Bobak, I., Jensen, L., & Zalar, M. (1989). *Maternity and gynecologic nursing* (pp. 760–762). St. Louis: Mosby.

Breener W., Edelman, D., & Hendricks, C. (1978). Characteristics of patients with placenta previa and results of "expectant management". *American Journal of Obstetrics and Gynecology 132*, 180–184.

Clark, S., Koonings, P., & Phelan, J. (1985). Placenta previa/accreta and prior cesarean section. *Obstetrics and Gynecology 66*, 89–92.

Clark, S., & Phelan, J. (1984, August). Surgical control of OB hemorrhage. *Contemporary Ob/Gyn*, p. 70.

Clark, S. (1986). Amniotic fluid embolism. *Clinics in Perinatology 13*(4), 801–811.

Clark, S. (1990). New concepts of amniotic fluids embolism: A review. *Obstetrical and Gynecological Survey, 45*, 360–368.

Comeau J., Shaw, L., & Marcell, C. (1983). Early placenta previa and delivery outcome. *Obstetrics and Gynecology, 61*, 577–580.

Cotton, D., Read, J., & Paul, R. (1980). The conservative aggressive management of placenta previa. *American Journal of Obstetrics and Gynecology, 137*, 687–695.

Cunningham, F., MacDonald, P., & Gant, N. (1989). *Williams obstetrics* (18th ed.). Norwalk, CT: Appleton & Lange.

Darby, M., Caritis, S., & Shen-Schwarz, S. (1989). Placental abruption in the preterm gestation: An association with chorioamnionitis. *Obstetrics and Gynecology, 74*(1), 88–92.

D'Angelo L., & Irwin, L. (1984). Conservative management of placenta previa: A cost-benefit analysis. *American Journal Obstetrics and Gynecology, 149*:320–326.

Duff, P. (1984, August). Defusing dangers of amniotic fluid embolism. *Contemporary Ob/Gyn, 127–134*.

Gianopoulos, J., Carver, T., & Tomich, P. (1987). Diagnosis of vasa previa with ultrasonography. *Obstetrics and Gynecology, 69:*488–492.

Gottesfeld, K. (1983, December). When the patient has placenta previa. *Contemporary Ob/Gyn 17,* 17–22.

Green, J. (1984). Placental abnormalities: Placenta previa and abruptio placentae. In R. Creasy & R. Resnik (Eds.), *Maternal-fetal medicine: Principles and practice* (pp. 539–559). Philadelphia: Saunders.

Hayashi, R. (1986). Hemorrhagic shock in obstetrics. *Clinics in Perinatology, 13*(4), 755–763.

Higgins, S. (1984). Essentials of fluid resuscitation and blood transfusion. *Contemporary Ob/Gyn,* 102–110.

Kouyoumdjian, A. (1980). Velamentous insertion of the umbilical cord. *Obstetrics and Gynecology, 56,* 737–742.

Ladewig, P., London, M., & Olds, S. (1990). *Essentials of maternal-newborn nursing* (2nd ed.) (pp. 309–310). Redwood City, CA: Addison-Wesley Nursing.

Lavery, J. (1987). *The human placenta: Clinical perspectives* (pp. 250–251). Rockville, MD: Aspen.

Lavery, J. (1982, July). When coagulopathy threatens the pregnant patient. *Contemporary Ob/Gyn,* 191–199.

Lockwood, C. (1990, January). Placenta previa and related disorders. *Contemporary Ob/Gyn,* 47–68.

Montiel, M. (1984, August). Tips for controlling hemorrhage diatheses. *Contemporary Ob/Gyn,* 87.

Naeye, R. (1978). Placenta previa predisposing factors and effects on the fetus and surviving infants. *American Journal of Obstetrics and Gynecology, 52*(5), 521–524.

Pelligra, R., & Sandberg, E. (1979). Control of intractable abdominal bleeding by external counterpressure. *Journal of the American Medical Association, 241:*708–713.

Poole, J. (1988). Getting perspective on HELLP syndrome. *Maternal Child Nursing, 13,* 432–437.

Quilligan, E. (1983). Third-trimester bleeding. In E. Quilligan (Ed.), *Current therapy in obstetrics and gynecology* (pp. 8–10). Philadelphia: Saunders.

Schmidt, J. (1984). Hemorrhagic complications of pregnancy. *NAACOG Update Series, 1*(15).

Silver, R., Depp, R., & Sabbagha, R. (1984). Placenta previa: Aggressive expectant management. *American Journal of Obstetrics and Gynecology, 150:*15–22.

Weckstein, L., Masserman, J., & Garite, T. (1987). Placenta accreta: A problem of increasing clinical significance. *Obstetrics and Gynecology, 69:*480–482.

Weinstein, L. (1982). Syndrome of hemolysis, elevated liver enzymes, and low platelet count. *American Journal of Obstetrics and Gynecology, 142:*159–163.

Weiner, C. (1986). The obstetric patient and disseminated intravascular coagulation. *Clinics in Perinatology, 13*(4):705–717.

Wexler P., & Gottesfeld, K. (1979). Early diagnosis of placenta previa. *Obstetrics and Gynecology,* 54:231–234.

Kathleen A. Kalb

Endocrine and Metabolic Disorders

Objectives

1. Describe maternal and fetal complications associated with endocrine and metabolic disorders in pregnancy

2. Recognize alterations in pregnancy associated with various endocrine and metabolic disorders

3. Identify signs and symptoms associated with endocrine and metabolic disorders that may be diagnosed preconceptually or during gestation and that require specific nursing interventions and care for the childbearing woman

4. Evaluate significant clinical signs and symptoms characterized by various endocrine and metabolic disorders during the childbearing period

5. Plan nursing assessments and interventions essential in caring for the childbearing woman with an endocrine or metabolic disorder

6. Prescribe specific educational content and strategies to empower the childbearing woman with an endocrine or metabolic disorder to knowledgeably participate in her plan of care throughout the childbearing experience

Diabetes Mellitus

Introduction

A. Definition

1. Chronic, systemic endocrine disorder
2. Caused by a lack of insulin secretion or increased cellular resistance to insulin
3. Characterized by an abnormal metabolism of carbohydrates, proteins, fats, and electrolytes
4. Results in hyperglycemia and other metabolic disturbances
5. Associated with severe neurological, cardiovascular, ocular, and renal complications

B. Symptoms

1. Excessive thirst and hunger

2. Frequent urination
3. Blurred vision
4. Weight loss
5. Recurrent infections
6. Often asymptomatic in its early stages

C. Classification

1. Insulin-dependent diabetes mellitus (IDDM), also called type I diabetes
   a. Usually appears before the age of 30 years
   b. Has an abrupt onset of symptoms requiring prompt medical treatment with insulin
   c. Approximately 10% of all individuals diagnosed with diabetes have IDDM
2. Noninsulin-dependent diabetes mellitus (NIDDM), also called type II diabetes
   a. NIDDM is diagnosed primarily in adults older than 30 years of age
   b. Disease is typically symptom-free for many years, with slow onset and progression of symptoms
   c. Incidence of NIDDM increases with age, accounting for about 90% of all diagnosed cases of diabetes
   d. Disease is managed with diet, exercise, oral hypoglycemic medications, or insulin
3. Gestational diabetes mellitus (GDM)
   a. Onset or first recognition of symptoms occurs during pregnancy
   b. Estimated to occur in approximately 3% of pregnancies
   c. Usually disappears after delivery
   d. Women diagnosed with GDM are at increased risk for developing diabetes at a later date
   e. Symptoms are generally mild and not life-threatening to the pregnant woman
   f. Maternal hyperglycemia is associated with increased fetal morbidity; therefore, maintenance of normal glucose levels is required
4. Impaired glucose tolerance (IGT)
   a. Characterized by hyperglycemia at a level lower than that which qualifies as a diagnosis of diabetes
   b. Symptoms of diabetes are absent

D. Metabolic changes in pregnancy

1. Changes in carbohydrate, protein, and fat metabolism in normal pregnancy are profound, mediated by the developing fetus and production of placental hormones
2. First half of pregnancy is considered an anabolic phase
   a. In pregnant women without diabetes, this is associated with increased estrogen and progesterone secretion leading to increased beta-cell activity and insulin production
   b. Increased insulin production leads to an increased tissue response to insulin and increased storage of glycogen and fat in the liver and other tissues
3. Second half of pregnancy is characterized by a catabolic phase with increased insulin resistance due to diabetogenic hormones produced by the placenta; in women who cannot meet the increasing demands for insulin production, this leads to progressive hyperglycemia
   a. Increased production of human placental lactogen (HPL)
   b. Elevated levels of estrogen, progesterone, blood triglycerides, free fatty acids, and serum cortisol
   c. Tendency for increased lipolysis and ketone production
4. Developing fetus continuously removes glucose and amino acids from the maternal circulation
   a. Glucose and amino acids are readily transported across the placenta, insulin is not

   b. Maternal hyperglycemia leads to fetal beta-cell hyperplasia and fetal hyper-insulinemia
      (1) Fetal hyperinsulinism functions as a growth hormone for the developing fetus
      (2) Fetal hyperinsulinism contributes to macrosomia, which leads to a decrease in surfactant production and development of respiratory distress syndrome in the neonate
   5. The constant drain on maternal glucose levels across the placenta leads to hypoglycemia and explains the low fasting blood glucose levels observed during normal pregnancy

E. Primary goals in the treatment of diabetes and pregnancy

   1. Achieve and maintain normal maternal glucose levels
   2. Note: normal blood glucose levels are lower during pregnancy than in the nonpregnant state because of the drain on maternal blood glucose levels by the fetus (Table 29–1)

Clinical Practice

PREGESTATIONAL DIABETES

A. Assessment

   1. Introduction
      a. Incidence of pregestational insulin treated diabetes is approximately 0.2 to 0.3% of all pregnancies
      b. Pregnant women with pregestational diabetes are categorized according to the classic system of White with some minor modifications (Table 29–2.)
      c. Distinctions between IDDM (type 1) and NIDDM (type II) may not be critical in the actual management of diabetes during pregnancy
      d. The quality of the metabolic regulation throughout pregnancy and presence or absence of serious complications of diabetes, especially nephropathy, hypertension, and heart disease, account for most of the risks associated with diabetes in pregnancy rather than the genetic characteristics of the maternal diabetes
   2. History
      a. Preconceptual assessments
         (1) Classification of diabetes in pregnancy
         (2) Blood glucose control, Hgb A1c (glycosylated hemoglobin), and frequency of self blood glucose monitoring
         (3) Presence of vascular complications and current vascular status
         (4) Adequacy of current diet and plans for dietary regulation in pregnancy
         (5) Current insulin regimen
         (6) Current method of contraception and family planning
      b. Gestational assessments

Table 29–1
BLOOD GLUCOSE VALUES IN PREGNANCY

	Ideal*	Goal
Fasting blood glucose	55–60 mg/dl	<90 mg/dl
1 hour postprandial	120–140 mg/dl	<140 mg/dl
Mean blood glucose	84 mg/dl	<100 mg/dl
Hemoglobin A1c	2–5%	<7%

* These values are demonstrated in women with neither diabetes nor carbohydrate intolerance during pregnancy.

Table 29–2
MODIFIED WHITE'S CLASSIFICATION OF DIABETES IN PREGNANCY

Class		Age of Onset		Duration	Vascular Disease	Treatment
A		Any		Any	None	Diet alone
	A1	During pregnancy			None	Diet alone
	A2	During pregnancy			None	Insulin
B		≥20		<10	None	Insulin
C		10–19	or	10–19	None	Insulin
D		≤10	or	>20	Benign (hypertension, background retinopathy)	Insulin
F		Any		Any	Nephropathy	Insulin
R		Any		Any	Proliferative retinopathy	Insulin
H		Any		Any	Cardiac disease	Insulin
T		Any		Any	Renal transplant	Insulin

(1) Dietary regulation and intake
(2) Glucose monitoring
    (a) Frequency and method of testing
    (b) Pattern and recorded results of self-monitoring of blood glucose levels
    (c) Response to changing pattern of blood glucose results in adjustment of insulin requirements
    (d) Hgb A1c, usually each trimester
(3) Insulin administration and intensified insulin therapies
    (a) Multiple injections, usually a mixture of regular and intermediate acting insulins administered in the morning in a 1:2 ratio and in the evening in a 1:1 ratio
    (b) Continuous subcutaneous insulin infusion by an insulin pump
    (c) Dosage adjustments according to changing insulin requirements during pregnancy to maintain euglycemia
(4) Urinalysis (UA) and urine culture (UC) usually each trimester or if client has symptoms
(5) Evaluation of fetal status
    (a) Ultrasound testing
        (i) Pregnancy dating
        (ii) Fetal growth and development
        (iii) Assessment of congenital anomalies
        (iv) Presence of macrosomia or intrauterine growth retardation (IUGR)
    (b) Maternal serum alpha-feto-protein (AFP)
    (c) Biophysical profile (BPP)
    (d) Nonstress testing (NST)
    (e) Contraction stress testing (CST)
    (f) Maternal assessment of fetal activity and fetal movement counts
    (g) Amniocentesis to assess fetal lung maturity and optimize timing of delivery
3. Physical findings
  a. Maternal effects
    (1) Altered insulin requirements during pregnancy
    (2) Possible acceleration of vascular disease secondary to diabetes including diabetic retinopathy, nephropathy, and neuropathy
    (3) Increased maternal mortality, associated with the following
        (a) Ischemic heart disease
        (b) Advanced vascular disease
        (c) Ketoacidosis

(d) Hypoglycemia

(e) Complications of cesarean section

(4) Hydramnios

(5) Pregnancy-induced hypertension (PIH)

(6) Increased risk of hypoglycemia, especially in first trimester

(7) Increased risk of ketoacidosis, especially in second trimester

(8) Dystocia (related to fetal macrosomia)

(9) Anemia

(10) Infections, especially urinary tract infections (UTIs)

b. Fetal and neonatal effects

(1) Increased incidence of congenital malformations and anomalies, including cardiac, skeletal, neurological, genitourinary, and gastrointestinal

(2) Respiratory distress syndrome

(3) Macrosomia and birth trauma (classes A to C, mothers without vascular disease)

(4) IUGR (classes D to T, mothers with vascular disease)

(5) Neonatal hypoglycemia

(6) Neonatal hypocalcemia

(7) Neonatal hyperbilirubinemia

(8) Neonatal polycythemia

4. Psychosocial findings

a. Presence of support system—partner or family

b. Occupational status

c. Financial concerns

d. Planned or unplanned pregnancy

e. Family's response to pregnancy

f. Feelings regarding high-risk status of pregnancy

5. Diagnostic procedures

a. Hgb A1c (blood test that reflects mean blood glucose levels during the previous 4 to 8 weeks)

b. Renal function tests

c. Ophthalmological examination

d. Cardiovascular assessment

B. Nursing Diagnoses

1. Alteration in metabolism of carbohydrates, proteins, fats, and electrolytes related to pre-existing diabetes and pregnancy

2. Anxiety related to potential for exacerbation of maternal vascular complications; anxiety related to pregnancy and its outcome

3. Powerlessness related to fetal outcome

4. Knowledge deficit related to self-monitoring and obstetrical management of diabetes during pregnancy

5. High risk for fetal injury related to fetal dependence on maternal glycemic states

6. Alteration in family systems related to demands of optimal diabetes and obstetrical care during pregnancy

C. Interventions/Evaluations

1. Alteration in metabolism of carbohydrates, proteins, fats, and electrolytes related to pre-existing diabetes and pregnancy

a. Interventions

(1) Monitor blood glucose levels and results of testing including Hgb A1c

(2) Assist with regulation of insulin dosage according to changing physiological needs and blood glucose levels in each trimester of pregnancy; *note:* may switch to human forms of insulin and intensify insulin regimen with multiple injections two to four times daily or initiate insulin pump therapy

        (3) Encourage urine testing for ketones for blood glucose levels of 240 mg/dl or over and during maternal illness

        (4) Review signs and symptoms for maternal hypoglycemia and ketoacidosis, which may be altered during pregnancy

    b. Evaluations

        (1) Blood glucose levels remain within individualized goals determined for optimal maternal and fetal outcome

        (2) Insulin dosages are regulated according to changing physiological needs and maternal blood glucose levels in each trimester of pregnancy

        (3) Urine is tested for ketones when blood glucose levels are 240 mg/dl or higher during maternal illness

        (4) Signs and symptoms of maternal hypoglycemia and ketoacidosis are promptly recognized and managed during pregnancy

2. Anxiety related to potential for exacerbation of maternal vascular complications; anxiety related to pregnancy and its outcome

    a. Interventions

        (1) Clinical assessments

           (a) Blood pressure monitoring

           (b) Presence of visual disturbances

           (c) Signs and symptoms of PIH and UTIs

        (2) Prompt identification of alterations in clinical assessments and referral for appropriate medical and obstetrical management

    b. Evaluations

        (1) Alterations in blood pressure, presence of visual disturbances, and signs and symptoms of PIH and UTIs are promptly assessed

        (2) Appropriate referrals for medical and obstetrical management of clinical alterations in pregnancy are obtained to minimize potential maternal and fetal complications

3. Powerlessness related to fetal outcome

    a. Interventions

        (1) Discuss strategies for maintenance of optimal glycemic control during pregnancy

        (2) Provide information about tests and procedures for fetal assessment

        (3) Encourage active participation in decision making and planning for medical and obstetrical care throughout pregnancy

        (4) Discuss feelings about pregnancy and self-monitoring practices for management of diabetes during pregnancy

    b. Evaluations

        (1) Client maintains optimal glycemic control during pregnancy

        (2) Client receives information about tests and procedures for fetal assessment

        (3) Client actively participates in decision making and planning for medical and obstetrical care throughout pregnancy

        (4) Client expresses her feelings about her pregnancy and self-monitoring practices for management of diabetes during pregnancy

4. Knowledge deficit related to self-monitoring and obstetrical management of diabetes during pregnancy

    a. Interventions

        (1) Discuss rationale for blood glucose control and importance of euglycemia before conception and during pregnancy

        (2) Review self-care practices

           (a) Blood glucose monitoring and frequency of testing

           (b) Insulin administration

           (c) Adjustment of insulin dosages based on blood glucose determinations

           (d) Dietary management during pregnancy

        (3) Refer for dietary counseling to ensure optimal diet for glycemic control and fetal growth and development

        (4) Discuss plan of care for obstetrical management and fetal assessment
    b. Evaluations
        (1) Client verbalizes rationale for blood glucose control and importance of euglycemia before conception and during pregnancy
        (2) Client demonstrates proper techniques and frequency for blood glucose monitoring and insulin administration, adjusts insulin dosages based on blood glucose determinations, and modifies dietary intake during pregnancy
        (3) Client receives dietary counseling to ensure optimal diet for glycemic control and fetal growth and development
        (4) Client verbalizes recommended plan of care for obstetrical management and fetal assessment
  5. High risk for fetal injury related to fetal dependence on maternal glycemic states
    a. Interventions
        (1) Monitor maternal glycemia
        (2) Assess fetal well-being, including results of NST, CST, BPP, and ultrasound testing
        (3) Encourage maternal assessment of fetal movement using daily fetal movement counts
    b. Evaluations
        (1) Client demonstrates dietary management, blood glucose monitoring, and insulin dosage adjustments to maintain euglycemia
        (2) Fetal status and well-being are monitored using NST, CST, BPP, and ultrasound testing
        (3) Client participates in assessment of fetal well-being using daily fetal movement counts and reports changes in pattern of fetal activity
  6. Alteration in family systems related to demands of optimal diabetes and obstetrical care during pregnancy
    a. Interventions
        (1) Assess alterations in maternal work or employment status and potential economic impact of pregnancy including financial concerns and expenses
        (2) Assess maternal support systems and the presence and involvement of significant others in assisting the client with self-monitoring practices and care
        (3) Encourage active participation of significant others in prenatal care and testing
        (4) Discuss family's responses to pregnancy
    b. Evaluations
        (1) Client expresses financial concerns related to alterations in maternal work/employment status during pregnancy
        (2) Client describes support systems and the presence and involvement of significant others in plan of self-monitoring and care during pregnancy
        (3) Client's significant others will actively participate in prenatal care and testing
        (4) Client discusses family's responses to pregnancy

Health Education

A. Preconceptual

1. Discussion of potential maternal and fetal risks associated with diabetes and pregnancy, effects of diabetes on pregnancy and pregnancy on diabetes
2. Referral of client for genetic counseling
3. Discussion of financial expenses and other demands related to increased surveillance of maternal and fetal status during pregnancy

4. Discussion of rationale for interdisciplinary team approach and role of each team member in the management of diabetes and pregnancy
5. Discussion of rationale for optimal blood glucose control before conception and during pregnancy, including need for contraception and family planning to ensure optimal timing of conception and early diagnosis of pregnancy; *note:* research has demonstrated that near-normal blood glucose levels at the time of conception and in the early weeks of gestation may significantly decrease the incidence of congenital anomalies associated with infants of mothers with diabetes
6. Review of self-care practices and self-monitoring expectations during pregnancy, including diet, intensification of insulin regimen, and plan for medical and obstetrical management

B. Pregnancy

1. Reinforcement of medical and obstetrical management plan during pregnancy
2. Ongoing assessment of blood glucose levels and adjustment of insulin requirements to ensure euglycemia
3. Minimization of potential maternal and fetal complications associated with diabetes and pregnancy

C. Postpartum

1. Precipitous decrease in insulin requirements in immediate postpartum period related to delivery of placenta and cessation of contra-insulin hormones associated with pregnancy; usually persists for at least 72 hours after delivery
2. Breastfeeding is usually encouraged in women with diabetes
   a. May be associated with decreased insulin requirements
   b. Necessitates continued dietary modifications to ensure adequate nutrition during lactation and milk production
   c. Insulin secreted in breast milk is digested by the infant and does not affect the infant's blood glucose levels
   d. Maternal hyperglycemia will sweeten the breast milk and may result in infant hyperinsulinemia; therefore, lactating mothers with diabetes are encouraged to maintain normal blood glucose levels

Gestational Diabetes Mellitus

Introduction

A. Definition

1. Carbohydrate intolerance of variable severity with onset or first recognition during the present pregnancy
2. Client may require insulin for treatment
3. Condition may persist after pregnancy
4. Glucose intolerance may have antedated the pregnancy

B. Incidence

1. Occurs in approximately 2 to 3% of all pregnant women
2. Affects 60,000 to 90,000 women per year

Clinical Practice

A. Assessment

1. History (associated risk factors)
   a. History of gestational diabetes in previous pregnancy
   b. Previous infant weighed over 9 lb (4000 g)
   c. Previous unexplained intrauterine fetal demise (IUFD)

      d. Previous infant with congenital anomaly

      e. Obesity

      f. Family history of diabetes

      g. Age 35 years or over

  2. Physical findings and associated risk factors

      a. Maternal effects

         (1) Development of polyhydramnios or suspected macrosomia or increased fundal height relative to dating of pregnancy

         (2) Persistent glycosuria

         (3) Urinary frequency after first trimester

         (4) Reported feelings or behaviors of excessive thirst or hunger

      b. Fetal and neonatal effects

         (1) Fetal macrosomia; associated with operative delivery, birth trauma, shoulder dystocia, and obesity

         (2) Neonatal hypoglycemia

         (3) Neonatal hypocalcemia

         (4) Neonatal polycythemia

         (5) Neonatal hyperbilirubinemia

         (6) Respiratory distress syndrome

         (7) Infants of mothers with fasting and postprandial hyperglycemia are at greatest risk for intrauterine death or neonatal mortality

         (8) Overall perinatal mortality has been reported to be 6.4% when GDM is untreated; recent studies suggest there is no increase in perinatal mortality when GDM is managed appropriately and maternal glucose levels are normal

         (9) Increased risk of childhood obesity

  3. Psychosocial findings

      a. Presence of support systems—partner or family

      b. Adequacy of coping responses associated with diagnosis of high-risk pregnancy

      c. Financial considerations related to need for more intensive monitoring of pregnancy and possible need for cesarean birth

      d. Occupational status

      e. Planned or unplanned pregnancy

      f. Family's response to pregnancy

      g. Feelings regarding high-risk status of pregnancy

  4. Diagnostic procedures

      a. Glucose screening test (GST)

         (1) All pregnant women should be screened for glucose intolerance during pregnancy; universal screening is recommended by the American Diabetes Association because selective screening based on clinical attributes or obstetrical history has been shown to be inadequate

         (2) Pregnant women who have not been identified as having glucose intolerance before the 24th week of gestation should have a GST performed between the 24th and 28th weeks of gestation

         (3) Administer 50 g of oral glucose, given without regard to time of the last meal or time of day

         (4) Measure venous plasma glucose 1 hour later; level should be below 140 mg/dl; a value of 140 mg/dl or above is recommended as a threshold to indicate need for a full diagnostic oral glucose tolerance test (OGTT)

      b. Oral glucose tolerance test

         (1) Diagnosis of GDM is based on results of the 100-g OGTT during pregnancy (interpreted according to the diagnostic criteria of O'Sullivan and Mahan)

         (2) Definitive diagnosis requires that two or more of the venous plasma (or serum) glucose concentrations be met or exceeded

            (a) Fasting, 105 mg/dl

      (b) 1 hour, 190 mg/dl
      (c) 2 hour, 165 mg/dl
      (d) 3 hour, 145 mg/dl

B. **Nursing Diagnoses**

1. Alteration in metabolism of carbohydrates, proteins, fats, and electrolytes related to pregnancy
2. Anxiety related to maternal diagnosis and implications for neonatal outcome
3. Altered self-concept related to diagnosis of high-risk pregnancy
4. High risk for fetal injury related to macrosomia associated with fetal dependence on maternal glycemic states
5. Knowledge deficit related to altered management plan and self-care activities required for glycemic assessment and control during pregnancy
6. Altered nutrition and diet for optimal management of maternal glycemia
7. Alteration in family systems related to demands of optimal diabetes and obstetrical care during pregnancy

C. **Interventions/Evaluations**

1. Alteration in metabolism of carbohydrates, proteins, fats, and electrolytes related to pregnancy
   a. Interventions
      (1) Monitor fasting and postprandial blood glucose levels
      (2) Assist client in self-monitoring of blood glucose levels and recording results
      (3) Discuss rationale for normalizing blood glucose levels during pregnancy, and review the effects of elevated blood glucose levels on fetal growth and development and neonatal outcome
      (4) Review normal changes in carbohydrate metabolism during pregnancy and significance of impaired glucose tolerance to developing fetus
   b. Evaluations
      (1) Alterations in fasting and postprandial blood glucose levels are recognized and managed with dietary modifications and insulin administration
      (2) Client demonstrates proper technique in self-monitoring of blood glucose and records results
      (3) Client verbalizes rationale for normalization of blood glucose levels during pregnancy and describes the effects of elevated blood glucose levels on fetal growth and development and neonatal outcomes
      (4) Client states normal changes in carbohydrate metabolism during pregnancy and significance of impaired glucose tolerance to developing fetus
2. Anxiety related to maternal diagnosis and implications for neonatal outcome
   a. Interventions
      (1) Provide information regarding effects of elevated blood glucose levels on developing fetus and rationale for normalizing maternal glucose levels
      (2) Discuss dietary modifications and self-monitoring of blood glucose levels to promote normalization of blood glucose levels
      (3) Encourage active participation in self-monitoring practices and decision making about plan for managing GDM
      (4) Discuss results of fetal assessment tests and procedures for evaluation of fetal status and well-being
   b. Evaluations
      (1) Client states effects of elevated blood glucose levels on developing fetus and rationale for normalizing maternal glucose levels
      (2) Client modifies her dietary intake and self-monitors blood glucose levels to promote normalization of blood glucose levels
      (3) Client actively participates in self-monitoring practices and decision making regarding the plan for managing GDM

(4) Client is informed of results of fetal assessment tests and procedures for evaluation of fetal status and well-being

3. Altered self-concept related to diagnosis of high-risk pregnancy
    a. Interventions
        (1) Encourage maternal expression of feelings and concerns related to diagnosis of GDM
        (2) Discuss alterations in anticipated plan for obstetrical care and provide support to minimize potential complications related to unexpected interventions necessitated in pregnancy
    b. Evaluations
        (1) Client expresses her feelings and concerns about the diagnosis of GDM
        (2) Client describes alterations in anticipated plan for obstetrical care and identifies sources of support to minimize potential complications related to unexpected interventions necessitated in pregnancy

4. High risk for fetal injury related to macrosomia associated with fetal dependence on maternal glycemic states
    a. Interventions
        (1) Monitor blood glucose levels
        (2) Monitor fetal status using NST, CST, BPP, and ultrasound testing
    b. Evaluations
        (1) Client participates in monitoring of blood glucose levels
        (2) Fetal status and development are monitored using NST, CST, BPP, and ultrasound testing

5. Knowledge deficit related to altered management plan and self-care activities required for glycemic assessment and control during pregnancy
    a. Interventions
        (1) Review rationale for normal blood glucose levels in pregnancy
        (2) Discuss plan for normalizing blood glucose levels, including dietary management, blood glucose monitoring, and possible insulin administration; *note:* insulin is usually prescribed if fasting or postprandial blood glucose levels are persistently elevated despite dietary modifications
    b. Evaluations
        (1) Client verbalizes rationale for normal blood glucose levels in pregnancy
        (2) Client demonstrates normalization of blood glucose levels through dietary management, blood glucose monitoring, and possible insulin administration if indicated

6. Altered nutrition and diet for optimal management of maternal glycemia
    a. Interventions
        (1) Refer client for dietary counseling to ensure proper diet for normalization of blood glucose levels and optimal fetal growth and development
        (2) Encourage client to record dietary intake and blood glucose results
    b. Evaluations
        (1) Client receives dietary counseling to ensure proper diet for normalization of blood glucose levels and optimal fetal growth and development
        (2) Client records dietary intake and blood glucose levels

7. Alteration in family systems related to demands of optimal diabetes and obstetrical care during pregnancy
    a. Interventions
        (1) Encourage client to express concerns related to plan for diabetes management during pregnancy and family support for adherence to dietary recommendations and glycemic control
        (2) Provide anticipatory guidance about the need for additional fetal assessment and frequency of prenatal appointments and testing for evaluation of maternal glycemic status
        (3) Assess impact of diagnosis of GDM on family
    b. Evaluations
        (1) Client expresses her concerns about the plan for diabetes management

during pregnancy and family support for adherence to dietary recommendations and glycemic control

    (2) Client receives anticipatory guidance about the need for additional fetal assessment and frequency of prenatal appointments and testing for evaluation of maternal glycemic status

    (3) Appropriate resources and support are available to family to minimize impact of diagnosis of GDM and its management on the family

Health Education

A. Breastfeeding should be encouraged in women with GDM

B. Women diagnosed with GDM should be closely observed postpartum to detect diabetes early in its course; initially, evaluation should occur at the first postpartum visit by a 2-hour OGTT with a 75-g glucose load

C. Approximately 40% of women diagnosed with GDM develop overt diabetes within 20 years of index pregnancy; maintaining ideal body weight, eating a healthful diet, and regular exercise may decrease the likelihood of developing overt diabetes or delay its onset

Hyperthyroidism (Graves' disease)

Introduction

A. Diagnosis and management of thyroid disease in pregnancy is complicated by the normal changes of pregnancy that mimic hyperthyroidism and a hypermetabolic state

B. Hyperdynamic symptoms are characteristic of both normal pregnancy and hyperthyroidism

1. Increased metabolic rate
2. Increased protein-bound iodine values
3. Increased iodine uptake

C. Various metabolic and hormonal changes that occur in pregnancy affect the thyroid gland

1. Presence of placental estrogen alters thyroid function studies such as the total thyroxine (T_4) and triiodothyronine resin uptake (T_3RU)
2. Other metabolic changes can be seen in thyroid function tests during pregnancy (Table 29–3)

Table 29–3
THYROID FUNCTION TESTS DURING PREGNANCY

Patient	Total T_4	Free T_4	FT_4I*	Total T_3	Free T_3	T_3RU†	TSH
Normal nonpregnant	Normal 5–13 μg/ 100 ml	Normal 2.70 μg/ 100 ml	Normal 4.5–12	Normal 70–150 μg/ 100 ml	Normal 1.5 μg/ 100 ml	Normal 0.8–1.15	Normal
Normal pregnant	Increased	Normal	Normal	Slight increase	Normal	Decreased	Normal
Pregnant hyperthyroid	Increased	Increased	Increased	Normal to slight increase	–	Increased	Normal
Pregnant hypothyroid	Decreased	Decreased	Decreased	Normal to slight decrease	–	Decreased	High

    * Free thyroxine index.
    † T_3 resin uptake.

D. Incidence of hyperthyroidism in pregnancy is approximately 0.2% (one in every 500 to 1000 pregnancies)

E. Graves' disease is the most common cause of hyperthyroidism during pregnancy

F. Fertility is generally not affected when mild to moderate hyperthyroidism occurs

G. Treatment of hyperthyroidism is complicated by the presence of the fetus

1. The fetus may be jeopardized by surgery or antithyroid medications used to control the overactivity of the sympathetic nervous system and the overactive thyroid gland
2. Drugs that inhibit synthesis of thyroid hormones such as propylthiouracil (widely preferred in pregnancy because it has been reported to have limited placental transfer) or methimazole are thiourias, which cross the placenta and pass freely into the fetal circulation, interfering with fetal thyroid function

H. Fetal synthesis of thyroid hormones

1. Synthesis begins at 10 to 12 weeks
2. Hormone production remains low in the fetus through the second trimester, increasing in the last trimester of pregnancy
   a. If drug treatment is not effective or if drug intolerance exists, partial thyroidectomy or total resection of the maternal thyroid gland is indicated
   b. Surgery is usually recommended after the first trimester to decrease the risk of spontaneous abortion

I. Associated with increased incidence of postpartum hemorrhage if not well controlled

J. When diagnosed during pregnancy, hyperthyroidism may be transient or permanent; spontaneous remissions may occur during pregnancy

Clinical Practice

A. Assessment

1. History
   a. Clinical symptoms
      (1) Weakness
      (2) Tremor
      (3) Heat intolerance and sensitivity
      (4) Increased appetite
      (5) Failure to gain weight or actual weight loss
      (6) Fatigue
      (7) Insomnia
      (8) Diarrhea
      (9) Nervousness
      (10) Excessive sweating
   b. Infertility
      (1) Anovulation and amenorrhea may occur if hyperthyroidism is not treated
      (2) When treated, hyperthyroidism is not usually associated with infertility
2. Physical findings
   a. Maternal effects
      (1) Resting pulse greater than 100 beats/min
      (2) Proximal muscle wasting
      (3) Separation of the distal nail from the nailbed
      (4) Eye signs
         (a) Stare with exophthalmus
         (b) Lid lag

(c) Lid retraction

(d) Chemosis

(5) Goiter—diffusely enlarged, soft gland

(6) Soft skin with fine hair

(7) Increased skin warmth

(8) Development of thyroid storm or thyrotoxic crisis

    (a) Presents clinically with high fever, tachycardia, severe dehydration, profuse sweating, restlessness, nausea and vomiting associated with abdominal pain, and possible pulmonary edema or congestive heart failure

    (b) Most commonly occurs in pregnant women in whom the hyperthyroidism has not been detected or is poorly controlled

    (c) Precipitating factors include infection, labor, and cesarean section

    (d) If untreated, thyroid storm is associated with increased perinatal mortality and maternal heart failure

(9) Increased incidence of PIH if not well controlled

(10) Side effects associated with antithyroid medications

  b. Fetal and neonatal effects

    (1) Increased incidence of preterm labor and delivery

    (2) Increased risk of small-for-gestational-age or low-birth-weight infants

    (3) Small increase in perinatal mortality

    (4) Mild fetal or neonatal hypothyroidism, goiter, or mental deficiencies associated with maternal use of antithyroid medication, which may impair fetal thyroid function and cause hypothyroidism

    (5) Hyperthyroidism is *not* associated with an increased incidence of spontaneous abortions or fetal anomalies in clients who are kept euthyroid

    (6) If hyperthyroidism is untreated, rates of spontaneous abortion, intrauterine death, and stillbirth increase

    (7) Rare occurrence of fetal thyrotoxicosis in presence of maternal thyroid storm

3. Psychosocial findings

  a. Presence of support systems—partner or family

  b. Adequate coping mechanisms

  c. Occupational status

  d. Financial concerns

  e. Planned or unplanned pregnancy

  f. Family's response to pregnancy

  g. Feelings regarding high-risk status of pregnancy

4. Diagnostic procedures

  a. Laboratory findings: elevated free thyroxine index (FT_4I), free T_4, T_3RU, and total T_4 (see Table 29–3)

  b. Maintaining fetus in euthyroid state, especially in last trimester, is recognized as essential for brain development; the FT_4I is a useful index of fetal thyroid status

  c. Neonates born to mothers with hyperthyroidism have serum thyroxine determinations performed at birth and are observed closely during the first 2 weeks of life for signs and symptoms of hyperthyroidism

B. Nursing Diagnoses

1. Anxiety related to maternal diagnosis, pregnancy, and its outcome

2. Knowledge deficit related to the therapeutic regimen to optimize maternal and fetal outcomes in pregnancy

3. High risk for injury to the fetus or neonate related to medical management with antithyroid drugs

C. Interventions/Evaluations

1. Anxiety related to maternal diagnosis, pregnancy, and outcome

  a. Interventions

(1) Assess maternal anxiety level, including behavioral and physiological changes

(2) Encourage maternal expression of feelings and concerns

(3) Inform the client of all procedures and expectations, presenting accurate information and answering her questions

(4) Encourage active participation in decision making about the therapeutic regimen

b. Evaluations

(1) Behavioral and physiological changes associated with maternal anxiety do not compromise the client's ability to participate in the therapeutic regimen prescribed during pregnancy

(2) Client expresses feelings and concerns about pregnancy and its outcome

(3) Client describes accurate information about procedures and expectations during pregnancy

(4) Client actively participates in decision-making process about implementation of the therapeutic regimen

2. Knowledge deficit related to therapeutic regimen to optimize maternal and fetal outcomes in pregnancy

a. Interventions

(1) Assess understanding of effects of hyperthyroidism on pregnancy and fetal development, including possible fetal goiter and hypothyroidism

(2) Discuss plan for frequent monitoring of total T_4 to ensure that lowest possible amount of antithyroid medication is administered for control of client's symptoms while minimizing fetal exposure to antithyroid medications

(3) Perform clinical assessment to determine adequacy of maternal response to antithyroid medications

(a) Pulse below 100

(b) Reflexes 2+ to 3+

(c) Loss of tremor

(d) Normal weight gain

(e) Normal fetal growth

(4) Review complications of antithyroid therapy

(a) Purpuric skin rash

(b) Pruritus

(c) Fever

(d) Nausea

(e) Rarely agranulocytosis may occur, usually after 1 to 2 months of therapy

(5) Instruct the client to report fever, sore throat, or other symptoms of infection

(6) Provide accurate information about all procedures, tests, and interventions planned during pregnancy and after birth of the infant

(7) Inform client of results of laboratory tests and provide information about fetal status and well-being

(8) Review dietary requirements in pregnancy to reinforce adequate nutritional intake and facilitate fetal growth and development; *note:* increased metabolic state requires increased calories and protein intake

(9) Instruct the client about the signs and symptoms of preterm labor

(10) Review the signs and symptoms of hyperthyroidism, the use of self-monitoring diaries, and self-assessment records

b. Evaluations

(1) Client verbalizes understanding of effects of hyperthyroidism on pregnancy and fetal development, including possible fetal goiter and hypothyroidism

(2) Client verbalizes plan for frequent monitoring of total T_4 levels to ensure lowest possible amount of antithyroid medication is adminis-

tered for control of her symptoms while minimizing fetal exposure to antithyroid medications

(3) Client demonstrates therapeutic response to antithyroid medications

(4) Client states possible complications of antithyroid therapy including skin rash, pruritus, fever, and nausea

(5) Client reports fever, sore throat, or other symptoms of infection, if present

(6) Client receives accurate information about all procedures, tests, and interventions planned during pregnancy and after birth of infant

(7) Client is informed of fetal status and well-being throughout pregnancy and at birth

(8) Client reports adequate nutritional intake during pregnancy

(9) Client verbalizes signs and symptoms of preterm labor

(10) Client actively participates in monitoring and recording signs and symptoms of hyperthyroidism during pregnancy

3. High risk for injury to the fetus or neonate related to medical management with antithyroid drugs

a. Interventions

(1) Monitor fetal growth and development through ultrasound testing and fundal height measurement

(2) Fetal heart rate (FHR) monitored in utero as metabolic guide for the following

(a) Fetal hyperthyroidism (FHR above 160)

(b) Fetal hypothyroidism (FHR below 120)

(3) Assess maternal serum total T_4 levels for possible adjustment of dosage for thiourea therapy

(a) The lowest possible amount is used to control symptoms; the client is kept mildly hyperthyroid or within the high end of the normal range of pregnancy to minimize potential detrimental effects to the fetus

(b) Keeping the fetus in euthyroid state, especially near term, is recognized as essential for brain and neurological development

(4) Assess client for signs and symptoms of preterm labor

(5) Perform fetal movement counts to assess fetal well-being

b. Evaluations

(1) Fetal growth and development and FHR are within normal parameters

(2) Maternal total T_4 levels are maintained in the prescribed range to control symptoms (the client may be mildly hyperthyroid)

(3) Signs and symptoms of preterm labor are promptly reported and managed to minimize incidence of preterm birth

(4) Fetal activity and movement indicate fetal well-being

Health Education

A. Preconceptual

1. Assessment of adequacy of antithyroid medications with baseline laboratory values

2. Discussion of potential maternal and fetal complications associated with hyperthyroidism in pregnancy, including thyroid storm

B. Prenatal

1. Careful history taking and physical assessment of the client's symptoms at each prenatal visit

2. Treatment with antithyroid drugs in pregnancy and close monitoring to determine minimal dosage required to control symptoms

3. Discussion of information regarding fetal status and potential maternal and fetal complications associated with hyperthyroidism in pregnancy

4. Explanation and discussion of the presence of congenital goiter or signs of

airway obstruction necessitating intubation at birth; evaluation of thyroid function of the newborn

5. Nutritional counseling to meet additional calorie requirements

C. **Postpartum:** clients taking antithyroid medications such as propylthiouracil may breastfeed if the infant's thyroid status is closely monitored (every 2 to 4 weeks); generally, infants exposed to small amounts of antithyroid medications do not become hypothyroid

Hypothyroidism

Introduction

A. Definition

1. Rare condition in pregnancy
2. Women with hypothyroidism ovulate irregularly and are frequently infertile or experience menstrual dysfunction or amenorrhea

B. Etiology

1. Primary hypothyroidism is due to the following
   a. Hashimoto's thyroiditis
   b. Therapy with antithyroid drugs
   c. Iodine deficiency
   d. Destruction of the thyroid gland
2. Secondary hypothyroidism is from pituitary-hypothalamic disease

C. Prognosis for the mother and fetus is good with successful hormone replacement

D. High fetal mortality and morbidity are characteristics of the hypothyroid state when replacement therapy is inadequate or not instituted during pregnancy

Clinical Practice

A. Assessment

1. History
   a. Fatigue and malaise, lack of energy
   b. Cold intolerance
   c. Lethargy
   d. Headache
   e. Constipation
   f. Paresthesias
   g. Infertility, if thyroid function is significantly impaired
   h. Possible increased rate of stillbirth (risk is doubled if maternal hypothyroidism is untreated)
   i. Increased incidence of spontaneous abortion (risk is doubled if maternal hypothyroidism is untreated)
2. Physical findings
   a. Maternal effects
      (1) Dry, scaly skin
      (2) Thin, brittle nails
      (3) Alopecia or hair loss
      (4) Poor skin turgor
      (5) Delayed deep tendon reflexes (slow relaxation phase)
      (6) Enlarged thyroid gland (goiter)

b. Fetal and neonatal effects
   (1) If mother is untreated, fetal loss is 50%
   (2) Increased risk of congenital goiter
   (3) Increased risk of true cretinism
   (4) Increased incidence of congenital anomalies (risk is tripled if maternal hypothyroidism is untreated)
3. Psychosocial findings
   a. Adaptation to chronic illness or diagnosis
   b. Presence of support systems—partner or family
   c. Adequate coping mechanisms
   d. Occupational status
   e. Financial concerns
   f. Planned or unplanned pregnancy
   g. Family's response to pregnancy
   h. Feelings regarding high-risk status of pregnancy
4. Diagnostic procedures
   a. Diagnosis is confirmed by the presence of low total T_4, free T_4, and T_3RU
   b. TSH is above normal (see Table 29–3)
   c. Screen newborn for T_4 level

B. Nursing Diagnoses

1. Anxiety related to maternal diagnosis, pregnancy, and its outcome
2. Knowledge deficit related to the therapeutic regimen to optimize maternal and fetal outcomes in pregnancy
3. High risk for injury to the fetus or neonate related to inadequate thyroid replacement therapy

C. Interventions/Evaluations

1. Anxiety related to maternal diagnosis, pregnancy, and its outcome
   a. Interventions
      (1) Assess maternal anxiety level, including behavioral and physiological changes
      (2) Encourage maternal expression of feelings and concerns
      (3) Inform the client of all procedures and expectations, presenting accurate information and answering her questions
      (4) Encourage active participation in decision making about the therapeutic regimen
   b. Evaluations
      (1) Behavioral and physiological changes associated with maternal anxiety do not compromise the client's ability to participate in therapeutic regimen prescribed during pregnancy
      (2) Client expresses her feelings and concerns about the pregnancy and its outcome
      (3) Client is accurately informed about procedures and expectations during pregnancy
      (4) Client actively participates in decision-making process about the implementation of the therapeutic regimen
2. Knowledge deficit related to the therapeutic regimen to optimize maternal and fetal outcomes in pregnancy
   a. Interventions
      (1) Assess client's understanding of effects of adrenal hyperfunction on pregnancy and fetal development
      (2) Provide accurate information about all procedures, tests, and interventions planned during pregnancy and after birth of the infant; *note:* thyroid hormones administered endogenously or exogenously do not cross the placenta in significant amounts

    (3) Inform the client of fetal status and well-being

    (4) Instruct the client in self-monitoring fetal activity using daily fetal movement counts

  b. Evaluations

    (1) Client verbalizes an understanding of pregnancy and normal growth and development of the fetus

    (2) Client receives accurate information about all procedures, tests, and interventions planned during pregnancy and after birth of the infant

    (3) Client is informed of fetal status and well-being throughout pregnancy and during birth

    (4) Client participates in assessment of fetal well-being by performing daily fetal movement counts

3. High risk for injury to the fetus or neonate related to inadequate thyroid replacement therapy

  a. Interventions

    (1) Monitor fetal growth and development by ultrasound screening

    (2) Assess maternal serum total T_4 and T_3RU levels for possible adjustment of dosage to keep within the normal range during pregnancy and to minimize detrimental effects to fetus

  b. Evaluations

    (1) Fetal growth and development is within normal parameters

    (2) Maternal serum free T_4 levels are maintained in the prescribed range to ensure a euthyroid state throughout pregnancy

Health Education

A. Preconceptual

1. Assessment of adequacy of thyroid replacement as indicated by the free-thyroxine index (plasma free-T_4 index) and achievement of clinical and biochemical euthyroidism
2. Assessment of fertility and ovulation
3. Discussion of potential maternal and neonatal complications associated with hypothyroidism in pregnancy; with adequate hormonal replacement, outcome for the mother and fetus is improved

B. Prenatal

1. Careful history taking and physical assessment of the client's symptoms at each prenatal visit
2. Treatment should begin as soon as possible with thyroid replacement medication
  a. During pregnancy, thyroid replacement must be adequate for maternal needs and for adequate fetal growth and development
  b. The plasma free-T_4 index (free-thyroxine index) is used to monitor the adequacy of replacement therapy during pregnancy
  c. Placental transfer of thyroid hormone replacement is negligible
  d. Long-term thyroxine replacement therapy usually continues at same dosage during pregnancy as before pregnancy
3. Information about fetal status and potential maternal and fetal complications associated with hypothyroidism in pregnancy should be discussed
4. Tests and procedures indicated during pregnancy and used for assessment of the neonate at birth should be explained and discussed with the client

C. Postpartum: long-term thyroxine replacement therapy usually continues at same dosage after pregnancy as before pregnancy

Adrenal Disorders

HYPERADRENOCORTICISM (CUSHING'S SYNDROME)

Introduction

A. General overview

1. Many parameters of adrenal function are altered during pregnancy
2. Normal physiological changes in pregnancy mimic adrenal disease
   a. Abdominal striae
   b. Edema
   c. Increased pigmentation
   d. Decreased glucose tolerance
3. Physiological hypercortisolism occurs in normal pregnancy, and is associated with the following
   a. Changes in circulating levels of adrenocorticotropic hormone (ACTH)
   b. Dexamethasone suppressibility

B. Definition

1. Adrenal hyperfunction is most commonly seen as Cushing's syndrome, a rare disorder of steroid overproduction that occurs with adrenal tumors or adenomas or with adrenal hyperplasia secondary to elevated ACTH secretion
2. Adrenal hyperfunction is also seen with exogenous steroid administration (women with this syndrome are generally infertile because of ovulatory failure; this condition is extremely rare in pregnancy)
3. In most cases, hypercortisolism is diagnosed during pregnancy and in the postpartum period

C. Effects on pregnancy

1. Maternal effects
   a. Excessive maternal morbidity has been reported in a review of 45 reported cases discussed in the literature
   b. Maternal complications
      (1) Abnormal glucose tolerance test (GDM)
      (2) Pulmonary edema (44%)
      (3) Hypertension (100%) associated with progression to the HELLP syndrome
   c. Data are limited regarding maternal prognosis in pregnancy since most women are infertile
   d. Poor wound healing, wound infection, and dehiscence are seen if cesarean delivery is performed
2. Fetal and neonatal effects
   a. Increased incidence of spontaneous abortions
   b. Increased stillbirths
   c. Increased premature births

Clinical Practice

A. Assessment

1. History
   a. Emotional lability
   b. Psychiatric disorders
   c. Glucose intolerance
   d. Excessive weight gain
2. Physical findings
   a. Centripetal obesity with muscle wasting and proximal myopathy

    b. Acne

    c. Striae

    d. Hirsutism

    e. Moon face, facial rounding

    f. "Buffalo hump" (increased fat over the dorsal vertebrae)

    g. Hypertension

3. Psychosocial findings

    a. Emotional lability

    b. Psychiatric disorders

    c. Presence of support system—partner; family

    d. Occupational status

    e. Financial concerns

    f. Planned or unplanned pregnancy

    g. Family's response to pregnancy

    h. Feelings regarding high-risk status of pregnancy

4. Diagnostic procedures

    a. Plasma cortisol level is elevated

    b. Dexamethasone suppression test is abnormal

    c. Ultrasonography may indicate adrenal tumors of the adrenal glands

B. Nursing Diagnoses

1. Anxiety related to maternal diagnosis, pregnancy, and its outcome
2. Knowledge deficit related to the therapeutic regimen to optimize maternal and fetal outcomes in pregnancy
3. High risk for injury to the fetus or neonate related to suppression of adrenal function and maternal hypertension

C. Interventions/Evaluations

1. Anxiety related to maternal diagnosis, pregnancy, and its outcome

    a. Interventions

        (1) Assess maternal anxiety level, including behavioral and physiological changes

        (2) Encourage maternal expression of feelings and concerns

        (3) Inform client of all procedures and expectations, presenting accurate information and answering her questions

        (4) Encourage active participation in decision making about the therapeutic regimen

    b. Evaluations

        (1) Behavioral and physiological changes associated with maternal anxiety do not compromise the client's ability to participate in the therapeutic regimen prescribed during pregnancy

        (2) Client expresses her feelings and concerns about the pregnancy and its outcome

        (3) Client is accurately informed about procedures and expectations during pregnancy

        (4) Client actively participates in decision-making process about the implementation of the therapeutic regimen

2. Knowledge deficit related to the therapeutic regimen to optimize maternal and fetal outcomes in pregnancy

    a. Interventions

        (1) Assess client's understanding of effects of adrenal hyperfunction on pregnancy and fetal development

        (2) Provide accurate information about all procedures, tests, and interventions planned during pregnancy and after birth of the infant

        (3) Inform client of fetal status and well-being

        (4) Instruct client regarding the signs and symptoms of preterm labor and self-monitoring of fetal activity with daily fetal movement counts

b. Evaluations
   (1) Client verbalizes understanding of the effects on pregnancy and normal growth and development of fetus
   (2) Client receives accurate information about all procedures, tests, and interventions planned during pregnancy and after birth of the infant
   (3) Client is informed of fetal status and well-being throughout pregnancy and at birth
   (4) Client reports any signs or symptoms of preterm labor and any decrease or significant change in fetal movement patterns
3. High risk for injury to the fetus or neonate related to suppression of adrenal function and maternal hypertension
   a. Interventions
      (1) Monitor fetal growth and development
      (2) Monitor signs and symptoms of preterm labor
   b. Evaluations
      (1) Fetal growth and development are within normal parameters
      (2) Preterm labor will be recognized early and management instituted promptly to minimize incidence of preterm birth

Health Education

A. Preconceptual

1. Assessment of fertility and ovulation
2. Discussion of potential maternal and neonatal complications associated with adrenal hyperfunction in pregnancy

B. Prenatal

1. Careful history taking and physical assessment of the client's symptoms at each prenatal visit
2. Endocrine consultation to determine the cause of syndrome
3. Information regarding fetal status and potential maternal and fetal complications associated with adrenal hyperfunction in pregnancy, including increased risk of preterm labor and stillbirth

Hypoadrenocorticism (Addison's Disease)

Introduction

A. Definition

1. Referred to as adrenal hypofunction, hypoadrenocorticism is most commonly associated with Addison's disease
2. Women with untreated Addison's disease rarely conceive
3. Diagnosis is usually established before pregnancy and the woman is on maintenance steroid replacement when conception occurs
4. Signs and symptoms of Addison's disease are unchanged by pregnancy

B. Effects on pregnancy

1. Maternal effects
   a. If Addison's disease is untreated, women are more likely to develop acute adrenal crisis (acute adrenal insufficiency)
   b. Risk of adrenal crisis increased in postpartum period because of the inability to mount an adrenal response to the stress of delivery
2. Fetal and neonatal effects
   a. Increased incidence of small-for-gestational age infants
   b. Depressed adrenal function related to maternal therapy with steroids

Clinical Practice

A. Assessment

1. History
   a. Weakness
   b. Fatigue
   c. Nausea and vomiting
   d. Anorexia
2. Physical findings (*note:* some of these signs and symptoms may occur in normal pregnancy; suspect adrenal insufficiency if the symptoms are unusually severe or persistent)
   a. Weight loss
   b. Hypotension
   c. Increased skin pigmentation
3. Psychosocial findings
   a. Presence of support system—partner or family
   b. Occupational status
   c. Financial concerns
   d. Planned or unplanned pregnancy
   e. Family's response to pregnancy
   f. Feelings regarding high-risk status of pregnancy
4. Diagnostic procedures
   a. Diagnosis is confirmed by low plasma cortisol for pregnancy: because plasma cortisol increases during gestation, this value may be in the normal, nonpregnant range and still represent a deficiency
   b. ACTH stimulation test may be performed
      (1) Baseline serum cortisol is drawn
      (2) 25 units of ACTH is administered intramuscularly
      (3) Repeat serum cortisol level is obtained in 1 hour
      (4) Normal results = doubled baseline value (minimum)

B. Nursing Diagnoses

1. Anxiety related to maternal diagnosis, pregnancy, and its outcome
2. Knowledge deficit related to the therapeutic regimen to optimize maternal and fetal outcomes in pregnancy
3. High risk for injury to the fetus or neonate related to maternal steroid replacement therapy

C. Interventions/Evaluations

1. Anxiety related to maternal diagnosis, pregnancy, and its outcome
   a. Interventions
      (1) Assess maternal anxiety level, including behavioral and physiological changes
      (2) Encourage maternal expression of feelings and concerns
      (3) Inform client of all procedures and expectations, presenting accurate information and answering her questions
      (4) Encourage active participation in decision making regarding therapeutic regimen
   b. Evaluations
      (1) Behavioral and physiological changes associated with maternal anxiety do not compromise the client's ability to participate in therapeutic regimen prescribed during pregnancy
      (2) Client expresses her feelings and concerns related to pregnancy and its outcome
      (3) Client is accurately informed about procedures and expectations during pregnancy
      (4) Client actively participates in decision-making process regarding implementation of therapeutic regimen

2. Knowledge deficit related to therapeutic regimen to optimize maternal and fetal outcomes in pregnancy
   a. Interventions
      (1) Assess understanding of effects of adrenal hypofunction on pregnancy and fetal development
      (2) Provide explanations regarding possible needs for altering or increasing dosage of adrenocortical hormones during pregnancy
         (a) Minor illnesses
         (b) Acute adrenal crisis
         (c) At time of delivery (either vaginal or cesarean birth)
         (d) In the postpartum period
      (3) Review signs and symptoms of acute adrenal crisis
         (a) Nausea and vomiting
         (b) Abdominal pain
         (c) Fever
         (d) Hypotension
         (e) Shock
      (4) Provide accurate information about all procedures, tests, and interventions planned during pregnancy and after birth of the infant
      (5) Inform client of fetal status and well-being
      (6) Review dietary requirements for adequate nutritional intake and to promote normal fetal growth and development during pregnancy
   b. Evaluations
      (1) Client verbalizes understanding of risks associated with adrenal hypofunction to self and fetus
      (2) Client states rationale and management plan for alterations in adrenocortical hormone therapy during pregnancy and childbirth
      (3) Client verbalizes the signs and symptoms of acute adrenal crisis
      (4) Client receives accurate information about all procedures, tests, and interventions planned during pregnancy and after birth of the infant
      (5) Client is informed of fetal status and well-being throughout pregnancy and at birth
      (6) Client verbalizes adequate nutritional intake during pregnancy
3. High risk for injury to the fetus or neonate related to maternal steroid replacement therapy
   a. Interventions
      (1) Monitor fetal growth and development
      (2) Assess adrenal function at birth
   b. Evaluations
      (1) Fetal growth and development are within normal parameters
      (2) Neonatal adrenal function is assessed at birth

Health Education

A. Preconceptual

1. Assessment of adequacy of adrenocortical hormone replacement as indicated by serum cortisol levels
2. Assessment of fertility and ovulation
3. Discussion of potential maternal and neonatal complications associated with adrenal hypofunction in pregnancy; with adequate steroid replacement, outcomes for the mother and neonate are improved

B. Prenatal

1. Careful history taking and physical assessment of the client's symptoms at each prenatal visit are important in the diagnosis of adrenal hypofunction (Addison's disease)
2. Treatment with steroid replacement should begin as soon as possible

3. Information regarding potential maternal and neonatal complications associated with adrenal hypofunction in pregnancy should be discussed, as well as alterations in dosage of prescribed adrenocortical hormones to minimize potential complications of acute adrenal crisis and to provide adequate glucocorticoid coverage during birth and in the postpartum period

Maternal Phenylketonuria

Introduction

A. Definition

1. Phenylketonuria (PKU), also known as hyperphenylalaninemia
2. Autosomal recessive genetic trait (defect) in which the body's ability to efficiently metabolize phenylalanine is impaired because of an enzyme (phenylalanine hydroxylase) deficiency
3. Phenylalanine is an essential amino acid found in all protein foods; deficiency of the enzyme prevents metabolization of phenylalanine and leads to severe mental retardation if untreated
4. In classic PKU, the absence of phenylalanine hydroxylase results in the accumulation of phenylalanine and its metabolites in the blood and urine, inhibiting normal brain development
5. When untreated, PKU causes severe mental, physical, and behavioral disabilities

B. Incidence

1. Incidence of PKU is reported to be 1 in 10,000 live births in the United States
2. About 200 infants with PKU are born each year in the United States

C. Management of classic PKU

1. Infants are placed on a low-phenylalanine diet
2. Diet has been highly successful in preventing mental retardation

D. Maternal PKU

1. Definition: because women identified as newborns with PKU have been successfully treated with dietary management and have reached childbearing age, the emergence of maternal PKU has been recognized as another form of PKU
2. Women with classic PKU and other forms of PKU classified as hyperphenylalaninemias face a significant risk of having infants with mental retardation, intrauterine and postnatal growth retardation, low birth weight, microcephaly, congenital heart defects, and/or other malformations
3. These defects are the result of the mother's elevated serum phenylalanine levels that cross the placenta and overwhelm the fetus' ability to metabolize it
   a. This occurs even in the presence of a normal genetic makeup in the fetus
   b. However, there is also a higher incidence of hyperphenylalaninemic infants born to mothers with PKU
4. Maternal PKU prevents the normal expression of liver phenylalanine hydroxylase during fetal development, creating phenotypic hyperphenylalaninemia
5. Management of maternal PKU
   a. Treatment with a low-phenylalanine diet after birth will not help these infants since the damage occurs in utero
   b. Key to successful management of maternal PKU is the institution of the specific low phenylalanine diet before conception; ideally the program of dietary therapy is coordinated in collaboration with a PKU clinic

E. Effects on pregnancy

1. Maternal effects
   a. None specific to pregnancy

   b. Requirements of low-phenylalanine diet and careful dietary management during pregnancy
2. Fetal and neonatal effects
   a. If maternal serum phenylalanine levels are elevated, infants are at greater risk for the following
      (1) Mental retardation
      (2) Intrauterine and postnatal growth retardation
      (3) Low birth weight
      (4) Microcephaly
      (5) Congenital heart defects
      (6) Other congenital malformations
   b. Fetal phenylalanine levels are about 50% higher than maternal levels
   c. Incidence of hyperphenylalaninemia among infants born to mothers with PKU is increased as a result of impaired expression of liver phenylalanine hydroxylase during fetal development
   d. Depending on the zygosity of the father for PKU, the infant either inherits the disease or is a carrier

Clinical Practice

A. Assessment

1. History
   a. Identification of childhood PKU, ideally before conception when woman is planning pregnancy
   b. Dietary assessment and counseling: a low-phenylalanine diet is mandatory before conception and during pregnancy to optimize pregnancy outcome
2. Physical findings: none are specific to maternal PKU, although serum phenylalanine levels may be elevated if diet is not restricted
3. Psychosocial findings
   a. Presence of support system—partner or family
   b. Planned or unplanned pregnancy
   c. Family's response to pregnancy
   d. Feelings regarding high-risk status of pregnancy due to maternal condition that may affect fetal growth and development
   e. Concerns about low-phenylalanine diet and adhering to it during pregnancy
   f. Access to clinic or health care provider specializing in care and support of women with maternal PKU
4. Diagnostic procedures
   a. Serum phenylalanine levels are carefully monitored during pregnancy
   b. Goal of dietary management is to maintain levels between 2 and 8 mg/dl

B. Nursing Diagnoses

1. High risk for fetal injury related to dependence on maternal phenylalanine levels
2. Anxiety related to maternal diagnosis, pregnancy, and its outcome
3. Knowledge deficit related to therapeutic regimen to minimize potential effects of PKU on developing fetus
4. Altered nutrition related to low-phenylalanine diet required before conception and during pregnancy

C. Interventions/Evaluations

1. High risk for fetal injury related to dependence on maternal phenylalanine levels
   a. Interventions
      (1) Monitor fetal growth and development

      (2) Assess maternal serum phenylalanine levels
        (a) The level considered safe for fetus is 4 to 10 mg/dl
        (b) Ideally, this level is achieved before conception
      (3) Refer client for genetic counseling
   b. Evaluations
      (1) Fetal growth and development are within normal parameters
      (2) Maternal serum phenylalanine levels are maintained in the prescribed range throughout pregnancy
      (3) Client receives information relevant to fetal outcome and genetic inheritance through genetic counseling

2. Anxiety related to maternal diagnosis, pregnancy, and its outcome
   a. Interventions
      (1) Assess client's anxiety level, including behavioral and physiological changes
      (2) Encourage client's expression of feelings and concerns
      (3) Inform client of all procedures and expectations, presenting accurate information and answering her questions
      (4) Encourage active participation in decision making about the therapeutic regimen
   b. Evaluations
      (1) Behavioral and physiological changes associated with maternal anxiety do not compromise the client's ability to demonstrate appropriate dietary management and to participate in the therapeutic regimen prescribed during pregnancy
      (2) Client expresses her feelings and concerns about the pregnancy and its outcome
      (3) Client is accurately informed about procedures and expectations during pregnancy
      (4) Client actively participates in decision-making process regarding implementation of the therapeutic regimen

3. Knowledge deficit related to therapeutic regimen to minimize potential effects of PKU on developing fetus
   a. Interventions
      (1) Assess understanding of low-phenylalanine diet and food-exchange lists
      (2) Refer to dietician for dietary counseling and adaptation of diet to ensure adequate dietary intake for pregnancy and normal growth and development of fetus
      (3) Provide accurate information about all procedures, tests, and interventions planned during pregnancy and after birth of the infant
      (4) Inform client of fetal status and well-being
   b. Evaluations
      (1) Client verbalizes understanding of low-phenylalanine diet and food-exchange lists
      (2) Client receives information about adequate dietary intake for pregnancy and normal growth and development of the fetus
      (3) Client receives accurate information about all procedures, tests, and interventions planned during pregnancy and after birth of the infant
      (4) Client is informed of fetal status and well-being throughout pregnancy and at birth

4. Altered nutrition related to low-phenylalanine diet required before conception and during pregnancy
   a. Interventions
      (1) Assess understanding of low-phenylalanine diet and food-exchange lists
      (2) Refer client to dietician for dietary counseling and adaptation of diet to

ensure adequate dietary intake for pregnancy and normal growth and development of fetus
(a) Diet combines low-protein foods (primarily fruits and vegetables) with special formulas containing all amino acids except phenylalanine
(b) Prenatal vitamins should not be prescribed because all except folic acid are provided in special dietary formulas used to treat PKU
(c) Folic acid supplements should be provided separately
(3) Monitor client's ability to follow dietary requirements and reported intake
(4) Monitor maternal weight gain and fetal growth during pregnancy
b. Evaluations
(1) Client verbalizes understanding of low-phenylalanine diet and food-exchange lists
(2) Client's dietary intake is adequate for pregnancy and normal growth and development of fetus
(3) Client verbalizes her ability to follow dietary requirements and to report prescribed dietary intake
(4) Client demonstrates adequate weight gain with appropriate fetal growth during pregnancy

Health Education

A. **Preconceptual:** ideally, refer the client to a PKU clinic, which can provide biochemical analysis, nutritional formulas, and support for management of women before and during pregnancy

1. Genetic assessment of risk to potential offspring for the inheritance of PKU and for genetic counseling
2. Initiation of low-phenylalanine diet before conception
3. Discussion of potential risks to offspring including inheritance of PKU, effects of elevated phenylalanine levels on fetal development, specific dietary treatment beginning before conception, and therapeutic regimen prescribed during pregnancy
4. Sex education, family planning, and contraceptive counseling; it is important that this information is also available to adolescents with childhood PKU so that unintentional pregnancy may be prevented and appropriate dietary requirements may be instituted preconceptually
5. Importance of early identification of pregnancy
6. Potential dangers to fetus from untreated maternal PKU and fetal protection offered by dietary treatment beginning before conception and throughout pregnancy

B. **Prenatal**

1. Importance of maintenance of low-phenylalanine diet to optimize pregnancy and neonatal outcomes
2. Ongoing explanations and education regarding rationale for prescribed tests and procedures to assess fetal growth and well-being

C. **Postpartum**

1. Assessment and screening of neonate to evaluate PKU status
2. Institution of low-phenylalanine diet for neonate with PKU (usually recommended to be initiated before 3 weeks of age)
3. Contraception counseling to prevent unintended pregnancy and encourage return to low-phenylalanine diet before conception; many centers specializing in the care of individuals with PKU recommend indefinite continuation of the PKU diet for women with PKU throughout their childbearing years

CASE STUDIES AND STUDY QUESTIONS

Mary Cochran is a 28-year-old, gravida 1, para 0 (G1,P0) woman with insulin-dependent diabetes mellitus of 12 years' duration. Mary is hospitalized at 9 weeks' gestation to regulate her blood glucose levels and to assess the adequacy of her current diabetes regimen. Mary describes this pregnancy as unplanned but states she is very excited and wants to "get my blood sugars in a normal range again as soon as possible." Mary is currently taking regular insulin and NPH insulin before breakfast and before supper. She self-monitors her blood glucose levels two or three times a day. She reports two night-time episodes of hypoglycemia during the past week. Mary states that she has had laser treatments in both eyes for proliferative retinopathy and was hospitalized 10 years ago for management of diabetic ketoacidosis.

1. The nurse assesses Mary's anxiety about the possible effects of diabetes on pregnancy and tells Mary that the most important factor in achieving a successful pregnancy with minimal complications is which of the following?

   a. The number of years that Mary has had diabetes and the age at which she was diagnosed.

   b. The absence of vascular complications.

   c. Maintenance of near-normal blood glucose levels throughout pregnancy.

   d. Frequency of self-monitoring of blood glucose levels.

2. According to the information initially obtained by the nurse, how is Mary classified using White's classification of diabetes in pregnancy?

   a. Class C diabetes.

   b. Class D diabetes.

   c. Class F diabetes.

   d. Class R diabetes.

3. The nurse prepares Mary for the laboratory work, clinical assessments, and consults that will be obtained during her hospitalization. These additional tests and referrals will include all of the following except

   a. Biophysical profile.

   b. Dietary counseling.

   c. UA and UC.

   d. Glycosylated hemoglobin (Hgb A1c).

4. Mary is concerned about the episodes of hypoglycemia that have occurred at night during the previous week. The nurse explains that this commonly occurs early in pregnancy for what reason?

   a. The fetus produces insulin that crosses the placenta and decreases maternal insulin requirements.

   b. The fetus is constantly using maternal glucose for its growth and development.

   c. The placenta produces hormones that decrease maternal insulin requirements during pregnancy.

   d. The metabolic changes associated with pregnancy predispose women with IDDM to experience decreased needs for insulin during pregnancy.

5. Strategies that Mary and the nurse discuss during Mary's hospitalization to normalize blood glucose levels include all of the following except

   a. Increasing the frequency of self-monitoring of blood glucose levels to at least four times daily, before meals and at bedtime.

   b. Adding additional protein for Mary's bedtime snack to decrease the likelihood of nocturnal hypoglycemia.

   c. Reviewing the plan for adjusting insulin dosages based on blood glucose levels and changing insulin requirements throughout pregnancy.

   d. Decreasing exercise and physical activity to minimize energy expenditures that alter insulin requirements.

6. Risk factors associated with gestational diabetes include all of the following except

   a. Previous history of IUGR.

   b. Family history of diabetes.

   c. Obesity.

   d. Maternal age over 35 years.

7. Infants born to women with gestational

diabetes are at increased risk for which of the following?

a. Fetal macrosomia.

b. Neonatal hyperglycemia.

c. Neonatal seizures.

d. Congenital anomalies.

8. Jane Jones presents to labor and delivery at 36 weeks' gestation with the possible diagnosis of thyroid storm. Which of the following signs and symptoms are characteristic of thyroid storm?

a. Fatigue, sudden weight loss, heat intolerance, extreme weakness.

b. Low blood pressure, bradycardia, lethargy, generalized interstitial edema.

c. Blurred vision, hypertension, epigastric pain, severe headache.

d. High fever, tachycardia, dehydration, profuse sweating, restlessness.

9. Christine Parker was diagnosed with Addison's disease 3 years ago. Since that time, she has been managed with prednisone for maintenance steroid replacement. She is admitted to labor and delivery at 40 weeks' gestation and is in labor. In addition to monitoring Christine's progress in labor and fetal status, what following clinical signs and symptoms should be closely monitored during labor, delivery, and in the immediate postpartum period?

a. Nausea and vomiting, abdominal pain, fever, hypotension, shock.

b. Hyperventilation, dehydration, odor of acetone on breath, impaired mental status.

c. High fever, tachycardia, dehydration, congestive heart failure.

d. Hypertension, central nervous system irritability, edema, proteinuria.

10. Why is the institution of a low-phenylalanine diet indicated before conception and during pregnancy in a woman with PKU?

a. To prevent the inheritance of this disease by the developing fetus.

b. To minimize the incidence of mental retardation, microcephaly, congenital heart defects, and growth retardation in the developing fetus.

c. To promote the fetus' ability to metabolize phenylalanine in utero.

d. To prevent the expression of liver phenylalanine hydroxylase during fetal development.

Answers to Study Questions

1. c	2. d	3. a
4. b	5. d	6. a
7. a	8. d	9. a
10. b		

REFERENCES

Abrams, R.S., & Coustan, D.R. (1990). Gestational diabetes update. *Clinical Diabetes, 8*(2), 120–124.

American Diabetes Association. (1990). Position statement: Gestational diabetes mellitus. *Diabetes Care, 13*(1), 1s, 5–6.

Bevan, J.S., Gough, M.H., Gillmer, D.G., & Burke, C.W. (1987). Cushing syndrome in pregnancy: The timing of definitive treatment. *Clinical Endocrinology, 27*(2), 225–233.

Dickinson, J.E., & Palmer, S.M. (1990). Gestational diabetes: Pathophysiology and diagnosis. *Seminars in Perinatology, 14*(1), 2–11.

Freinkel, N., Dooley, S.L., & Metzger, B.E. (1985). Care of the pregnant woman with insulin-dependent diabetes mellitus. *New England Journal of Medicine, 313*(2), 96–101.

Gabbe, S.G. (1985). Management of diabetes mellitus in pregnancy. *American Journal of Obstetrics and Gynecology, 153*(8), 824–828.

Ghavami, M., Levy, H.L., & Erbe, R.W. (1986). Prevention of fetal damage through dietary control of maternal hyperphenylalaninemia. *Clinical Obstetrics and Gynecology, 29*(3), 580–585.

Hickey, C.A., & Covington, C. (1990). Maternal phenylketonuria: Case management as a preventive approach to a chronic condition affecting pregnancy. *NAACOG'S Clinical Issues in Perinatal and Women's Health Nursing, 1*(2), 214–225.

Karacic, B. (1986). Antepartal nursing management of Graves' disease. *Journal of Obstetric, Gynecologic, and Neonatal Nursing, 15*(3), 214–218.

Landon, M.B., & Gabbe, S.G. (1990). Antepartum surveillance and delivery timing in diabetic pregnancies. *Clinical Diabetes, 8*(3), 1, 36, 38–40, 43, 46.

Lott, J.W. (1988). PKU: A nursing update. *Journal of Pediatric Nursing, 3*(1), 29–34.

Metzger, B.E., & Freinkel, N. (1990). Diabetes and pregnancy: Metabolic changes and management. *Clinical Diabetes, 8*(1), 1–10.

Meyer, B.A., & Palmer, S.M. (1990). Pregestational diabetes. *Seminars in Perinatology, 14*(1), 12–23.

Rotondo, L.M. (1990). Diabetes mellitus: Impact on pregnancy. *NAACOG's Clinical Issues in Perinatal and Women's Health Nursing, 1*(2), 133–145.

Smith, J.E. (1990). Pregnancy complicated by thyroid disease. *Journal of Nurse-Midwifery, 35*(3), 143–149.

Thomas, R., & Reid, P.L. (1987). Thyroid disease and reproductive dysfunction: A review. *Obstetrics and Gynecology, 70*(5), 789–798.

Sheila Sanning Shea and Gary Sparger

Trauma in Pregnancy

Objectives

1. State the normal physiological changes that potentially affect the evaluation of a pregnant trauma patient

2. Identify the major mechanisms of injury that affect the pregnant trauma patient

3. Describe the components of the primary and secondary survey for a pregnant trauma patient

4. List interventions to prevent maternal and fetal mortality resulting from trauma

5. Develop a plan of care for a pregnant patient experiencing blunt or penetrating trauma

6. Assimilate knowledge about the physiological changes of pregnancy and the specific mechanisms of injury in the assessment, diagnosis, planning, intervention, and evaluation of a pregnant trauma patient and her fetus

7. Interpret physiological assessment and diagnostic findings to establish priorities for the care of the pregnant trauma patient and her fetus

Introduction

A. Incidence and epidemiology

1. Trauma is the leading cause of maternal death in women of childbearing age
2. Contemporary pregnant women continue to work and engage in recreational activities well into the third trimester or to term
3. Pregnant women are exposed to risks associated with an overall increase in violence in our society that may result in injuries due to gunshot wounds, stabbings, assaults, or major falls
4. Poverty and overcrowding are linked to assaults on pregnant women
5. An estimated 7% of pregnant women experience some type of trauma during their pregnancy
6. The incidence of injury increases throughout the pregnancy
   a. First trimester: 8.8%
   b. Second trimester: 40%
   c. Third trimester: 52% (Fort & Harlin, 1970)

7. Deaths due to trauma account for 22% of all nonobstetrical deaths and are at least equal to the number of deaths caused by pre-eclampsia and eclampsia
8. Anatomical and physiological changes predispose the pregnant woman to accidental injury
   a. Easy fatigability predisposes the woman to fainting in the first trimester
   b. The enlarged uterus alters the woman's gait and balance, leading to clumsiness
   c. Loosening of pelvic joints causes pelvic tilt and increased lordosis, leading to altered balance
   d. The enlarged uterus is an anterior presenting part that is susceptible to force of impact

B. Mechanism of injury

1. Motor vehicle accidents
   a. Motor vehicle accidents are the leading cause of death for women 15 to 44 years of age
   b. Ten times more fatalities occur from vehicular crashes than from any other mechanisms during the reproductive years
   c. In severe collisions, death is most often caused by major head injury and multiple life-threatening injuries
   d. Fetal death is frequently proportional to the severity of the maternal injury
   e. The most common cause of fetal death is the death of the mother
2. Falls
   a. Falls are a significant threat to the pregnant woman
   b. Minor falls usually do not result in serious injury to the woman or fetus
   c. Maternal head injury and fractures are the most frequently occurring injuries from major falls
   d. The occurrence of pelvic fracture greatly increases the incidence of injury to the gravid uterus
3. Assaults
   a. The enlarged abdomen reduces mobility and increases susceptibility to harm; the protuberant abdomen is frequently involved in assaults
   b. Incidents of domestic violence indicate pregnant women are at greater risk for being injured
4. Burns
   a. Burn injuries account for less than 2% of all injuries to pregnant women
   b. Fetal survival is greatly influenced by gestational age and severity of maternal injury
   c. Effects of carboxyhemoglobin are more severe in the fetus; elevated fetal carboxyhemoglobin levels can exist in the face of nonlethal maternal levels
   d. Lethal maternal burn injuries generally lead to spontaneous delivery of the fetus before the mother dies
5. Gunshot wounds
   a. The enlarged uterus acts as a protective shield for mother and is the most frequently injured abdominal organ
   b. Projectiles fired from low-velocity weapons commonly lose momentum and remain in the intrauterine cavity
   c. Maternal death rarely occurs from gunshot injury to the pregnant uterus
   d. Fetal injury and mortality rate are significant with ballistic injury to the abdomen; therefore, emergency laparotomy is indicated
   e. The severity of injury depends on the following
      (1) Velocity of missile
      (2) Type of bullet
      (3) Production of secondary missiles
      (4) Range or distance from assailant to victim
6. Stab wounds
   a. Abdominal stab wounds have an associated risk of injury to intra-

abdominal organs and the gravid uterus, but they are less serious than ballistic injuries

b. Minor fetal injuries may lead to in utero bleeding, resulting in higher maternal survival than fetal survival

Clinical Practice

A. Assessment

1. History
   a. Mechanism of injury
      (1) Blunt injury
         (a) Motor vehicle accident
            (i) Position in vehicle (driver, passenger, front, rear)
            (ii) Restraints used (shoulder harness, lap belt, three-point restraint)
            (iii) Speed the vehicle was traveling; combined speed of collision
            (iv) Ejection from vehicle; extrication required
         (b) Assault
            (i) Offending object
            (ii) Loss of consciousness
         (c) Fall
            (i) Height of fall
            (ii) Surface victim landed on
            (iii) Body part impacted
      (2) Penetrating injury
         (a) Stab wound
            (i) Offending object, type
            (ii) Length and width of blade
            (iii) Direction of assault
         (b) Ballistic or gunshot wound
            (i) Type and caliber of weapon
            (ii) Velocity and mass
            (iii) Distance from weapon to victim, range
            (iv) Trajectory
      (3) Burns
         (a) Type (thermal, chemical, electrical, or radiation)
         (b) Extent of burn (total body surface area burned)
         (c) Depth of burn (partial or full thickness)
         (d) Carbon monoxide exposure
   b. Focused obstetrical history
      (1) Gestational age (estimated date of confinement [EDC] or first day of last normal menstrual period)
      (2) Multiple fetus
      (3) Number of pregnancies, live births, and abortions
      (4) Delivery history
      (5) Rh factor
      (6) Prenatal complications
      (7) Vaginal bleeding and/or clots
      (8) Abdominal pain and/or uterine contractions
   c. Medical history (AMPLE mnemonic)
      (1) A: allergies
      (2) M: current medications
      (3) P: previous medical problems or chronic illness
      (4) L: time of last meal or oral intake
      (5) E: events preceding injury
2. Physical findings
   a. Primary survey: rapid, brief assessment of the client to identify any life-

threatening problem requiring immediate intervention; a brief history is obtained if possible to include chief complaint, circumstances, and mechanism of injury

(1) Airway
  (a) Open and clear
    (i) Client is able to speak
    (ii) No stridor
    (iii) No visible foreign matter in the upper airway
  (b) Obstructed
    (i) Client is unable to speak
    (ii) Stridor or noisy respirations
    (iii) Cyanosis and dusky mucous membranes and nail beds
    (iv) Substernal and intercostal retractions
    (v) Decreased level of consciousness
    (vi) Vomitus, teeth, blood, secretions, or debris in upper airway
    (vii) Soft tissue damage to the face and neck
    (viii) Absent respirations

(2) Breathing
  (a) Effective
    (i) Spontaneous rise and fall of chest
    (ii) Unlabored respirations
    (iii) Equal chest expansion
    (iv) No accessory muscle use
  (b) Ineffective
    (i) Apnea or agonal respirations less than 10/min
    (ii) Shallow, ineffective respirations
    (iii) Cyanosis and dusky mucous membranes and nailbeds
    (iv) Severe retractions
    (v) Decreased level of consciousness
    (vi) Unequal or absent breath sounds; asymmetry of chest wall expansion
    (vii) Tracheal shift or distended neck veins
    (viii) Obvious chest wounds such as an open pneumothorax; impaled object in chest; multiple rib fractures

(3) Circulation
  (a) Effective
    (i) Palpable major and peripheral pulses between 60 and 100 beats/min
    (ii) Normal capillary refill time (less than 2 seconds)
    (iii) Pink, warm, and dry skin
    (iv) Client alert and oriented
    (v) Fetal heart tones within normal limits
  (b) Ineffective
    (i) Unable to palpate major pulses
    (ii) Obvious external hemorrhage
    (iii) Delayed capillary refill (more than 2 seconds)
    (iv) Decreased level of consciousness
    (v) Pale, cool, moist skin
    (vi) Possible abnormal or absent fetal heart rate

(4) Neurological
  (a) AVPU method
    (i) A: alert
    (ii) V: responds to verbal stimuli
    (iii) P: responds to painful stimuli
    (iv) U: unresponsive
  (b) Glasgow coma scale: see Table 30–1

b. Secondary survey (brief but thorough head-to-toe survey is performed to determine all injuries, both obvious and hidden)

Table 30–1
GLASGOW COMA SCALE

Finding	Score
Eye opening	
Spontaneous	4
To voice	3
To pain	2
None	1
Best verbal response	
Oriented	5
Confused	4
Inappropriate words	3
Incomprehensible sounds	2
None	1
Best motor response	
Obey command	6
Purposeful movement (pain)	5
Withdrawal (pain)	4
Flexion (pain)	3
Extension (pain)	2
None	1

(1) Additional data are collected about the details and mechanism of injury and medical history
(2) Any clothing not removed during the primary survey must be removed at this time
    (a) Clothes should be cut off for two considerations
        (i) In the interest of time
        (ii) If the client is unstable, particularly with a suspected spinal injury
    (b) Cover the client with warm blankets or radiant warmers to prevent hypothermia
(3) The secondary survey uses inspection, palpation, percussion, and auscultation skills
(4) General overview
    (a) Complete vital signs
        (i) Auscultated blood pressures in both arms if chest injuries are suspected
        (ii) Apical pulse
        (iii) Respiratory rate
    (b) General appearance of client
        (i) Abnormal posturing
        (ii) Other unusual body positioning
        (iii) Unusual odors
(5) Head and face
    (a) Surface wounds, ecchymosis, edema, deformity
    (b) Pupil size, equality, and reactivity
    (c) Raccoon eyes (periorbital ecchymosis caused by dissection of blood from a basilar skull fracture)
    (d) Blood or clear drainage from nose or ears
    (e) Battle sign (ecchymosis over mastoid process behind the ear)
    (f) Nasal deformity or tenderness
(6) Neck
    (a) Surface wounds and edema
    (b) Tracheal deviation
    (c) Distended neck veins
    (d) Subcutaneous emphysema
(7) Chest
    (a) Surface wounds

        (b) Impaled objects

        (c) Ecchymosis

        (d) Subcutaneous emphysema

        (e) Bilateral and symmetrical chest rise

        (f) Accessory muscle use

        (g) Breath sounds and heart sounds

        (h) Pain on palpation, crepitus, deformity

    (8) Abdomen and flanks

        (a) Bowel signs auscultated (before palpation of abdomen to prevent false-positive findings)

        (b) Surface wounds

        (c) Seat belt marks

        (d) Impaled objects

        (e) Ecchymosis

        (f) Distension, rigidity

        (g) Evisceration (exposed internal organs)

    (9) Pelvis and genitalia

        (a) Surface wounds

        (b) Ecchymosis and edema of perineum or genitalia

        (c) Instability or tenderness on palpation of anterior iliac crests and/or symphysis pubis

        (d) Bleeding from the urinary meatus, vagina, or rectum

        (e) Pain and/or urge to void

    (10) Extremities

        (a) Surface wounds

        (b) Edema and/or ecchymosis

        (c) Deformities: open or closed

        (d) Bony crepitus on palpation

        (e) Skin color, temperature, and presence of distal pulses

        (f) Spontaneous motor function of all extremities

        (g) Gross sensory function of all extremities

    (11) Posterior

        (a) Observe cervical spine precautions and log roll client to assess for presence of injuries on posterior body

        (b) Surface wounds of back, flanks, buttocks, or thighs

        (c) Pain or deformity on palpation of entire spinal column

        (d) Pain, masses, bruising of costovertebral (CVA) angle

  c. Fetal assessment

    (1) Fetal heart rate is the best indicator of fetal condition

    (2) Auscultate fetal heart tones with stethoscope or Doppler; normal fetal heart rate is 120 to 160 beats/min

    (3) Electronic fetal monitoring is ideal for essential ongoing fetal assessment

    (4) Fundal height

        (a) Measure distance from symphysis pubis to top of the uterus

        (b) Measurement in centimeters approximates weeks of gestation

    (5) Labor status

        (a) Cervical dilatation

        (b) Rupture of membranes

        (c) Effacement

        (d) Station

    (6) Specific responses to trauma

        (a) Premature rupture of membranes

        (b) Abruptio placentae

        (c) Uterine rupture

        (d) Fetal distress

3. Psychosocial findings

  a. Anxiety or fear about life of fetus

b. Anxiety or fear about client's own well-being and ability to care for infant
c. Guilt about being injured and causing potential harm to fetus
4. Diagnostic procedures
   a. Laboratory
      (1) Complete blood count (CBC), differential, platelet count (normal hematocrit is 30 to 35%; WBC count is approximately 20,000)
      (2) Blood type and Rh factor with crossmatch
      (3) Sodium, potassium, chloride, and carbon dioxide
      (4) Blood urea nitrogen (BUN) and creatinine clearance
      (5) Glucose
      (6) Clotting factors: prothrombin time (PT), partial thromboplastin time (PTT)
      (7) Fibrinogen
         (a) Normal is 80 to 180 ml/dl; this rises to 400 to 500 ml/dl at term
         b. An apparently normal level can actually reflect a low level and impending disseminated intravascular coagulation (DIC), which can follow placental abruption
      (8) Amylase
      (9) Urinalysis (dip for blood at bedside)
      (10) Arterial blood gases
      (11) Possible toxicology studies
   b. Radiological studies
      (1) Perform studies as indicated for diagnosis of any trauma client; radiation risk to fetus should not interfere with life-saving interventions for mother
         (a) Chest x-ray: radiograph: 1 millirad per examination
         (b) Pelvis x-ray: radiograph: 210 millirad per examination
      (2) Protect client from unnecessary exposure
      (3) Uterus should be shielded with lead apron whenever possible
      (4) IV pyelogram (IVP) dye does not cross placenta
   c. Computerized axial tomography (CT) scan
      (1) Using sequential slices of tissue with small gaps between cuts decreases radiation exposure
      (2) Assess for bleeding and solid organ injury
      (3) Magnetic resonance imaging (MRI) may be used because of its advantages over CT scans
         (a) Magnetic resonance imaging uses no ionizing radiation
         (b) Vascular structures can be evaluated without the need to inject iodinated contrast medium
         (c) Imaging of deep pelvic structures is not dependent on a urine-filled bladder
   d. Ultrasound testing
      (1) Is a readily available bedside study
      (2) Can identify fetal cardiac activity and detect fetal heart tones or fetal death
      (3) Determines
         (a) Gestational age
         (b) Fetal position
         (c) Amount of amniotic fluid
         (d) Multiple gestations
         (e) Placental location
         (f) Possible placental abruption (not 100% accurate)
      (4) May detect free fluid in maternal peritoneal cavity
      (5) B-mode or gray-scale unit is an accurate method to determine fetal size and maturity, placental location, and retroplacental or pelvic hematomas
   e. Amniocentesis

(1) Tests for fetal compromise and fetal lung maturity

(2) Assesses for presence of RBCs to rule out intrauterine bleeding or for meconium staining

(3) Lecithin/sphingomyelin (L/S) ratio and presence of phosphatidylglycerol can determine fetal lung maturity if delivery is deemed imminent

(4) Can be done only in second and third trimesters

f. Diagnostic peritoneal lavage (DPL)

(1) Reliable surgical technique to diagnose intraperitoneal injury with 94 to 99% accuracy; not contraindicated in pregnancy

(2) Useful for clients with the following conditions:

(a) Depressed level of consciousness

(b) Drug-impaired state or unexplained shock

(c) Inability to be monitored because of the effects of general anesthesia

(3) Will not detect extraperitoneal or diaphragmatic injury

(4) Nasogastric tube and urinary drainage catheter are placed before procedure

(5) Procedure

(a) Mini-laparotomy incision made under xiphoid and peritoneal dialysis lavage catheter introduced into peritoneum

(b) Aspiration of more than 20 ml of frank blood is considered positive

(c) If aspiration is negative, 1 liter of warmed lactated Ringer's solution or normal saline solution is infused over 10 to 15 minutes into peritoneal cavity

(d) The solution bag is lowered to gravity drainage and specimens are obtained for evaluation

(6) Positive DPL requires surgical intervention as evidenced by the following

(a) Aspiration of blood

(i) 100,000 RBCs/mm^3 (blunt trauma)

(ii) 1000 to 100,000 RBCs/mm^3 (penetrating trauma)

(iii) More than 500 WBCs/mm^3

(b) Amylase greater than 175 Somogyi units

(c) Presence of bile, fecal material, or bacteria

g. Ongoing fetal monitoring by auscultation of fetal heart tones or electronic monitoring

B. Nursing Diagnoses

1. Ineffective airway clearance
2. Impaired gas exchange
3. Ineffective breathing pattern
4. Alteration in cardiovascular tissue perfusion
5. Decreased cardiac output
6. Fluid volume deficit
7. Alteration in cerebral tissue perfusion
8. Anticipatory grief related to potential loss of fetus or maternal fears for own well-being
9. Alteration in fetal tissue perfusion

C. Interventions/Evaluations

1. Ineffective airway clearance

a. Interventions

(1) Open airway with jaw thrust or chin lift keeping head in neutral, midline position

(2) Clear airway with fingersweep or gentle suction

(3) Maintain open airway with appropriate adjunct (oropharyngeal or nasopharyngeal airway, esophageal obturator airway, tracheal intubation, cricothyroidotomy)

(4) Immobilize cervical spine
   (a) Manual stabilization (Fig. 30–1)
   (b) Rigid cervical collar
   (c) Use sandbags, IV bags, or rolled towels
   (d) Tape across forehead (avoid tape across chin, which may cause airway obstruction)
   (e) Backboard
(5) Control bleeding or swelling
(6) Consider insertion of nasogastric tube for gastric decompression and airway protection
b. Evaluations
   (1) Airway is open and clear; client is able to speak
   (2) Client exhibits no stridor
   (3) No foreign matter is visible in the upper airway
   (4) Cervical spine precautions are maintained
2 and 3. Impaired gas exchange; ineffective breathing pattern
   a. Interventions
      (1) If client is not breathing
         (a) Positive-pressure ventilation with bag-valve-mask device and 100% oxygen
         (b) Obtain arterial blood gases
      (2) If breathing is present but ineffective
         (a) Administer oxygen by mask at 10 to 15 liters/min and assist ventilations as necessary
         (b) Identify and intervene for specific life-threatening injuries
            (i) Tension pneumothorax
               ● Severe respiratory distress, tracheal shift, distended neck veins, absent breath sounds
               ● Immediate needle thoracostomy on affected side
            (ii) Open pneumothorax
               ● Sucking or gurgling chest wound, severe respiratory distress, or cyanosis
               ● Seal wound with sterile occlusive dressing; monitor for development of tension pneumothorax
            (iii) Flail chest
               ● Severe respiratory distress, cyanosis, paradoxical chest wall movement
               ● Assist with intubation and mechanical ventilation
               ● Prevent IV fluid overload
            (iv) Massive hemothorax
               ● Severe respiratory distress, signs of hypovolemic shock (prior conditions ruled out)
               ● Assist with insertion of large-bore chest tube on affected side at fifth or sixth intercostal space
               ● Anticipate autotransfusion

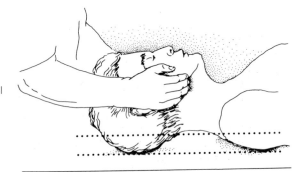

Figure 30–1
Manual stabilization of the cervical spine.

b. Evaluations
  (1) Rise and fall of chest is spontaneous
  (2) Respirations are unlabored
  (3) Chest wall expansion is equal and symmetrical
  (4) No accessory muscle is used
  (5) Skin is pink, warm, and dry
  (6) Client is alert and oriented
4, 5, and 6. Alteration in cardiovascular tissue perfusion; decreased cardiac output; fluid volume deficit
  a. Interventions
    (1) If pulse is absent
      (a) Begin cardiopulmonary resuscitation
      (b) Prepare for emergency open thoracotomy to control intrathoracic hemorrhage
      (c) Prepare for autotransfusion
      (d) Consider use of pneumatic antishock garment (Fig. 30–2) to increase peripheral vascular resistance
        (i) Inflate only legs to prevent poor perfusion to uterus
        (ii) Use is controversial during pregnancy

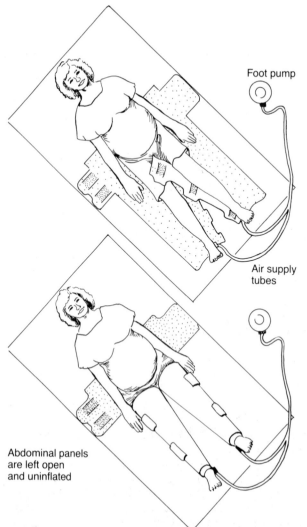

Foot pump

Air supply
tubes

Abdominal panels
are left open
and uninflated

Figure 30–2
Application of the MAST suit during
pregnancy.

      (2) If pulse is present but ineffective
         (a) Administer oxygen at 10 to 15 liters/min by mask; assist ventilations as necessary
         (b) Control obvious external hemorrhage by direct pressure, or elevation of extremities (consider clamping or tourniquet if client is *in extremis*)
         (c) Establish venous access
           (i) Establish two 14- to 16-gauge IV lines with Y-type blood administration tubing
           (ii) Assist with possible placement of central line or cutdown
         (d) Aggressive fluid resuscitation
           (i) Warmed crystalloid solution (lactated Ringer's solution or normal saline), titrated to hemodynamic status
           (ii) Infusion of 300 ml of fluid for each 100 ml of estimated blood loss may be needed to maintain adequate circulating volume
           (iii) Burn injury fluid resuscitation
              • Four milliliters of crystalloid solution × the percentage of body surface area burned × client weight in kilograms given over first 24 hours
              • Half of the total volume is given in first 8 hours after burn injury
           (iv) Administer uncrossmatched, O-negative blood if client is in profound hypovolemic shock at 1 ml for each 1 ml of estimated blood loss
           (v) Replacement of clotting factors must be considered when packed cells are given
         (e) Obtain blood for type and crossmatch, determine hemoglobin and hematocrit values and arterial blood gases, and conduct other ordered studies
         (f) Consider using pneumatic antishock garment
         (g) Initiate continuous cardiac monitoring (heart rate increases 15 to 20 beats/min during pregnancy)
         (h) Place client in left lateral position to prevent supine hypotension syndrome; may need to manually displace uterus or place supports under client's right hip to tilt client 30° to the left side
         (i) Insert indwelling urinary catheter to monitor hourly output; urinary output is a sensitive indicator of tissue perfusion status and of the adequacy of fluid replacement
         (j) Monitor for oozing from puncture sites, gastrointestinal or genitourinary tract, vagina, or wounds
  b. Evaluations
    (1) Client has improved level of consciousness
    (2) Skin is pink, warm, and dry
    (3) Urinary output is greater than 30 ml/hr
    (4) Distal pulses are present and strong
    (5) Capillary refill time is less than 2 seconds
    (6) Respiratory rate is between 14 and 20 breaths/min without accessory muscle use
    (7) Pulse pressure is 40 points, and systolic blood pressure is above 100 mm Hg
    (8) PaO_2 is above 80 torr in room air; $PaCO_2$ is between 35 and 45 torr
7. Alteration in cerebral tissue perfusion
  a. Interventions
    (1) Consider administration of naloxone (Narcan), glucose, or thiamine to rule out drug intoxication, hypoglycemia, or nutritional deficits as cause of decreased level of consciousness
    (2) Prevent increased intracranial pressure (ICP)

(a) Administer oxygen at 10 to 15 liters/min by mask

(b) Maintain head in midline position to facilitate venous drainage

(c) Elevate head of bed 30° if not contraindicated

(d) Assist with intubation if indicated and hyperventilate to maintain $PaCO_2$ of 26 to 30 torr; elevated $PaCO_2$ causes cerebral vessel dilation and increases ICP

(e) Obtain arterial blood gases

(f) Avoid IV fluid overload

(g) Cover open wounds with sterile dressings

(h) Do not stem flow of possible cerebrospinal fluid leaks; place sterile dressing under nose or over ear

(i) Tetanus prophylaxis for any open wound

b. Evaluations

(1) Client is alert and oriented

(2) PaO_2 is greater than 80 torr on room air

(3) $PaCO_2$ is between 35 and 45 torr (26 to 30 torr if client is being hyperventilated)

(4) No seizures or abnormal posturing noted

(5) Wound care management performed

8. Anticipatory grief related to potential loss of fetus or maternal fears for own well-being

a. Interventions

(1) Establish trusting relationship by being nonjudgmental; stay with client and explain all procedures and interventions

(2) Provide periodic updates on maternal and fetal status

(3) Actively listen to client's questions and responses

(4) Involve significant others; permit others to be present if client is stable

(5) Involve religious leader, social worker, or mental health nurse in care

(6) Answer questions regarding fetus honestly and realistically

b. Evaluations

(1) Client exhibits appropriate grieving behavior

(2) Client verbalizes feelings and fears

(3) Significant others are involved in care

(4) Support and reassurance are provided to the client and her significant others

9. Alteration in fetal tissue perfusion

a. Interventions

(1) Aggressive maternal resuscitation (leading cause of fetal death is maternal death)

(2) Emergency (crash) cesarean section for a fetus of viable gestational age

(a) Indications

(i) Fetal distress

- Late and ominous decelerations of fetal heart rate, severe bradycardia or tachycardia
- Blood on amniocentesis
- Positive Kleihauer-Betke (K-B) stain in maternal blood (evaluation of fetal hemoglobin)

(ii) Improve surgical field exposure by emptying uterus to save the mother

(iii) Ruptured diaphragm

(iv) Unstable pelvic or spinal fractures at term

(v) Placental abruption of at least 50%

(vi) Uterine rupture

(vii) Uncontrolled hemorrhage

(viii) Maternal death (postmortem cesarean section)

(b) Factors affecting fetal survival of postmortem cesarean section

(i) Fetal gestational age

(ii) Fetal health before maternal death

(iii) Maternal cause of death (e.g., severe hemorrhage)

(iv) Adequacy of resuscitation

(v) Time interval between maternal death and fetal delivery

(c) Newborn resuscitation required (see Chapter 21 on newborn resuscitation)

(3) Admit all pregnant clients with viable fetuses and with major injuries to the hospital or observe them in the emergency department for continuous monitoring after resuscitation and stabilization for 24 to 48 hours

Health Education

A. Prevention

1. Wearing of three-point seat belt properly during pregnancy to prevent ejection or serious injury from collision with steering wheel or dashboard (Fig. 30–3)
   a. Wear seat belt with shoulder strap positioned between breasts and above dome of uterus
      (1) Lap belt is worn under the uterus and across the anterior spines of the pelvis
      (2) A small, soft pillow may be placed between the body and seat belt for comfort
   b. Three-point restraints help prevent rapid-deceleration, forward-flexion injuries that can cause shearing forces on the uterus

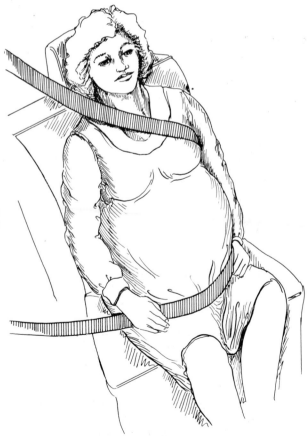

Figure 30–3
Three-point auto restraint positioned correctly for use by a pregnant woman.

   c. Lap belts used alone may cause injury to enlarged gravid uterus, especially if worn loose enough to ride up over abdomen
     (1) A pregnant client should be advised that use of only a lap belt is preferable to using no restraint
     (2) However, it is then preferable that she ride in the back seat
  2. Referral to public education programs regarding danger to mother and fetus when seat belt is not worn; omission of seat belt for all persons increases chance of ejection, which increases chance of death by 20 times
  3. Enforcement of current laws to require seat belt use

B. Education

  1. Prenatal care to include information about normal anatomical changes that predispose pregnant women to accidents
  2. Encouragement of frequent rest breaks
  3. Safety measures in the home and workplace such as avoiding climbing on chairs and ladders
  4. Counseling regarding possibility of spousal or partner abuse during pregnancy

---

CASE STUDY AND STUDY QUESTIONS

1. In trauma, the most common cause of fetal death is:

  a. Death of the mother.

  b. Placental abruption.

  c. Uterine rupture.

  d. Penetrating injury to the fetus.

2. The primary survey in multisystem trauma focuses on:

  a. In-depth management and definitive care interventions.

  b. Life-threatening priorities.

  c. A thorough head-to-toe assessment.

  d. Chief complaint, past medical history, and allergies.

3. Of the following IV solutions, which is preferred in the initial resuscitation of a pregnant trauma client?

  a. D5½ normal saline at 100 ml/hr.

  b. Warm normal saline or lactated Ringer's solution titrated to the hemodynamic status of the client.

  c. 500 ml of colloid solution over 2 hours.

  d. Two to four units of packed RBCs.

4. In the severely head-injured client, initial interventions aimed at reducing increased intracranial pressure include:

  a. Vigorous suctioning to clear the airway.

  b. Hypoventilation.

  c. Maintenance of PCO_2 at 26 to 30 torr.

  d. Trendelenburg position.

5. Tissue perfusion is considered adequate if all of the following are present except:

  a. Client is alert and oriented.

  b. Capillary refill time is less than 2 seconds.

  c. Skin is pink, warm, and dry.

  d. Urinary output is less than 20 ml/hr.

Lisa Marshall, 26 years old and 36 weeks pregnant, was involved in a motor vehicle accident while on her way to visit her mother. She was the driver of a compact car that was broadsided on the driver's side by a delivery van that had run a red light. On arrival at the scene, the police found moderate damage to Lisa's car.

Lisa was wearing a seat belt that included a shoulder harness and lap belt in the proper position. The paramedics found her to be alert, but she continued to ask, "What happened?" The field primary survey revealed a patent airway, no respiratory distress, and slightly pale, diaphoretic skin. Lisa's chief complaint was abdominal pain "all over"; she had what appeared to be a seat belt contusion across the lower abdomen. Her vital signs were heart rate, 92 beats/min; respirations 24/min; and blood pressure, 92/64. Oxygen was applied at 15 liters/min by mask as full spinal immobilization was instituted. En route to the nearest trauma center, two 16-gauge IV lines were established in each forearm.

On arrival to the emergency department, Lisa was evaluated by the trauma team with the assistance of the obstetrical and neonatal intensive care unit (NICU) teams. Oxygen was continued and cervical spine precautions maintained. Lisa remained alert but confused about the circumstances of the accident and the date.

After it had been determined that Lisa's airway, breathing, and circulation were intact, the secondary survey was performed. A thorough head-to-toe assessment revealed only a small laceration on the left parietal area of the head, abdominal contusions, pain on palpation of the anterior iliac crests, and superficial abrasions to both anterior knees. Lisa was completely undressed and covered with warm blankets.

Baseline laboratory studies were obtained; diagnostic radiographs of the cervical spine, chest, and pelvis were negative for injury. Continuous electronic fetal monitoring was instituted and revealed regular uterine contractions every 2 to 3 minutes and fetal heart tones of 136 beats/min. A urinary drainage catheter was inserted and was negative for blood by dipstick testing.

Soon after the initial evaluation of Lisa, a change in baseline was noted as the fetal heart tones revealed a tachycardia of 180 to 200 beats/min. Lisa's vital signs were now heart rate, 134 beats/min; respirations, 28/min; blood pressure, 88 and palpable. An emergency cesarean section and exploratory laparotomy were performed immediately. The operation revealed both a ruptured spleen and partial placental detachment from the uterine wall. A boy was delivered without evidence of distress, and a splenectomy was performed.

Lisa was discharged home on postoperative day 6 without complications. Her son had not been injured in the accident and had been discharged to the maternal grandmother on day 3 in good condition.

6. Ongoing assessment of the adequacy of resuscitation efforts includes:

   a. Vital signs every 5 to 15 minutes until stable.

   b. Urinary output every 30 to 60 minutes.

   c. Frequent level of consciousness evaluations.

   d. All of the above.

7. Because of Lisa's mechanism of injury, a complete neurological examination must be completed. This evaluation includes assessment of her:

   a. Level of consciousness.

   b. Motor and sensory responses.

   c. Pupil size, equality, and reactivity to light.

   d. All of the above.

8. Additional information regarding the mechanism of injury in the above accident may include the following except:

   a. The need for extrication.

   b. The speed at which the vehicles were traveling.

   c. The intersection at which the accident occurred.

   d. Passenger space intrusion.

9. The most appropriate position for Lisa to be placed in is:

   a. Flat with her legs elevated and her uterus displaced to the left.

   b. Semi-Fowler's position to facilitate breathing.

   c. Head down, left lateral position to prevent vomiting and possible aspiration.

   d. Trendelenburg position to improve blood flow to the brain.

10. The least appropriate actual nursing diagnosis for Lisa is:

   a. Anticipatory grief.

   b. Ineffective breathing pattern.

   c. Decreased cardiac output.

   d. Fluid volume deficit.

Carol Simon was brought by private car to the emergency department after being involved in a drive-by gang-related shooting in front of her home. She was 17 years old and 32 weeks pregnant with her second child. Carol had received no prenatal care for this pregnancy.

The emergency department staff removed Carol from the back seat of the car; she had no pulse and was not breathing. She had an obvious gunshot wound to the upper back between the shoulder blades, and no apparent exit wound was seen. Cardiopulmonary resuscitation was begun, and the trauma team was assembled immediately.

On arrival in the trauma room, Carol underwent as immediate open thoracotomy to identify the extent of her internal injuries, to perform internal cardiac massage, and to crossclamp the aorta. The pericardium was opened, and no blood was found. The heart was in ventricular fibrillation. A simultaneous emergency cesarean section was done. A boy was delivered, and the development of some palpable pulse was noted before transfer to the NICU.

Despite vigorous volume resuscitation and manual cardiac compression, Carol died in the emergency department. Her baby remained in the NICU in critical condition because of respiratory failure and probable cerebral anoxia.

11. In addition to the emergency trauma staff, who else should the nurse immediately notify?

a. Labor and delivery staff.

b. NICU physician and nurses.

c. Blood bank staff.

d. All of the above.

12. Factors affecting fetal survival of a postmortem cesarean section include which of the following?

a. Time interval between maternal death and fetal delivery.

b. Fetal gestational age.

c. Adequacy of resuscitation.

d. All of the above.

13. Priorities in the initial care of Carol include:

a. Applying the pneumatic antishock garment and inflating the legs and abdominal compartments.

b. Establishing a patent airway and ventilating the client by endotracheal intubation and administration of 100% oxygen.

c. Amniocentesis to determine fetal lung maturity.

d. Administration of crystalloid solution at a 3 : 1 ratio for estimated volume lost.

14. In addition to maternal death, indications for a crash cesarean section include all of the following except:

a. All pelvic fractures.

b. Uterine rupture.

c. Severe placental abruption.

d. Late and ominous decelerations of fetal heart rate.

15. The best choice of volume resuscitation for Carol is:

a. Infusion of 100 ml of crystalloid solution for each 100 ml of estimated blood loss.

b. Uncrossmatched, O-negative blood, 1 ml for each 1 ml of estimated blood loss.

c. Administration of 500 ml of colloid solution to improve volume expansion rapidly.

d. Rapid crystalloid solution infusion until complete type and crossmatch is completed to avoid possible transfusion reaction.

Answers to Study Questions

1. a	2. b	3. b
4. c	5. d	6. d
7. d	8. c	9. a
10. b	11. d	12. d
13. b	14. a	15. b

REFERENCES

Baker, D. (1982). Trauma in the pregnant patient. *Surgical Clinics of North America, 62*(2), 275–289.

Bocka, J., Courtney, J., Pearlman, M., Tintinalli, J., Lorenz, R., Swor, R., Krome, R., Glover, J. (1988). Trauma in pregnancy. *Annals of Emergency Medicine, 17*(8), 829–834.

Bojanowski, C., Hill, K., & Martin, D. (1988). Assessment of the pregnant trauma patient. *Dimensions of Critical Care Nursing, 7*(6), 356–362.

Bremer, C., & Cassata, L. (1986). Trauma in pregnancy. *Nursing Clinics of North America, 21*(4), 705–716.

Buschbaum, H. (1979). *Trauma in pregnancy.* Philadelphia: Saunders.

Committee on Trauma Research, Commission on Life Sciences, National Research Council and the Institute of Medicine (1985). *Injury in America: A continuing public health problem.* Washington, DC: National Academy Press.

Crosby, W. (1983). Traumatic injuries during pregnancy. *Clinical Obstetrics and Gynecology, 26*(4), 902–912.

Dees, G., & Fuller, M. (1989). Blunt trauma in the pregnant patient. *Journal of Emergency Nursing, 15*(6), 495–499.

Drost, T., Rosemurgy, A., Sherman, H., Scott, L., & Williams, J. (1990). Major trauma in pregnant women: Maternal/fetal outcome. *Journal of Trauma, 30*(5), 574–578.

Fort, A., & Harlin, R. (1970). Pregnancy outcome after noncatastrophic maternal trauma during pregnancy. *Obstetrics and Gynecology, 35*(10), 912.

Foster, C. (1984). The pregnant trauma patient. *Nursing 84, 14*(11), 58–63.

Higgins, S., & Garite, T. (1984). Late abruptio placentae in trauma patients: Implications for monitoring. *Obstetrics and Gynecology, 63*(3), 10S–12S.

Higgins, S. (1988). Perinatal protocol: Trauma in pregnancy. *Journal of Perinatology, 8*(3), 288–292.

Morkovin, V. (1986). Trauma in pregnancy. In R.G. Farrell (Ed.), *OB/GYN emergencies: The first 60 minutes* (pp. 71–86). Rockville, MD: Aspen.

Neufeld, J., Moore, E., Marx, J., & Rosen, P. (1987). Trauma in pregnancy. *Emergency Medicine Clinics of North America, 5*(3), 623–640.

O'Keeffe, D. (1985). When the accident victim is pregnant. *Contemporary Obstetrics and Gynecology, 26*(1), 148–164.

Pearse, C., Magrina, J., & Finley, B. (1984). Use of MAST suit in obstetrics and gynecology. *Obstetrical Gynecological Survey, 39*(6), 416–422.

Peckman, C., & King, R. (1963). A study of intercurrent conditions observed during pregnancy. *American Journal of Obstetrics and Gynecology, 87,* 609–624.

Reedy, N., & Brucker, M. (1991). Obstetrics and gynecologic emergencies. In S. Kitt & J. Kaiser (Eds.), *Emergency nursing: A physiologic and clinical perspective* (pp. 339–345). Philadelphia: Saunders.

Rice, D., & MacKenzie, E. (1989). *Cost of injury in the United States: A report to Congress.* San Francisco: Institute for Health and Aging, University of California and Injury Prevention Center, The Johns Hopkins University.

Sheehy, S., Marvin, J., & Jimmerson, C. (1989). Special considerations for the traumatized pregnant patient. In Baxt, W.G. (Ed.), *Manual of clinical trauma care: the first hour.* St. Louis: Mosby.

Smith, L. (1988). The pregnant trauma patient. In V. Cardona, P. Hurn, M. Bastnagel, P. Scanlon-Schilpp, & S. Veise-Berry (Eds.), *Trauma nursing: From resuscitation through rehabilitation* (pp. 643–663). Philadelphia: Saunders.

Stafford, P. (1981). Protection of the pregnant woman in the emergency department. *Journal of Emergency Nursing, 7*(3), 97–102.

Stauffer, D. (1986). The trauma patient who is pregnant. *Journal of Emergency Nursing, 12*(2), 89–93.

Tringa, G. (1980). Medical aspects of seatbelt usage. *Journal of Traffic Medicine, 8*(37), 38–39.

Vander Veer, J., Jr. (1984). Trauma during pregnancy. *Topics in Emergency Medicine, 6*(1), 72–77.

Karen Foster-Anderson

Surgery in Pregnancy

Objectives

1. Recognize the potential risks of anesthesia to the pregnant client
2. Distinguish surgical risks to the pregnant client and the fetus in the first, second, and third trimesters
3. Analyze alterations in the pregnant client's physiology and the risks associated with anesthesia
4. Identify optimal timing for elective surgery when performed during pregnancy
5. Identify potential complications to the pregnant surgical client
6. Assess the client's response to surgery and potential for preterm labor
7. Recognize symptoms of the pregnant client with acute cholecystitis
8. Recognize symptoms of appendicitis in the pregnant client
9. Recognize the client at risk for cervical imcompetence
10. Define the function of the cervical cerclage
11. Recognize risk factors in the potential placement of the cerclage
12. Select appropriate nursing actions based on acquired knowledge of the alterations in the pregnant client's physiology and integrate that knowledge into her preoperative, intraoperative, and postoperative care
13. Recognize psychosocial stressors affecting the pregnant client undergoing surgery
14. Integrate the care of the pregnant surgical client and her family based on the analysis of the client's needs in an emotionally and physically stressful situation
15. Formulate nursing interventions to prevent postoperative surgical complications in the pregnant surgical client

Introduction

A. Incidence of nonobstetrical surgery performed during pregnancy is 1.6% of all pregnancies or up to 50,000 procedures/year (Shnider & Webster, 1965)

B. Types of procedures

1. Ovarian tumors and acute appendicitis are the most common surgical complications requiring surgery in pregnancy
2. Cervical cerclage (correction for incompetent cervix)
3. Cholecystectomy

C. Anesthesia

1. Effects on altered maternal physiology must be considered
2. Effects on developing fetus must be considered in the timing of surgery and anesthesia

D. Factors that optimize outcome

1. Preoperative, intraoperative, and postoperative care
2. Knowledge of maternal physiology and fetal growth and development
3. Assessment of pregnant surgical client's needs
4. Assessment of fetal well-being
5. Knowledgeable and well-planned nursing care significantly contributes to optimal outcome for mother and fetus

Clinical Practice

ANESTHESIA

A. Introduction

1. Anesthetic management priorities
   a. Maternal safety
   b. Avoidance of teratogenic drugs
   c. Avoidance of fetal asphyxia
   d. Prevention of preterm labor (Shnider & Levinson, 1987)
2. Pregnancy-induced changes to maternal physiology
   a. Cardiopulmonary changes
   b. Respiratory changes
   c. Gastrointestinal changes
3. Effects on fetus
   a. Gestational age of lowest risk
   b. Anesthesia of choice
      (1) Varies according to type of surgery
      (2) Varies according to gestational age
4. Objectives of care for pregnant surgical client
   a. Evaluation of mother (client)
   b. Evaluation of fetus

B. Assessment

1. History
   a. Gestational age (by date of last menstrual period (LMP) or ultrasound test)
   b. Urgency related to the need for surgery
   c. Presence of underlying illness
   d. Known maternal drug allergies
   e. Current medications
   f. Surgical history: previous responses to anesthesia
   g. Previous obstetrical history
   h. Pain evaluation: location, intensity, characteristics, and duration
2. Physical examination
   a. Gestational age: uterine size, fundal height
   b. Vital signs

(1) Temperature
(2) Pulse
(3) Respiration
(4) Blood pressure
c. Evaluation of fetal heart rate (FHR): Doppler or continuous fetal monitoring
d. Evaluation of uterine activity
(1) Palpation
(2) Continuous fetal monitoring
e. Respiratory status: dyspnea, evidence of distress, fever, and congestion
f. Client's response to illness: pain evaluation
3. Psychosocial responses
a. Stress factors
(1) Anxiety
(2) Fear of pregnancy loss or of harm to fetus
(3) Fear of harm to self
b. Behavioral factors
(1) Difficulty communicating: confusion
(2) Response to pain
(3) Open expression of fears and anxieties
4. Diagnostic procedures
a. Ultrasonography
b. Fetal monitoring
c. Preoperative laboratory evaluation: complete blood count (CBC), urinalysis (UA), type and crossmatch of blood products
d. Palpation of uterus
e. Electrocardiogram (ECG), chest x-ray film (shielded), if indicated

C. Nursing Diagnoses

1. Alteration in maternal tissue perfusion
2. Alteration in fetal tissue perfusion
3. Anxiety related to potential alteration in client and fetal health
4. Alteration in pain or comfort

D. Interventions/Evaluations

1. Alteration in maternal tissue perfusion
a. Interventions: preoperative care
(1) Monitor vital signs
(a) Temperature
(b) Pulse
(c) Respiration
(d) Blood pressure
(2) IV hydration
(a) Maintenance by 16- or 18-gauge intracatheter infusion of 900- to 1000 ml of nondextrose crystalloid solution (Ringer's lactate or normal saline)
(3) Left lateral positioning in the second and third trimesters (the enlarging uterus compresses the vena cava in the supine position, thereby decreasing uteroplacental blood flow); if left lateral position is not possible, place a wedge (pillow or rolled blanket) under right hip to displace uterus to the left
(4) FHR monitoring: Doppler or external fetal monitor
(5) Preoperative laboratory tests
b. Interventions: postoperative care (in addition to above)
(1) Anesthetic agents: at present, no anesthetic drug—premedicant, IV induction agent, inhalation agent, or local anesthetic—has been proven to be teratogenic in humans (Shnider & Levinson, 1987); however, lack of sufficient data suggests that elective surgery should be delayed until

after pregnancy and that the first trimester should be avoided if at all possible

(a) Regional anesthesia: spinal or epidural administration allows much less fetal exposure but may not allow for adequate anesthesia for the required surgery

(i) Major side effect includes a hypotensive effect from peripheral vasodilatation

(ii) Increased fluid and lateral positioning may improve this transient effect

(b) General anesthesia

(i) If administration is necessary during first trimester, there is no proof that any one technique is superior to another

(ii) In no study has any one anesthetic agent been found to be associated with a higher or lower incidence of preterm delivery (Shnider & Levinson, 1987)

(2) Maintenance of adequate oxygenation: oxygen given via face mask (8 to 10 l/min), especially with general anesthetic agents

(3) Intake and output (I&O) monitoring and recording

(4) Assessment of thrombosis/phlebitis (Homans' sign)

(5) Antiembolic stockings

(6) Avoidance of vasoconstrictors (may decrease uteroplacental blood flow)

c. Evaluations

(1) Client's vital signs remain stable

(2) Client maintains adequate oxygenation and circulation intraoperatively and postoperatively

(3) Client maintains adequate intake and output

(4) Client avoids thromboembolic phenomenon

2. Alteration in fetal tissue perfusion

a. Interventions: preoperative care and postoperative care

(1) Monitor maternal vital signs

(a) Temperature

(b) Pulse

(c) Respiration

(d) Blood pressure

(2) Monitor FHR and uterine contractions (UCs)

(3) Use of continuous fetal monitoring intraoperatively (if possible) and postoperatively

(4) Left lateral positioning of mother

(5) Adequate oxygenation of mother

(6) IV hydration of mother

(7) Maternal medication: avoidance of vasoconstrictors and medication that increases maternal hypotension

b. Evaluations

(1) Mother's vital signs remain stable

(2) FHR remains stable

(3) Mother experiences minimal uterine contractibility, which is recognized and treated appropriately

3. Anxiety related to potential alteration in client and fetal health

a. Interventions: preoperative and postoperative care

(1) Assess client's coping status and abilities

(2) Assess social support system and integrate into client care

(3) Provide opportunity for verbalization of fears, anxieties, and concerns

(4) Facilitate discussion with anesthesiologist, client, and her family to discuss options of anesthetic agents

(5) Teach stress reduction techniques, and reinforce client's ability to implement techniques

(6) Integrate mental health care team with client care, if appropriate

b. Evaluations
   (1) Client demonstrates positive coping strategies
   (2) Social support system is involved with client care
   (3) Client demonstrates stress reduction techniques
   (4) Client demonstrates knowledge of anesthetic choices, risks and benefits, and recommendations
4. Alteration in pain or comfort
   a. Interventions: preoperative and postoperative care
      (1) Assess quality of pain: location, duration, aggravating and alleviating factors
      (2) Provide comfort measures: positioning, use of pillows
      (3) Monitor client's vital signs with FHR
      (4) Administer analgesia: acetaminophen or narcotic analgesia, as ordered
   b. Evaluations
      (1) Client experiences a reduction in postoperative discomfort
      (2) Client's vital signs and FHR remain stable

SURGERIES

Cholecystectomy

A. Introduction

1. Incidence is 1/4000 to 5000 pregnancies (Scott, 1990)
2. Previous pregnancies predispose to cholecystitis
3. Surgical management is used only if medical management unsuccessful or if rupture of gallbladder or pancreatitis is evident
4. Optimal timing of surgery is during second trimester (after highest risk for spontaneous abortion and organogenesis has passed and before enlarging uterus impairs surgical exposure)
5. Maternal mortality (15%) and fetal loss (60%) have been associated with secondary pancreatitis
6. Surgery should not be delayed if urgently indicated
7. Second-trimester risk of surgery is primarily preterm labor

B. Assessment

1. History
   a. Assessment of pain: stabbing, colicky, or steady pain midepigastrium that radiates to the right upper quadrant, right flank, or right shoulder
   b. Excessive flatulence, heartburn, or fatty food intolerance
   c. Increased discomfort after meals
   d. Nausea or vomiting
   e. Medical and surgical history
   f. Obstetrical history
   g. Gestational age by LMP or ultrasonography
2. Physical examination
   a. Abdominal examination
      (1) Palpation: rebound tenderness, rigidity, and uterine contractions
      (2) Auscultation: bowel sounds
         (a) Peristaltic rushes (borborygmi) may indicate an intestinal obstruction (Scott, 1990)
   b. Vital signs
      (1) Temperature
      (2) Pulse
      (3) Respiration
      (4) Blood pressure
   c. FHR

   d. Presence or absence of vaginal bleeding: the client should not experience bleeding with a diagnosis of cholecystitis
   e. Cervical examination to differentiate pain from preterm labor contractions
3. Psychosocial factors
   a. Anxiety
   b. Fear of loss of pregnancy
   c. Fear of personal harm
4. Diagnostic procedures
   a. Laboratory tests
      (1) CBC with differential
         (a) WBC of 15,000 to 20,000 mm^3 may be normal in pregnancy
         (b) Hemoglobin level should be stable (>10.0 g/dl)
      (2) UA and urine culture to differentiate cholecystitis from pyelonephritis or cystitis
      (3) Electrolytes, liver function tests, bilirubin
         (a) Serum amylase level may be increased fourfold during pregnancy (serial elevated amylase levels may be associated with pancreatitis [Cunningham, MacDonald, & Gant, 1989])
         (b) Serum alkaline phosphatase value may be increased to twice that of nonpregnant values (even higher values may be seen in cholecystitis [Simon, 1983])
   b. Ultrasonography: fetus and gallbladder (stones)
   c. Fetal monitoring to rule out preterm labor (see Chapter 34 for further discussion)
   d. Chest x-ray film (shielded)

Ovarian tumors: Ovarian Cystectomy or Oophorectomy

A. Introduction

1. Hazard of ovarian tumors
   a. Malignancy
   b. Torsion
   c. Obstruction in labor (Brundnell & Wilds, 1984)
2. Corpus luteum cysts
   a. Corpus luteum cyst most common during first trimester; supports pregnancy during that time
   b. After first trimester, decreased risk of spontaneous abortion from removal (Brundnell & Wilds, 1984)
3. Benign ovarian tumors
   a. Dermoids
   b. Serous cystadenomas
   c. Mucinous cystadenomas
4. Malignant ovarian tumors
   a. Dysgerminomas
   b. Granulosa cell tumors (Scott, 1990)
5. Ultrasound test most useful tool for diagnosis and evaluation
6. Surgical intervention indicated if tumor is
   a. Solid
   b. Bilateral
   c. Hormonally active
   d. Symptomatic
   e. Increasing in size (Scott, 1990)

B. Assessment

1. History
   a. Pain: onset, location, and quality
   b. Presence of vaginal bleeding

    c. Gestational age by date of LMP or ultrasound test

    d. Presence of adnexal mass: palpation or ultrasound test

    e. Medical and surgical history: previous gynecological surgery

    f. Obstetrical history: previous pregnancies or complications

    g. Ability to urinate: as tumor enlarges, may be urinary obstruction

2. Physical examination

    a. Presence of adnexal mass confirmed by pelvic examination, ultrasound test, or both

    b. FHR

    c. Vital signs

      (1) Temperature

      (2) Pulse

      (3) Respiration

      (4) Blood pressure

    d. Palpation of uterine contractions

    e. Presence of vaginal bleeding

    f. Cervical status: presence of dilation

    g. Fundal height: approximate for gestational age or increasing as tumor enlarging

    h. Abdominal examination: presence of ascites and distended bladder

3. Psychosocial factors

    a. Anxiety

    b. Fear of harm to fetus and loss of pregnancy

    c. Fear of harm to personal well-being

    d. Fear of loss of future fertility

4. Diagnostic procedures

    a. Ultrasound test: fetal and adnexal mass evaluation (solid or cystic and size)

    b. Fetal monitoring to rule out preterm labor preoperatively and postoperatively and assess FHR

    c. Laboratory tests: CBC, UA, type and crossmatch blood products

    d. Chest x-ray film (shielded)

Appendectomy

A. Introduction

1. Incidence

    a. Is most common surgical complication of pregnancy

    b. Occurs 1 in every 1500 to 2000 pregnancies (Scott, 1990)

    c. Occurs with equal frequency in all trimesters

2. Symptoms

    a. Enlarged uterus makes interpretation of physical signs difficult (Brundnell & Wilds, 1984)

    b. Right flank pain versus right lower quadrant pain (classic sign)

    c. Symptoms confused with

      (1) Preterm labor

      (2) Pyelonephritis

    d. No cervical change

3. Peritonitis increases the incidence of preterm labor, and the client should be treated with tocolytic agents (Brundnell & Wilds, 1984)

B. Assessment

1. History

    a. Gestational age by date of LMP or ultrasound

    b. Medical condition: existence of acute or chronic health problems

    c. Previous surgeries

    d. Obstetrical history

e. Symptoms
(1) Nausea and vomiting
(2) Fever
(3) Periumbilical pain
(4) Right flank pain
(5) Anorexia
(6) Constipation
(7) Diarrhea
f. Assessment of pain: location, duration, quality, aggravating or alleviating factors
2. Physical examination
a. Abdominal examination
(1) Rebound tenderness
(2) Uterine contractions
b. Vital signs
(1) Temperature
(2) Pulse
(3) Respiration
(4) Blood pressure
c. FHR
d. Evidence of vaginal bleeding
e. Cervical examination for labor status
3. Psychosocial factors
a. Anxiety related to pain of potentially unknown etiology
b. Fear of loss of pregnancy
c. Fear for personal well-being
4. Diagnostic procedures
a. Fetal monitoring
b. Laboratory tests
(1) CBC with differential
(a) Hemoglobin level should be greater than 10.0
(b) WBC may not be helpful since values of 15,000 to 20,000 are seen in pregnancy and labor; however, a shift to the left (differential count of greater than 80% polymorphonuclear leukocytes) is a significant finding (Dornhoffer & Calkins, 1988)
(2) UA and urine culture
(a) Help to differentiate urinary tract infection from the clinical picture
(b) In the second half of pregnancy, pyuria was found in 20% of patients with appendicitis; sterile pyuria may result from the proximity of the appendix to the ureter or renal pelvis (Dornhoffer & Calkins, 1988)
c. Ultrasonography: to assess fetal well-being, as well as signs of placental abruption
d. Chest x-ray film (shielded): if respiratory evaluation required

Cervical Cerclage

A. Introduction

1. Cervical incompetence
a. Painless dilation of cervix during second trimester
b. Repeated second-trimester abortion in absence of contractions (Shortle & Jewelewicz, 1989)
2. Surgical technique that closes or supports cervix at level of internal os is done to support pregnancy to viability (Shortle & Jewelewicz, 1989)
a. McDonald's suture: mersilene suture placed at cervicovaginal junction and removed for labor (Shortle & Jewelewicz, 1989)
b. Shirodkar procedure: mersilene tape encircles the cervix, passed under the

mucosa; may remove for labor or perform cesarean section and leave intact (Scott, 1990)
3. Optimal timing: after first trimester, most practitioners choose between 14 and 18 weeks of gestation
4. Tocolytic therapy is an adjunctive therapy to treat preterm labor or uterine irritability

B. Assessment

1. History
   a. Gestational age by date of LMP or ultrasound test
   b. Obstetrical history of second-trimester losses
   c. Previous gynecological surgery and cervical laceration
   d. Medical illness
   e. Second-trimester dilation of cervix in previous pregnancies
   f. History of premature rupture of membranes (PROM) in previous pregnancies
   g. History of vaginal bleeding
   h. Diethylstilbestrol (DES) exposure
2. Physical examination
   a. Pelvic examination
      (1) Cervical dilation ($\leq$3 to 4 cm to be candidate for cerclage)
      (2) Evidence of infection (treat infection before cerclage)
      (3) Status of membranes (must be intact for cerclage)
   b. FHR: presence (viability)
3. Psychosocial factors
   a. Anxiety
   b. Fear of loss of pregnancy
   c. Fear for personal well-being
4. Diagnostic procedures
   a. Ultrasonography: gestation, cervical length, and internal os dilation
   b. Fetal monitoring
   c. Preoperative laboratory tests: CBC, UA
   d. Palpation of uterus to assess uterine activity or use of external fetal monitor

C. Nursing Diagnoses

1. Alteration in cardiopulmonary fetal tissue perfusion
2. Alteration in comfort or pain
3. Anxiety related to potential alteration in client and fetal health

D. Interventions/Evaluations

1. Alteration in cardiopulmonary fetal tissue perfusion
   a. Interventions: preoperative care
      (1) Monitor maternal vital signs and blood pressure
      (2) Apply fetal monitor in the second and third trimesters to assess fetal well-being and to evaluate contractions
      (3) Begin or maintain IV infusion with an intracatheter (16 or 18 gauge) of Ringer's lactate or normal saline
      (4) Maintain and record accurate intake and output
      (5) Lateral positioning of mother, especially in second and third trimesters
         (a) The enlarging uterus places increased pressure on the vena cava in the supine position, thereby decreasing blood return
         (b) The lateral position (especially on left) allows for greater uteroplacental perfusion
         (c) If left lateral position is not possible, placing a wedge (of pillow or rolled blanket) under right hip displaces the uterus appropriately
      (6) With cervical cerclage, position the client in slight Trendelenburg position to decrease cervical pressure

(7) Perioperative laboratory results of CBC and UA
b. Interventions: postoperative care (in addition to above)
   (1) Administer oxygen via face mask at 8 to 10 l/min, or maintain endotracheal or nasotracheal airway, if needed
   (2) Monitor incision for bleeding or evidence of dehiscence
   (3) Monitor vaginal bleeding for amount, color, and clotting
   (4) Apply antiembolic stockings
   (5) Provide incentive spirometer and instruct in use
   (6) Teach and ensure turning, coughing, and deep-breathing exercises
   (7) Administer analgesics, as ordered
   (8) Avoid use of teratogenic drugs or vasoconstrictors (which may decrease uteroplacental perfusion)
   (9) Administer tocolytic drugs as needed (see Chapter 34 for further discussion of dosages and administration routes)
   (10) Monitor and interpret laboratory values, especially stability of hemoglobin and hematocrit values
   (11) Assess Homans' sign
c. Evaluations
   (1) Client's vital signs remain within normal limits
   (2) FHR remains within normal limits, with no signs of distress
   (3) Accurate intake and output is maintained
   (4) Client remains in lateral or Trendelenburg position
   (5) Incision is without signs of bleeding, infection, or dehiscence
   (6) Antiembolic stockings are in place
   (7) Client uses incentive spirometer and performs coughing and deep-breathing exercises and lungs remain clear
   (8) Client and fetus show no untoward effects of analgesia
   (9) Client has no uterine contractions
2. Alteration in comfort or pain
a. Interventions: preoperative care and postoperative care
   (1) Assess quality, location, characteristics of pain, aggravating and alleviating factors, duration, and associated events
   (2) Assess and monitor maternal vital signs
      (a) Temperature
      (b) Pulse
      (c) Respiration
      (d) Blood pressure
   (3) Apply fetal monitor (after 20 to 24 weeks) and assess FHR and uterine contractions
   (4) Provide IV hydration
   (5) Ensure bedrest in left lateral position (Trendelenburg position for cervical cerclage)
   (6) Provide comfort measures
      (a) Positioning with use of pillows
      (b) Narcotic analgesia: narcotics are not known teratogens in adult humans when administered in recommended adult doses
         (i) May decrease beat-to-beat variability of FHR or cause fetal bradycardia
         (ii) Administer minimal effective dose for a minimal amount of time
   (7) Nasogastric suction is often the initial conservative management before decision for surgery (cholecystectomy); may also be used postoperatively for comfort
   (8) Tocolytic agents are indicated if uterine contractility is present
b. Evaluations
   (1) Client's vital signs and FHR remain stable
   (2) Client experiences a minimal amount of uterine contractility, which is recognized and treated appropriately

(3) Client experiences a reduction in preoperative and postoperative pain

3. Anxiety related to potential alteration in client and fetal health
    a. Interventions: preoperative and postoperative care
        (1) Evaluate client's coping abilities
        (2) Assess social support network
        (3) Allow for verbalization of fears, anxieties, and concerns
        (4) Recognize significance of previous fetal losses: offer positive encouragement and reinforcement of therapeutic regimen
        (5) Teach stress reduction techniques (relaxation, breathing, visualization, and imagery), and reinforce client's ability to implement these techniques
        (6) Integrate mental health team in care per client needs
    b. Evaluations
        (1) Client demonstrates appropriate coping techniques
        (2) Support system (family/friends) are involved in client care
        (3) Client demonstrates and uses stress reduction techniques

Health Education

A. Involve client in care

1. Surgical options
2. Anesthetic choices
3. Analgesics
4. Postoperative care

B. Teach signs and symptoms of preterm labor (see Chapter 34 for further information)

C. Discharge instructions include

1. Follow-up care as ordered by physician
2. Medications
3. Reporting of signs and symptoms of infection
    a. Pain
    b. Fever
    c. Vaginal bleeding
4. Reporting of signs and symptoms of preterm labor
5. Discussion of importance of client's awareness of and cooperation with the following
    a. Antiembolic or support stockings
    b. Progressive ambulation and activity (or restrictions)
    c. Diet and fluid intake
    d. Adequate rest
    e. Avoidance of heavy lifting (including lifting children)
    f. Avoidance of constipation
6. Review of medications: dose, route, frequency, and side effects

D. Stress need for social support and increased assistance at home

CASE STUDIES AND STUDY QUESTIONS

A 25-year-old gravida 1, para 0 (G1,P0) at 26 weeks of gestation arrives in the emergency room with a 2-day history of right flank pain, nausea and vomiting, and anorexia. She denies urinary frequency, urgency, or burning and states her last bowel movement was 24 hours previous to admission. On examination, pain is elicited with deep palpation at the right flank and right lower quadrant. The uterus is soft and nontender. The pelvic examination reveals a long cervix without dilation and the adnexae are not palpable.

Vital signs: oral temperature, 38.3°C (101°F); pulse of 92; respiratory rate of 18 breaths/min; blood pressure, 124/72; FHR 140 beats/min. Admission laboratory values: hemoglobin, 12.4 g/dl; WBC, 24,000/mm³; UA, clear. Client is sent for an ultrasound test that reveals a viable, singleton pregnancy, at 26 weeks' gestation, with no evidence of separation of the placenta. An appendectomy was performed and her postoperative course was without complication. She delivered a healthy infant without complication at term.

Answer the following questions true or false.

1. In the presence of appendicitis at 26 weeks of gestation, the cervix dilates.

2. Surgery is the treatment of choice for appendicitis during pregnancy.

3. Narcotics may not be used for postoperative analgesia.

4. Vaginal bleeding usually accompanies acute appendicitis.

5. Palpating for uterine contractions is an effective method to evaluate for preterm labor postoperatively.

6. The left lateral position in the postoperative period improves uteroplacental perfusion for the client.

7. General anesthesia presents an increased risk for preterm labor.

8. Pyelonephritis may also present as flank pain during pregnancy.

A 30-year-old gravida 4, para 1 (G4,P1) at 16 weeks' gestation has arrived at the antenatal clinic. Her obstetrical history is significant because of a preterm birth at 32 weeks' gestation, and two midtrimester losses at 18 and 22 weeks, respectively.

Pelvic examination: cervix, 25% effaced and 1-cm dilated; intact membranes. Vital signs: oral temperature 37°C (98.6°F); pulse of 90; respiratory rate of 20; blood pressure, 120/68; FHR of 132 beats/min. Diagnostic ultrasound test reveals a singleton, 16-week viable intrauterine pregnancy. The client is scheduled for surgery (placement of cervical cerclage) next week.

Answer the following questions true or false.

9. This client's obstetrical history and current physical status are not consistent with incompetent cervix.

10. This client presents at optimal timing for placement of the cerclage.

11. Placing the client in the Trendelenburg position decreases cervical pressure.

12. The cerclage may be placed if the amniotic membranes are ruptured.

13. The first trimester is the optimal timing for placement of the cerclage.

14. Maternal physical exercise increases the risk of incompetent cervix.

15. Use of the fetal monitor is an effective way to evaluate uterine irritability or contractility.

16. Medication to prevent preterm labor (tocolytic therapy) may be given postoperatively to increase uterine relaxation.

Answers to Study Questions

1. False	2. True	3. False
4. False	5. True	6. True
7. False	8. True	9. False
10. True	11. True	12. False
13. False	14. False	15. True
16. True		

REFERENCES

Brown, S. (1986). The pregnant patient: Postanesthetic considerations. *Journal of Post Anesthesia Nursing, 1*(1), 17–22.
Brundnell, M., & Wilds, P. (1984). *Medical problems in obstetrics and gynecology.* Bristol, England: Wright.
Cunningham, G., MacDonald, P., & Gant, N. (1989). *Williams obstetrics* (18th ed.). Norwalk, CT: Appleton & Lange.
Datta, S., & Ostheimer, G. (1987). *Common problems in obstetric anesthesia.* Chicago: Year Book.

Delaney, A. (1983). Anesthesia in the pregnant woman. *Clinical Obstetrics and Gynecology, 26*(4), 795–800.

Dornhoffer, J., & Calkins, J. (1988). Appendicitis complicating pregnancy. *Kansas Medicine, 89*(5), 139–142.

James, F., & Wheeler, A. (1982). *Obstetric anesthesia: The complicated patient.* Philadelphia: Davis.

Kerswani, R. (1984). Acute appendicitis complicating pregnancy. *Journal of the Indian Medical Association, 82*(9), 316–318.

Olds, S., London, M., & Ladewig, P. (1992). *Maternal newborn nursing* (4th ed.) Menlo Park, CA: Addison-Wesley.

Scott, J. (ed.) (1990). *Danforth's obstetrics and gynecology.* (6th ed.). Philadelphia: Lippincott.

Shnider, S., & Levinson, G. (1987). *Anesthesia for obstetrics* (2nd ed.). Baltimore: Williams & Wilkins.

Shnider, S., & Webster, G. (1965). Maternal and fetal hazards of surgery during pregnancy. *American Journal of Obstetrics and Gynecology, 92,* p. 891.

Shortle, B., & Jewelewicz, R. (1989). Cervical incompetence. *Fertility and Sterility, 52*(2), 181–188.

Simon, J. (1983). Biliary tract disease and related surgical disorders during pregnancy. *Clinical Obstetrics and Gynecology, 26*(4), 810–820.

Barbara A. Moran

Substance Abuse in Pregnancy

Objectives

1. Discuss the scope of substance abuse in pregnancy

2. Recognize signs of substance abuse

3. Describe the effects of drug use during pregnancy on the developing fetus

4. Instruct pregnant women about the effects of drugs on their pregnancy

5. Elicit appropriate history and pertinent information from the client

6. Formulate a plan of care based on a client's history of substance abuse

7. Analyze psychosocial problems of the client and refer her to the appropriate agency

8. Recognize the teaching needs of the pregnant substance abuser

Substance Abuse

Introduction

A. Major public health issue

1. Drug use has increased in the general population, and therefore it has increased during pregnancy

2. The incidence of cocaine use has increased rapidly among young, adult, childbearing women

3. High school students favor cocaine second only to marijuana.

B. Estimated statistics

1. Fifty-nine percent of women in urban populations consume alcohol

2. Forty-four percent of women smoke cigarettes

3. Twenty-eight percent use marijuana

4. Seventeen percent use cocaine

5. Ten to 20 million Americans have used some form of cocaine

6. Four to six million Americans use it regularly

7. Every day another 5000 people try cocaine for the first time

8. Between 1 in 10 and 1 in 50 women in the United States uses cocaine at some time during pregnancy.

9. Polydrug use, such as alcohol and tobacco with marijuana or cocaine, has become more common

C. Effects relate to the following

1. Lifestyle of mother
   a. Poor compliance
   b. Poor nutrition
   c. Sexually transmitted diseases (STDs)
   d. Inadequate housing
   e. Late prenatal care
2. Direct effect of drug on mother and fetus

D. Outcomes relate to the following

1. Adequacy of prenatal care
2. Presence of obstetrical or maternal complications
3. Abuse of multiple drugs

E. Effects on fetus

1. Generalized growth retardation and its associated complications
2. Increased in the frequency of sudden infant death syndrome (SIDS)

F. Methadone hydrochloride

1. Is available to treat the pregnant drug abuser
2. Blocks the craving of withdrawal
3. Is longer acting and therefore is thought to stabilize the environment for the fetus, sustaining the addict and avoiding withdrawal
4. Advantages
   a. Decreased maternal complications
   b. Decreased prematurity and low birth weight
5. Disadvantages
   a. Increased incidence of low Apgar scores
   b. Increased withdrawal symptoms as compared with infants of heroin-addicted mothers
   c. Increased incidence of seizures

G. Variables

1. Multiple-drug use
2. Client reporting is unreliable
3. Oral administration may reduce the drug's ability to cross the placenta
4. Drugs taken IV and intranasally more readily cross the placenta

Clinical Practice

A. Assessment

1. History
   a. Erratic appetite
   b. Fatigue
   c. Late prenatal care, missed appointments
   d. Poor nutrition
   e. Maternal tachycardia
   f. Inappropriate behavior
   g. History of child abuse, neglect, sexual abuse
   h. Deterioration in personal hygiene
   i. Prior stillbirths or miscarriages
   j. Drug use: kind of drugs used, setting of abuse, duration, frequency and route of administration, and symptoms experienced during withdrawal
   k. Allergies

    l. STDs
    m. Placenta abruption
    n. Previous fetal death
    o. Hepatitis
    p. Acquired immune deficiency syndrome (AIDS)
    q. Loss of sense of smell
    r. Irregular menses, amenorrhea
2. Physical findings (Table 32–1)
    a. Bloodshot eyes
    b. Slurred speech
    c. Dilated or constricted pupils
    d. Restlessness
    e. Shortness of breath
    f. Poor dental hygiene
    g. Rhinitis, nasal or sinus irritation, septal erosion

Table 32–1
SIGNS OF RECENT USE OF OR WITHDRAWAL FROM SUBSTANCES*

	Signs of Recent Use	Signs of Withdrawal
Sedatives Beer, wine, wine coolers, liquor, Xanax, Valium, Librium, sleeping pills, Dalmane, Halcion, Restoril	Odor of fresh or stale alcohol Unsteady gait Slurred speech Nystagmus Hangover	Tremors at rest or on exertion Reflexes of +2 or above Diaphoresis—palms, forehead, generalized Elevated vital signs, especially temperature and blood pressure Nausea and vomiting Seizures and delirium tremens
Opiates Codeine, heroin, Dilaudid, Percodan, Demerol, Methadone, Darvon, Talwin	Track or needle marks (including the breast, axilla) Pinpoint pupils Nodding Depressed mood Abscess or skin popping (especially on abdomen and legs)	Sniffing, yawning Tearing of eyes Gooseflesh (especially on chest) Diarrhea Nausea Abdominal cramps Increased pupil size Decreased pupillary response Complaints of muscle or joint pain
Stimulants Preludin, cocaine, uppers, amphetamines, caffeine, nicotine	Track or needle marks Nasal irritation Anxiety Paranoia Frequent purposeless movements (e.g., foot tapping) Picking at skin	Irritability Complaining of sleep disturbance (hyper/hypo) Anxiety GI upset Headaches Excoriated areas from scratching Depression/ suicidal tendencies
Hallucinogens LSD, PCP, mescaline, marijuana	Paranoia Anxiety Thought disorders Impaired judgment	Withdrawal symptoms (subtle and variable)

* Medical problems associated with substance abuse: history of pelvic infections; problem pregnancies; irregular periods, amenorrhea, or sexually transmitted diseases HIV-positive; history of hepatitis, abscesses.

Courtesy of Catherine Wilson, R.N., M.Ed., The Center for Perinatal Addiction.

    h. Hepatomegaly
    i. Subcutaneous abscesses or cellulitis
    j. Needle marks, ecchymotic spots or scars, phlebitis
    k. Jaundice secondary to liver failure
    l. Distended neck veins secondary to liver failure
    m. Unsteady walk
    n. Impaired coordination
    o. Slowed reflexes
    p. Elevated blood pressure
    q. Tachycardia
    r. Altered moods and perceptions
    s. Nausea
    t. Dizziness
    u. Shortness of breath
    v. Odor of substance on clothing
    w. Burns on fingertips or singed eyebrows or eyelashes
  3. Psychosocial findings
    a. Low self-esteem
    b. Depression
    c. Chronic anxiety
    d. Inability to maintain close relationships
    e. Family disorganization
    f. Manipulativeness
    g. Hostility or anger
    h. Unplanned pregnancy
    i. Denial
  4. Diagnostic studies
    a. Complete blood count (CBC) and urinalysis (UA)
    b. Toxicological urine screening (detects cocaine ingestion within past 24 hours)
    c. Venereal Diseases Research Laboratory test (VDRL)
    d. Cervical culture for gonorrhea and chlamydia
    e. Papanicolaou's test (Pap smear)
    f. Hepatitis profile
    g. Human immunodeficiency virus (HIV) testing
    h. Sonography (to detect intrauterine growth retardation [IUGR])
    i. Tuberculin (TB) skin test

B. **Nursing Diagnoses**

1. Knowledge deficit related to substance abuse and its effect on self and pregnancy
2. Altered nutrition: Less than body requirements related to pregnancy and drug abuse
3. Altered family process related to developmental transition of pregnancy
4. Anxiety related to drug use during pregnancy
5. Noncompliance related to difficulty in following prenatal recommendations
6. High risk for injury to self and fetus related to drug use during pregnancy
7. Alteration in health maintenance related to lack of prenatal care
8. High risk for altered parenting related to effects of drugs
9. Self-esteem disturbance related to need for drugs

C. **Interventions/Evaluations**

1. Knowledge deficit related to substance abuse and its effect on self and pregnancy; see Tables 32–2 and 32–3 and Figure 32–1 for the effects of cocaine on maternal, fetal, and neonatal systems and commonly reported teratogenic effects of abused drugs
    a. Interventions

Table 32–2
OBSTETRICAL COMPLICATIONS ASSOCIATED
WITH THE ADDICTED PATIENT

Complications of mothers

Abruptio placentae
Anemia
Cellulitis
Low birth weight
Maternal hypertension
Placental insufficiency
Postpartum hemorrhage
Pre-eclampsia
Premature rupture of membranes
Preterm labor/delivery
Septic thrombophlebitis
Spontaneous miscarriage
Sexually transmitted disease
Stillbirths
Urinary tract infection

Complications of newborns

Detrimental maternal–infant bonding
Exaggerated startle response
Generalized growth retardation
Hypoglycemia
Increased frequency of sudden infant death syndrome
Intracranial hemorrhage
Intrauterine growth retardation
Low birth weight
Meconium aspiration
Neurobehavioral abnormalities (altered sleep patterns, irritability, jitteriness, tremors, depressed sucking)
Pneumonia
Possible seizures
Respiratory distress syndrome
Small head circumference

(1) Give accurate and specific information on complications associated with drug use and the increase in morbidity and mortality in a nonjudgmental way
(2) Explain that quitting or decreasing drugs at any time in pregnancy improves obstetrical outcome
(3) Explain dangers of operating vehicles or machinery while under influence of drugs
(4) Reinforce client's understanding with printed material at a level she can understand
b. Evaluations
(1) Client verbalizes effects of substance abuse on self and developing fetus
(2) Client avoids substance abusive behavior
2. Altered nutrition: Less than body requirements related to pregnancy and drug abuse
a. Interventions
(1) Provide supplemental vitamins
(2) Provide ferrous sulfate
(3) Provide folic acid if folate levels are low
(4) Provide nutritional counseling, emphasizing protein intake
(5) Reinforce information with printed material to take home
(6) Use a variety of teaching methods to reinforce material
b. Evaluations
(1) Client avoids further nutritional decline

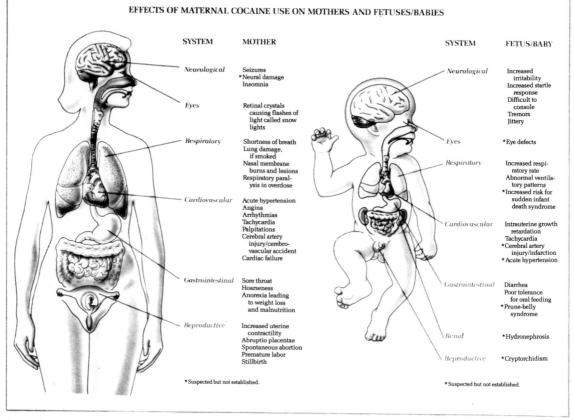

Figure 32–1
Effects of maternal cocaine use on mothers and fetuses (*left*) and on infants (*right*). (From Smith, J. [1988]. The dangers of prenatal cocaine use. *MCN*, *13*, 175. By permission of Network Graphics.)

        (2) Client has appropriate uterine growth for gestational age
        (3) Client goes to a nutritionist on referral
  3. Altered family process related to developmental transition of pregnancy
    a. Interventions
        (1) Assess client's perception of her pregnancy and her role as a new mother
        (2) Assist client in identifying support systems
        (3) Use an interdisciplinary team approach in a nonjudgmental and sensitive manner
        (4) Assist family to support patient in a nonjudgmental and supportive fashion
        (5) Help client identify stresses in her family life
        (6) Promote attachment by recommending attendance at childbirth preparation and parenting classes
        (7) Provide reading material on pregnancy, parenting, and newborn care
        (8) Encourage verbalization of fears and concerns
    b. Evaluations
        (1) Client identifies support system
        (2) Client verbalizes acceptance of pregnancy
        (3) Client maintains support from significant others
        (4) Client expresses her feelings freely and appropriately

Table 32–3
COMMONLY REPORTED TERATOGENIC EFFECTS OF ABUSED DRUGS

Special Fetal Effects	Opiates	Alcohol	Other Sedative-Hypnotic Drugs	Cocaine	Other Stimulants	Hallucinogens	Marijuana	Nicotine
Structural nonspecific growth retardation	X	X	—	X	—	—	X	X
Specific dysmorphic effects	—	X	—	X	—	—	—	—
Behavioral	X	X	X	X	X	X	X	X
Neurobiochemical (abstinence syndrome)	X	X	X	—	—	—	—	—
Increased fetal and perinatal mortality	X	X	—	X	—	—	—	X
Women reporting use in pregnancy (varies with population)	5%	>50%	<5%	<20%	<5%	<5%	5–34%	>50%

From Hoegerman, G., Wilson, C.A., Thurmond, E., Schnoll, S.H. (1990). Drug-exposed neonates. *Western Journal of Medicine, 152*(5), 559–564.

(5) Client and her family express understanding of pregnancy and role transition

4. Anxiety related to drug use during pregnancy
   a. Interventions
      (1) Establish trusting relationship by providing consistent care
      (2) Present as many options as possible for increased control over situation
      (3) Involve significant others in prenatal care
      (4) Be patient, repeat explanations, and be concrete
      (5) Phrase questions positively to elicit honest responses (i.e., "To care for you and your baby, I need to know . . ." or "I noticed track marks and I'm concerned for you and your baby and need to know . . .")
   b. Evaluations
      (1) Client verbalizes concerns and issues in the supportive environment
      (2) Client verbalizes decrease in anxiety

5. Noncompliance related to difficulty in following prenatal recommendations
   a. Interventions
      (1) Provide information on effects of drugs on self and infant repeatedly and in a variety of teaching methods
      (2) Educate the client and her family regarding importance of follow-up prenatal visits
      (3) Refer the client to social services and other supportive agencies
      (4) Explore with the client ways to reduce barriers to compliance
   b. Evaluations
      (1) Client acknowledges the need for importance of prenatal care
      (2) Client keeps appointments
      (3) Client participates actively in health care maintenance

6. High risk for injury to self and fetus related to drug use during pregnancy
   a. Interventions
      (1) Identify substance abuse in client
      (2) Teach, review, reinforce information on a level the client understands
      (3) Monitor maternal and fetal withdrawal
      (4) Instruct the client to monitor fetal activity
      (5) Help family members or significant other develop skills necessary to support the client
      (6) Refer the client to appropriate counseling or rehabilitation
   b. Evaluations
      (1) Client minimizes potential for further injury by decreasing substance abuse
      (2) Family or significant other supports the client

7. Alteration in health maintenance related to lack of prenatal care
   a. Interventions
      (1) Determine the client's capability of maintaining health
      (2) Provide anticipatory guidance on common concerns of pregnancy
      (3) Encourage self-care measures (i.e., sleep, nutrition, and exercise)
   b. Evaluations
      (1) Client maintains current health status
      (2) Client recognizes normal physiological pregnancy changes

8. High risk for altered parenting related to effects of drugs
   a. Interventions
      (1) Encourage verbalization of the client's feelings about her pregnancy
      (2) Involve significant others in prenatal care and discussion
      (3) Encourage listening to fetal heart rate by the mother and significant other at each visit
      (4) Show sonogram to the client so she can visualize the fetus
      (5) Provide information on fetal growth and development
      (6) Help the client to identify major areas in her life that will be affected by the new infant

    b. Evaluations
       (1) Client accepts pregnancy
       (2) Client begins attachment behaviors
       (3) Client develops role identity as a parent
       (4) Client has a knowledge base for effective parenting
9. Self-esteem disturbance related to need for drugs
    a. Interventions
       (1) Provide a nonjudgmental, concerned, and empathetic environment
       (2) Encourage the client to express her feelings and concerns about herself, her drug use, and her unborn child
       (3) Assist the client in identifying factors that decrease her self-esteem
       (4) Assist the client in identifying ways that will restore her self-esteem
    b. Evaluations
       (1) Client verbalizes positive and realistic statements about herself
       (2) Client verbalizes factors that decrease her self-esteem
       (3) Client actively participates in restorative activities

Health Education

A. Prevention

1. Dispel myths that cocaine is harmless; educate client on the potential dangers of drug use to both mother and baby
2. Inform client of contraindication of drug use while breastfeeding (include alcohol, amphetamines, cocaine, heroin, marijuana, and nicotine)

B. Referral to community

1. Refer pregnant women to specialized programs that address the medical, obstetrical, psychological, and neonatal and pediatric needs of women and their babies
2. Resources
    a. Cocaine hotline: 1–800–COCAINE
    b. National Institute on Drug Abuse: 1–800–662–HELP (301) 443–1124
    c. Pregnancy Environmental Hotline: (617) 786–4957
    d. Local methadone programs
    e. National Association for Perinatal Addiction Research and Education (NAPARE): (312) 329–2512
    f. March of Dimes Birth Defects Foundation: (914) 428–7100
    g. Institute on Black Chemical Abuse (IBCA): (612) 871–7878
    h. National Self-Help Clearinghouse: (212) 840–1258
    i. National Center for Education in Maternal and Child Health (NCEMCH): (202) 625–8400
    j. Healthy Mothers, Healthy Babies (HMHB): (202) 863–2458
    k. National Clearinghouse for Alcohol and Drug Information (NCADI): (301) 468–2600
    l. National Institute of Child Health and Human Development (NICHD): (301) 496–5133
    m. Center for Perinatal Addiction: (804) 371–6685
    n. National Perinatal Association: (813) 971–1008
    o. Office for Substance Abuse Prevention: (301) 443–5266

Tobacco

Introduction

A. U.S. Surgeon General's Report

1. Smoking is the chief, single avoidable cause of death

2. It is the most important public health issue
3. It is the major health hazard for women

B. **Statistics**

1. Thirty percent of women in the United States of reproductive age smoke cigarettes
2. The effect of maternal smoking on fetal development (fetal tobacco syndrome [FTS]) has been investigated for 30 years
   a. Spontaneous abortions
   b. Stillbirths
   c. Decreased maternal weight gain
   d. Lower-birth-weight infants
3. Passive smoking is associated with lower birth weights
4. The child of a mother who smokes half a pack per day is twice as likely to be of low birth weight

C. **Compounds in cigarettes are readily absorbed, causing maternal vasoconstriction and reduced oxygen availability**

1. Carbon monoxide
2. Nicotine
3. Cyanide

D. **Opportunity for nurses to affect the health of mothers and children**

1. Identification
2. Health education
3. Support

Clinical Practice

A. **Assessment**

1. History
   a. Prior tobacco use
   b. Current use
   c. Quantity of cigarettes smoked daily
   d. Family members who smoke
2. Physical findings
   a. Cough
   b. Congestion
   c. Tobacco air (smell) surrounding patient
3. Psychosocial findings
   a. Anxiety
   b. Guilt
   c. Denial
   d. Hostility or anger
4. Diagnostic procedure: ultrasonography (to detect IUGR)

B. **Nursing Diagnoses**

1. Knowledge deficit related to effects of smoking on self and pregnancy
2. Alteration in nutrition: Less than body requirements related to smoking during pregnancy
3. High risk for injury related to smoking during pregnancy
4. Ineffective individual coping

C. **Interventions/Evaluations**

1. Knowledge deficit related to effects of smoking on self and family
   a. Interventions
      (1) Provide the client with factual information about the health hazard of smoking to herself

       (a) Hemorrhage (from abruptio placentae and placenta previa)

       (b) Sepsis (from ruptured membranes)

       (c) Bronchitis

       (d) Lung cancer

       (e) Hypertension and cardiovascular disease

       (f) Spontaneous abortion

       (g) Depletion of vitamin C level, which is needed to produce collagen and which enhances absorption of iron

    (2) Provide the client with factual information about the health hazard of smoking to the unborn child

       (a) Reduction in uteroplacental flow that may impair oxygen exchange across the placenta

       (b) Abortion, stillbirth, and prematurity

       (c) IUGR

       (d) Low birth weight (200 to 400 g [7 to 14 oz] smaller)

       (e) SIDS occurs twice as frequently in children of smokers

       (f) Low Apgar scores

       (g) Neurobehavioral effects

       (h) Increased frequency of apnea

    (3) Emphasize that the earlier a pregnant woman gives up smoking, the lower her risk of having a low-birth-weight infant

    (4) Use a variety of teaching techniques to meet learning needs

    (5) Provide written information at appropriate level for the client to take home

    (6) Involve the client's family and friends in the learning process

  b. Evaluations

    (1) Client verbalizes the effects of smoking on herself and her unborn child

    (2) Client expresses a desire to quit smoking

2. Alteration in nutrition: Less than body requirements related to smoking during pregnancy

  a. Interventions

    (1) Provide supplemental vitamins

    (2) Provide ferrous sulfate

    (3) Provide folic acid

    (4) Provide nutritional counseling

  b. Evaluations

    (1) Client avoids further nutritional decline

    (2) Client has appropriate uterine growth for gestational age

3. High risk for injury related to smoking during pregnancy

  a. Interventions

    (1) Teach, review, and reinforce information

    (2) Provide specific suggestions for decreasing cigarette use

       (a) Assess when the client is smoking (i.e., with meals, at social occasions, when bored)

       (b) Decrease client's intake by one cigarette per day

       (c) Substitute a healthy behavior for a cigarette (i.e., a walk, a nutritious snack)

       (d) Advise the client to brush her teeth when she has an urge to smoke

  b. Evaluation: client reduces the potential for further injury by decreasing the number of cigarettes she smokes per day

4. Ineffective individual coping

  a. Interventions

    (1) Assist the client in identifying stressors that trigger smoking

    (2) Help the client identify alternative ways of coping (i.e., relaxation or substitution of fruits or vegetables in place of cigarettes)

    (3) Refer the client to appropriate programs for stress reduction and smoking cessation

  b. Evaluations

(1) Client uses other coping mechanisms appropriately
(2) Client develops skills to reduce stress and anxiety
(3) Client identifies stressors that trigger smoking

Health Education

A. Referral to specialized programs for smoking cessation

B. Referral to organizations for information

1. American Cancer Society: (212) 599–8200
2. American Lung Association: (212) 315–8700
3. Stop Teenage Addiction to Tobacco (STAT): (413) 567–7587
4. March of Dimes Birth Defects Foundation: (914) 428-7100
5. American Heart Association: (214) 750–5300

Alcohol

Introduction

A. Characteristics

1. Most commonly used drug
2. Mind- and mood-altering drug
3. Central nervous system (CNS) depressant

B. Statistics

1. There is an estimated 2 to 70% consumption rate during pregnancy
2. Five or more drinks a day or binge drinking risks having a child with fetal alcohol syndrome
3. As few as one or two drinks a day will decrease birth weight
4. If a previous child is diagnosed with fetal alcohol syndrome, the incidence rate is higher
5. No safe limit of consumption of alcohol during pregnancy has been defined

C. Fetal alcohol syndrome (FAS)

1. Identified in the United States in 1973
2. Leading cause of mental retardation
3. Pattern of mental, physical, and behavioral defects in children (Table 32–4)

Table 32–4
POSSIBLE FETAL ALCOHOL
SYNDROME MANIFESTATIONS

Cardiac defects
Cleft lip or palate
Delayed motor and language development
Fusion of cervical vertebrae
Increased infections
Increased irritability
Indistinct philtrum (groove above the upper lip)
Kidney defects
Microcephaly
Mild-to-moderate mental retardation
Poor suck
Prenatal and postnatal growth retardation
Retarded bone growth
Short palpebral fissures (small eye openings)
Strabismus, ptosis, myopia

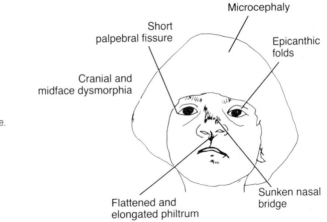

Figure 32–2
Fetal alcohol syndrome.

a. Prenatal and postnatal growth deficiency
b. Facial malformations (Figs. 32–2 and 32–3)
   (1) Small head circumference
   (2) Cranial and midface dysmorphia
   (3) Sunken nasal bridge
   (4) Flattened and elongated philtrum (groove between the nose and upper lip)
   (5) Short palpebral fissures (the opening between the margins of the upper and lower lids)
   (6) Epicanthic folds (vertical fold of skin over the angle of the inner canthus of eye)
   (7) CNS dysfunction
   (8) Varying degrees of major organ system malfunctions

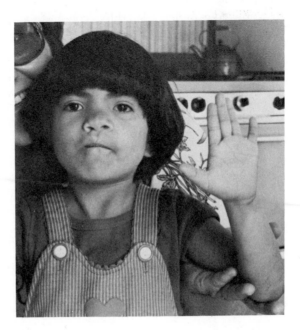

Figure 32–3
Fetal alcohol syndrome. (Courtesy of the March of Dimes Birth Defects Foundation, White Plains, NY.)

Clinical Practice

A. Assessment

1. History
   a. Disorientation
   b. Clumsy
   c. Hepatic disease
   d. Family history
   e. Alcohol history of client to include type, amount of daily intake, and whether other substances were taken with alcohol
   f. Allergies
2. Physical findings
   a. Possibly poor nutritional and hygiene status
   b. Hepatomegaly
   c. Tremors
   d. Edema
   e. Agitated behavior
   f. Memory difficulty
3. Psychosocial findings
   a. Low self-esteem
   b. Anxiety and fear
   c. Depression
   d. Family disorganization
   e. Hostility or anger
   f. Denial
   g. Possibly unplanned pregnancy
4. Diagnostic studies
   a. Blood alcohol level (to establish presence of alcohol in system); a blood alcohol level of 0.10 is legally defined as intoxication in most of the U.S.
   b. CBC
   c. Serum electrolytes
   d. Serial sonograms to detect IUGR
   e. VDRL
   f. Hepatitis profile

B. Nursing Diagnoses

1. Knowledge deficit related to alcohol use and its effect on pregnancy
2. Alteration in nutrition: Less than bodily requirements related to pregnancy and alcohol use
3. Anxiety related to alcohol effects on pregnancy and self
4. Altered family processes related to developmental transition of pregnancy
5. Noncompliance related to difficulty in following prenatal recommendations
6. High risk for injury related to use of alcohol during pregnancy
7. High risk for altered parenting related to alcohol use

C. Interventions/Evaluations

1. Knowledge deficit related to alcohol use and its effect on pregnancy
   a. Interventions
      (1) Provide factual information about health hazards of alcohol to women and developing fetus
         (a) Fetal risk factors
            (i) CNS involvement (including mental retardation)
            (ii) Facial dysmorphia
            (iii) Growth retardation (before and after birth)
            (iv) Spontaneous abortion
            (v) Stillbirth

(b) Maternal risk factors
    (i) Cirrhosis
    (ii) Increased obstetrical complications
    (iii) Infertility
    (iv) Malnutrition
    (v) Withdrawal
(2) Inform the client that decreasing and stopping alcohol intake at any point during pregnancy will improve the outcome
(3) Give written information at a level the mother will understand

b. Evaluations
    (1) Client verbalizes the effects of alcohol on the developing fetus
    (2) Client decreases alcohol intake

2. Alteration in nutrition: Less than bodily requirements related to pregnancy and alcohol use
a. Interventions
    (1) Provide supplemental vitamins
    (2) Provide ferrous sulfate
    (3) Provide folic acid
    (4) Provide nutritional counseling and reinforce information with printed material

b. Evaluations
    (1) Client avoids further nutritional decline
    (2) Client has appropriate uterine growth for gestational age
    (3) Client has nutritionist intervention

3. Anxiety related to alcohol effects on pregnancy and self
a. Interventions
    (1) Establish trusting relationship with the client
    (2) Involve the client's significant other in prenatal care
    (3) Provide careful and repeated information on alcohol effects and potential for improvement with decreased intake
    (4) Provide the client with options to allow for increased control over situation
    (5) Give information in a positive manner so as not to promote guilt
    (6) Express questions in a matter-of-fact, nonjudgmental and open-minded way

b. Evaluation: client verbalizes decreased anxiety about the future

4. Altered family processes related to developmental transition of pregnancy
a. Interventions
    (1) Assess family's ability to support the client in a nonjudgmental and supportive fashion and involve them in counseling, referral, and treatment
    (2) Use interdisciplinary team approach in a nonjudgmental and sensitive manner
    (3) Recommend attendance at childbirth preparation and parenting classes
    (4) Provide written material about pregnancy, parenting, and newborn care

b. Evaluations
    (1) Client identifies support systems
    (2) Significant other is involved in a supportive manner
    (3) Client is referred for appropriate treatment
    (4) Client verbalizes impact of alcoholism on herself and her family

5. Noncompliance related to difficulty in following prenatal recommendations
a. Interventions
    (1) Provide information repeatedly
    (2) Provide information in a nonthreatening and nonjudgmental manner
    (3) Help the client identify reasons for noncompliance

b. Evaluations

(1) Client verbalizes the importance of and attends follow-up visits
(2) Client identifies factors that act as barriers to compliance
(3) Client uses support systems to help with compliance
6. High risk for injury related to use of alcohol during pregnancy
  a. Interventions
    (1) Identify alcohol use and its severity
    (2) Teach, review, and reinforce information
    (3) Give specific suggestions for controlling alcohol intake
      (a) Measure alcohol
      (b) Avoid two-liquor mixes
      (c) Never gulp down drinks
      (d) Learn to refuse a drink and substitute an alternative such as juice
      (e) Don't drink on an empty stomach
    (4) Help family members and significant others develop skills necessary to support the client
    (5) Refer the client to appropriate counseling and rehabilitation
  b. Evaluation: client minimizes potential for further injury by decreasing alcohol intake
7. High risk for altered parenting related to alcohol use
  a. Interventions
    (1) Provide environment to encourage verbalization of feelings regarding pregnancy
    (2) Involve significant others in prenatal care and discussions
    (3) Encourage listening to fetal heart rate by the client and significant others at each visit
    (4) Show sonogram to the client so she can visualize the fetus
    (5) Provide information on fetal growth and development
    (6) Help the client to identify major components in her life that will be affected by the new infant
  b. Evaluations
    (1) Client accepts her pregnancy
    (2) Client begins attachment behaviors
    (3) Client develops role identity as a parent
    (4) Client has knowledge base for effective parenting

Health Education

A. Prevention

1. Dispel myths about alcohol intake during pregnancy through public education programs and at initial prenatal visit
2. Inform the client that use of alcohol may decrease milk-ejection reflex

B. Resources

1. American Medical Society on Alcoholism and Other Drug Dependencies: (212) 206–6770
2. National Association of State Alcohol and Drug Abuse Directors (NASADAD): (202) 783–6868
3. National Association for Children of Alcoholics (NACA): (714) 499–3889
4. National Association of Native American Children of Alcoholics (NANACA): (202) 324–9360
5. National Council on Alcoholism, Inc.: 800–NCA–CALL
6. March of Dimes Birth Defects Foundation: (914) 428–7100
7. National Self-Help Clearinghouse: (212) 840–1258
8. National Clearinghouse for Alcohol and Drug Information
9. Alcoholics Anonymous

CASE STUDIES AND STUDY QUESTIONS

Substance Abuse

Margie Greer is a 29-year-old G2, P0 who is 18 weeks pregnant. She is married and very excited about the pregnancy. On her third prenatal visit, you notice that she has nasal congestion and slightly slurred speech. There is no odor of alcohol. You suspect she might be using cocaine.

1. A toxicological urine screen can detect cocaine ingestion within the past

   a. 10 hours.

   b. 24 hours.

   c. 1 week.

   d. 2 hours.

2. A possible result of cocaine use would be

   a. IUGR.

   b. Polyhydramnios.

   c. Polydipsia.

   d. Post-term pregnancy.

3. It is probable that Margie is using cocaine intranasally. What is the significance of this?

   a. It may reduce its ability to cross the placenta.

   b. It more readily crosses the placenta.

   c. It does not reach the placenta because it is exhaled immediately.

4. Answer the following true or false.

   a. Stillbirths are associated with the addicted patient.

   b. Both premature rupture of membranes (PROM) and abruptio placentae are associated with drug abuse during pregnancy.

   c. Cocaine will not cause ill effects to fetus if used only in second trimester.

   d. Maternal–infant bonding may be enhanced by some drug use because of the relaxation effect.

   e. SIDS is not associated with addiction.

Smoking

Maureen Vance is an 18-year-old G1 whose last menstrual period was 21 weeks earlier. Her history is unremarkable except for the fact that she smokes a pack of cigarettes a day. She believes smoking helps her control her weight and also helps her relax. She has been told that smoking will not harm the baby. On examination, Maureen has gained 908 g (2 lb) since the beginning of her pregnancy. Her blood pressure is 118/72, the fetal heart rate is 140. She has not noticed fetal movement.

5. What three detrimental compounds are found in cigarettes?

   a. Carbon monoxide.

   b. Nicotine.

   c. Cyanide.

   d. Tar.

   e. Tannic acid.

6. All of the following are major effects of smoking on pregnancy **except:**

   a. Maternal vasoconstriction and reduced oxygen availability.

   b. Reduced oxygen-carrying capacity of RBCs.

   c. Fetal bradycardia.

7. Which of the following are maternal risks due to smoking?

   a. Abruptio placentae.

   b. Vitamin C depletion.

   c. Excessive weight gain.

   d. Bronchitis.

8. Answer the following true or false.

   a. Impaired uteroplacental blood flow decreases oxygen exchange across the placenta.

   b. Babies born to mothers who smoke will not have weight problems.

   c. SIDS occurs less frequently in babies of mothers who smoke.

   d. It is not important if a mother quits smoking in the second trimester, since the damage is already done.

Alcohol

Janice Nealy is a 29-year-old who delivered a 3203-g (7 lb, 1 oz) baby boy 24 hours earlier. Janice says that she had been concerned during her pregnancy because she drank heavily in her first trimester before knowing she was pregnant. She begins to ask questions.

9. Answer the following true or false.

 a. Growth retardation may result from alcohol ingestion.

 b. Spontaneous abortions occur more frequently in mothers who drink heavily.

 c. Drinking after the first trimester is acceptable.

10. Features of fetal alcohol syndrome are all the following **except:**

 a. CNS damage.

 b. Flattened philtrum.

 c. Cardiac defects.

 d. Short fingers.

11. When counseling a woman who is pregnant, what should you tell her?

 a. Alcohol in the third trimester will not affect the fetus.

 b. One glass of wine is considered safe.

 c. There is no safe limit of alcohol during pregnancy.

Answers to Study Questions

1. b
2. a
3. b
4. a. True b. True c. False d. False e. False.
5. a, b, c.
6. c
7. a, b, d.
8. a. True b. False c. False d. False.
9. a. True b. True c. False.
10. d
11. c

REFERENCES

Aaronson, L. (1989). Perceived and received support: Effects on health behavior during pregnancy. *Nursing Research, 38*(1), 4.
Adams, C., Eyler, C.D., & Behnke, M. (1990). Nursing interventions with mothers who are substance abusers. *Journal of Perinatal and Neonatal Nursing, 3*(4), 43–52.
Alexander, L.L. (1987). The pregnant smoker: Nursing implications. *Journal of Obstetric, Gynecologic, and Neonatal Nursing, 16*(3), 167–173.
Alexander, L. (1988). Patient smoking cessation: Treatment strategies. *Nurse Practitioner, 13*(10), 27.
Berget, A., & Weille, B. (1988). Cigarette smoking and alcohol consumption during pregnancy by Danish women and their spouses: A potential source of fetal morbidity. *American Journal of Drug and Alcohol Abuse, 14*(3), 405.
Bernstein, L., Pike, M.C., Lobo R.A., Depue, R.H., Ross R.K., & Henderson, B.E. (1989). Cigarette smoking in pregnancy results in marked decrease in maternal HCG and oestradio levels. *British Journal of Obstetric and Gynecology, 96*(1), 92–6.
Briggs, G.G., Freeman, R.K., & Yaffe, S.J. (1986). *Drugs in pregnancy and lactation.* Baltimore: Williams & Wilkins.
Brooten, D., Peters, M.A., Glatts, M., Gaffney, S. E., Knapp, M., Cohen, S., et al. (1987). A survey of nutrition, caffeine, cigarette and alcohol intake in early pregnancy in an urban clinic population. *Journal of Nurse-Midwifery, 32*(2), 85.
Chasnoff, I.J. (1986). *Drug use in pregnancy: Mother and child.* Boston: MTP.
Chasnoff, I.J. (1988). *Drugs, alcohol, pregnancy, and parenting.* Boston: Academic.
Chasnoff, I. (1988). Drug use in pregnancy: Parameters of risk. *Pediatric Clinics of North America, 25*(6), 1403.
Chasnoff, I.J., & Griffith, D. (1989). Cocaine: Clinical studies of pregnancy and the newborn. *Annals of the New York Academy of Science, 562,* 260.
Chasnoff, I.J., Griffith, D., MacGregor, S., Dinkes, K., & Burns, K. (1989). Temporal patterns of cocaine use in pregnancy. *Journal of the American Medical Association, 26*(12), 1741.
Chatterjee, M., Abdel-Rahman, M., Bhandal, A., Klein, P., & Bogden, J. (1988). Amniotic fluid cadmium and thiocyanote in pregnancy women who smoke. *Journal of Reproductive Medicine, 33*(5), 417.
Cherukuri, R., Minkoff, H., et al. (1988). A cohort study of alkaloidal cocaine ("crack") in pregnancy. *Obstetrics and Gynecology, 72*(2), 147.

Chisum, G.M. (1990). Nursing interventions with the antepartum substance abuser. *Journal of Perinatal and Neonatal Nursing, 3*(4), 26–33.

Chychula, N.M. (1990). The cocaine epidemic: A comprehensive review of use abuse and dependence. *Nurse Practitioner, 15*(7), 31.

Doyle, D. (1986). Teratology: A primer. *Neonatal Network, 5*(2), 24–29.

Eleason, M., & Williams, J.K. (1990). Fetal alcohol syndrome and the neonate. *Journal of Perinatal and Neonatal Nursing, 3*(4), 64–72.

Edelin, K.C., Gurganieus, L., Golar, K., Oellerich, D., Kyei-Aboagye, K., Adel, H. (1988). Methadone maintenance in pregnancy: Consequences to care and outcome. *Obstetrics and Gynecology, 3*(71), 399.

Ernhart, C., Sokol, R., Ager, J., Tlucak, M., & Martier, S. (1989). Alcohol-related birth defects: Assessing the risk. *Annals of the New York Academy of Science, 562*, 159–72.

Ershoff, D.H., Mullen, P.D., & Quinn, V.P. (1989). A randomized trial of a serialized self-help smoking cessation program for pregnant women in an HMO. *American Journal of Public Health, 79*(2), 182.

Fingerhut, L.A., Kleinman, J.C., & Kendrick, J.S. (1990). Smoking before, during, and after pregnancy. *American Journal of Public Health, 80*(5), 541–544.

Flandermeyer, A. (1987). A comparison of the effects of heroin and cocaine abuse upon the neonate. *Neonatal Network, 5*(12), 42–48.

Frank, D.A., Zuckerman, B.S., Amaro, H., Aboagye, K., Bauchner, H., Cabral, H., Fried, L., et al. (1988). Cocaine use during pregnancy: Prevalence and correlates. *Pediatrics, 82*(6), 888–95.

Fried, P. (1989). Postnatal consequences of maternal marijuana use in humans. *Annals of the New York Academy of Science, 562*, 123–132.

Godin, G., & Lepage, L. (1988). Understanding the intentions of pregnant nullipara to not smoke cigarettes after childbirth. *Journal of Drug Education, 18*(2), 115–124.

Haglund, B., & Cnattingius, S. (1990). Cigarette smoking as a risk factor for sudden infant death syndrome: A population-based study. *American Journal of Public Health, 801*(1), 29–32.

Hebel, J., et al. (1988). Dose response of birth weight to various measures of maternal smoking during pregnancy. *Journal of Clinical Epidemiology, 41*(5), 483–489.

Hoegerman, G., Wilson, C.A., Thurmond, E., Schnoll, S.H., (1990). Drug-exposed neonates. *Western Journal of Medicine, 152*(5), 559.

Horowitz, J. (1988). Anesthetic implications of substance abuse in the parturient. *Journal of the Association of Nurse Anesthetists, 56*(6), 510–514.

House, M.A. (1990). Cocaine. *American Journal of Nursing, 90*(4), 41.

Howard, J. (1990). Cocaine and its effect on the newborn. *Neonatal Intensive Care, 3*(2), 38.

Kennard, M.J. (1990). Cocaine use during pregnancy: Fetal and neonate effects. *Journal of Perinatal and Neonatal Nursing, 3*(4), 53–63.

Little, B., Snell, L.M., Gilstrap, L.C., Gant, N.F., & Rosenfeld, C. (1989). Alcohol abuse during pregnancy: Changes in frequency in a large urban hospital. *Obstetrics and Gynecology, 74*(4), 547–50.

Little, B., Snell, L., Klein, V.R., & Gilstrap, L.C. (1989). Cocaine abuse during pregnancy: Maternal and fetal implications. *Obstetrics and Gynecology, 73*(2), 157–160.

Little, R., Anderson, K., Ervin, C., Roberts, B., & Clarres, S.S. (1989). Maternal alcohol use during breastfeeding and infant mental and motor development at one year. *New England Journal of Medicine, 321*(7), 425.

MacArthur, C., & Knox, E.G. (1988). Smoking in pregnancy: Effects of stopping at different stages. *British Journal of Obstetrics and Gynecology, 95*, 551–555.

MacGregor, S.N., Keith, L.G., Bachicha, J.A., & Chasnoff, I.J. (1989). Cocaine abuse during pregnancy: Correlation between prenatal care and perinatal outcome. *Obstetrics and Gynecology, 74*(6), 882.

Messimer, S.R., Hickner, J.M., Henry, R.C. (1989). A comparison of two antismoking interventions among pregnant women in eleven private primary care practices. *Journal of Family Practice, 28*(3), 283.

Mohler, S. (1987). Passive smoking: A danger to children's health. *Journal of Pediatric Health Care, 1*,(6), 298–304.

Morrow, R., Ritchie, J.W., & Bull, S. (1988). Maternal cigarette smoking: The effects of umbilical and uterine blood flow velocity. *American Journal of Obstetrics and Gynecology, 159*(5), 1069.

Morrow-Tlucak, M., Ernhart, C.B., Sokol, R.J., Martier, S., & Ager, J. (1989). Underreporting of alcohol use in pregnancy: Relationship to alcohol problem history. *Alcoholism: Clinical and Experimental Research, 13*(3), 399–401.

Petitti, K., & Coleman, C. (1990). Cocaine and the risk of low birthweight. *American Journal of Public Health 80*(1), 25.

Povenmire, K.I. (1990). Recognizing the cocaine addict. *Nursing '90, 20*(5), 46.

Rosett, H., & Weiner, L. (1984). *Alcohol and the fetus.* New York: Oxford University.

Schnoll, S.H., & Karan, L.D. (1989). Substance abuse. *Journal of the American Medical Association, 261*(19), 2890–2892.

Smith, J. (1988). The dangers of perinatal cocaine use. *MCN: American Journal of Maternal Child Nursing, 13*(3), 174–179.

Sokol, R.S., Miller, S.I., & Martier, S. (1981). Identifying the alcohol abusing obstetric/gynecologic patient. *Professional Educational Reprints,* No. (ADM) 81–1163, March of Dimes.

Stephens, C. (1981). The fetal alcohol syndrome: Cause for concern. *MCN: American Journal of Maternal Child Nursing, 6*(4), 251–256.

Stern, L. (1984). *Drug use in pregnancy.* Boston: Adis.

Sullivan, K.R. (1990). Maternal implications of cocaine use during pregnancy. *Journal of Perinatal and Neonatal Nursing, 3*(4), 12–25.

Vanderveen, E. (1989). Public health policy: Maternal substance use and child health. *Annals of the New York Academy of Science, 562,* 255.

Warren, K.R. (1988). Alcohol-related birth defects. *Public Health Reports, 103*(6), 638.

Weiner, L., Morse, B.A., & Garrido, P. (1989). FAS/FAE: Focus in prevention on women at risk. *International Journal of the Addictions, 24*(5), 385–395.

Williamson, D., Serdula, M., Kendrick, J., & Binkin, N. (1989). Comparing the prevalence of smoking in pregnant and non-pregnant women, 1985–1986. *Journal of the American Medical Association, 261*(1), 70–74.

Zuckerman, B.K., Frank, D.A., Hingson, R., Amaro, H., & Levenson, S.M. (1989). Effects of maternal marijuana and cocaine use on fetal growth. *New England Journal of Medicine, 320*(12), 762–768.

Harriet Gillerman

Other Medical Complications

Objectives

1. Review the anatomical and physiological changes in the cardiovascular, respiratory, renal, hematological, gastrointestinal, and hepatic systems in pregnancy

2. Describe the data to be documented in obtaining a history from pregnant clients with cardiac, respiratory, renal, hematological, gastrointestinal, and hepatic complications

3. Select nursing diagnoses appropriate for obstetrical clients with cardiac, respiratory, renal, hematological, gastrointestinal, and hepatic complications

4. Describe the fetal implications for pregnant clients with medical complications

5. Describe the signs and symptoms and laboratory data that indicate cardiac, respiratory, renal, hematological, gastrointestinal, and hepatic complications of pregnancy

6. Formulate a nursing care plan (consisting of nursing diagnoses, interventions, and evaluations based on nursing history and assessments) for the obstetrical client with cardiovascular, respiratory, renal, hematological, gastrointestinal, and hepatic complications

7. Design a plan to teach principles necessary for maintenance of health for obstetrical clients with cardiac, respiratory, renal, hematological, gastrointestinal, and hepatic complications

Cardiac Complications

Introduction

Because pregnancy brings about many alterations in the maternal cardiovascular system, pregnant clients must accommodate many physiological changes.

A. Pregnant clients with normal cardiac function are able to adapt to these changes without difficulty, but clients with significant heart disease face potential decompensation and death

B. It is possible that clients would not have experienced problems with the cardiac condition until the stresses of pregnancy caused exacerbation of the disease

C. Cardiac complications occur in approximately 1% of all pregnant women; whether these women have favorable outcomes depends on numerous factors

1. The functional capacity of the heart
2. The presence of other factors that increase the cardiac workload
3. The health care support they receive

Clinical Practice

A. Assessment

1. History
   a. Specific forms of heart disease
      (1) Anatomical or structural
         (a) Women born with anatomical or structural congenital heart anomalies are now surviving to childbearing age in increasing numbers
         (b) Some have had surgical corrections and others have not
         (c) Those who have not may have residual hemodynamic defects that expose them to bacterial endocarditis and other risks with childbearing
         (d) The most common anatomical and structural forms are idiopathic hypertrophic subaortic stenosis (IHSS) and mitral valve disease
      (2) Physiological
         (a) Arrhythmias, bradyarrhythmias, and tachyarrhythmias are not usually treated unless they significantly compromise maternal hemodynamics
         (b) Pulmonary hypertension is increased vascular resistance in the pulmonary circulation
         (c) Pulmonary edema results from a failure of the left side of the heart to pump blood forward, with resultant backward congestion of fluid into the lungs
         (d) Peripartum cardiomyopathy is a disorder that usually develops in the last month of pregnancy or the first 6 months postpartum in a woman without previous cardiac disease or any other cause of cardiac failure: signs and symptoms are those of right- and left-sided congestive heart failure (CHF) including cardiomegaly
2. Physical findings
   a. Normal pregnancy is associated with many changes that can mimic the signs and symptoms of cardiac disease; Table 33–1 illustrates the signs and

Table 33–1
SIGNS AND SYMPTOMS COMMON TO NORMAL PREGNANCY COMPARED WITH SIGNS AND SYMPTOMS OF ACTUAL CARDIAC DISEASE IN PREGNANCY

Signs and Symptoms Suggestive of Heart Disease That Are Common to Normal Pregnancy	Signs and Symptoms of Actual Heart Disease
Chest discomfort	Chest discomfort with myocardial ishcemia
Dyspnea	Severe dyspnea that limits activity; paroxysmal nocturnal dyspnea
Orthopnea	Progressive orthopnea
Palpitations	Cardiac arrhythmia
Easy fatiguability	Fatigue with chest pain and syncope
Dizzy spells	Dizzy spells plus other actual signs and symptoms
Syncope	Syncope with exertion
Systolic murmurs	Loud harsh systolic murmurs: grade III intensity, diastolic murmurs
Dependent edema	Dependent plus nondependent edema
Rales in lower lung fields	Rales that do not clear with deep inspiration; hemoptysis
Visible neck veins	Persistent neck vein distension
Cardiomegaly	Cardiomegaly plus hepatomegaly and ascites

symptoms suggestive of heart disease associated with pregnancy versus those of actual heart disease

b. The New York Heart Association cardiac disease classification is based on clinical function (Table 33–2); these same classes are used to describe the pregnant client with cardiac disease

c. This classification has been replaced by some systems that use criteria such as cause and anatomical diagnosis

d. Signs and symptoms of cardiac decompensation

  (1) Right-sided CHF

    (a) Neck vein distension

    (b) Hepatomegaly

    (c) Dependent and nondependent edema

    (d) Weight gain

  (2) Left-sided CHF

    (a) Dyspnea

    (b) Orthopnea

    (c) Rales

    (d) Cough

    (e) Extreme fatigue

    (f) Chest pain

    (g) Syncope

    (h) Pallor

    (i) Cyanosis

    (j) Cardiac arrhythmias

e. Fetal assessment

  (1) Fetal health depends on an adequate and continuous supply of oxygenated maternal blood to the uterus: if this oxygenated blood supply is limited because of cardiac disease, the risk of abnormal fetal development or death is significantly increased

  (2) Methods of fetal assessment

    (a) Ultrasound testing

    (b) Nonstress testing (NST)

    (c) Biophysical profile

    (d) Fetal heart rate (FHR) tracings

  (3) The fetus is at risk for hypoxia because of maternal hypoxemia

  (4) The incidence of prematurity is increased because of maternal hypoxemia

  (5) The incidence of intrauterine growth retardation (IUGR) and small-for-gestational age infants is increased

  (6) The incidence of spontaneous abortion and stillbirth is increased

Table 33–2
NEW YORK HEART ASSOCIATION CARDIAC DISEASE CLASSIFICATION

Class	Description
I	Clients with cardiac disease and no limitation of physical activity. Clients in this class do not have symptoms of cardiac insufficiency, nor do they experience pain.
II	Clients with cardiac disease and slight limitation of physical activity. They are comfortable at rest, but if ordinary physical activity is undertaken, discomfort results in the form of excessive fatigue, palpitation, dyspnea, or anginal pain.
III	Clients with cardiac disease and marked limitation of physical activity. They are comfortable at rest, but less-than-ordinary activity causes discomfort in the form of excessive fatigue, palpitation, dyspnea, or anginal pain.
IV	Clients with cardiac disease and inability to perform any physical activity without discomfort. Symptoms of cardiac insufficiency or of the anginal syndrome may occur even at rest, and if any physical activity is undertaken, discomfort is increased.

(7) If parents have congenital heart disease, the chance that the offspring will inherit the anomaly is 1 to 4%

(8) If the mother has a cyanotic congenital heart disease, the fetus is at increased risk of hypoxia

B. Nursing Diagnoses

1. Decreased cardiac output related to diseased maternal heart
2. Activity intolerance related to decreased cardiac output and tissue malnutrition
3. Anxiety and fear related to complicated pregnancy
4. Self-care deficit related to inability to perform activities of daily living (ADL) secondary to bed rest or fatigue
5. High risk for alteration in family process related to maternal complications of pregnancy and hospitalization
6. Knowledge deficit related to diagnosis of heart disease complicating pregnancy

C. Interventions/Evaluations

1. Decreased cardiac output related to diseased maternal heart
   a. Interventions
      (1) Support cardiac functioning by limiting cardiac demands (stress, too much activity)
      (2) Decrease the risks of further complications
      (3) Maintain client in left lateral or semi-Fowler's position when on bed rest
      (4) Maintain client's diet for low sodium intake: 2 g sodium or lower as necessary
      (5) Weigh client daily: observe for increasing weight indicating fluid retention
      (6) Assess edema: if client is on fluid restriction, regulate IV and oral (PO) fluids as ordered
      (7) Monitor intake and output (I&O)
      (8) Auscultate breath sounds; encourage turning, coughing, and deep breathing
      (9) Administer prescribed cardiotonics and diuretics
      (10) Administer potassium replacement as indicated by laboratory work
      (11) Administer antiarrhythmics as ordered
      (12) Monitor vital signs and increase frequency when unstable
      (13) Keep client comfortable in labor and delivery to decrease pain and therefore cardiac workload
      (14) Aid client in avoiding a long, difficult labor
      (15) Aid client in avoiding lengthy pushing in the second stage of labor especially use of closed glottis pushing (see Chap. 15 for discussion of alternative pushing methods)
      (16) Observe client for signs and symptoms of fluid overload immediately after delivery of the placenta and in the postpartum period
   b. Evaluation: the cornerstone of evaluation is to ensure that the client does not experience cardiac failure
      (1) Client has no edema
      (2) Client has no adventitious breath sounds
      (3) Client's respirations are normal in rate, rhythm, and depth
      (4) Client has normal urine output (30 to 60 cc/hr)
      (5) Client has no fatigue with normal activity
      (6) Client has normal skin color and pulses
      (7) Client is oriented to person, place and time
      (8) Client has no visual disturbances
2. Activity intolerance related to decreased cardiac output and tissue malnutrition

    a. Interventions
      (1) Assess activity tolerance
      (2) Assist client in modifying schedule and spacing activities to allow for more rest
      (3) Maintain client's activity level short of fatigue
      (4) Provide long periods for sleep at night and frequent rest periods during the day
      (5) Assist client with ADL and ambulation
    b. Evaluation: client tolerates progressive activities as evidenced by the following
      (1) Normal vital signs
      (2) Decreased dizziness, light-headedness, and weakness
3. Anxiety and fear related to complicated pregnancy
    a. Interventions
      (1) Discuss client's fears and concerns about her pregnancy and its outcome
      (2) Provide reassurance and comfort
      (3) Obtain and begin involvement of medical social worker (MSW) and other health team members
      (4) If possible and appropriate, have client's friends and family visit frequently; instruct them about visiting hours
      (5) Encourage client to ask questions about tests, medicines, treatments, and physician orders
      (6) Explain all procedures and their purpose
      (7) Acknowledge client's feelings and respond in a manner appropriate to her needs
      (8) Encourage client's interest in diversional activities (e.g., crafts, books, music)
      (9) Maintain clean, orderly, quiet, and stress-free environment
     (10) Assess family members' level of anxiety and knowledge of disease process; assess them as a support system for client
     (11) Arrange for infant special care staff to visit with client; orient client to realistic expectations
     (12) Encourage client to use visualization exercises, music, and crafts for relaxation
    b. Evaluations
      (1) Client verbalizes her fears and concerns about her pregnancy
      (2) Client feels supported and listened to
      (3) Client is able to relax and sleep
4. Self-care deficit related to inability to perform ADL secondary to bed rest or fatigue
    a. Interventions
      (1) Assess client's level of self-care with ADL
      (2) Assist client with all ADL
        (a) Personal hygiene
        (b) Feeding
        (c) Dressing
        (d) Positioning
      (3) Assess and use equipment for special needs of client
      (4) Involve family with client's care
      (5) Contact home health nurses and have them evaluate client to make visits at home after discharge
      (6) Consult with MSW if appropriate or at client's request
    b. Evaluation: client assists with her daily care without evidence of fatigue or irritability and with no change in her vital signs
5. High risk for alteration in family process related to maternal complications of pregnancy and hospitalization

   a. Interventions

     (1) Allow client and her family members to ventilate fears about pregnancy outcome

     (2) Assess client's and family members' responses to complicated pregnancy

       (a) Presence of unresolved guilt, blame, hostility, or jealousy

       (b) Inability to problem solve adequately

       (c) Ineffective patterns of communication

       (d) Observe client's interactions with other family members

     (3) Assess level of financial burden on family

     (4) Discuss affects of prolonged hospitalization on the family process

     (5) Encourage client and her family to participate in support groups and education programs

     (6) Utilize outside resources

       (a) MSW

       (b) Clinical nurse specialist

       (c) Clinical psychologist

       (d) Lay support and self-help groups

       (e) Home health care

       (f) Financial assistance programs

     (7) Assist family in reorganizing roles at home and setting priorities to maintain family integrity and to reduce stress

     (8) Aid family members in changing their expectations of the client in a realistic manner

     (9) Encourage frequent visits by family members

    (10) Make sure family members are oriented to visiting hours, bathrooms, cafeteria, gift shop, etc.

    (11) Prepare client and her family members for signs of depression, anxiety, and dependency

    (12) Meet the physical needs of the client

    (13) Assess client's spiritual needs and help her to meet those needs

   b. Evaluations: client and her family demonstrate a functional system of mutual support for each other as evidenced by the following

     (1) Seeking appropriate external resources when needed

     (2) Engaging in open communication with the health team

     (3) Participating in care of the hospitalized family member

6. Knowledge deficit related to diagnosis of heart disease complicating pregnancy

   a. Interventions

     (1) Assess client's and family members' readiness and ability to learn

     (2) Determine client's knowledge of her illness, its treatment, and preventive measures

     (3) Assess client's adherence to prescribed behavior and its effect on her lifestyle

     (4) Begin client and family education regarding what cardiac disease is and the effects it has on the mother and fetus

     (5) Provide information to enable the pregnant woman with cardiac complications to obtain proper support and care

     (6) Discuss signs and symptoms to report

       (a) Shortness of breath

       (b) Dyspnea

       (c) Decreased ability to perform activities

       (d) Extreme fatigue

       (e) Edema

       (f) Anorexia

     (7) Explain the purpose of treatments, interventions, and tests

     (8) Teach client behavioral interventions

(a) Bed rest in lateral positions (explain physiological rationale)
(b) Observance of prescribed medication regimen
(c) Maintenance of as quiet and stress-free an environment as possible
(9) Explain to client the rationale and procedure for the following
(a) NST
(b) Contraction stress testing (CST)
(c) Biophysical profile
(d) Amniocentesis
b. Evaluations
(1) Client verbalizes an understanding of cardiac disease and its effect on the fetus
(2) Client is able to describe the cardiac disease process, causes, signs and symptoms, and interventions for disease control

Health Education

A. Preconceptual counseling

1. Discuss the risk of pregnancy to the mother and the fetus
2. Discuss contraception with low-dose estrogen compounds, diaphragms and condoms
3. Discuss potentially teratogenic cardiovascular drugs (warfarin, propranolol, thiazide diuretics)
4. Discuss the advances in medical and surgical therapy, fetal surveillance, and neonatal care that have improved the outcome for women with cardiac disease

B. Encourage client to be in the care of an obstetrician and a cardiologist

C. Discuss the importance of regular and frequent medical supervision

D. Teach client about rationale for modifying her diet and activities, and of taking prescribed medications

E. Teach client to avoid exposure to infection

F. Ensure that client obtains antibiotic prophylaxis before dental and surgical procedures

G. Teach client to restrict activity to that which is just short of fatigue

H. Teach client to get adequate rest with frequent rest periods

I. Teach client to modify diet; no added salt or about 2 g/day (more stringent with CHF)

J. Teach client to avoid excessive weight gain

K. Teach client to maintain normal hemoglobin levels with proper nutrition and supplements

L. Ensure that client keeps appointments with her cardiologist and obstetrician

Renal Complications

Introduction

Women who have pre-existing but minimal renal disease tolerate pregnancy well but must be carefully monitored.

A. Studies have shown that pregnancy does not have an adverse effect on long-term renal function and underlying renal disease as long as blood pressure is controlled.

B. The outlook can be ominous, however, when high blood pressure occurs with simultaneous deterioration of renal function early in pregnancy

C. In many patients, renal disease may not be diagnosed until after conception because the glomerular filtration rate (GFR) may not have increased enough to produce symptoms before conception

D. The risks of fetal death as well as neonatal mortality and morbidity associated with growth retardation and prematurity are increased in pregnancies complicated by renal disease

Clinical Practice

A. Assessment

1. History
   a. Incidence of urinary tract infections (UTIs): anatomical and physiological changes of pregnancy result in the following
      (1) Stasis of urine
      (2) Delayed emptying
      (3) Increased risk of infection
   b. Incidence and duration
      (1) Acute renal disease
      (2) Chronic renal disease
      (3) Nephrotic syndrome
      (4) Renal failure
      (5) Renal transplantation
2. Physical findings
   a. Signs and symptoms and studies diagnostic of renal disease
      (1) Urinalysis
         (a) Proteinuria, the loss of protein into the urine from the intravascular compartment, indicates glomerular damage
         (b) Hematuria with red cell casts indicates glomerular inflammation and injury
         (c) Pyuria indicates inflammation or infection
         (d) Polyuria and nocturia may be signs of inability to concentrate urine
         (e) Urine cultures should be done frequently because of susceptibility to infection
      (2) Other laboratory and diagnostic studies for renal disease
         (a) Creatinine
         (b) Blood urea nitrogen (BUN)
         (c) Uric acid
         (d) Radiological studies to rule out obstruction
         (e) Renal biopsy
   b. Signs and symptoms of UTI
      (1) Dysuria
      (2) Frequency
      (3) Urgency
      (4) Fever
      (5) Chills
      (6) Hematuria
      (7) Lower abdominal pain
   c. Signs and symptoms of pyelonephritis
      (1) UTI signs and symptoms
      (2) Costovertebral angle (CVA) tenderness
      (3) Fever (increased over that in UTI) and chills
   d. Fetal assessment: because of the strong association of renal disease with IUGR, fetal surveillance is important
      (1) Antepartum FHR testing
      (2) Ultrasound testing
      (3) Fetal lung maturity assessment

B. Nursing Diagnoses

1. High risk for infection related to anatomical and physiological changes of the renal system in pregnancy
2. Fluid volume excess or deficit related to inability of the kidney to regulate fluid balance
3. Alteration in comfort related to bladder spasm or renal colic
4. Activity intolerance related to anemia
5. Anxiety and fear related to complicated pregnancy
6. Knowledge deficit related to pregnancy complicated by renal disease
7. High risk for alteration in family process related to maternal complications and hospitalization

C. Interventions/Evaluations

1. High risk for infection related to anatomical and physiological changes of the renal system in pregnancy
   a. Interventions: observe for signs and symptoms of infection
      (1) Fever
      (2) Chills
      (3) Abdominal and CVA pain
      (4) Skin lesions
   b. Evaluation: client exhibits no fever, chills, abdominal or CVA pain, or skin lesions
2. Fluid volume excess or deficit related to inability of the kidney to regulate fluid balance
   a. Interventions
      (1) Observe for signs and symptoms of improvement and deterioration in condition by observing the following parameters
         (a) Urinalysis reports
         (b) Kidney function tests: creatinine, BUN, uric acid
         (c) Complete blood count (CBC)
         (d) Urine output
         (e) Proteinuria
         (f) Blood pressure values
         (g) Amount of edema in the legs, arms, hands, and sacral area
         (h) Daily weight
         (i) Positioning in left lateral position when on bed rest
         (j) Administering prescribed medications
         (k) Assessing skin turgor, color, and temperature
         (l) Observing for signs and symptoms of superimposed pre-eclampsia and UTI
         (m) Administering intake as indicated
            (i) Observe fluid restrictions
            (ii) Encourage fluids
            (iii) Force fluids
      (2) Observe and record color, amount, and consistency of urine
      (3) Observe for signs and symptoms of renal failure
         (a) Increased BUN
         (b) Increased creatinine
         (c) Nausea and vomiting
         (d) Systemic edema
         (e) Anorexia
         (f) Urticaria
         (g) Stomatitis
         (h) Anemia
         (i) Elevated blood pressure
         (j) Fatigue

(k) Headache

(l) Fluid and electrolyte imbalance (sodium, potassium, calcium, phosphorus)

b. Evaluations: the cornerstone of evaluation is to ensure that the client is free of renal insufficiency and failure, hypertension, and superimposed preeclampsia

(1) Urinalysis within normal limits

(2) BUN, creatinine, uric acid, CBC within normal limits

(3) Urine output 30 to 60 cc/hr

(4) Vital signs, especially blood pressure, within normal limits for client

(5) Absence of edema, hyper-reflexia, and proteinuria

(6) Normal weight gain or loss

(7) Good skin turgor

3. Alteration in comfort related to bladder spasm or renal colic

a. Interventions

(1) Assess pain-precipitating factors and document deviation from baseline

(a) Quality

(b) Region radiation

(c) Severity

(d) Duration

(e) Relieving factors

(2) Have client evaluate pain intensity on a 1 to 10 scale (10 being most severe)

(3) Observe, report, and record verbal and nonverbal expressions of pain, fear, and anxiety

(4) Provide and encourage rest periods and a restful environment

(5) Medicate client with analgesics, antispasmodics, and antibiotics as ordered

(6) Assess effectiveness of pain medications

(7) Provide comfort measures

(a) Reposition client

(b) Provide client with skin care

(c) Assist client with ambulation and movement in bed

(d) Splint client and assist her with coughing and deep breathing

(8) Teach client and her family about factors that contribute to pain experience

(9) Assess client's urgency and frequency of urination and nocturia

(10) Palpate client's bladder for distension

b. Evaluations

(1) Client verbalizes decreased pain intensity (using a scale of 1 to 10) in response to analgesics or other interventions within 1 hour of administration

(2) Client maintains pain control or absence of pain as evidenced by the following

(a) Client's statement

(b) Decreased use of analgesics

(c) Increased activity

4. Activity intolerance related to anemia

a. Interventions

(1) Assess activity tolerance

(2) Assist client in modifying her schedule and spacing her activities to allow for more rest

(3) Maintain client's activity level just short of fatigue

(4) Provide long periods for sleep at night and frequent rest periods during the day

(5) Assist client with ADL and ambulation

   b. Evaluations: Client tolerates progressive activities as evidenced by the following
      (1) Normal vital signs
      (2) Normal I&O
      (3) Absence of pain
5. Anxiety and fear related to complicated pregnancy
   a. Interventions
      (1) Discuss client's fears and concerns about her pregnancy and its outcome
      (2) Provide reassurance and comfort
      (3) Obtain and begin involvement of MSW and other health team members
      (4) If possible and appropriate, have client's friends and family visit frequently; instruct them about visiting hours
      (5) Encourage client to ask questions about tests, medicines, treatments, and physician orders
      (6) Explain all procedures and their purpose
      (7) Acknowledge client's feelings and respond in a manner appropriate to her needs
      (8) Encourage client's interest in diversional activities (e.g., crafts, books, music)
      (9) Maintain clean, orderly, quiet, and stress-free environment
      (10) Assess family members' level of anxiety and knowledge of disease process; assess them as a support system for client
      (11) Arrange for infant special care staff to visit with client; orient client to realistic expectations
      (12) Encourage client to use visualization exercises, music, and crafts for relaxation
   b. Evaluations
      (1) Client verbalizes her fears and concerns about her pregnancy
      (2) Client feels supported and listened to
      (3) Client is able to relax and sleep
6. Knowledge deficit related to pregnancy complicated by renal disease
   a. Interventions
      (1) Assess client's and family members' readiness and ability to learn
      (2) Determine client's knowledge of her illness, its treatment, and preventive measures
      (3) Assess client's adherence to prescribed behavior and its effect on her lifestyle
      (4) Begin client and family education regarding what renal disease is and the effects it has on the mother and fetus
      (5) Provide information to enable the pregnant woman with renal complications to obtain proper support and care
      (6) Discuss signs and symptoms to report
         (a) Dysuria, frequency, urgency
         (b) Fever and chills
         (c) Hematuria
         (d) Lower abdominal pain
         (e) Decreased urine output
         (f) Shortness of breath
         (g) Dyspnea
         (h) Decreased ability to perform activities
         (i) Increasing pain
         (j) Fatigue
         (k) Edema
         (l) Anorexia
         (m) Confusion
      (7) Explain the purpose of treatments, interventions, and tests

(8) Teach client behavioral interventions
    (a) Bed rest in lateral positions (explain physiological rationale)
    (b) Observance of prescribed medication regimen
    (c) Maintenance of as quiet and stress-free an environment as possible
(9) Explain to client the rationale and procedure for the following:
    (a) NST   (c) Biophysical profile
    (b) CST   (d) Amniocentesis

b. Evaluations
  (1) Client verbalizes an understanding of renal disease and its effect on the fetus
  (2) Client is able to describe the renal disease process, causes, signs, and symptoms, and interventions for disease control

7. High risk for alteration in family process related to maternal complications and hospitalization

a. Interventions
  (1) Allow client and her family members to ventilate their fears about pregnancy outcome
  (2) Assess client's and family members' responses to complicated pregnancy
    (a) Presence of unresolved guilt, blame, hostility, or jealousy
    (b) Inability to problem solve adequately
    (c) Ineffective patterns of communication
    (d) Observe client's interactions with her family members
  (3) Assess level of financial burden on family
  (4) Discuss effects of prolonged hospitalization on the family process
  (5) Encourage client and her family to participate in support groups and education programs
  (6) Use outside resources
    (a) MSW
    (b) Clinical nurse specialist
    (c) Clinical psychologist
    (d) Lay support and self-help groups
    (e) Home health care
    (f) Financial assistance programs
  (7) Assist family in reorganizing roles at home and setting priorities to maintain family integrity and to reduce stress
  (8) Aid family members in changing their expectations of the client in a realistic manner
  (9) Encourage frequent visits by family members
  (10) Make sure family members are oriented to visiting hours, bathrooms, cafeteria, gift shop, and so forth
  (11) Prepare client and her family members for signs of depression, anxiety, and dependency
  (12) Meet the physical needs of the client
  (13) Assess client's spiritual needs and help her to meet those needs

b. Evaluations: client and family demonstrate a functional system of mutual support for each other as evidenced by the following
  (1) Seeking appropriate external resources when needed
  (2) Engage in open communication between family members and health team
  (3) Participating in care of hospitalized family member

Health Education

A. Preconceptual counseling

1. Discuss increased risk of fetal loss and pre-eclampsia with clients already demonstrating proteinuria and hypertension

2. Discuss increased incidence of anovulation, menstrual irregularities, loss of libido, and decreased fertility among clients with underlying chronic renal disease
3. Discuss effects of pregnancy on chronic renal disease

B. **Teach client self-monitoring of weight gain, edema, and blood pressure**

C. **Teach client to avoid exposure to infection**

D. **Plan with client how she can get adequate sleep and take frequent rests**

E. **Ensure adequate nutrition with prescribed diet and fluid intake**

F. **Instruct client to keep appointments with her nephrologist and obstetrician**

G. **Teach proper perineal hygiene**

H. **Teach all women to recognize the symptoms of UTI**

1. Dysuria
2. Frequency
3. Urgency
4. Chills
5. Low-grade fever
6. Hematuria
7. Lower abdominal pain

I. **Teach signs and symptoms of premature labor and increased uterine irritability**

Respiratory Complications

Introduction

Pregnancy brings about alterations in respiratory physiology because of the increase in abdominal girth and hormonal change.

A. **These physiological changes can cause clients with a previously compromised respiratory status to decompensate and to require support of their respiration**

B. **The outcomes of pregnant clients with respiratory complications depend on the adequacy of ventilation and oxygenation and the early detection of decompensation**

C. **Hypoxia is the major threat to the fetus**

D. **Specific forms of respiratory disease**

1. Asthma is the most common form of obstructive lung disease in pregnancy
   a. Pregnancy appears to have no consistent effect on asthma; it is unlikely that a pregnant woman's asthma will become worse during pregnancy provided she is given adequate treatment and she avoids stimuli that provoke an attack
   b. Most medications used to treat chronic asthma are considered safe to use during pregnancy
2. Tuberculosis is caused by infection with the acid-fast bacillus *Mycobacterium tuberculosis*
   a. The incidence of tuberculosis is rising, especially among the Southeast Asian population in the United States
   b. Treatment with antituberculosis drugs has improved management in general as well as in pregnancy
   c. Ethambutol and isoniazid are considered safe to use in pregnancy
3. Respiratory insufficiency and failure

   a. Basis for respiratory insufficiency
      (1) Obstruction of the tracheobronchial tree
      (2) Decreased movement of gases to and from the lungs
      (3) Abnormality of blood flow in the pulmonary capillaries
      (4) Impairment in the alveolar membrane permeability
   4. Respiratory insufficiency occurs when the exchange of O_2 and CO_2 is not adequate to meet the needs of the body during normal activities
   5. Respiratory failure occurs when ventilation is not sufficient to achieve gas exchange that meets the needs of the body even at rest

E. **Dyspnea, which is experienced by most women at some time during a normal pregnancy, may suggest lung disease or may be the result of normal physiological changes of pregnancy**

Clinical Practice

A. **Assessment**

1. History
   a. Duration and severity of shortness of breath and dyspnea
   b. Degree of exercise and activity limitations
   c. Type of cough
   d. Amount of hemoptysis
   e. Amount, color, and consistency of sputum
   f. Duration and severity of wheezing and chest tightness
   g. Duration and severity of fever, chills, and night sweats
2. Physical findings
   a. Rate, rhythm, and depth of respirations
   b. Auscultation of the lungs
   c. Skin color
   d. Blood pressure and pulse
   e. Level of consciousness
   f. I & O
   g. Fetal assessment for signs and symptoms of hypoxia
      (1) FHR tracing
      (2) Biophysical profile
      (3) NST
3. Diagnostic procedures
   a. Arterial blood gases
   b. Chest x-ray (with abdominal shield)
   c. CBC
   d. Pulmonary function tests

B. **Nursing Diagnoses**

1. Alteration in respiratory function related to the pathophysiology of the respiratory structures
2. Impaired gas exchange related to the pathophysiology of respiratory structures or functions
3. Ineffective airway clearance related to thickened mucous secretions
4. Activity intolerance related to hypoxia
5. Anxiety and fear related to complicated pregnancy
6. Knowledge deficit related to pregnancy complicated by respiratory disease
7. High risk for alteration in family process related to maternal complications and hospitalization

C. **Interventions/Evaluations**

1. Alteration in respiratory function related to the pathophysiology of the respiratory structures; impaired gas exchange related to the pathophysiology of

respiratory structures or functions; ineffective airway clearance related to thickened mucous secretions

a. Interventions

    (1) Position in semi- or high-Fowler's position with lateral tilt and supported arms for adequate breathing and decreased dyspnea

    (2) Auscultate lung fields for baseline and monitor frequently

    (3) Observe respiration for rate, rhythm, and regularity

    (4) Administer prescribed medications and respiratory treatments

        (a) Bronchodilators

        (b) Antibiotics

        (c) Antituberculosis drugs

        (d) Corticosteroids as indicated

    (5) Assess for productive and nonproductive cough

    (6) Turn client, assist her in coughing and deep breathing, administer incentive spirometer, and note effectiveness of treatment

    (7) Prevent increased oxygen consumption related to painful contractions by medicating the patient adequately during labor

    (8) Prevent client from hyperventilating during labor by providing coaching and support

b. Evaluations: the cornerstone of evaluation is to ensure that the client has an absence of respiratory distress

    (1) Normal arterial blood gas values, CBC, and chest x-ray

    (2) Respirations of normal rate, rhythm, and depth

    (3) No adventitious breath sounds

    (4) No fatigue with normal activity

    (5) Normal skin color and pulses

    (6) Oriented to person, place, and time

2. Activity intolerance related to hypoxia

a. Interventions

    (1) Assess activity tolerance

    (2) Assist client in modifying her schedule and spacing her activities to allow for more rest

    (3) Maintain client's activity level just short of fatigue

    (4) Provide long periods for sleep at night and frequent rest periods during the day

    (5) Assist client with ADL and ambulation

b. Evaluations: client tolerates progressive activities as evidenced by the following

    (1) Normal vital signs with rest and activity

    (2) Normal depth and clarity of respirations

    (3) Decreased weakness

3. Anxiety and fear related to complicated pregnancy

a. Interventions

    (1) Discuss client's fears and concerns about pregnancy and outcome

    (2) Provide reassurance and comfort

    (3) Obtain and begin involvement of MSW and other health team members

    (4) If possible and appropriate, have client's friends and family visit frequently; instruct them about visiting hours

    (5) Encourage client to ask questions about tests, medicines, treatments, and physician orders

    (6) Explain all procedures and their purpose

    (7) Acknowledge client's feelings and respond in a manner appropriate to her needs

    (8) Encourage interest in diversional activities (e.g., crafts, books, music)

    (9) Maintain clean, orderly, quiet, and stress-free environment

    (10) Assess family members' level of anxiety and knowledge of disease process; assess them as a support system

(11) Arrange for infant special care staff to visit with client; orient client to realistic expectations

(12) Encourage client to use visualization exercises, music, and crafts for relaxation

b. Evaluations

(1) Client verbalizes her fears and concerns about her pregnancy

(2) Client feels supported and listened to

(3) Client is able to relax and sleep

4. Knowledge deficit related to pregnancy complicated by respiratory disease

a. Interventions

(1) Assess client's and family members' readiness and ability to learn

(2) Determine client's knowledge of illness, treatment, and preventative measures

(3) Assess client's adherence to prescribed behavior, and its effect on her lifestyle

(4) Begin client and family education regarding what respiratory disease is and the effects it has on the mother and fetus

(5) Provide information to enable the pregnant woman with respiratory complications to obtain proper support and care

(6) Discuss signs and symptoms to report

(a) Shortness of breath

(b) Dyspnea

(c) Rapid respirations

(d) Cough and congestion

(e) Fever and chills

(f) Decreased ability to perform activities

(g) Extreme fatigue

(7) Explain the purpose of treatments, interventions, and tests

(8) Teach client behavioral interventions

(a) Bed rest in the semi-Fowler's position (explain physiological rationale)

(b) Observance of prescribed medication regimen

(c) Maintenance of as quiet and stress-free an environment as possible

(9) Explain to client the rationale and procedure for the following

(a) NST

(b) CST

(c) Biophysical profile

(d) Amniocentesis

b. Evaluations

(1) Client verbalizes an understanding of respiratory disease and its effect on the fetus

(2) Client is able to describe the respiratory disease process, causes, signs and symptoms, and interventions for disease control

5. High risk for alteration in family process related to maternal complications and hospitalization

a. Interventions

(1) Allow client and her family members to ventilate their fears about pregnancy outcome

(2) Assess client's and family members' responses to complicated pregnancy

(a) Presence of unresolved guilt, blame, hostility, or jealousy

(b) Inability to problem solve adequately

(c) Ineffective patterns of communication

(d) Observe client's interactions with her family members

(3) Assess level of financial burden on family

(4) Discuss effects of prolonged hospitalization on the family process

(5) Encourage client and her family to participate in support groups and education programs

(6) Utilize outside resources
    (a) MSW
    (b) Clinical nurse specialist
    (c) Clinical psychologist
    (d) Lay support and self-help groups
    (e) Home health care
    (f) Financial assistance programs
(7) Assist family in reorganizing roles at home and setting priorities to maintain family integrity and to reduce stress
(8) Aid family members in changing their expectations of the client in a realistic manner
(9) Encourage frequent visits by family members
(10) Make sure family members are oriented to visiting hours, bathrooms, cafeteria, gift shop, etc.
(11) Prepare client and family members for signs of depression, anxiety, and dependency
(12) Meet the physical needs of the client
(13) Assess client's spiritual needs and help her to meet those needs
b. Evaluations: client and family demonstrate a functional system of mutual support as evidenced by the following
    (1) Seeking appropriate external resources when needed
    (2) Engaging in open communication between family members and health team
    (3) Participating in care of hospitalized family member

Health Education

A. Teach client to avoid exposure to antigens and infection

B. Help client plan to restrict her activity to that just short of fatigue

C. Help client plan how to get adequate sleep with frequent rest periods

D. Teach client to maintain normal hemoglobin levels by high iron intake

E. Ensure adequate nutrition and fluid intake

Connective Tissue Disorders of Pregnancy: Systemic Lupus Erythematosus (SLE)

Introduction

A. Systemic lupus erythematosus (SLE) is a chronic multisystem collagen vascular disease that is thought to be caused by an autoimmune process and that affects the body's connective tissue

1. The incidence is higher among Afro-Americans, females, and those with genetic predisposition
2. It is a disease of remissions and exacerbations

B. The clinical manifestations present during the course of SLE fall into categories

1. Constitutional symptoms
    a. Fatigue
    b. Fever
    c. Weight loss
2. Musculoskeletal
    a. Arthralgia
    b. Arthritis

3. Skin and mucous membrane
   a. Butterfly rash
   b. Discoid rash
   c. Mucosal ulcers
4. Gastrointestinal
   a. Anorexia
   b. Vomiting
   c. Abdominal pain
5. Liver
   a. Hepatomegaly
   b. Enzyme elevation
   c. Chronic hepatitis
6. Cardiac disease
   a. Pericarditis
   b. Myocarditis
   c. Ischemia
   d. Hypertension
7. Pulmonary
   a. Chest pain
   b. Pleural effusion
   c. Pneumonitis
8. Hematological
   a. Anemia
   b. Leukopenia
   c. Thrombocytopenia
9. Renal
   a. Nephritis
   b. Nephrotic syndrome
   c. Hypertension
10. Nervous system
    a. Seizures
    b. Psychosis

C. To standardize the classification of SLE, a committee of the American Rheumatism Association proposed a list of 11 criteria; four or more of these clinical manifestations should be present to make the diagnosis of SLE

1. Malar rash (butterfly rash)
2. Discoid rash
3. Photosensitivity
4. Oral ulcers (usually painless)
5. Arthritis (involving two or more peripheral joints)
6. Serositis (pleuritis or pericarditis)
7. Renal disorder (persistent proteinuria over 0.5 g or cellular casts)
8. Neurological disorder (seizure or psychosis)
9. Hematological disorder (hemolytic anemia, leukopenia, lymphopenia, or thrombocytopenia)
10. Immunological disorder (positive lupus erythematosus cell, anti-DNA, anti-SM, or false-positive serological test for syphilis)
11. Antinuclear antibody (ANA)

D. The fetus is considered to be at higher risk than the mother with SLE

1. With maternal SLE, there is an increased risk of the following
   a. Spontaneous abortion
   b. Stillbirth
   c. Prematurity
   d. Neonatal death
2. Perinatal mortality is high as a result of IUGR and prematurity

3. SLE complicated by exacerbation at time of conception and during pregnancy, renal involvement, and hypertension increases the risk of perinatal mortality

4. Fetal surveillance usually begins at about 28 weeks' gestation

E. Neonatal effects of maternal SLE include neonatal lupus and congenital heart block; the dermatological and cardiac abnormalities develop when immune complexes cross the placental barrier and are deposited in the skin and along the conduction system of the heart

Clinical Practice

A. Assessment

1. History
   a. Duration and presence of signs and symptoms listed by the American Rheumatism Association
   b. Race: higher incidence among Afro-Americans
   c. Family history of SLE
   d. Obstetrical history
      (1) Stillbirth
      (2) Miscarriage
      (3) Neonatal death
      (4) IUGR
      (5) Prematurity
   e. Response to previous pregnancies
   f. Duration of exacerbations and remissions
2. Physical findings
   a. Constitutional symptoms
      (1) Fatigue
      (2) Fever
      (3) Weight loss
   b. Musculoskeletal
      (1) Arthralgia
      (2) Arthritis
   c. Skin and mucous membrane
      (1) Butterfly rash
      (2) Discoid rash
      (3) Mucosal ulcers
   d. Gastrointestinal
      (1) Anorexia
      (2) Vomiting
      (3) Abdominal pain
   e. Liver
      (1) Hepatomegaly
      (2) Enzyme elevation
      (3) Chronic hepatitis
   f. Cardiac disease
      (1) Pericarditis
      (2) Myocarditis
      (3) Ischemia
      (4) Hypertension
   g. Pulmonary
      (1) Chest pain
      (2) Pleural effusion
      (3) Pneumonitis
   h. Hematological
      (1) Anemia
      (2) Leukopenia

       (3) Thrombocytopenia
     i. Renal
       (1) Nephritis
       (2) Nephrotic syndrome
       (3) Hypertension
     j. Nervous system
       (1) Seizures
       (2) Psychosis
  3. Diagnostic procedures
    a. Laboratory value abnormalities found in clients with SLE are
       (1) Anemia
       (2) Leukopenia
       (3) Thrombocytopenia
       (4) Positive direct Coombs' test
       (5) Positive ANA (antinuclear antibody) test
       (6) Lupus erythematosus cells
       (7) Decreased complement levels
       (8) Increase in gamma globulin
       (9) Positive rheumatoid factor
       (10) False-positive syphilis test
       (11) Positive lupus anticoagulant
       (12) Prolonged prothrombin and thrombin time
       (13) Positive anticardiolipin antibody
    b. Critical laboratory tests to be performed are
       (1) CBC
       (2) Platelet count
       (3) Electrolytes
       (4) BUN
       (5) Creatinine clearance
       (6) Urinalysis
       (7) Urine protein quantification
       (8) SGPT
       (9) SGOT
       (10) Bilirubin
       (11) Erythrocyte sedimentation rate (ESR)
       (12) Serum ANA and complement
       (13) ECG

B. Nursing Diagnoses

1. High risk for infection related to corticosteroid therapy
2. Activity intolerance related to bed rest and limited activity
3. Alteration in comfort related to joint and systemic pain secondary to disease process
4. Powerlessness related to unpredictable course of disease process
5. Ineffective individual coping related to unpredictable course of physical and emotional condition
6. Knowledge deficit related to disease process and drug therapy
7. Anxiety related to complicated pregnancy
8. High risk for alteration in family process related to maternal complications of pregnancy and hospitalization
9. High risk for complications: pregnancy complicated by SLE

C. Interventions/Evaluations

1. High risk for infection related to corticosteroid therapy
    a. Interventions
       (1) Use aseptic technique for all potential sites of infection
       (2) Perform and instruct client in proper handwashing

(3) Maintain client's hydration with fluids

(4) Observe skin, joints, and extremities for areas of redness and swelling

(5) Encourage client to maintain caloric and protein intake

(6) Observe type, amount, and odor of discharge or drainage

(7) Assess client each shift for

    (a) Fundal tenderness

    (b) Pain, burning, and frequency of urination

    (c) Flank pain

(8) Assess for hyperthermia signs and symptoms

    (a) Fever

    (b) Chills

    (c) Client feels hot

(9) Monitor vital signs, especially temperature, every 4 hours and as needed

(10) Space activities and encourage adequate rest

(11) Monitor laboratory results, especially WBC

(12) Instruct client to avoid exposure to persons with known infectious processes

b. Evaluations

  (1) Client has no signs and symptoms of infection and remains afebrile

  (2) Client identifies signs and symptoms of infection in a timely manner

  (3) Client obtains appropriate medical and nursing intervention for infection

  (4) Client responds to treatment for infection in a timely manner

2. Activity intolerance related to bed rest and limited activity

a. Interventions

  (1) Assess activity tolerance

  (2) Assist client in modifying her schedule and spacing her activities to allow for more rest

  (3) Instruct client to maintain an activity level that is just short of fatigue

  (4) Provide long periods for sleep at night and frequent rest periods during the day

  (5) Assist client with ADL and ambulation

b. Evaluation: client tolerates progressive activities as evidenced by the following

  (1) Normal vital signs

  (2) Decreased dizziness, light-headedness, and weakness

3. Alteration in comfort related to joint and systemic pain secondary to disease process

a. Interventions

  (1) Assess pain-precipitating factors, quality, region radiation, severity, duration, and relieving factors; document deviation from baseline

  (2) Have client evaluate pain intensity on a 1 to 10 scale (10 being most severe)

  (3) Observe, report, and record verbal and nonverbal expressions of pain, fear, and anxiety

  (4) Provide and encourage rest periods and a restful environment

  (5) Medicate client with analgesics as ordered

  (6) Assess effectiveness of pain medications

  (7) Provide comfort measures

    (a) Reposition

    (b) Give skin care

    (c) Assist with ambulation and movement in bed

    (d) Splint client and assist her with coughing and deep breathing

  (8) Teach client and family about factors that contribute to pain experience

b. Evaluations

  (1) Client verbalizes decreased pain intensity (using a scale of 1 to 10) in

response to analgesics or other interventions within 1 hour of administration

(2) Client maintains pain control or absence of pain as evidenced by the following
   (a) Client's statement
   (b) Decreased use of analgesics
   (c) Increased activity

4. Powerlessness related to unpredictable course of disease process
   a. Interventions
      (1) Allow client opportunities to express her concerns and feelings
      (2) Provide a specific time during the shift when the client knows she can ask questions and discuss subjects of her choice
      (3) Inform client about her condition, treatment, and results
      (4) Point out the positive changes in the client's condition
      (5) Contact self-help support groups
      (6) Offer options when possible
         (a) Room arrangements
         (b) Daily plan of activities
         (c) Food choices
         (d) Short- and long-term goals
   b. Evaluations
      (1) Client identifies factors that she can control
      (2) Client makes decisions about her care, treatment, and activities

5. Ineffective individual coping related to unpredictable course of physical and emotional condition
   a. Interventions
      (1) Assist client in improving her self-esteem
      (2) Discuss the illness as a pathological process
      (3) Maintain a positive attitude to communicate that the client can overcome her physical and emotional problems
      (4) Assist client in communicating with self-help groups
      (5) Assist client in using alternative coping strategies: relaxation techniques, meditation
      (6) Set short-term coping goals with client
   b. Evaluations
      (1) Client verbalizes the need for continued treatment
      (2) Client expresses a sense of hope in dealing with the disease process and her future
      (3) Client uses alternative coping mechanisms to deal with stress

6. Knowledge deficit related to disease process and drug therapy
   a. Interventions
      (1) Assess client's and family members' readiness and ability to learn
      (2) Determine client's knowledge of her illness, its treatment, and preventive measures
      (3) Assess client's adherence to prescribed behavior, and its effect on her lifestyle
      (4) Begin client and family education regarding what connective tissue disease is and the effects it has on the mother and fetus
      (5) Provide information to enable the pregnant woman with connective tissue disease complications to obtain proper support and care
      (6) Discuss signs and symptoms to report
         (a) Chest pain
         (b) Bleeding
         (c) Confusion
         (d) Decreased ability to perform activities
         (e) Fever
         (f) Extreme fatigue

        (g) Edema

        (h) Anorexia

        (i) Vomiting

        (j) Abdominal pain

        (k) Weight loss

    (7) Explain the purpose of treatments, interventions, and tests

    (8) Teach client behavioral interventions

        (a) Bed rest in the lateral position (explain physiological rationale)

        (b) Observance of prescribed medication regimen

        (c) Maintenance of as quiet and stress-free an environment as possible

    (9) Explain to client the rationale and procedure for the following

        (a) NST

        (b) CST

        (c) Biophysical profile

        (d) Amniocentesis

  b. Evaluations

    (1) Client verbalizes an understanding of connective tissue disease and its effect on the fetus

    (2) Client is able to describe the disease process, causes, signs and symptoms, and interventions for disease control

7. Anxiety related to complicated pregnancy

  a. Interventions

    (1) Discuss client's fears and concerns about her pregnancy and its outcome

    (2) Provide reassurance and comfort

    (3) Obtain and begin involvement of MSW and other health team members

    (4) If possible and appropriate, have client's friends and family visit frequently; instruct about visiting hours

    (5) Encourage client to ask questions about tests, medicines, treatments, and physician orders

    (6) Explain all procedures and their purpose

    (7) Acknowledge client's feelings and respond in a manner appropriate to her needs

    (8) Encourage interest in diversional activities (e.g., crafts, books, music)

    (9) Maintain clean, orderly, quiet, and stress-free environment

    (10) Assess family members' level of anxiety and knowledge of disease process; assess them as a support system for client

    (11) Arrange for infant special care staff to visit with client; orient client to realistic expectations

    (12) Encourage client to use visualization exercises, music, and crafts for relaxation

  b. Evaluations

    (1) Client verbalizes her fears and concerns about her pregnancy

    (2) Client feels supported and listened to

    (3) Client is able to relax and sleep

8. High risk for alteration in family process related to maternal complications of pregnancy and hospitalization

  a. Interventions

    (1) Allow client and her family members to ventilate their fears about pregnancy outcome

    (2) Assess client's and family members' responses to complicated pregnancy

        (a) Presence of unresolved guilt, blame, hostility, or jealousy

        (b) Inability to problem solve adequately

        (c) Ineffective patterns of communication

        (d) Observe client's interactions with her family members

    (3) Assess level of financial burden on family

(4) Discuss effects of prolonged hospitalization on the family process

(5) Encourage client and her family to participate in support groups and education programs

(6) Utilize outside resources

   (a) MSW

   (b) Clinical nurse specialist

   (c) Clinical psychologist

   (d) Lay support and self-help groups

   (e) Home health care

   (f) Financial assistance programs

(7) Assist family in reorganizing roles at home and setting priorities to maintain family integrity and reduce stress

(8) Aid family members in changing their expectations of the client in a realistic manner

(9) Encourage frequent visits by client's family members

(10) Make sure family members are oriented to visiting hours, bathrooms, cafeteria, gift shop, etc.

(11) Prepare client and her family members for signs of depression, anxiety, and dependency

(12) Meet the physical needs of the client

(13) Assess client's spiritual needs and help her to meet those needs

b. Evaluations: client and family demonstrate a functional system of mutual support as evidenced by the following

(1) Seeking appropriate external resources when needed

(2) Engaging in open communication between family members and health team

(3) Participating in care of hospitalized family member

9. High risk for complications: pregnancy complicated by SLE

a. Interventions

(1) Prevent further complications for the SLE client

   (a) Identify the many signs and symptoms and forms of SLE

   (b) Alleviate the symptoms of SLE

   (c) Monitor the pregnant SLE client for placental competency and fetal well-being

(2) Observe for varied signs and symptoms indicating exacerbation of SLE

(3) Distinguish between the symptoms of SLE and pre-eclampsia

(4) Monitor client closely for pre-eclampsia

(5) Administer prescribed medications and observe for side effects of

   (a) Corticosteroids

   (b) Salicylates

   (c) Nonsteroidal anti-inflammatory agents

   (d) Analgesics

   (e) Antipyretics

   (f) Immunosuppressants

(6) Educate client about the drugs being administered and their side effects

(7) Protect client from infection

(8) Observe client's vital signs for small changes and trends that can indicate systemic disease

(9) Observe client for signs and symptoms of glucose intolerance due to corticosteroids

(10) Observe client for signs and symptoms of deteriorating cardiovascular and renal status

(11) Observe client closely for worsening condition in the postpartum period

(12) Observe client for early signs and symptoms of psychosis

   (a) Restlessness

   (b) Distractibility

    (c) Emotional sensitivity
    (d) Confusion
    (e) Vague personality changes
    (f) Disorientation
  b. Evaluations: client has remission or absence of signs and symptoms of SLE
    (1) Malar rash (butterfly rash)
    (2) Discoid rash
    (3) Photosensitivity
    (4) Oral ulcers (usually painless)
    (5) Arthritis (involving two or more peripheral joints)
    (6) Serositis (pleuritis or pericarditis)
    (7) Renal disorder (persistent proteinuria of more than 0.5 g or cellular casts)
    (8) Neurological disorder (seizure or psychosis)
    (9) Hematological disorder (hemolytic anemia, leukopenia, lymphopenia, or thrombocytopenia)
    (10) Immunological disorder (positive lupus erythematosus cell, anti-DNA, anti-SM, or false positive serologic test for syphilis)
    (11) Antinuclear antibody (ANA)

Health Education

A. Discuss the increased incidence of spontaneous abortions, stillbirths, IUGR, and perinatal complications

B. Discuss the increased incidence of maternal nephritis, placental insufficiency, and pre-eclampsia

C. Discuss the need for close monitoring of client's condition during pregnancy

D. Encourage client to keep appointments with her internist or rheumatologist and her obstetrician or perinatologist

E. Teach client importance of frequent monitoring of creatinine clearance, proteinuria, and hematological parameters

F. Teach self-monitoring of weight gain, edema, and blood pressure

G. Teach clients about SLE signs and symptoms, prescribed medications, and side effects

H. Teach client to avoid exposure to infection

I. Teach client to get adequate sleep with frequent rest periods

J. Ensure adequate nutrition with prescribed diet and fluid intake

K. Teach the client that corticosteroids, a strong immunosuppressant, can mask the symptoms of infection

L. Teach client to avoid exposure to persons with known infectious processes

M. Plan with client how she can avoid periods of fatigue or stress

Hematological Complications

Introduction

A. The anemias

1. Depending on the group studied, about 20 to 50% of pregnant women are anemic

2. Pregnant women with anemia have a higher incidence of puerperal complications than do women with normal hemoglobin values
3. The most common cause of anemia in pregnancy is iron deficiency, the diagnosis of which is best made through laboratory studies
   a. Hemoglobin below 11 g/dl or hematocrit below 35%
   b. Signs and symptoms
      (1) Pallor
      (2) Fatigue
      (3) Decreased exercise tolerance
      (4) Anorexia
      (5) Weakness
      (6) Malaise
      (7) Dyspnea
      (8) Edema
4. Folic acid deficiency produces anemia of the megaloblastic type in pregnancy
   a. Caused by increased folate demands of pregnancy and decreased GI absorption
   b. Usually found in combination with iron deficiency
5. Sickle cell anemia
   a. Recessive, hereditary, familial, hemolytic anemia
      (1) Occurs when the gene for the production of S hemoglobin is inherited from both parents
      (2) When S hemoglobin gene is transmitted from only one parent, offspring usually has the sickle cell trait, not the anemia
   b. Defect in the hemoglobin causes erythrocytes to be shaped like a sickle
   c. Stimulators of the sickling process
      (1) Hypoxia
      (2) Hypertension
      (3) Acidosis
      (4) Dehydration
      (5) Exertion
      (6) Infection
   d. Characteristics of the disorder
      (1) Chronic anemia
      (2) Increased susceptibility to infection
      (3) Intermittent episodes of vascular occlusion by the abnormal erythrocytes
   e. Occurs most commonly in people of Afro-American or Mediterranean ancestry
   f. Pregnant women with sickle cell anemia are prone to other disorders
      (1) Pyelonephritis
      (2) Urinary tract infection
      (3) Leg ulcers
      (4) Bone infection
      (5) Cardiopathy
   g. Signs and symptoms of sickle cell crisis and of exacerbation of the disease
      (1) Pain in the abdomen, chest, vertebrae, or extremities
      (2) Sudden anemia
      (3) Marked pallor
      (4) Cardiac failure
6. Thalassemia (Mediterranean or Cooley's anemia) is an anemia in which an insufficient amount of hemoglobin is produced to fill the RBCs; it is a hereditary disease that involves abnormal synthesis of the alpha or beta chains of hemoglobin, which leads to premature RBC death
   a. Thalassemia minor produces a mild but persistent anemia, but the RBC count may be normal and there usually are no systemic problems
   b. The thalassemias occur most commonly in people of Mediterranean, Middle Eastern, Southeast Asia, or Chinese descent

B. Thrombocytopenia

1. Thrombocytopenia can be a consequence of the following
   a. Inadequate production of platelets
   b. Increased peripheral consumption of platelets
   c. Destruction of platelets
2. Numerous drugs, chemicals, and physical agents can influence platelet production
3. The body can develop an antiplatelet antibody that is responsible for destruction of platelets; this immune process is called idiopathic thrombocytopenia purpura
4. The signs and symptoms of thrombocytopenia include the signs and symptoms of bleeding
   a. Petechiae
   b. Oozing from the IV site or wound
   c. Hematuria
   d. Hematemesis
   e. Hemoptysis
   f. Signs of cerebral hemorrhage
5. Laboratory tests diagnostic of thrombocytopenia
   a. Low platelet count
   b. Prolonged bleeding time

C. Thrombophlebitis

1. During pregnancy, there is an increased potential for thromboses resulting from increased levels of coagulation factors and decreased fibrinolysis
2. Clients at high risk for thromboembolic disease during pregnancy include those with the following
   a. History of pulmonary embolus
   b. Deep vein thrombosis
   c. Artificial heart valves
   d. Primary hypercoagulable disorders
   e. Obesity
   f. Operative delivery
   g. Prolonged immobilization
3. Common signs and symptoms of deep vein thrombosis
   a. Pain
   b. Tenderness
   c. Edema
   d. Change in limb color
   e. Calf pain with passive dorsiflexion (Homans' sign)

D. Fetal Implications

1. Chronic anemia limits the amount of oxygen available for fetal oxygenation and increases the risk for the following
   a. Abortion
   b. Premature birth
   c. Small-for-gestational age neonates
2. With idiopathic thrombocytopenia purpura (ITP), the fetus is at risk for hemorrhage in utero or after birth because the antiplatelet antibodies are actively transported across the placenta, causing thrombocytopenia

Clinical Practice

A. Assessment

1. History
   a. Iron-deficiency anemia: specifically investigate evidence of decreased dietary iron intake

592   Core Curriculum for Maternal-Newborn Nursing

      b. Sickle cell anemia
        (1) Family history
        (2) Afro-American or Mediterranean ancestry
      c. Thalassemia: Mediterranean, Middle Eastern, Southeast Asian, or Chinese descent
      d. Thrombocytopenia: family history
      e. Thrombophlebitis
        (1) Pulmonary embolus
        (2) Deep vein thrombosis
        (3) Artificial heart valve
        (4) Hypercoagulable disorder
        (5) Prolonged immobilization
        (6) Obesity
2. Physical findings: signs and symptoms specific to the diagnosed hematologic disorder
      a. Iron-deficiency anemia
        (1) Pallor
        (2) Fatigue
        (3) Decreased exercise tolerance
        (4) Anorexia
        (5) Weakness
        (6) Malaise
        (7) Dyspnea
        (8) Edema
      b. Sickle cell anemia or sickle cell crisis
        (1) Pain in the abdomen, chest, vertebrae, joints, or extremities
        (2) Sudden anemia
        (3) Marked pallor
        (4) Cardiac failure
      c. Thalassemia: mild persistent anemia with no unusual systemic problems
      d. Thrombocytopenia: signs and symptoms of bleeding
        (1) Petechiae
        (2) Oozing from IV site or wound
        (3) Hematuria
        (4) Hemoptysis
        (5) Signs of cerebral hemorrhage
      e. Thrombophlebitis
        (1) Pain
        (2) Tenderness
        (3) Edema
        (4) Change in limb color
        (5) Calf pain with dorsiflexion (Homans' sign)
3. Diagnostic procedures: evaluate laboratory data for indicators or presence of specific disorder
      a. Iron-deficiency anemia
        (1) Hemoglobin below 11 g/dl
        (2) Hematocrit less than 35%
      b. Sickle cell anemia: defective red blood cells shaped like a sickle
      c. Thalassemia
        (1) Mild persistent anemia
        (2) Normal RBC count
      d. Thrombocytopenia
        (1) Low platelet count
        (2) Prolonged bleeding time
      e. Thrombophlebitis
        (1) Increased WBC count
        (2) Larger calf or thigh circumference

f. Fetal assessment
(1) Ultrasound testing
(2) Antepartal FHR testing
(3) Fetal lung maturity if need for delivery is imminent

B. Nursing Diagnoses

1. Alteration in tissue perfusion related to deep vein thrombosis or thrombophlebitis
2. Alteration in comfort related to sickling process
3. Activity intolerance related to fatigue and malaise
4. High risk for infection related to decreased systemic resistance secondary to loss of antibodies
5. Knowledge deficit related to disease process and drug therapy
6. Anxiety related to complicated pregnancy
7. High risk for alteration in family process related to maternal complications and hospitalization
8. High risk for bleeding

C. Interventions/Evaluations

1. Alteration in tissue perfusion related to deep vein thrombosis or thrombophlebitis
   a. Interventions
      (1) Assess extremity
         (a) Temperature
         (b) Color
         (c) Pulses
         (d) Capillary refill
         (e) Swelling sensation
         (f) Movement
         (g) Strength
      (2) Elevate or position leg on pillows or use foot cradle as indicated
      (3) Reduce or remove external compression that impedes flow: pillows, leg crossing
      (4) Change client's position every 2 hours while she is on bed rest
      (5) Measure and record calf and thigh circumference
      (6) Assess skin integrity
      (7) Assess for complications of deep vein thrombosis
         (a) Sudden chest pain
         (b) Cough
         (c) Dyspnea
         (d) Change in level of consciousness
      (8) Administer anticoagulant medications as ordered
      (9) Give instructions to client concerning medications and side effects of bleeding
      (10) Assess for signs and symptoms of bleeding if client is on anticoagulants
         (a) Petechiae
         (b) Hematemesis
         (c) Hematuria
         (d) Epistaxis
         (e) Blood in stool
         (f) Bleeding from gums
         (g) Hematocrit
         (h) Platelets
   b. Evaluations
      (1) Adequate circulation to lower extremities maintained
         (a) Warmth
         (b) Pink color

          (c) Palpable pulses

          (d) No swelling

          (e) Immediate capillary refill

          (f) Movement

          (g) Sensation

          (h) Strength

          (i) Tone intact

          (j) Skin integrity

      (2) Client has no symptoms of bleeding

          (a) Hematuria

          (b) Hematemesis

          (c) Epistaxis

          (d) Hemoptysis

          (e) Blood in stool

          (f) Vaginal bleeding

      (3) Client has no evidence of complications of deep vein thrombosis

  2. Alteration in comfort related to sickling process

    a. Interventions

      (1) Assess pain-precipitating factors, quality, region radiation, severity, duration, and relieving factors; document deviation from baseline

      (2) Have client evaluate pain intensity on a 1 to 10 scale (10 being most severe)

      (3) Observe, report, and record verbal and nonverbal expressions of pain, fear, and anxiety

      (4) Provide and encourage rest periods and a restful environment

      (5) Medicate with analgesics as ordered

      (6) Assess effectiveness of pain medications

      (7) Provide comfort measures

          (a) Reposition

          (b) Give skin care

          (c) Assist with ambulation and movement in bed

          (d) Splint client and assist her with coughing and deep breathing

      (8) Teach client and her family about factors that contribute to pain experience

      (9) Monitor CBC, hemoglobin, hematocrit, and platelets

     (10) Maintain hydration and nutrition with adequate fluid and food intake

     (11) Assess extremities

          (a) Pain

          (b) Edema

          (c) Pulses

          (d) Temperature

          (e) Color

          (f) Sensation

          (g) Tone

          (h) Movement

     (12) Force fluids to ensure adequate hydration in sickle cell crisis

    b. Evaluations

      (1) Client verbalizes decreased pain intensity (using a scale of 1 to 10) in response to analgesics or other interventions within 1 hour of administration

      (2) Client maintains pain control or absence of pain as evidenced by the following

          (a) Client's statement

          (b) Decreased use of analgesics

          (c) Increased activity

  3. Activity intolerance related to fatigue and malaise

    a. Interventions

(1) Assess activity tolerance
(2) Assist client in modifying her schedule and spacing her activities to allow for more rest
(3) Maintain client's activity level just short of fatigue
(4) Provide long periods for sleep at night and frequent rest periods during the day
(5) Assist client with ADL and ambulation
b. Evaluation: client tolerates progressive activities as evidenced by the following
(1) Normal vital signs
(2) Decreased dizziness, light-headedness, and weakness
4. High risk for infection related to decreased systemic resistance secondary to loss of antibodies
a. Interventions
(1) Use aseptic technique for all potential sites of infection
(2) Perform and instruct client in proper handwashing
(3) Maintain client's hydration with fluids
(4) Observe skin, joints, and extremities for areas of redness and swelling
(5) Encourage client to maintain caloric and protein intake
(6) Observe type, amount, and odor of discharge or drainage
(7) Assess client each shift for the following
(a) Fundal tenderness
(b) Pain, burning, and frequency of urination
(c) Flank pain
(8) Assess for hyperthermia signs and symptoms
(a) Fever
(b) Chills
(c) Patient feels hot
(9) Monitor vital signs, especially temperature, every 4 hours and as needed
(10) Space client's activities and encourage adequate rest
(11) Monitor laboratory results especially WBC count
(12) Instruct client to avoid exposure to persons with known infectious processes
b. Evaluations
(1) Client has no signs and symptoms of infection and remains afebrile
(2) Client identifies signs and symptoms of infection in a timely manner
(3) Client obtains appropriate medical and nursing intervention for infection
(4) Client responds to treatment for infection in a timely manner
5. Knowledge deficit related to disease process and drug therapy
a. Interventions
(1) Assess client's and family members' readiness and ability to learn
(2) Determine client's knowledge of her illness, its treatment, and preventive measures
(3) Assess client's adherence to prescribed behavior, and its effects on her lifestyle
(4) Begin client and family education regarding what hematological disease is and the effects it has on the mother and fetus
(5) Provide information to enable the pregnant woman with hematological complications to obtain proper support and care
(6) Discuss signs and symptoms to report
(a) Shortness of breath
(b) Dyspnea
(c) Decreased ability to perform activities
(d) Extreme fatigue
(e) Edema

           (f) Anorexia

           (g) Pain or swelling in joints or extremities

       (7) Explain the purpose of treatments, interventions, and tests

       (8) Teach client behavioral interventions

           (a) Bed rest in the lateral position (explain physiological rationale)

           (b) Observance of prescribed medication regimen

           (c) Maintenance of as quiet and stress-free an environment as possible

       (9) Explain to client the rationale and procedure for the following

           (a) NST

           (b) CST

           (c) Biophysical profile

           (d) Amniocentesis

  b. Evaluations

       (1) Client verbalizes an understanding of hematological disease and its effect on the fetus

       (2) Client is able to describe the hematological disease process, causes, signs and symptoms, and interventions for disease control

6. Anxiety related to complicated pregnancy

  a. Interventions

       (1) Discuss client's fears and concerns about her pregnancy and its outcome

       (2) Provide reassurance and comfort

       (3) Obtain and begin involvement of MSW and other health team members

       (4) If possible and appropriate, have client's friends and family visit frequently; instruct them about visiting hours

       (5) Encourage client to ask questions about tests, medicines, treatments, and physician orders

       (6) Explain all procedures and their purpose

       (7) Acknowledge client's feelings and respond in a manner appropriate to her needs

       (8) Encourage interest in diversional activities (e.g., crafts, books, music)

       (9) Maintain clean, orderly, quiet, and stress-free environment

      (10) Assess family members' level of anxiety and knowledge of disease process; assess them as a support system for the client

      (11) Arrange for infant special care staff to visit with client; orient client to realistic expectations

      (12) Encourage client to use visualization exercises, music and crafts for relaxation

  b. Evaluations

       (1) Client verbalizes her fears and concerns about her pregnancy

       (2) Client feels supported and listened to

       (3) Client is able to relax and sleep

7. High risk for alteration in family process related to maternal complications and hospitalization

  a. Interventions

       (1) Allow client and her family members to ventilate their fears about pregnancy outcome

       (2) Assess client's and family members' responses to complicated pregnancy

           (a) Presence of unresolved guilt, blame, hostility, or jealousy

           (b) Inability to problem solve adequately

           (c) Ineffective patterns of communication

           (d) Observe client's interactions with her family members

       (3) Assess level of financial burden on family

       (4) Discuss effects of prolonged hospitalization on the family process

       (5) Encourage client and her family to participate in support groups and education programs

       (6) Use outside resources
         (a) MSW
         (b) Clinical nurse specialist
         (c) Clinical psychologist
         (d) Lay support and self-help groups
         (e) Home health care
         (f) Financial assistance programs
       (7) Assist family in reorganizing roles at home and setting priorities to maintain family integrity and to reduce stress
       (8) Aid family members in changing their expectations of the client in a realistic manner
       (9) Encourage frequent visits by family members
      (10) Make sure family members are oriented to visiting hours, bathrooms, cafeteria, gift shop, and so forth
      (11) Prepare client and her family members for signs of depression, anxiety, and dependency
      (12) Meet the physical needs of the client
      (13) Assess client's spiritual needs and help her to meet those needs
  b. Evaluations: client and family demonstrate a functional system of mutual support for each other as evidenced by the following
      (1) Seeking appropriate external resources when needed
      (2) Engage in open communication between family members and health team
      (3) Participating in care of hospitalized family member
8. High risk for bleeding
  a. Interventions
      (1) Monitor client's vital signs every 4 hours or more frequently as indicated
      (2) Observe for and report signs and symptoms of bleeding
         (a) Epistaxis
         (b) Hematemesis
         (c) Hematuria
         (d) Petechiae
         (e) Bleeding gums
         (f) Increased vaginal bleeding
         (g) Wound drainage
         (h) Hematomas
      (3) Monitor bleeding time, CBC, and platelets
      (4) Observe color, consistency, and amount of stool and urine
      (5) Administer blood products per physician order following hospital protocol
  b. Evaluations
      (1) Client demonstrates no evidence of bleeding as shown by absence of the following
         (a) Epistaxis
         (b) Hematemesis
         (c) Hematuria
         (d) Petechiae
         (e) Blood in the stool
         (f) Hemoptysis
         (g) Bleeding gums
         (h) Increased vaginal bleeding
      (2) Client verbalizes signs and symptoms of bleeding
      (3) Client has a return to optimal blood levels of CBC, platelets, and bleeding time in 1 week

Health Education

Educate the client about nutrition, medications, lifestyle, activity, and rest to prevent and treat hematological disorders of pregnancy

A. Encourage client to keep appointments with her internist or hematologist and obstetrician

B. Teach client how to prevent conditions that cause sickling and other exacerbations of hematological disorders

C. Teach client to avoid exposure to people with infection

D. Teach client to avoid periods of fatigue or stress

E. Plan with client how she can get adequate sleep and take frequent rests

F. Ensure adequate nutrition with prescribed diet and fluid intake

G. Teach client about her condition: the signs and symptoms, prescribed medications, and side effects

H. Counsel client preconceptually when indicated

I. Teach client about contraceptive measures

Gastrointestinal Complications of Pregnancy

Introduction

A. Hyperemesis gravidarum—pernicious nausea and vomiting of pregnancy— is more common in Western civilizations

1. This severe nausea and vomiting occurs as a result of nutritional deficiency and fluid and electrolyte imbalance
2. In severe cases, weight loss, acetonuria, and ketosis may occur with potential neurological, hepatic, and renal damage
3. The cause of this condition is a combination of psychological and physiological factors
4. Table 33–3 describes hyperemesis according to the useful laboratory tests, potential results, and rationale

B. Inflammatory bowel disease affects primarily the age group that includes women of childbearing years; inflammatory bowel disease includes disorders such as regional enteritis, ulcerative colitis, and Crohn's colitis

Table 33–3
DESCRIPTION OF HYPEREMESIS

Laboratory Test Serum Electrolyte	Result	Rationale
K	Hypokalemia	Loss of electrolytes with vomiting
Na	Hyponatremia	
Cl	Hypochloremia	
Acid base and pH	Combined acid–base disorder	
	Acidosis	Acidosis—starvation, ketosis
	Alkalosis	Alkalosis—secondary to loss of hydrogen and potassium in vomitus
Kidney function		
Creatinine	Elevated	Decreased renal function
BUN	Elevated	

1. The effects of inflammatory bowel disease on pregnancy and vice versa are not significant in incidence, but the disorder is harder to recognize and treat
   a. X-ray study is usually contraindicated, and signs and symptoms may be confusing
   b. Ultrasound testing is considered to be safe and helpful
2. Spontaneous abortion rates are higher in clients with Crohn's disease
3. The incidence of prematurity and congenital deformity, however, does not increase with gastrointestinal (GI) disturbances

Clinical Practice

A. Assessment

1. History
   a. The following factors should be obtained from the client for inclusion in the data base
      (1) Abdominal pain or distension
      (2) Nausea and vomiting
      (3) Diarrhea
      (4) Indigestion
   b. Signs and symptoms that accompany precipitating factors
2. Physical findings
   a. Signs and symptoms of GI disturbances
      (1) Anorexia
      (2) Nausea and vomiting
      (3) Indigestion
      (4) Abdominal pain or distension
      (5) Diarrhea
   b. Signs and symptoms of fluid and electrolyte imbalance and nutritional deficiencies
      (1) Dry mucous membranes
      (2) Poor skin turgor
      (3) Malaise
      (4) Low blood pressure
   c. Symptoms of severe fluid and electrolyte imbalance and nutritional deficiency
      (1) Weight loss
      (2) Acetonuria
      (3) Ketosis
3. Diagnostic procedures: laboratory studies (see Table 33–3)—electrolytes, acid–base studies, renal function studies

B. Nursing Diagnoses

1. Fluid volume deficit related to decreased fluid intake and nausea, vomiting, or diarrhea
2. Alteration in comfort related to abdominal pain or nausea and vomiting
3. Activity intolerance related to nutritional, fluid, and electrolyte imbalance
4. Alteration in nutrition: less than body requirements related to anorexia, nausea, vomiting, or diarrhea
5. Anxiety related to complicated pregnancy
6. Knowledge deficit related to GI disturbance , complicated pregnancy
7. High risk for alteration in family process related to maternal complications and hospitalization

C. Interventions/Evaluations

1. Fluid volume deficit related to decreased fluid intake and nausea, vomiting, or diarrhea

a. Interventions
   (1) Monitor client's vital signs
   (2) Hydrate client adequately
   (3) Monitor client's I&O
   (4) Assess client's skin turgor, color, and temperature
   (5) Observe client's urine for color, consistency, and amount
   (6) Assess amount, color, and consistency of client's vomitus and stool
   (7) Assess client's oral mucous membranes
   (8) Assess level of consciousness
   (9) Weigh client daily, noting loss or gain
   (10) Assess client for edema of the legs, arms, hands, or sacral region
   (11) Auscultate client's lungs every shift and as needed
   (12) Observe client for cough, dyspnea, tachypnea, and sputum
   (13) Administer parenteral fluids, electrolytes, antiemetics, and supplements as prescribed and as needed
b. Evaluations: client responds to treatment to correct alteration in fluid volume as evidenced by the following
   (1) Balanced I&O
   (2) Maintenance of normal weight
   (3) Absence of edema
   (4) Clear lungs
   (5) Vital signs within normal limits
   (6) Normal laboratory values
   (7) Good skin turgor
   (8) Normal level of consciousness
   (9) Moist mucous membranes
2. Alteration in comfort related to abdominal pain or nausea and vomiting
   a. Interventions
      (1) Assess pain-precipitating factors, quality, region radiation, severity, duration, relieving factors; document any deviation from baseline
      (2) Have client evaluate pain intensity on a 1 to 10 scale (10 being most severe)
      (3) Observe, report, and record verbal and nonverbal expressions of pain, fear, and anxiety
      (4) Provide and encourage rest periods and a restful environment
      (5) Medicate client with analgesics or antiemetics as ordered
      (6) Assess effectiveness of pain medications
      (7) Provide comfort measures
         (a) Reposition
         (b) Give skin care
         (c) Assist with ambulation and movement in bed
         (d) Splint client and assist her with coughing and deep breathing
      (8) Teach client and her family about factors that contribute to pain experience
   b. Evaluations
      (1) Client verbalizes decreased pain intensity (using a scale of 1 to 10) in response to analgesics or other interventions within 1 hour of administration
      (2) Client maintains pain control or absence of abdominal pain and nausea and vomiting as evidenced by the following
         (a) Client's statement
         (b) Decreased use of analgesics
         (c) Increased activity
3. Activity intolerance related to nutritional, fluid, and electrolyte imbalance
   a. Interventions
      (1) Assess client's activity tolerance
      (2) Assist client in modifying her schedule and spacing her activities to allow for more rest

(3) Maintain client's activity level just short of fatigue

(4) Provide long periods for sleep at night and frequent rest periods during the day

(5) Assist client with ADL and ambulation

b. Evaluation: client tolerates progressive activities as evidenced by the following

(1) Normal vital signs

(2) Decreased dizziness, light-headedness, and weakness

4. Alteration in nutrition: less than body requirements related to anorexia, nausea, vomiting, or diarrhea

a. Interventions

(1) Assess client's nutritional status and fluid balance stability by monitoring the following

(a) Weight

(b) Condition of mucous membranes

(c) Skin turgor

(2) Discuss pregnancy changes in first trimester

(a) Morning sickness

(b) Small, frequent, meals of dry foods

(c) Toast and crackers before rising in the morning

(3) Discuss signs and symptoms of hypoglycemia

(a) Shaking

(b) Fast heartbeat

(c) Sweating

(d) Tingling

(e) Personality change

(f) Dizziness

(g) Hunger

(h) Blurred vision

(i) Nervousness

(j) Excitedness

(k) Pale and moist skin

(l) Drowsiness

(m) Headache

(n) Fatigue

(o) Irritability

(4) Maintain odor-free, well-ventilated room

(5) Assess the client's affect and response to her family, environment, and pregnancy

(6) Reduce or eliminate factors that contribute to anorexia, nausea, vomiting, and diarrhea

(7) Consult with nutritionist and dietician

(8) Obtain history of client's food allergies, likes and dislikes, and usual diet

(9) Administer progressive diets according to the client's tolerance

(a) Small frequent feedings

(b) Liquids at effective times before or after a meal

(10) Help client maintain good oral hygiene before and after ingestion of food

(11) Give client instructions according to proper diet

(a) Foods and liquids to avoid

(b) Specific times to eat specific foods

(c) Alternate sources of foods

(12) Initiate health teaching and referrals as indicated

b. Evaluations: client maintains adequate nutrition as evidenced by the following

(1) Adequate weight gain

(2) Eating a well-balanced diet

(3) An understanding of her condition

(4) An ability to choose a proper diet

5. Anxiety related to complicated pregnancy
   a. Interventions
      (1) Discuss client's fears and concerns about her pregnancy and its outcome
      (2) Provide reassurance and comfort
      (3) Obtain and begin involvement of MSW and other health team members
      (4) If possible and appropriate, have client's friends and family visit frequently; instruct them about visiting hours
      (5) Encourage client to ask questions about tests, medicines, treatments, and physician orders
      (6) Explain all procedures and their purpose
      (7) Acknowledge client's feelings and respond in a manner appropriate to her needs
      (8) Encourage interest in diversional activities (e.g., crafts, books, music)
      (9) Maintain clean, orderly, quiet, and stress-free environment
      (10) Assess family members' level of anxiety and knowledge of disease process; assess them as a support system for the client
      (11) Arrange for infant special care staff to visit with patient; orient client to realistic expectations
      (12) Encourage client to use visualization exercises, music, and crafts for relaxation
   b. Evaluations
      (1) Client verbalizes her fears and concerns about her pregnancy
      (3) Client feels supported and listened to
      (3) Client is able to relax and sleep
6. Knowledge deficit related to GI disturbance, complicated pregnancy
   a. Interventions
      (1) Assess client's and family members' readiness and ability to learn
      (2) Determine client's knowledge of her illness, its treatment, and preventive measures
      (3) Assess client's adherence to prescribed behavior and its effect on her lifestyle
      (4) Begin client and family education regarding what GI disease is and the effects it has on the mother and fetus
      (5) Provide information to enable the pregnant woman with GI complications to obtain proper support and care
      (6) Discuss signs and symptoms to report
         (a) Anorexia
         (b) Nausea
         (c) Vomiting
         (d) Weight loss
         (e) Abdominal pain or distension
         (f) Diarrhea
         (g) Decreased ability to perform activities
         (h) Extreme fatigue
         (i) Decreased urine output
         (j) Dry mucous membranes
         (k) Poor skin turgor
      (7) Explain the purpose of treatments, interventions, and tests
      (8) Teach client behavioral interventions
         (a) Bed rest in the lateral position (explain physiological rationale)
         (b) Observance of prescribed medication regimen
         (c) Maintenance of as quiet and stress-free an environment as possible
      (9) Explain to client the rationale and procedure for the following
         (a) NST

        (b) CST
        (c) Biophysical profile
        (d) Amniocentesis
  b. Evaluations
    (1) Client verbalizes an understanding of GI disease and its effect on the fetus
    (2) Client is able to describe the GI disease process, its causes, signs and symptoms, and interventions for disease control

7. High risk for alteration in family process related to maternal complications and hospitalization
  a. Interventions
    (1) Allow client and her family members to ventilate their fears about pregnancy outcome
    (2) Assess client's and family members' responses to complicated pregnancy
        (a) Presence of unresolved guilt, blame, hostility or jealousy
        (b) Inability to problem solve adequately
        (c) Ineffective patterns of communication
        (d) Observe client's interactions with her family members
    (3) Assess level of financial burden on family
    (4) Discuss effects of prolonged hospitalization on the family process
    (5) Encourage client and her family to participate in support groups and education programs
    (6) Use outside resources
        (a) MSW
        (b) Clinical nurse specialist
        (c) Clinical psychologist
        (d) Lay support and self-help groups
        (e) Home health care
        (f) Financial assistance programs
    (7) Assist family in reorganizing roles at home and setting priorities to maintain family integrity and to reduce stress
    (8) Aid family members in changing their expectations of the client in a realistic manner
    (9) Encourage frequent visits by family members
    (10) Make sure family members are oriented to visiting hours, bathrooms, cafeteria, gift shop, and so forth
    (11) Prepare client and her family members for signs of depression, anxiety, and dependency
    (12) Meet the physical needs of the client
    (13) Assess client's spiritual needs and help her to meet those needs
  b. Evaluations: client and family demonstrate a functional system of mutual support for each other as evidenced by the following
    (1) Seeking appropriate external resources when needed
    (2) Engage in open communication between family members and health team
    (3) Participating in care of hospitalized family member

Health Education

A. Give specific diet and nutritional information and directions: amount, type, and time for food and liquid

B. Teach danger signs and symptoms of pregnancy to report to physician

C. Plan with the client how she can get adequate sleep and take frequent rests

D. Teach client to avoid fatigue or stress

Hepatic Complications of Pregnancy

Introduction

A. Acute fatty liver disease of pregnancy, a rare and severe disease of unknown cause, occurs in the third trimester, or at about the 36th week of gestation

1. Characteristics of affected women
   a. Usually primigravidas
   b. Increased frequency in twin gestation
   c. Incidence is 1/13,000
2. For diagnosis, the physician rules out other disorders
   a. Acute viral hepatitis
   b. Cholestasis of pregnancy
   c. Pre-eclampsia
3. Usual treatment
   a. Stabilization of the client
   b. Immediate delivery
   c. Intensive medical and nursing support
4. Major signs and symptoms
   a. Abdominal pain
   b. Nausea and vomiting
   c. Jaundice
   d. Hypoglycemia
   e. Coma

B. The client's condition can deteriorate rapidly

1. Poor prognosis and high mortality rates (approximately 20%)
2. Associated problems
   a. Hepatic failure
   b. Hepatic coma
   c. Coagulopathy
3. Associated with a high incidence of stillbirth

Clinical Practice

A. Assessment

1. History
   a. Gestation age (disease of third trimester)
   b. Gravida (primigravida)
   c. Possible multiple gestation
2. Physical findings
   a. Nausea and vomiting
   b. Malaise
   c. Fatigue
   d. Abdominal pain
   e. Jaundice
   f. Petechiae
   g. Signs and symptoms of pre-eclampsia
   h. Altered sensorium; coma in advanced cases
   i. Ascites
   j. Preterm labor
   k. Vaginal bleeding
3. Diagnostic procedures: evaluate laboratory studies for the following
   a. Elevated amylase, ammonia, creatinine, and transamylase levels
   b. Hyperbilirubinemia
   c. Hyperuricemia

d. Decreased antithrombin III
 e. Thrombocytopenia
 f. Hypofibrinogenemia
 g. Hypoglycemia
 h. Proteinuria
 i. Increased fibrin split products
 j. Prolonged prothrombin time
 k. Anemia
 l. Leukocytosis

B. Nursing Diagnoses

1. Activity intolerance related to malaise and lethargy
2. Anxiety related to complicated pregnancy
3. Ineffective individual and family coping related to poor progress and seriousness of condition
4. High risk for alteration in family process related to maternal complications of pregnancy and hospitalization
5. High risk for infection related to systemic disease and lowered resistance
6. Knowledge deficit related to pregnancy complicated by hepatic disease
7. Alteration in nutrition related to anorexia, nausea, vomiting, and diarrhea
8. Powerlessness related to the unpredictable course of the disease process
9. Self-care deficit related to lethargy, malaise, or confusion
10. Alteration in thought processes related to confusion
11. High risk for complications: systemic response related to diseased liver

C. Interventions/Evaluations

1. Activity intolerance related to malaise and lethargy
   a. Interventions
      (1) Assess client's activity tolerance
      (2) Assist client in modifying her schedule and spacing her activities to allow for more rest
      (3) Maintain client's activity level just short of fatigue
      (4) Provide long periods for sleep at night and frequent rest periods during the day
      (5) Assist client with ADL and ambulation
   b. Evaluation: client tolerates progressive activities as evidenced by the following
      (1) Normal vital signs
      (2) Decreased dizziness, light-headedness, and weakness
2. Anxiety related to complicated pregnancy
   a. Interventions
      (1) Discuss client's fears and concerns about her pregnancy and its outcome
      (2) Provide reassurance and comfort
      (3) Obtain and begin involvement of MSW and other health team members
      (4) If possible and appropriate, have client's friends and family visit frequently; instruct them about visiting hours
      (5) Encourage client to ask questions about tests, medicines, treatments, and physician orders
      (6) Explain all procedures and their purpose
      (7) Acknowledge client's feelings and respond in a manner appropriate to her needs
      (8) Encourage interest in diversional activities (e.g., crafts, books, music)
      (9) Maintain clean, orderly, quiet, and stress-free environment
      (10) Assess family members' level of anxiety and knowledge of disease process; assess them as a support system for the client

        (11) Arrange for infant special care staff to visit with the client; orient client to realistic expectations

        (12) Encourage client to use visualization exercises, music, and crafts for relaxation

    b. Evaluations

        (1) Client verbalizes her fears and concerns about her pregnancy

        (2) Client feels supported and listened to

        (3) Client is able to relax and sleep

3. Ineffective individual and family coping related to poor progress and seriousness of condition

    a. Interventions

        (1) Assist client in improving her self-esteem

        (2) Discuss the illness as a pathological process

        (3) Maintain a positive attitude to communicate that the client can overcome her physical and emotional problems

        (4) Assist client in communicating with self-help groups

        (5) Assist client in using alternative coping strategies: relaxation techniques, meditation

        (6) Set short-term coping goals with client

    b. Evaluations

        (1) Client verbalizes the need for continued treatment

        (2) Client expresses a sense of hope in dealing with the disease process and her future

        (3) Client uses alternative coping mechanisms to cope with stress

4. High risk for alteration in family process related to maternal complications of pregnancy and hospitalization

    a. Interventions

        (1) Allow client and her family members to ventilate fears about pregnancy outcome

        (2) Assess client's and family members' responses to complicated pregnancy

            (a) Presence of unresolved guilt, blame, hostility, or jealousy

            (b) Inability to solve problems adequately

            (c) Ineffective patterns of communication

            (d) Observe client's interactions with her family members

        (3) Assess level of financial burden on family

        (4) Discuss effects of prolonged hospitalization on the family process

        (5) Encourage client and her family to participate in support groups and education programs

        (6) Utilize outside resources

            (a) MSW

            (b) Clinical nurse specialist

            (c) Clinical psychologist

            (d) Lay support and self-help groups

            (e) Home health care

            (f) Financial assistance programs

        (7) Assist family in reorganizing roles at home and setting priorities to maintain family integrity and to reduce stress

        (8) Aid family members in changing their expectations of the client in a realistic manner

        (9) Encourage frequent visits by family members

        (10) Make sure family members are oriented to visiting hours, bathrooms, cafeteria, and gift shop

        (11) Prepare client and her family members for signs of depression, anxiety, and dependency

        (12) Meet the physical needs of the client

        (13) Assess client's spiritual needs and help her to meet those needs

   b. Evaluations: client and her family demonstrate a functional system of mutual support for each other as evidenced by the following
   - (1) Seeking appropriate external resources when needed
   - (2) Engaging in open communication between family members and health team
   - (3) Participating in care of hospitalized family member
5. High risk for infection related to systemic disease and lowered resistance
   a. Interventions
   - (1) Use aseptic technique for all potential sites of infection
   - (2) Perform and instruct client about proper handwashing
   - (3) Maintain client's hydration with fluids
   - (4) Observe client's skin, joints, and extremities for areas of redness and swelling
   - (5) Encourage client to maintain caloric intake
   - (6) Observe type, amount, and odor of discharge or drainage
   - (7) Assess client each shift for the following
     - (a) Localized pain
     - (b) Signs of inflammation
   - (8) Assess for hyperthermia signs and symptoms
     - (a) Fever
     - (b) Chills
     - (c) Client feels hot
   - (9) Monitor vital signs, especially temperature, every 4 hours and as needed
   - (10) Space activities and encourage adequate rest
   - (11) Monitor laboratory results, especially WBC
   - (12) Instruct client to avoid exposure to persons with known infectious processes
   b. Evaluations
   - (1) Client has no signs and symptoms of infection and remains afebrile
   - (2) Client identifies signs and symptoms of infection in a timely manner
   - (3) Client obtains appropriate medical and nursing intervention for infection
   - (4) Client responds to treatment for infection in a timely manner
6. Knowledge deficit related to pregnancy complicated by hepatic disease
   a. Interventions
   - (1) Assess client's and family members' readiness and ability to learn
   - (2) Determine client's knowledge of her illness, its treatment, and preventive measures
   - (3) Assess client's adherence to prescribed behavior and its effect on her lifestyle
   - (4) Begin client and family education regarding what hepatic disease is and the effects it has on the mother and fetus
   - (5) Provide information to enable the pregnant woman with hepatic complications to obtain proper support and care
   - (6) Discuss signs and symptoms to report
     - (a) Abdominal pain
     - (b) Altered sensorium
     - (c) Decreased ability to perform activities
     - (d) Extreme fatigue
     - (e) Edema
     - (f) Anorexia, nausea, vomiting
     - (g) Jaundice, petechiae
   - (7) Explain the purpose of treatments, interventions, and tests
   - (8) Teach client behavioral interventions
     - (a) Bed rest in the lateral position (explain physiological rationale)
     - (b) Observance of prescribed medication regimen

          (c) Maintenance of as quiet and stress-free an environment as possible
- (9) Explain to client the rationale and procedure for the following
  - (a) NST
  - (b) CST
  - (c) Biophysical profile
  - (d) Amniocentesis
- b. Evaluations
  - (1) Client verbalizes an understanding of hepatic disease and its effect on the fetus
  - (2) Client is able to describe the hepatic disease process, its causes, signs and symptoms, and interventions for disease control
7. Alteration in nutrition related to anorexia, nausea, vomiting, and diarrhea
   - a. Interventions
     - (1) Assess client's nutritional status and fluid balance stability by monitoring the following
       - (a) Weight
       - (b) Condition of mucous membranes
       - (c) Skin turgor
     - (2) Discuss pregnancy changes in first trimester
       - (a) Morning sickness
       - (b) Small, frequent meals of dry foods
       - (c) Toast and crackers before rising in the morning
     - (3) Discuss signs and symptoms of hypoglycemia
       - (a) Shaking
       - (b) Fast heartbeat
       - (c) Sweating
       - (d) Tingling
       - (e) Personality change
       - (f) Dizziness
       - (g) Hunger
       - (h) Blurred vision
       - (i) Nervousness
       - (j) Excitedness
       - (k) Pale and moist skin
       - (l) Drowsiness
       - (m) Headache
       - (n) Fatigue
       - (o) Irritability
     - (4) Maintain odor-free, well-ventilated room
     - (5) Assess the client's affect and response to her family, environment, and pregnancy
     - (6) Reduce or eliminate factors contributing to anorexia, nausea, vomiting, and diarrhea
     - (7) Consult with nutritionist and dietician
     - (8) Obtain history of client's food allergies, likes and dislikes, and usual diet
     - (9) Administer progressive diets according to client's tolerance
       - (a) Small frequent feedings
       - (b) Liquids at effective times before or after a meal
     - (10) Help client maintain good oral hygiene before and after ingestion of food
     - (11) Give client instructions according to proper diet
       - (a) Foods and liquids to avoid
       - (b) Specific times to eat specific foods
       - (c) Alternate sources of foods
     - (12) Initiate health teaching and referrals as indicated
   - b. Evaluations: client maintains adequate nutrition

          (1) Adequate weight gain

          (2) Eating a well-balanced diet

          (3) An understanding of her condition

          (4) An ability to choose proper diet

  8. Powerlessness related to the unpredictable course of the disease process

    a. Interventions

        (1) Allow client opportunities to express her concerns and feelings

        (2) Provide a specific time during the shift that the client knows she can ask questions and discuss subjects of her choice

        (3) Inform client about her condition, treatment, and results

        (4) Point out the positive changes in the client's condition

        (5) Contact self-help support groups for the client

        (6) Offer client options when possible

          (a) Room arrangements

          (b) Daily plan of activities

          (c) Food choices

          (d) Short- and long-term goals

    b. Evaluations

        (1) Client identifies factors that she can control

        (2) Client makes decisions about her care, treatment, and activities

  9. Self-care deficit related to lethargy, malaise, or confusion

    a. Interventions

        (1) Assess client's level of self-care with ADL

        (2) Assist client with all ADL if needed

          (a) Personal hygiene

          (b) Feeding

          (c) Dressing

          (d) Positioning

        (3) Procure and use equipment for client's special needs

        (4) Involve family with client's care

        (5) Contact home health nurses and have them evaluate client to make visits at home after discharge

        (6) Consult with MSW if appropriate or at client's request

    b. Evaluation: client assists with her daily care without evidence of the following

        (1) Fatigue

        (2) Irritability

        (3) Change in vital signs

 10. Alteration in thought processes related to confusion

    a. Interventions

        (1) Correlate physical assessment, laboratory values, and confused state

        (2) Have all persons caring for the client introduce themselves

        (3) Discuss current events

        (4) Assess reality orientation to person, place, and time

        (5) Use safety measures as necessary

        (6) Encourage verbalization

        (7) Listen carefully to client's communication

        (8) Reorient client as necessary to person, place, and time

        (9) Space client's activities to ensure adequate sleep and rest

       (10) Explain all procedures simply and clearly

       (11) Approach client in slow, calm manner

       (12) Give client simple directions and explanations

       (13) Reduce unessential stimuli: physical surroundings, personnel

       (14) Encourage client's family to bring her familiar objects from home

         (a) Pictures of family

         (b) Calendar

         (c) Clock

b. Evaluation: client demonstrates the ability to evaluate reality, as evidenced by orientation to person, place, and time

11. High risk for complications: systemic response related to a diseased liver
    a. Interventions
        (1) Maintain a patent airway and effective ventilation and oxygenation
        (2) Orient client to person, place, and time
        (3) Administer prescribed diet to client: no protein, high glucose
        (4) Check to make sure that administered medications are not metabolized in the liver
        (5) Assist client with correction of her electrolyte and metabolic disturbances
        (6) Assist client with identification and correction of her coagulation defects
        (7) Prevent, observe for, and document signs and symptoms of infection
        (8) Minimize the risk of complications: hemorrhage, infection
        (9) Observe for multisystem disease as indicated by the following conditions
            (a) Hepatic failure
            (b) Hepatic encephalopathy
            (c) Renal failure
            (d) UTI
            (e) Hemorrhage
            (f) Anemia
            (g) GI bleeding
            (h) Hypoxia
            (i) Pneumonitis
    b. Evaluations: indications that the client's condition is stabilizing, as evidenced by the following criteria within normal limits
        (1) Level of consciousness and orientation to person, place, and time
        (2) Skin color
        (3) CBC
        (4) Electrolyte values
        (5) Liver function tests
        (6) Coagulation factors
        (7) Urinalysis
        (8) Kidney function tests

Health Education

A. Assist family in coping with the client's condition, progress, and treatment

B. Explain all procedures and laboratory tests to the client and her family

C. Teach the client to avoid exposure to infection

D. Plan with the client how she can get adequate sleep and take frequent rests

E. Instruct client to keep appointments with her internist and obstetrician

CASE STUDIES AND STUDY QUESTIONS

Sylvia Lohr is a 31-year old gravida, 1 para 0 (G1,P0) woman admitted to a level III labor and delivery unit for preterm labor at 32 weeks' gestation. Up to this time, her pregnancy has been normal, with the exception of increasing dyspnea and fatigue. Her medical history is normal with the exception of a tonsillectomy at age 5, an appendectomy at age 7, scarlet fever at age 9, and a series of other systemic infections. She had the usual childhood diseases of measles and chickenpox.

Sylvia's vital signs at admission are temperature 98.6°F (37°C), pulse 112, respirations 24, and blood pressure 130/70. Part of her assessment reveals the following: 2+ edema of lower extremities, no proteinuria, dyspnea with breath sounds clear in upper lobes and crackles that do not clear with deep inspiration.

1. The most significant event in Sylvia's history that might contribute to a diagnosis of cardiac complications of pregnancy is which of the following?

   a. Appendectomy at the age of 7 years.

   b. Childhood diseases, measles, and chickenpox.

   c. Scarlet fever at the age of 9 years.

   d. Tonsillectomy at the age of 5 years.

2. The most significant factor in the assessment is which of the following?

   a. Dyspnea with persistent lower lobe crackles.

   b. Respirations 24.

   c. Blood pressure 130/70.

   d. 2+ edema of lower extremities.

Further assessment of Sylvia in the first 24 hours of her admission reveals that she is very tired after eating part of her meals, experiences palpitations after talking for 10 minutes, has an increase in her respirations from 22 to 26 after talking for 5 minutes, and is comfortable when resting.

3. According to the New York Association Cardiac Disease Classification, Sylvia would be categorized as which of the following?

   a. Class I.

   b. Class II.

   c. Class III.

   d. Class IV.

4. Which of the following assessments indicate an increase in severity in Sylvia's cardiac condition?

   a. Weight gain with limited fluids.

   b. Chest pain at rest.

   c. Nausea and vomiting.

   d. Joint pain with bed rest.

5. The major risk to the fetus of a pregnancy complicated by cardiac disease is which of the following?

   a. Inherited cardiac anomaly.

   b. Increased risk of infection.

   c. Abnormal limb formation.

   d. IUGR.

Clarisse Dunn is a 21-year-old gravida 2, para 0 (G2,P0) woman at 28 weeks' gestation by ultrasound testing who is admitted to the high-risk unit with a diagnosis of UTI and possible right pyelonephritis and abdominal pain. She is positive for CVA and abdominal tenderness with no rebound tenderness. Clarisse states she has had three UTIs in this pregnancy, with the last being treated during her second trimester. At that time, she was treated with oral erythromycin, 500 mg daily for 1 week, without further incidence.

Her vital signs are temperature 101°F (38.3°C), pulse 104, respirations 20, and blood pressure 138/74.

6. Which of the following laboratory values should the nurse anticipate with a diagnosis of pyelonephritis?

   a. Elevated hemoglobin and hematocrit.

   b. Elevated creatinine.

   c. Decreased BUN.

   d. Decreased WBC count.

7. In addition to the laboratory tests, further diagnosis and assessment would include which of the following?

   a. Renal biopsy.

   b. Intravenous pyelogram.

   c. Fetal ultrasound testing.

   d. Amniocentesis.

8. Pyelonephritis may cause further complications, which include all except which of the following?

   a. Preterm labor.

   b. Renal insufficiency.

   c. Chorioamnionitis.

   d. Septicemia.

9. In observing for fluid volume excess or deficit, the nurse should assess for all ex-

cept which of the following?

a. Edema of hands and feet.

b. Ecchymotic areas of skin.

c. Skin turgor, color, and temperature.

d. Color, consistency, and amount of urine.

Shanda King is a 28-year-old Afro-American gravida 3, para 0 (G3, P0) woman at 24 weeks' gestation. She is admitted to the high-risk unit with generalized malaise, fatigue, anorexia, and knee and ankle pain. She has a history of feeling ill for 2 weeks and has lost 3 pounds in that time. Her other two pregnancies ended with miscarriages at 12 and 16 weeks' gestation, respectively. Shanda has experienced occasional periods of these signs and symptoms in the past and each time was treated for flu syndrome. She complains of a sensitivity to sunlight.

Her vital signs on admission are temperature 99.4°F (37.4°C), pulse 80, respirations 20, and blood pressure 140/84. Some significant laboratory findings on admission are hemoglobin 9.8, hematocrit level 30, WBCs 4500; and proteinuria of 3+. Shanda is diagnosed with systemic lupus erythematosus.

10. Which of the following complaints by Shanda indicate an increase in the severity of her condition?

a. "I can't remember if my husband was here today, and I feel confused."

b. "My knees and ankles are still hurting."

c. "Please close the curtains; I am having difficulty with the noise."

d. "I am very concerned for the future of this pregnancy."

11. The nurse anticipates which of the following laboratory tests to be ordered in response to the above symptoms?

a. CBC.

b. Liver enzymes.

c. Electrolyte values.

d. L/S ratio.

12. At 28 weeks' gestation, Shanda expresses the following symptoms. Which symptoms are indicative of further complications of SLE?

a. Headache and blurred vision.

b. Fatigue and feeling easily tired.

c. Increased appetite and bloated feeling.

d. Muscle cramps in legs.

13. Which common complication of SLE causes the symptoms identified in the last question?

a. Paralytic ileus.

b. Pre-eclampsia.

c. Calcium deficiency.

d. Flu syndrome.

Answers to Study Questions

1. c	2. a	3. c
4. b	5. d	6. b
7. c	8. c	9. b
10. a	11. b	12. a
13. b		

REFERENCES

Bobak, I., Jensen, M., & Zalar, M. (1989). *Maternity and gynecologic care* (4th ed.). St. Louis: Mosby.

Burrow, G., & Ferris, T. (1988). *Medical complications during pregnancy* (3rd ed.). Philadelphia: Saunders.

Carpentio, L. (1987). *Nursing diagnosis: Application to clinical practice.* Philadelphia: Lippincott.

Clark, S., Phelan, J., & Cotton, D. (1987). *Critical care obstetrics.* Oradell, NJ: Medical Economics Books.

Creasy, R., & Resnik, R. (1984). *Maternal-fetal medicine.* Philadelphia: Saunders.

Pritchard, J., McDonald, P., & Gant, N. (1987). *Williams' obstetrics.* (18th ed.). Norwalk, CT: Appleton-Century-Crofts.

Reeder, S., & Martin, L. (1987). *Maternity nursing.* Philadelphia: Lippincott.

Dorothy A. Austin

Labor and Delivery at Risk

Objectives

1. Identify risk factors in a client's prenatal history that put her at risk for preterm labor

2. Describe important assessment parameters for clients who are at high risk for preterm labor

3. Summarize treatments for the client in preterm labor

4. Discuss side effects of tocolytic therapy

5. Identify early signs and symptoms of chorioamnionitis

6. List potential complications for the client with premature rupture of the membranes

7. Describe methods commonly used for pregnancy dating

8. Define post-term pregnancy

9. Differentiate between the post-term pregnancy and the postmature infant

10. Discuss physical findings that lead to a diagnosis of intrauterine fetal demise

11. Describe the stages of grief

12. Differentiate between perinatal grief and other grieving responses

13. List potential bleeding or coagulation complications associated with intrauterine fetal demise

14. Explain the pathophysiology of amnoitic fluid embolism

15. Describe the signs and symptoms that lead to a diagnosis of amniotic fluid embolism

16. Discuss the mortality and morbidity associated with amniotic fluid embolism

17. Identify clients at high risk for uterine rupture

18. Discuss life-threatening complications that may result from uterine rupture

19. Classify the types of uterine rupture

20. Rank emergency actions in order of priority for a client presenting with traumatic uterine rupture

Preterm Labor

Introduction

A. Preterm labor is defined as regular uterine contractions and cervical dilation before the 37th week of gestation

B. Factors such as uterine anomalies, multiple gestation, polyhydramnios, and urinary tract infections (UTIs) are associated with a higher incidence of preterm labor

C. Familiarity with risk factors and prudent client education are the keys to early diagnosis and successful treatment

Clinical Practice

A. Assessment

1. History
   a. Signs and symptoms of uterine contractions
   b. Increased vaginal discharge or bloody show
   c. Presence of risk factors associated with preterm labor
      (1) Uterine anomalies
      (2) Multiple gestation
      (3) Polyhydramnios
      (4) Maternal age below 16 years or over 40 years
      (5) Smoking
      (6) Alcohol or drug abuse
      (7) Low socioeconomic status
      (8) Poor nutrition
      (9) Prior episode of preterm labor during this or in a previous pregnancy
   d. Signs and symptoms of UTI
      (1) Urinary frequency
      (2) Urgency
      (3) Dysuria
      (4) Flank pain
   e. Low back pain
   f. Pelvic pressure
   g. Gastrointestinal (GI) upset
      (1) Nausea
      (2) Vomiting
      (3) Diarrhea
2. Physical findings
   a. Uterine contractions palpable or evident on external fetal monitor
   b. Cervical changes: softening, effacement, or dilation
   c. Engagement of fetal presenting part
   d. Elevated temperature may indicate dehydration or infection
   e. Fetal heart rate (FHR): tachycardia may indicate maternal infection
3. Psychosocial findings
   a. Stress factors
      (1) Anxiety
      (2) Fear of pregnancy loss
      (3) Fear of unknown
   b. Behavioral response
      (1) Confusion, disorganization, difficulty communicating
      (2) Expresses fears
4. Diagnostic procedures
   a. Complete blood count (CBC): elevated WBC count may indicate infection (WBC count is normally elevated in pregnancy and in labor, but a WBC count above 18,000 is considered significant for infection)

b. Urinalysis: note presence of WBCs, RBCs, or bacteria
c. Urine culture and sensitivity testing
d. Amniotic fliud
   (1) Gram's stain
   (2) Culture and sensitivity
   (3) Amniotic fluid for lecithin-sphingomyelin (L/S) ratio to assess fetal lung maturity
e. Cervical cultures
   (1) Group B streptococcus
   (2) Chlamydia
   (3) Gonorrhea
f. Ultrasound examination
   (1) Assessment of presenting part
   (2) Gestational age
   (3) Multiple gestation
   (4) Amniotic fluid volume

B. Nursing Diagnoses

1. Alteration in comfort: pain related to uterine contractions
2. Anxiety related to unknown pregnancy outcome
3. Anticipatory grieving related to threatened pregnancy loss
4. Knowledge deficit related to preterm labor

C. Interventions/Evaluations

1. Alteration in comfort: pain related to uterine contractions
   a. Interventions
      (1) Hydrate client with oral (PO) or IV fluids (uterine contractions or irritability may result from dehydration)
      (2) Maximize uterine blood flow by placing client on bed rest in the left lateral position
      (3) Continuous external fetal monitoring for
         (a) FHR pattern
         (b) Frequency, duration, and approximate intensity of uterine contractions
      (4) Palpate client's abdomen to assess strength of uterine contractions
      (5) Administer tocolytic agents as ordered
         (a) Magnesium sulfate ($MgSO_4$)
            (i) Dosage and administration
               • Loading dose: 4 to 6 g intravenous piggyback (IVPB) over 20 to 30 minutes
               • Maintenance dose: 1 to 3 g/hr IVPB
               • Medication should be administered by infusion pump
            (ii) Side effects
               • Sweating
               • Flushing
               • Nausea and vomiting
               • Depressed deep tendon reflexes
               • Flaccid paralysis
               • Hypocalcemia
               • Depressed cardiac function
               • Respiratory depression
            (iii) Nursing actions
               • Monitor vital signs
               • Monitor deep tendon reflexes (DTRs) (generally graded on a scale of 0 to 4+) (Bates, 1987)
                  □ 4+: Very brisk, hyperactive; associated with clonus
                  □ 3+: Brisker than average
                  □ 2+: Average; normal reflex response

□ 1+: Diminished
□ 0: Absent
□ The patellar tendon is most commonly used to assess reflexes, since it is easiest to elicit, but biceps or triceps reflexes may also be used
- Monitor serum magnesium levels
- Although laboratory values may vary slightly from one institution to another, approximate values are as follows
  □ Therapeutic: 4 to 6 mEq/l
  □ Loss of DTRs: 10 mEq/l
  □ Respiratory depression: 15 mEq/l
  □ Cardiac arrest: 25 mEq/l
- Discontinue $MgSO_4$ in the presence of elevated serum levels or of signs and symptoms of central nervous system (CNS) or cardiovascular depression
- Administer antidote, calcium gluconate, if necessary

(b) Ritodrine hydrochloride
  (i) Dosage and administration
  - IV dosage
    □ 0.05 to 0.30 mg/min titrated according to uterine activity
    □ Increase by 0.05 mg/min every 10 minutes until contractions subside
    □ May be given more slowly to minimize side effects
  - PO dosage: 10 to 20 mg titrated to maintain suppression of uterine activity without unwanted side effects
  - IV medication must be given by infusion pump
  (ii) Side effects
  - Elevated heart rate
  - Widening of pulse pressure
  - Nausea and vomiting
  - Nervousness
  - Tremors
  - Transient elevation of blood and urine glucose levels
  - Cardiac arrhythmias
  - Pulmonary edema
  (iii) Contraindications
  - Placental abruption
  - Chorioamnionitis
  - Pre-viable gestation
  - Fetal demise
  - Fetal anomalies incompatible with life
  (iv) Relative contraindications
  - Maternal diabetes
  - Severe pregnancy-induced hypertension (PIH)
  - Intrauterine growth retardation (IUGR)
  - Maternal cardiac disease
  - Hyperthyroidism
  (v) Nursing actions
  - Baseline electrocardiogram (ECG) is recommended
  - Monitor pulse rate: hold next dose for rates above 120 beats/min

(c) Terbutaline sulfate
  (i) Dosage and administration
  - IV dosage
    □ 5 to 25 mcg/min titrated according to uterine activity
    □ Increase by 5 mcg/min every 20 minutes
  - Subcutaneous (SQ) dosage: 0.25 to 0.50 mg

- PO dosage: 2.5 to 5 mg every 2 to 8 hours
(ii) Side effects
  - Elevated heart rate
  - Nervousness
  - Tremors
  - Nausea and vomiting
  - Transient elevation in blood and urine glucose levels
  - Decrease in serum potassium level
  - Cardiac arrhythmias
  - Pulmonary edema
(iii) Contraindications: same as for ritodrine
(6) Explain side effects of tocolytic agent to client (as noted above)
(7) Monitor vital signs and FHR
(8) Monitor intake and output (I&O); avoid volume overload
b. Evaluations
(1) Decreased uterine activity; pain eliminated or decreased as evidenced by the following
    (a) Absence of uterine activity on external fetal monitor
    (b) Absence of decreased abdominal cramping as perceived by client
    (c) No further cervical dilation or effacement
(2) If cervix changes or uterine activity continues, re-evaluate tocolytic agent and dose
2. Anxiety related to unknown pregnancy outcome
a. Interventions
(1) Encourage client to verbalize her feelings and assist her in identifying specific concerns
(2) Provide information about preterm labor/delivery
(3) Provide information about premature infants; be as specific as possible, giving information related to her gestation
(4) Visit neonatal intensive care unit (NICU) with client to familiarize her with that environment
b. Evaluations
(1) Client demonstrates decreased signs of anxiety
(2) Client's questions and concerns are appropriate and realistic
3. Anticipatory grieving related to threatened pregnancy loss (refer to Chap. 25 on grief and loss for more information)
a. Interventions
(1) Encourage verbalization of client's feelings
(2) Assist client and her family in identifying their own best coping mechanisms
(3) Be realistic with information given
(4) Allow client and her family to participate in plan of care whenever possible
b. Evaluations
(1) Client and her family continue to exhibit bonding behaviors
(2) Client and her family do not express unrealistic expectations
4. Knowledge deficit related to preterm labor
a. Interventions
(1) Identify and explain to client her particular risk factors for preterm labor
(2) Teach client all signs and symptoms of preterm labor
(3) Demonstrate palpation of uterine contractions to client
(4) Explain how to accurately assess and record the frequency and duration of uterine contractions
(5) Provide client with written instructions for follow-up care should uterine activity occur; provide emergency phone numbers
b. Evaluations

(1) Client is able to describe risk factors and signs and symptoms of preterm labor
(2) Client demonstrates proper technique of abdominal palpation of uterine contractions
(3) Client can discuss plan of action in the event of significant uterine activity

Health Education

A. Teach client to recognize signs and symptoms of preterm labor

1. Uterine contractions, cramping, and low back pain
2. Feeling of pelvic pressure or fullness
3. Change in amount or character of vaginal discharge
4. Bloody show
5. GI upset: nausea, vomiting, diarrhea
6. General sense of discomfort or unease

B. Teach client how to palpate uterine contractions

1. Tell client to sit up from a reclining position and to immediately palpate her abdomen (this will usually induce a uterine contraction)
2. Client may also palpate the sensation of a muscular contraction by placing her hand over her biceps and flexing her arm
3. Describe contraction intensity; compare the feeling of firmness to the following
   a. Tip of nose: mild
   b. Tip of chin: moderate
   c. Forehead: strong

C. Review timing of contractions with the client; time contractions from onset to onset

D. Client should call health care provider or come to the hospital if contractions are coming regularly

E. Discuss treatment routines with the client

1. Bed rest in the left lateral position (mild uterine activity may subside with increased uterine blood flow)
2. Maintain adequate hydration: (uterine activity or irritability may result from dehydration)
3. If uterine activity persists, the client should call her health care provider or come to the hospital for further evaluation

Post-Term Pregnancy

Introduction

A. Normal human gestation is 40 weeks; post-term pregnancy as described by Creasy and Resnik (1989) is gestation past 294 days or 42 weeks

B. The ability of the placenta to continue to effectively provide the fetus with oxygen and nutrition is thought to be compromised after this point

Clinical Practice

A. Assessment

1. History: pregnancy dating
   a. Naegele's rule: add 7 days to the first day of the last menstrual period and count back 3 months

    b. Ultrasound examination: pregnancy can also be dated by ultrasound examination, by estimating fetal weight; by measuring fetal biparietal diameter, femur length, abdominal circumference, or chest circumference; or by using a formula involving the ratio of these values. Ultrasound dating is most accurate when done in the second trimester of pregnancy

2. Physical findings
    a. Gestational age by ultrasound examination
    b. Fundal height
        (1) Measurement from symphysis to top of fundus correlates approximately with the number of weeks of gestation (e.g., 22 cm indicates approximately 22 weeks' gestation)
        (2) If fetal presenting part is engaged, the fundal height is not as accurate
    c. Placental calcifications
        (1) Identified by ultrasound examination
        (2) May indicate postmature placenta
        (3) Some institutions use placental grading scales to quantify calcifications
    d. Amniotic fluid volume (AFV): may decrease in response to uteroplacental insufficiency
    e. Physical findings in the newborn
        (1) Long, lean bodies
        (2) Long fingernails
        (3) Abundant hair growth
        (4) Parchment-like skin (dry, peeling) (postmaturity occurs in only 20% of post-term pregnancies and diagnosis is not made until the time of delivery [Cohen, 1985])
    f. Higher incidence of meconium aspiration and asphyxia
3. Psychosocial findings
    a. Stress factors
        (1) Anxiety
        (2) Fear of unknown: expectations of delivery by estimated date of confinement (EDC) have not been fulfilled
    b. Behavioral response: impatience with normal discomforts of pregnancy
4. Diagnostic procedures: antepartum testing (see Chap. 11 on antepartum testing)
    a. Nonstress test (NST)
    b. Contraction stress test (CST)
    c. Biophysical profile

B. Nursing Diagnoses

1. Anxiety related to unknown pregnancy outcome
2. High risk for impaired tissue perfusion related to decreased placental function

C. Interventions/Evaluations

1. Anxiety related to unknown pregnancy outcome
    a. Interventions
        (1) Provide information to client on post-term pregnancy
        (2) Explain effects of postmaturity on the fetus
            (a) Potential decrease in amount of oxygen and nutrients to the fetus due to decreased placental perfusion
            (b) Loss of vernix caseosa causes fetal skin to appear dry and peeling
            (c) Decreased placental perfusion may also lead to fetal asphyxia and passage of meconium into the amniotic fluid
        (3) Encourage verbalization of feelings and help client to identify specific concerns and questions
        (4) Assist client in identifying her own best coping mechanism for dealing with stress
        (5) Allow client to participate in her plan of care whenever possible

b. Evaluations
(1) Client does not demonstrate high level of anxiety
(2) Client demonstrates understanding of her plan of care and is coping effectively
(3) Client can explain why she and the fetus are at risk with post-term pregnancy
2. High risk for impaired tissue perfusion related to decreased placental function
a. Interventions
(1) Maintain client in the left lateral position as much as possible to maximize placental blood flow
(2) Monitor FHR
(a) Antepartum testing protocols (NST, CST, biophysical profiles)
(b) Continuous fetal monitoring during labor and delivery
(3) Keep client well hydrated to maximize placental perfusion
(4) Prepare client for possibility of induction of labor
(a) Explain procedure to client
(b) Discuss indications and risks
(5) Prostaglandin gel may be used for cervical ripening
(a) Explain procedure to client
(b) Discuss indications and risks
(c) Assist with insertion of prostaglandin gel intracervically
(d) Continuous fetal monitoring should be done after client receives prostaglandin gel to observe for uterine contractions and to monitor FHR pattern
b. Evaluation
(1) FHR tracing shows no evidence of uteroplacental insufficiency such as late decelerations or loss of variability
(2) Client demonstrates understanding of labor induction process

Health Education

A. Define terms of normal gestation

B. Explain function of placenta

1. Delivery of oxygen and gas exchange
2. Delivery of nutrients for fetal growth
3. Decreased efficiency after 40th week

C. Review fetal growth and development

1. Organ development and maturation complete by 36th week
2. Last 4 weeks of gestation is primarily for weight gain
3. Vernix caseosa, the oily substance that protects the fetal skin in utero, begins to disappear after the 36th week, making the infant's skin appear dry and peeling

D. Discuss physiology of labor

1. Initiating mechanism for onset of labor is unknown
2. Cervix may require ripening with prostaglandin gel
a. Gel is inserted intracervically to induce softening and effacement
b. Continuous fetal monitoring is recommended after the insertion of prostaglandin gel since it may induce uterine contractions; assess for uterine activity and FHR patterns
3. Induction or augmentation of labor may be necessary and is most commonly done with oxytocin (Pitocin); it should not be done without continuous FHR monitoring

E. Discuss effect of post-term pregnancy on the fetus

1. Meconium passage into the amniotic fluid occurs with higher frequency in post-term pregnancy

2. Meconium aspiration at delivery causes a chemical pneumonitis and alveolar obstruction in newborn lungs
   a. Infant will be aggressively suctioned at delivery
   b. Infant will most likely be intubated and suctioned after delivery to make every attempt to avoid aspiration of meconium into lungs

Premature Rupture of the Membranes

Introduction

A. Premature rupture of the membranes (PROM) refers to the spontaneous rupture of the amniotic membrane before the onset of labor; this may occur at or before term

B. Gestational age, however, usually determines the plan and intervention

C. If the client is at term, she will most likely be delivered within 48 hours

D. Induction or augmentation may be necessary

E. For the purpose of this section, PROM refers to the rupture of membranes (ROM) before term

Clinical Practice

A. Assessment

1. History
   a. Gestational age
      (1) By last menstrual period (LMP)
      (2) By ultrasound dating
   b. Date and time of rupture of membranes
   c. Any pain, cramping, or feeling of pelvic pressure associated with PROM
   d. Any event that immediately preceded ROM (e.g., trauma)
   e. History of UTI: signs and symptoms of urinary frequency, urgency, dysuria, or flank pain
   f. History of vaginal or pelvic infection; signs and symptoms of change in vaginal discharge, pelvic pain
2. Physical findings
   a. Sterile speculum examination findings
      (1) Pooling of fluid in vaginal vault
      (2) Nitrazine test positive
      (3) Fern test positive
      (4) Appearance of cervix
      (5) Any discharge
      (6) Inflammation or lesions
      (7) Protrusion of membranes
      (8) Presenting part
      (9) Umbilical cord prolapse
   b. Amount, color, and consistency of fluid
      (1) Odor
      (2) Presence of vernix, blood, or meconium in fluid
   c. Vital signs: elevation of temperature may indicate presence of infection
   d. CBC: elevated WBC count may indicate presence of infection
   e. External fetal monitoring
      (1) Uterine contractions
      (2) Uterine irritability
      (3) FHR tachycardia
3. Psychosocial findings

a. Stress factors
  (1) Anxiety
  (2) Fear of pregnancy loss
  (3) Feeling unprepared for delivery
  (4) Guilt
b. Behavioral factors
  (1) Difficulty communicating
  (2) Expression of fears
  (3) Coping mechanisms
4. Diagnostic procedures
  a. Nitrazine test: paper turns blue in the presence of amniotic fluid
  b. Ferning: amniotic fluid on a slide crystallizes into a fern pattern that can be viewed under a microscope
  c. Amniotic fluid volume: as measured by ultrasound examination, AFV may help to confirm a questionable diagnosis of ROM (decreased if membranes are ruptured)
  d. Amniocentesis
    (1) Gram's stain: positivity indicates infection
    (2) Culture and sensitivity testing to identify specific organisms
    (3) Fetal maturity studies
      (a) L/S ratio
      (b) Foam stability index (FSI)
      (c) Shake test (if tests indicate fetal pulmonary maturity, delivery may be considered)

B. Nursing Diagnoses

1. High risk for infection related to break in amniotic membrane barrier and proximity to vaginal and enteric flora
2. Alteration in tissue perfusion related to umbilical cord compression due to decrease in fluid volume
3. Anxiety related to possible preterm delivery
4. Knowledge deficit related to PROM

C. Interventions/Evaluations

1. High risk for infection related to break in amniotic membrane barrier and proximity to vaginal and enteric flora
  a. Interventions
    (1) Monitor maternal vital signs: elevated temperature or increased pulse rate may indicate infection
    (2) Monitor CBC values: elevation in WBC count may indicate infection
    (3) Observe amniotic fluid for purulence or odor
    (4) Observe vaginal discharge: purulence or foul odor may indicate infection
    (5) Monitor FHR: observe for fetal tachycardia, which may develop with maternal infection
    (6) Monitor uterine activity; note contractions or uterine irritability
    (7) Palpate abdomen to assess for uterine tenderness
    (8) Do not perform any vaginal examinations
    (9) Administer antibiotics as ordered
  b. Evaluations
    (1) Client remains afebrile
    (2) WBC count is within normal limits
    (3) Client is free from malodorous vaginal discharge or amniotic fluid drainage
    (4) FHR pattern is within normal limits; fetus remains active with accompanying FHR accelerations
    (5) Client remains free of uterine contractions, irritability, or uterine tenderness

2. Alteration in tissue perfusion related to cord compression due to decreased amniotic fluid
   a. Interventions
      (1) Bed rest with FHR monitoring
         (a) Recommend continuous fetal monitoring for first 48 hours
         (b) Then bed rest with fetal heart check every 4 hours and daily NST
      (2) Evaluate fetal presenting part by Leopold's maneuver or ultrasound examination
         (a) Nonvertex presentations are at higher risk for umbilical cord prolapse
         (b) Client with nonvertex presentations may be put in a slight Trendelenberg position to decrease the chance of umbilical cord prolapse
      (3) Observe for evidence of cord compression: variable decelerations seen on fetal monitor
      (4) If severe variables are observed, institute amnioinfusion if ordered according to institutional protocol (See Chap. 16 for suggested protocols)
   b. Evaluations
      (1) FHR patterns remain within normal limits with no variable decelerations
      (2) Client does not experience prolapse of umbilical cord
3. Anxiety related to possible preterm delivery
   a. Interventions
      (1) Provide client with as much information as possible about PROM
      (2) Discuss fetal growth and development and focus on gestational age of this fetus
      (3) Visit NICU if possible to prepare client for intensive care environment
      (4) Include client in plan of care and decision making whenever possible
      (5) Encourage verbalization of client's feelings and help her to identify specific concerns
      (6) Identify coping mechanisms most helpful during times of stress
      (7) Identify client's support system
      (8) Contact social service if necessary to assist client
   b. Evaluations
      (1) Client demonstrates knowledge of fetal stages of development
      (2) Client has realistic expectations for baby delivered at this gestational age
      (3) Client understands possible need for delivery before term
      (4) Client demonstrates effective coping mechanisms and appropriate use of support persons
      (5) Lessening degree of anxiety accompanies client's increase in knowledge and use of social systems
4. Knowledge deficit related to PROM
   a. Interventions
      (1) Review anatomy and physiology with client; describe fetal membranes
      (2) Discuss potential complications and their treatments
         (a) Development of infection usually necessitates delivery
         (b) FHR variable decelerations warrant continuous fetal monitoring, possible amnioinfusion, and delivery for fetal distress
         (c) Prolapse of umbilical cord requires emergency cesarean section (C/S)
   b. Evaluations
      (1) Client can discuss gestational age of fetus and related fetal development
      (2) Client can list signs and symptoms of infection
      (3) Client demonstrates awareness of potential complications related to PROM and discusses their treatments

Health Education

A. Review anatomy and physiology of pregnancy

1. Enlarging uterus: appropriate to gestational age
2. Function of placenta: to provide oxygen and nutrients to the fetus

3. Umbilical cord: attaches fetal placental unit to mother
4. Fetal membranes
   a. Provide protective barrier to fetus
   b. Contain amniotic fluid to provide cushioning and flotation for fetus
   c. Eliminate compression of any fetal part, including the umbilical cord

B. **Fetal growth and development**

1. Use growth charts to give client a realistic idea of fetal size
2. Focus on key landmarks of fetal development
   a. Twenty-eight weeks: fetal anatomical development complete; maturity needed
   b. Thirty-four weeks: approaching pulmonary maturity
3. Discuss care in the NICU

C. **Teach client signs and symptoms of infection; instruct her to report any of the following symptoms**

1. Elevated temperature
2. Foul-smelling amniotic fluid
3. Significant increase in vaginal discharge
4. Abdominal pain or tenderness
5. Onset of uterine contractions

D. **Instruct client to come to the hospital immediately for prolapse of umbilical cord; explain significance of such and the need for emergency C section**

Multiple Gestation

Introduction

A. **Multiple-gestation pregnancies are seen more commonly now because of the increased use of ovulation-stimulating drugs**

B. **The incidence of multiple pregnancy in the United States is approximately 1.5% of all births**

C. **About one-third of these are monozygotic (i.e., originating from one zygote), whereas the other two-thirds are dizygotic (i.e., resulting from the fertilization of two ova)**

D. **Pregnancy risk factors, such as discordant growth and twin-to-twin transfusion syndromes, arise from carrying more than one fetus**

E. **The client with a multiple gestation is also at higher risk for many of the common complications of pregnancy such as PIH, abruptio placentae, preterm labor, and IUGR**

Clinical Practice

A. **Assessment**

1. History
   a. Pregnancy dating: diagnosis is often preceded by the observation that size is greater than dates
   b. Fertility enhancement: use of ovulation-stimulating drugs
   c. Family history of twins
2. Physical findings
   a. Fundal height measurement greater than number of weeks of gestation
   b. Leopold's maneuver may distinguish more than one fetus
   c. Auscultation of more than one heartbeat
   d. Ultrasound examination gives evidence of more than one fetus or gestational sac

e. Laboratory data
   (1) Beta-human chorionic gonadotropin (HCG) greatly elevated
   (2) Maternal serum alpha-fetoprotein (AFP) is elevated
f. Once the diagnosis of multiple gestation is made, the client should be considered at risk; assessment for pregnancy complications should include the following
   (1) Preterm labor
   (2) Maternal anemia
   (3) Abruptio placentae
   (4) PIH
   (5) Polyhydramnios
   (6) Congenital anomalies
   (7) IUGR
g. Assessment for complications specific to multiple gestation
   (1) Discordant growth
   (2) Twin-to-twin transfusion syndrome
3. Psychosocial responses
   a. Stress factors
      (1) Fear related to high-risk pregnancy
      (2) Fear of pregnancy loss
      (3) Anxiety related to parenting more than one infant
   b. Behavioral factors
      (1) Fear of upcoming events
      (2) Compulsiveness in preparing for children
4. Diagnostic procedures
   a. Ultrasound examination
      (1) Most reliable test for making diagnosis
      (2) Used to estimate fetal weight and diagnose discordance
      (3) Serial ultrasound scans follow fetal growth curves
      (4) Assessment of congenital anomalies
      (5) Assessment of AFV: polyhydramnios is more common in multiple gestation pregnancies
   b. Amniocentesis to diagnose chromosomal anomalies
   c. Antepartum surveillance for early detection of risks
      (1) NST
      (2) CST
      (3) Biophysical profile

B. Nursing Diagnoses

1. Alteration in health maintenance related to multiple gestation pregnancy
2. Anxiety related to high-risk pregnancy and delivery
3. Alteration in parenting related to delivery of more than one infant

C. Interventions/Evaluations

1. Alteration in health maintenance related to multiple-gestation pregnancy
   a. Interventions
      (1) Increase client's caloric intake to support growth and development of multiple gestation
      (2) Nutritional consult to evaluate specific dietary needs and assist client in plan to meet these
      (3) Monitor hemoglobin levels and hematocrit for maternal anemia
      (4) Discuss importance of additional rest
      (5) Observe for signs and symptoms of preterm labor
         (a) Premature contractions
         (b) Uterine cramping
         (c) Pelvic pain and pressure
         (d) Bloody show
      (6) Observe for signs and symptoms related to pregnancy complications

(a) Excessive weight gain
(b) Proteinuria
(c) Nondependent edema
(d) Vaginal bleeding

b. Evaluations
(1) Weight gain is appropriate throughout pregnancy
(2) Fetal growth remains on normal growth curve for each fetus
(3) Maternal hemoglobin levels and hematocrit remain within normal limits: hemoglobin above 11 mg/dl and hematocrit above 33%
(4) Client does not exhibit signs and symptoms of excessive fatigue
(5) Client does not demonstrate signs and symptoms of preterm labor
(6) Client is free from other complications of pregnancy (as noted above)

2. Anxiety related to high-risk pregnancy and delivery
a. Interventions
(1) Explain reasons for risk factors to client
(a) Increased placental demands for two or more developing fetuses
(b) Overdistension of uterus may lead to uterine irritability or premature contractions
(2) List signs and symptoms for client to be aware of and to report immediately
(3) Review delivery room practices and added precautions for multiple gestation
(a) Double set-up: having C section equipment available and ready in the room at the time of delivery
(b) Extra personnel are likely to be present at delivery to attend to needs of each newborn (especially if preterm)
(c) C section: many times is standard practice for multiple gestation pregnancies greater than two (i.e., triplets, quadruplets) and may be necessary for twins
(d) C section may be necessary for the second twin even after successful vaginal delivery of the first
(e) Ultrasound examination is often done after the delivery of twin A to reassess position of twin B, as well as to guide external version if needed to facilitate vaginal delivery
(f) Oxytocin administration may be necessary to augment uterine activity and to enhance descent of the second twin
(g) Twin B is at considerably higher risk for delivery-related complications such as umbilical cord prolapse, malpresentation, and abruptio placentae; therefore, intensive monitoring must be continued until twin B is delivered
(h) Each baby is individually stabilized, resuscitated as necessary, and identified; cord blood or other laboratory work needed is ordered
(4) Visit NICU if possible to prepare client for intensive care environment
(5) Encourage verbalization and assist client in identifying specific concerns
(6) Assist client in identifying support system and other resources available

b. Evaluations
(1) Client can list signs and symptoms of preterm labor
(2) Client identifies significant signs and symptoms of pregnancy complications that need to be reported immediately
(3) Client can discuss interventions specifically relating to multiple gestation that may be made either during pregnancy or during delivery
(4) Client has a realistic expectation of vaginal delivery
(5) Client can discuss components of NICU care as appropriate
(6) Client has developed a plan to use all resources and support services available to her

3. Alteration in parenting related to delivery of more than one infant
a. Interventions

(1) Provide list of resources and services available (e.g., Mothers of Twins support group, or lactation consultants)
(2) Discuss aspects of normal newborn infant care; assess learning needs
(3) Explore client's specific concerns
  b. Evaluation
(1) Client can identify resources available
(2) Client demonstrates appropriate techniques for infant bathing and feeding
(3) Client can discuss her specific concerns relating to the parenting role

Health Education

A. Twins

1. Monozygotic: identical twins—originated from one zygote that divided around the end of the first week of pregnancy
   a. Accounts for one-third of all twins
   b. Genetically identical: very similar in appearance
   c. No tendency to repeat in families (ACOG, 1989)
2. Dizygotic: fraternal twins—results from the fertilization of two ova
   a. Accounts for two-thirds of all twins
   b. Tends to repeat in families
   c. Increased risk with advancing maternal age
   d. May result from induction of ovulation by fertility drugs

B. Other multiple births

1. Triplets occur once in every 8100 pregnancies
2. Multiple births of more than three babies are extremely rare

C. Nutritional requirements

1. Caloric intake must be greatly increased to support the growth of multiple fetuses
2. Outline dietary plan for client

D. Inform client of high-risk status

E. Instruct client to be aware of any developing symptoms of complications

1. Preterm labor
   a. Uterine contractions, cramping, low back pain
   b. Feeling of pelvic pressure or fullness
   c. Change in amount or character of vaginal discharge
   d. GI upset: nausea, vomiting, or diarrhea
2. PROM: report any leaking of fluid
3. Precautionary measures
   a. Increase client's rest periods
   b. Have client lie in the left lateral position to maximize blood flow to the uterus
   c. Teach client to palpate uterine contractions (see Health Education in Preterm Labor section)

Intrauterine Fetal Demise

Introduction

A. Perinatal death, whether it occurs before delivery as an intrauterine fetal demise or after delivery as a neonatal death, presents a unique set of physical and psychosocial problems

B. The developmental task of attachment and preparing for parenthood is abruptly interrupted; parents are shocked and confused, and suddenly find themselves faced with issues of grief and mourning

C. The physical process of labor and delivery, as well as the handling of the infant after delivery, requires extreme sensitivity on the part of the nurse

Clinical Practice

A. Assessment

1. History
   a. Loss of fetal movement
   b. Diminishing signs of pregnancy
      (1) Maternal weight gain ceases
      (2) Mother may even lose weight
      (3) Breast changes begin to reverse
   c. Associated high-risk factors
      (1) Advanced diabetes in pregnancy
      (2) Systemic vascular disease
      (3) Collagen vascular disease
      (4) Previous unexplained loss of fetus
2. Physical findings
   a. Absence of FHR as determined by auscultation
   b. Absence of cardiac activity: as documented by ultrasound examination
   c. Abdominal rigidity or pain: present in clients with abruption
   d. Vaginal examination: observe for the following
      (1) Bleeding
      (2) Umbilical cord prolapse
      (3) Rupture of membranes: amniotic fluid often appears cloudy and brownish red if the fetus has been dead for several days
      (4) Note any cervical dilation or effacement
      (5) Note fetal presenting part or presence of any softening or overlapping of skull bones
3. Psychosocial findings
   a. Stress factors
      (1) Fear for self
      (2) Anxiety related to labor and delivery process
      (3) Confusion
   b. Behavioral factors
      (1) Difficulty in communicating
      (2) Shock and numbness (first stage of grief)
      (3) Demonstration of some attachment behaviors
      (4) Expression of significance of this pregnancy
      (5) Expression of significance of this loss
      (6) Expression of guilt
4. Diagnostic procedures
   a. Ultrasound examination: most accurate to identify absence of fetal cardiac activity
   b. Radiological signs of fetal death
      (1) Significant overlap of skull bones (process takes several days to develop)
      (2) Exaggerated curvature of the fetal spine (depends on the degree of maceration of sacral ligaments)
      (3) Evidence of gas in the fetus (uncommon but reliable sign)
   c. Palpation of collapsed fetal skull through the cervix
   d. Disseminated intravascular coagulopathy (DIC) screen: look for coagulation abnormalities since DIC is a complication related to intrauterine fetal demise

B. Nursing Diagnoses

1. Grieving related to fetal demise
2. High risk for alteration in tissue perfusion related to DIC

C. Interventions/Evaluations

1. Grieving related to fetal demise
    a. Interventions
        (1) Encourage client and her family to verbalize feelings
        (2) Discuss the grieving process with the client and her family (see Health Education section)
        (3) Allow client choices relating to labor and delivery (e.g., induction of labor immediately after diagnosis is made or waiting until the spontaneous onset of labor; clients often benefit from having a few days to deal with this issue before going through delivery)
        (4) Discuss the use of oxytocin or prostaglandin
            (a) Induction with oxytocin is most often used for fetuses at 28 weeks' gestation or beyond
            (b) Prostaglandin suppositories are often preferred for fetuses at earlier gestational stages
            (c) Discuss side effects of prostaglandin
                (i) Nausea
                (ii) Vomiting
                (iii) Diarrhea
        (5) Analgesia or anesthesia
            (a) More liberal use is possible when there is no consideration of drug effect on the fetus
            (b) Avoid oversedation because it may interfere with the grieving process
        (6) Offer client and her family the opportunity to see, touch, and hold the infant
        (7) Provide tangible remembrances (e.g., photographs, footprints, baby identification bands, locks of hair)
        (8) Offer support from clergy members
        (9) Offer baptism or blessing
        (10) Discuss autopsy with client and her family; explain its benefits
        (11) Discuss plans for funeral or memorial services
        (12) Prepare client and her family for appearance of the infant
        (13) Provide client and her family with information about support groups
        (14) Provide reading materials to the client and her family to take home since information may be overwhelming during hospitalization
        (15) Provide materials or references to address specific areas of grieving, such as siblings' responses, grandparents' responses, and so forth
        (16) Follow-up after delivery may be done by a bereavement counselor, a social worker, or the nurse who cared for the client; it should assess the progress of the client and her family in the grieving process after discharge and should continue to provide support
    b. Evaluations
        (1) Client and her family are able to verbalize their feelings and can identify specific ares of concern
        (2) Client and her family can discuss steps in the grieving process
        (3) Client and her family participate in plan of care whenever possible and feel a part of the decision-making process
        (4) Client is comfortable during labor and delivery
        (5) Client and her family see, touch, and hold the infant if they desire
        (6) Client and her family have tangible memories of the infant

(7) Client and her family are aware of available clergy support, as well as options such as baptism and blessing

(8) Client and her family demonstrate understanding of autopsy

(9) Client and her family are aware of options for funeral or memorial services

(10) Client and her family have information on support groups and services available

(11) Client and her family demonstrate appropriate grief response

2. High risk for alteration in tissue perfusion related to DIC (see Chap. 28)

a. Interventions

(1) Assess client for signs and symptoms of DIC

(a) Bleeding from puncture sites

(b) Oozing through surgical incision (if one is present)

(c) Bleeding from gums

(d) Hematuria

(2) Check laboratory values (or obtain order from physician to have coagulation studies done)

(a) Hemoglobin and hematocrit: may be low, reflecting blood loss

(b) Platelet count: may be low in DIC

(c) Prothrombin time (PT) and activated partial thromboplastin time (APTT): elevation indicates clotting dysfunction

(d) Clotting time: prolonged in DIC

(e) Bleeding time: prolonged in DIC

(f) Serum fibrinogen: elevated in DIC

(g) Fibrin split products: elevated in DIC

(3) Assess vital signs to estimate blood loss and its effect

(4) Administer blood and blood products as ordered

b. Evaluation

(1) Client has no signs or symptoms of DIC

(2) Client's vital signs remain within normal limits

Health Education

A. Stages of grief (see Chap. 25 on grief and loss)

1. Shock and numbness
2. Searching (includes anger)
3. Disorientation
4. Reorganization

B. Normal grief responses

1. Preoccupation with the dead infant
2. Guilt and self-blame
3. Anger and hostility
4. Parents may grieve at a different pace and, therefore, parents may seem not to be available to each other for support
5. Strange dreams related to the baby
6. Aching arms
7. Hearing a baby cry
8. Still feeling the baby move

C. Appearance of dead infant

1. Maceration (peeling) of the skin
2. Discoloration of areas that had pressure on them, which look grossly ecchymotic
3. Areas of swelling and fluid retention
4. Discussion of any specific abnormalities

5. Amniotic fluid often appears reddish brown and more viscous than normal
6. Delivery may cause trauma more readily (e.g., skull bones may collapse and cause unusual facial appearance)

Amniotic Fluid Embolism

Introduction

A. Entry of amniotic fluid into the maternal circulatory system is a rare but extremely dangerous obstetrical complication; incidence is approximately 1/65,000

B. It results in severe pulmonary vascular obstruction, especially when meconium is present in the fluid

C. Clinically, a tumultuous labor is followed by an acute onset of respiratory distress and circulatory collapse (often during the delivery process) and then, by a rapid onset of severe coagulopathy

D. The mortality rate for this complication has been reported to be as high as 80%

Clinical Practice

A. Assessment
1. History
   a. Rapid, vigorous labor
   b. Evidence of abruptio placentae
2. Physical findings
   a. Acute onset of respiratory distress, often during delivery process
      (1) Dyspnea
      (2) Chest pain
      (3) Cyanosis
      (4) Loss of consciousness
      (5) Pulmonary edema
   b. Acute onset of circulatory collapse
      (1) Severe hypotension
      (2) Severe hypoxia
      (3) If client does not die from the initial respiratory insult, she needs to overcome the severe hemorrhage and coagulopathy that follow
   c. Acute onset of coagulopathy
      (1) Uterine bleeding at delivery not easily controlled
      (2) Oozing may begin from puncture sites
3. Psychosocial findings
   a. Fear of death
   b. Fear on the part of the family in response to the rapid onset of life-threatening complications
4. Diagnostic procedures
   a. The diagnosis of amniotic fluid embolism must be made from the clinical picture
   b. The only way to make a definitive diagnosis is through the identification of amniotic fluid and particulate debris (e.g., meconium, vernix, lanugo, or mucin) that are obstructing the pulmonary vasculature
   c. This diagnostic procedure, however, is done only on autopsy

B. Nursing Diagnoses
1. Alteration in tissue perfusion related to pulmonary obstruction by particulate amniotic fluid
2. Fear related to life-threatening emergency

C. Interventions/Evaluations

1. Alteration in tissue perfusion related to pulmonary obstruction by particulate amniotic fluid
   a. Interventions
      (1) Recognize life-threatening diagnosis
      (2) Ensure IV access; if client does not have an IV line, start one immediately, since a delay of even a few minutes may result in circulatory collapse and make IV access impossible
      (3) Initiate cardiopulmonary rescusitation (CPR) if indicated
      (4) Administer oxygen at a rate of at least 8 l/min
      (5) Prepare for and assist with intubation and ventilation if client loses consciousness
      (6) Administer IV fluids rapidly if client is hypotensive; if blood pressure is maintained, do not overload with fluids since it could result in pulmonary edema
      (7) Monitor vital signs frequently
      (8) Observe for signs and symptoms of shock
      (9) Observe for signs and symptoms of coagulopathy (inability to control intrapartum or immediate postpartum vaginal bleeding or bleeding from IV site or puncture or trauma sites)
      (10) Send laboratory work
          (a) CBC
          (b) Platelet count
          (c) Arterial blood gases
          (d) Fibrinogen
          (e) Fibrin split products
          (f) PT and APTT
      (11) Prepare for and assist with placement of central line (a pulmonary artery catheter may be useful for further hemodynamic management)
      (12) Administer blood or volume expanders as ordered
   b. Evaluations
      (1) Client survives incident
      (2) Client survives resulting complications
          (a) Client is hemodynamically stable
          (b) CBC is within normal limits
          (c) Coagulation studies are within normal limits
          (d) Oxygen saturation is within normal limits
      (3) Client does not develop adult respiratory distress syndrome (ARDS)
2. Fear related to life-threatening emergency
   a. Interventions
      (1) Inform and reassure client as much as possible during crisis
      (2) After life-threatening emergency has resolved, allow client to verbalize her feelings
   b. Evaluations
      (1) Client does not experience panic during episode
      (2) Client resolves her fear once the crisis has passed

Health Education

A. Amniotic fluid embolism is so rare an obstetrical complication that there is no need to prepare a client for its possibility

B. After a client has survived such an incident, the nurse may explain to her what is known about amniotic fluid embolism

1. Composition of amniotic fluid
   a. Particulate matter leads to embolism
      (1) Fetal squamous cells (from exfoliation of skin)

(2) Vernix caseosa

(3) Lanugo

(4) Meconium

    (a) When amniotic fluid embolism accompanies other complications, such as abruptio placentae, there is a much higher incidence of fetal distress and resultant passage of meconium

    (b) Maternal pulmonary vascular obstruction is most severe when there is meconium in the fluid

2. Access to the maternal circulation

    a. Amniotic fluid is usually contained within the uterine cavity and is separated from the maternal circulatory system

    b. Introduction of amniotic fluid into the maternal circulation may occur in the following instances

        (1) The amnion and the chorion are open, such as occurs with rupture of the amniotic sac

        (2) There are open uterine or cervical veins, such as occurs with placental separation

        (3) There is a pressure gradient high enough to force the amniotic fluid into the maternal circulation, such as occurs in a very vigorous labor or with the tetanic contractions that result from abruptio placentae

3. Emboli: obstruction of the pulmonary vessels and interruption of the gas exchange is the same mechanism that occurs in any embolism

Uterine Rupture

Introduction

A. Uterine rupture is a rare occurrence, with an incidence of 1/1500, but is considered an obstetrical emergency

B. The most common cause is previous C section or major uterine surgery

C. Stimulation with oxytocin is also considered a cause

D. A normal uterus with no prior surgery and that is contracting spontaneously is unlikely to rupture unless there is significant trauma

E. With more and more clients choosing a trial of labor after a previous C section, it is important for the nurse to be familiar with the signs and symptoms of uterine rupture

Clinical Practice

A. Assessment

1. History

    a. Pregnancies, viable pregnancies, and estimated date of confinement (EDC)

    b. Previous C section and indication

    c. Types of uterine incision

        (1) Low transverse: considered to be the safest for subsequent stress of uterine contractions

        (2) Classical: considered to be the highest risk for rupture with the stress of uterine contractions

    d. Type of uterine activity: contraction frequency, duration, and intensity

    e. Pain

    f. Uterine anomalies

    g. Abdominal trauma: sharp or blunt

    h. Previous uterine trauma, such as perforation at the time of dilatation and curettage (D&C) or instrumented abortion

        i. Intrauterine administration of hypertonic saline

        j. Aggressive administration of oxytocin or prostaglandin

  2. Physical findings

    a. Abdominal examination: observe for any rigidity or tenderness

    b. Leopold's maneuver (position of fetus): observe for any unusual feeling of fetal parts since fetus could be outside of the uterus

    c. FHR tracing: observe for fetal distress; if uterus ruptures, placental circulation will be interrupted and result in acute fetal hypoxia

  3. Psychosocial findings

    a. Stress factors

      (1) Anxiety

      (2) Fear related to pain

      (3) Fear of the unknown

    b. Behavioral responses

      (1) Expression of fear

      (2) Difficulty in communicating

B. **Nursing Diagnoses**

1. High risk for injury: maternal shock related to blood loss secondary to uterine rupture
2. High risk for injury: fetal distress secondary to impaired uteroplacental blood flow
3. Alteration in comfort: pain related to uterine rupture
4. Fear related to life-threatening complication
5. Fear related to threatened loss of baby

C. **Interventions/Evaluations**

1. High risk for injury: maternal shock related to blood loss secondary to uterine rupture

    a. Interventions

      (1) Monitor maternal vital signs: observe for hypotension and tachycardia, which may indicate hypovolemic shock

      (2) Observe any blood loss and estimate amount as accurately as possible

      (3) Maintain IV access with large-bore IV

      (4) Prepare for emergency C section if there is any evidence of uterine rupture

        (a) Alert operating room and anthesiologist

        (b) Alert client's physician

        (c) Alert neonatal team or pediatrician

        (d) Perform abdominal shave and skin prep

        (e) Insert Foley catheter

        (f) Have client sign consent forms

      (5) Monitor hemoglobin and hematocrit levels

      (6) Administer blood and blood products as ordered

    b. Evaluation: client shows no evidence of hypovolemic shock

2. High risk for injury: fetal distress related to impaired uteroplacental blood flow

    a. Interventions

      (1) Maintain continuous FHR monitoring: observe for any indications of fetal distress, especially late decelerations or prolonged bradycardia

      (2) Maintain client on her left side to maximize uterine blood flow

    b. Evaluation: client is delivered of a viable infant with no irreversible damage

3. Alteration in comfort: pain related to uterine rupture

    a. Interventions

      (1) Continuous monitoring in labor for FHR and to record uterine activity; it is preferable to have an intrauterine pressure catheter in place to document intensity of uterine contractions accurately

      (2) Analgesics or anesthesia may be used for pain control if there is no evidence of abnormal uterine activity indicating rupture

(a) If the client has had analgesics or anesthesia, the pain associated with rupture may be masked

(b) The nurse must, therefore, be acutely aware of any changes in uterine activity patterns

b. Evaluations

(1) Client does not experience intolerable pain during labor

(2) Analgesics are not given when there is evidence of uterine rupture

4. Fear related to life-threatening complication

a. Interventions

(1) Encourage client to verbalize her feelings and to identify specific concerns

(2) Provide as much information as possible to the client

(3) Reassure client as often as possible during any emergency procedures

b. Evaluation: client does not have unreasonable fears

5. Fear related to threatened loss of fetus

a. Interventions: if there is a uterine rupture, every effort is made to deliver the fetus immediately by C section; a client's fear of losing the fetus at this point is a valid one

(1) Perform all tasks as quickly as possible

(2) Solicit help to minimize time it takes to prepare client for delivery

(3) Stay calm and reassure client that health care team is doing everything possible to save the fetus

b. Evaluation: client does not become uncooperative or hysterical as a result of fear

Health Education

A. Definitions

1. Uterine rupture is classified as complete or incomplete

2. It is defined by *Williams Obstetrics* (Pritchard, MacDonald, & Gant, 1987) as follows

a. Complete uterine rupture: laceration communicates directly with the peritoneal cavity

b. Incomplete uterine rupture: laceration is separated from the peritoneal cavity by the visceral peritoneum

c. Uterine scar dehiscence: previous scar begins to separate; this usually happens gradually, and if the fetal membranes are intact, there is no protrusion of fetal parts into the peritoneal cavity

B. Type of scar

1. Low transverse

a. Incision into the lower uterine segment

b. Because of the way the muscle fibers are arranged, low transverse scars are under relatively little tension when the uterus contracts

2. Classical incision

a. Uterine scar is vertically placed on the body of the uterus, up as far as the fundus

b. This area is under a great deal of stress with contractions

c. Classical incisions are done if a C section is indicated before term, because the lower uterine segment is not yet well enough developed, but they may also be done for an urgent C section; this is why it is important to ask the patient the reason for a previous C section

CASE STUDIES AND STUDY QUESTIONS

Connie Rudolph is a 22-year-old gravida 3, para 2 (G3,P2) woman. She was delivered of her first child spontaneously at 34 weeks' gestation and the child has subsequently done well. Her second child was born by C section at 29 weeks and died 10 days later from complications of prematurity. Connie is currently at 25 ⅔ weeks' gestation and has been feeling pelvic pressure and a vague sense of cramping since this morning at 7:00 A.M. It is now 11:00 A.M., and she has called the labor and delivery unit because of concerns about her cramping.

1. Which of the following is your best response to Connie?

   a. Maintain bed rest in the left lateral position and drink plenty of fluids.

   b. Come to the hospital immediately for further evaluation.

   c. Do not be concerned since the cramping is probably Braxton Hicks contractions and is normal at this gestational stage.

2. Connie is at risk for preterm labor because of which of the following?

   a. She is a young multipara.

   b. She has had a previous C section.

   c. She has had previous preterm labors and births.

   d. She is not at risk for preterm labor.

Post-term Pregnancy

Cherie Lane is a 26-year-old gravida 1, para 0 (G1,P0) woman. She has had no prenatal care but her last menstrual period puts her at 42 ⅔ weeks' gestation. She came into the hospital with possible rupture of membranes. She is not sure whether her membranes have ruptured because, although she felt a gush, she saw only a small amount of brownish fluid.

3. The labor and delivery nurse is concerned about Cherie because of which of the following?

   a. She is probably in preterm labor.

   b. Her history indicates oligohydramnios and the probable presence of meconium.

   c. She is at risk because she is an elderly primipara.

   d. She is in active labor at this time.

After Cherie has been on the external fetal monitor for 40 minutes, the tracing shows minimal FHR variability, but no evidence of decelerations. There is no fetal movement and no spontaneous FHR accelerations.

4. Appropriate nursing interventions at this time include which of the following?

   a. Preparing Cherie for an emergency C section.

   b. Allowing Cherie to ambulate to stimulate the onset of contractions.

   c. Maintain Cherie on bed rest in left lateral position, starting an IV, and continuing the FHR monitoring.

   d. Discharging Cherie home to return when contractions are 5 minutes apart.

Premature Rupture of Membranes

Lisa Scott is a 30-year-old gravida 3, para 2 (G3,P2) woman at 31 weeks' gestation. She presents to the labor and delivery suite complaining of leaking fluid for the past couple of hours. Her vital signs are blood pressure 108/60, pulse 70, respirations 20, and 97.6°F (36.4°C) temperature. She is monitored for 1 hour, and the FHR tracing is in the range of 130 to 145, showing average variability and no decelerations. No uterine contractions are perceived by Lisa or recorded on the monitor.

5. Lisa is a candidate for expectant management because of which of the following?

   a. She is afebrile and has no other symptoms of infection.

   b. Her fetus is in the vertex position.

   c. There is still a normal amount of amniotic fluid by ultrasound examination.

   d. She is not a candidate for expectant management.

6. In your initial assessment of Lisa, you note that she is nitrazine-negative but positive for vaginal pooling and ferning. This would lead you to believe that she is which of the following?

   a. Probably not ruptured, since nitrazine is the most accurate test.

   b. Most likely ruptured since there are many factors that may interfere with nitrazine testing.

   c. Definitely ruptured since ferning is 100% accurate.

d. Most likely infected since that causes a positive fern test.

Multiple Gestation

Sondra Genardo is a 33-year-old gravida 1, para 0 (G1,P0) woman. She has a history of infertility for 4 years and conceived while taking fertility drugs. She is carrying twins at 34 weeks' gestation and presents to the labor and delivery unit with complaints of cramping and a feeling of pelvic pressure. After 30 minutes on the fetal monitor, you note that Sondra has mild uterine contractions every 5 to 6 minutes. Her cervical examination reveals a long, closed posterior cervix.

7. Uterine activity at 34 weeks is particularly significant for Sondra because of which of the following?

   a. She is at high risk for preterm labor.

   b. She has been contracting and her cervix has not changed.

   c. She is at high risk for chorioamnionitis.

   d. There is no reason for concern; uterine contractions are common at this gestational age.

8. Sondra is also at high risk for which other pregnancy complications?

   a. PIH.

   b. Abruptio placentae.

   c. Premature rupture of membranes.

   d. All of the above.

Intrauterine Fetal Demise

Terri Oka is a 34-year-old gravida 3, para 1 (G3,P1) class C diabetic. She had a previous stillborn at 36 weeks' gestation with an undetermined cause of the fetal death. She is currently at 35 ³/₇ weeks' gestation. She has had an uneventful pregnancy so far but now calls the labor and delivery unit because she has not felt the baby move since early this morning. It is now 1:00 P.M.

9. Your best response to Terri is to tell her which of the following?

   a. To come in to labor and delivery as soon as possible for further evaluation.

   b. To wait at least 10 to 12 hours, then call her physician if she still has not felt movement.

   c. That her anxiety is most likely related to her previous loss at this gestation and therefore there is no need for concern.

   d. To maintain bed rest in the left lateral position.

10. When Terri arrives in the labor and delivery unit, you are unable to ascultate fetal heart tones. You suspect she may have an intrauterine fetal demise. The most definitive way to confirm this diagnosis is to do which of the following?

    a. Document the absence of fetal cardiac activity by ultrasonography.

    b. Send her for pelvic radiographs.

    c. Find an elevation in serum fibrinogen.

    d. Obtain an L/S ratio.

Amniotic Fluid Embolism

Nan Neuhaus is a 25-year-old gravida 1, para 0 (G1,P0) woman at term who arrives in the labor and delivery unit at 2:00 A.M. Her contractions started at midnight, and their frequency and intensity increased so rapidly that Nan could no longer tolerate the pain and came into the hospital. On examination, her cervix is 6 cm dilated and completely effaced. The presenting part is at zero station. Nan continues in very active labor with uterine contractions every 1 ½ to 2 minutes over the next 30 minutes, at the end of which she is completely dilated and effaced. She pushes for 10 minutes and is prepared for delivery.

11. Immediately after the delivery of the infant, Nan complains of dyspnea and shortness of breath. Within minutes, she becomes cyanotic and lethargic, and seems to be losing consciousness. Recognizing this clinical picture as most likely an amniotic fluid embolism, appropriate nursing actions are to do which of the following?

    a. Prepare a loading dose of magnesium sulfate for seizure precaution.

    b. Open Nan's IV line and also administer oxygen at high concentrations.

    c. Notify the NICU and prepare for possible neonatal transfer because the newborn is at great risk for respiratory distress syndrome (RDS).

d. Perform an abdominal shave and skin preparation to get Nan ready for emergency surgery.

12. Nan is intubated and ventilated by the anesthesiologist for 10 miniutes. She is fighting the endotracheal tube and breathing on her own. Blood for laboratory work is drawn, and her arterial blood gas values are within normal limits. Nan is extubated and she resumes spontaneous respirations. Her color is good, but nasal oxygen is kept on at 10 l/min. Her oxygen saturation is 96 to 97%. Nan has survived the initial insult of an amniotic fluid embolism. She is still at great risk for which subsequent complication?

a. Pre-eclampsia.

b. Adult respiratory distress syndrome.

c. Postpartum endometritis.

d. Deep vein thromboembolism.

Uterine Rupture

Paula Dunworthy is a 30-year-old gravida 2, para 1 (G2,P1) class B diabetic who is at term. She had a previous C section at 27 weeks' gestation for an abruptio placentae 6 years earlier.

13. Paula is not a candidate for trial of labor because of which of the following?

a. This baby is likely to be much bigger than her previous one.

b. She is a diabetic and therefore requires another C section.

c. A C section done at 28 weeks' gestation was likely to have been a classical incision.

d. She _is_ a good candidate for trial of labor.

14. If Paula arrived in the labor and delivery unit and told you she had been having contractions for the past 8 hours and now the pain "just won't go away," you might consider the possibility of uterine rupture. Other assessment parameters consistent with uterine rupture are which of the following?

a. Systolic hypertension.

b. Tachycardia.

c. Abdominal rigidity.

d. Excess fetal movement.

Answers to Study Questions

1. b	2. c	3. b
4. c	5. a	6. b
7. a	8. d	9. a
10. a	11. b	12. b
13. c	14. c	

REFERENCES

American College of Obstetricians and Gynecologists (1989). Multiple gestation. *ACOG Technical Bulletin, 131.*

Bates, B. (1987). *A guide to physical examination and history taking* (4th ed.). Philadelphia: Lippincott.

Clark, S.L., Phelan, J.P., Cotton, D.B. (1987). *Critical care obstetrics.* Oradell, NJ: Medical Economics.

Cohen, V. (1985). Postmaturity in pregnancy. *NAACOG Update Series, 3*(25), 1–8.

Creasy, R.K., & Resnick, R. (1989). *Maternal-fetal medicine: Principles and practice* (2nd ed.). Philadelphia: Saunders.

Dunn, L.K. (1982). Postmaturity pregnancy. In R. H. Schwarz & J. Schneider (Eds.). *Perinatal medicine* (pp. 304–311). Baltimore: Williams & Wilkins.

Fitzgerald, G.S. (1984). Preterm labor. Part 2: Management. *NAACOG Update Series, 1*(3), 1–8.

Freeman, R.K., Garite, T.J., Nageotte, M.P. (1991). *Fetal heart rate monitoring* (2nd ed.). Baltimore: Williams & Wilkins.

Garite, T.J. (1984). Premature rupture of the membranes. *Current Problems in Obstetrics and Gynecology, 7*(8), 4–45.

Herron, M. (1984). Preterm labor. Part 1: Preventing preterm births. *NAACOG Update Series, 1*(2), 1–8.

Leaphart, E.C. (1985). Perinatal loss: Strategies to facilitate bereavement. *NAACOG Update Series, 3*(2), 1–8.

Limbo, R., & Wheeler, S. (1986). *When a baby dies: A handbook for healing and helping.* LaCrosse, WI: Resolve Through Sharing.

Moore, K.L. (1974). *Before we are born* (2nd ed.). Philadelphia: Saunders.

Pritchard, J.A., MacDonald, P.C., & Gant, N.F., (1987). *Williams obstetrics* (18th ed.). Norwalk, CT: Appleton-Century-Crofts.

Patricia Higgins

Postpartum Complications

Objectives

1. Identify four different types of postpartum complications

2. Recognize the causes of postpartum complications

3. Select appropriate nursing actions to reduce postpartum complications

4. Define specific treatments for postpartum complications

5. Assess risk factors for women who are prone to postpartum complications

6. Design health education strategies to prevent postpartum complications

7. Appraise postpartum complications based on selected case studies

8. Analyze assessment data for postpartum complications based on risk factors presented by women

9. Interpret alterations in adaptation to maternal illness in the puerperium

10. Analyze alterations in maternal psychological adaptation in the puerperium

11. Formulate nursing interventions to prevent disequilibrium in transition to parenthood and implement the nursing process to promote a healthy outcome

12. Apply the nursing process to provide care to the high-risk postpartum client and her family based on analysis and synthesis of the client's needs in her particular situation

Postpartum hemorrhage

INTRODUCTION

A. **Approximately one-third of maternal deaths are related to postpartum hemorrhage, which is defined as a blood loss greater than 500 ml in the first 24 hours after delivery**

1. Immediate postpartum hemorrhage occurs in the first 24 hours after delivery, and late postpartum hemorrhage occurs after the first 24 hours after delivery, usually at 7 to 14 days of the postpartum period

2. The major causes of postpartum hemorrhage are uterine atony, lacerations,

hematomas, retained placental fragments, uterine inversion, and coagulation disorders

   a. The most frequent cause of bleeding in the puerperium arises from interference with involution of the uterus
   b. Uterine atony occurs early after delivery in 75 to 85% of the postpartum cases
   c. Late postpartum hemorrhage is often caused by retained placental fragments
3. The overall incidence of postpartum hemorrhage is 4% of deliveries

B. Hematoma, a cause of postpartum hemorrhage, is a collection of blood in the pelvic tissue due to damage to a vessel wall without laceration of the tissue
1. This trauma can result from forceps' manipulation, pressure of the presenting part on pelvic structures, or excessive fundal pressure on the uterus

C. Disseminated intravascular coagulation (DIC) can cause postpartum hemorrhage by altering the blood clotting mechanism; abruptio placentae, fetal demise, or amniotic fluid embolism may be the underlying cause of DIC (see Chapter 28 for a complete discussion of hemorrhagic disorders)

CLINICAL PRACTICE

A. Assessment
1. History
   a. Precipitous or prolonged first or second stages of labor, or both
   b. Overstretching of the uterus (suggests a large fetus, hydramnios, or multiple gestation)
   c. Drugs (general anesthesia, oxytocin, and magnesium sulfate)
   d. Toxins (amnionitis and intrauterine fetal demise)
   e. Use of forceps or other intravaginal manipulations, such as internal podalic version
   f. Previous postpartum hemorrhage, uterine rupture, or uterine surgery (cesarean section or dilatation and curettage)
   g. Past placenta previa, placenta increta, or placenta percreta
   h. Uterine malformation
   i. Maternal exhaustion
   j. Defects in the decidua (outer layer of the endometrium that sloughs off as lochia)
   k. Manipulation of the placenta which occurs when the placenta is not delivered intact and manual extraction is necessary
   l. Rapid fetal descent
   m. Coagulation disorders, such as idiopathic thrombocytopenia, purpura, von Willebrand's disease
2. Physical findings
   a. Uterine atony
      (1) Boggy, large uterus
      (2) Expelled clots
      (3) Bleeding (bright red blood) visible and evident
   b. Lacerations
      (1) Firm uterus with bright red blood
      (2) Steady stream or trickle of unclotted blood
   c. Hematoma
      (1) Firm uterus with bright red blood
      (2) Extreme perineal or pelvic pain
      (3) Bluish bulging area just under the skin surface
      (4) Difficultly in voiding
      (5) Unexplained tachycardia

       (6) Hypotension
       (7) Anemia
  d. Retained placental fragments
       (1) Placenta is not delivered intact
       (2) Uterus remains large
       (3) Bleeding is painless and blood is bright red in color
  e. DIC
       (1) Petechiae
       (2) Ecchymosis
       (3) Prolonged bleeding from gums and venipuncture sites
       (4) Uncontrolled bleeding during childbirth
       (5) Tachycardia
       (6) Oliguria
       (7) Signs of acute renal failure
       (8) Convulsions
       (9) Coma
  f. Decreased systolic blood pressure
  g. Reduced pulse pressure and delayed capillary filling time
  h. Cold, clammy skin
  i. Profound hypotension
  j. Signs of metabolic acidosis
  k. Signs of shock do not appear until hemorrhage is advanced because of increased fluid and blood volume of pregnancy
3. Psychosocial response
  a. Fear
  b. Anxiety and restlessness
  c. Fatigue
4. Diagnostic procedures
  a. Complete blood count (CBC)
  b. Type and crossmatching of blood products for transfusion
  c. Blood work-up to determine reduced platelets, prolonged prothrombin time, fibrinogen depression, normal clotting time, and prolonged partial thromboplastin time

B. Nursing Diagnoses

1. Fluid volume deficit: high risk for complications related to postpartum hemorrhage
2. Fatigue related to blood loss
3. Fear related to acute hemorrhage

C. Interventions/Evaluations

1. Fluid volume deficit: high risk for complications related to postpartum hemorrhage
  a. Interventions
       (1) After initial postdelivery assessment, assess the height and midline position of the fundus at least each shift
          (a) If uterus is soft and boggy, perform manual uterine massage
          (b) For mild uterine bogginess, put baby to breast if mother is breastfeeding
       (2) Monitor lochia for color, odor, amount, consistency, clots, count or weight of used pads (1 g = 1 ml)
       (3) Keep accurate intake and output (I&O)
       (4) Monitor and record vital signs
       (5) Turn client when assessing postpartal bleeding so blood does not pool unnoticed underneath her
       (6) Keep client flat to supply blood to heart and brain
       (7) Set up for IV infusion of Ringer's lactate or saline solution

(8) Catheterization of distended bladder may assist uterine contraction and descent

(9) Check that crossmatching has been completed for blood replacement

(10) Administer oxytocin in 500 to 1000 ml of solution

(11) If uterus remains atonic, give ergonovine maleate (Ergotrate) or methylergonovine (Methergine) IV or IM, if ordered

(12) If bleeding persists, ask physician to consider prostaglandin therapy

(13) Have physician check for retained placental fragments

(14) Surgical intervention is last resort

(15) Provide bimanual compression if physician is not available or there are no standing orders for oxytocin

(16) Provide explanations to the client of all procedures

  b. Evaluations

(1) Fundus firm, midline, and at the level of the umbilicus or below

(2) Lochia is red, odorless, moderate in amount, and unclotted

(3) Vital signs are normal

(4) I&O is adequate

2. Fatigue related to blood loss

  a. Interventions

(1) Allow and schedule client rest periods that are undisturbed

(2) Assist client with activities of daily living

(3) Encourage client to monitor appropriate nutritional intake

(4) Work around client's schedule to conserve energy

(5) Organize work habits and tasks

(6) Encourage client to take vitamins and iron tablets

(7) Prevent orthostatic hypotension when getting client up

  b. Evaluations

(1) Client has enough energy to care for self and baby

(2) Client has support from family and friends to help with household tasks

(3) Client maintains optimal nutritional status

(4) Client has adequate sleep and rest

3. Fear related to acute hemorrhage

  a. Interventions

(1) Stay with client and use physical touch

(2) Offer client reassurance and support

(3) Give information to client in clear, brief statements

(4) Keep client's family informed

  b. Evaluations

(1) Client has positive support during a crisis situation

(2) Family is informed of client's progress and status

HEALTH EDUCATION

A. Teach client about involution process (where the client's fundus should be when she can no longer feel it)

B. Teach client about lochia changes (when bleeding should stop and how lochia should appear)

C. Teach client about perineal care (how to apply and change menstrual pads)

D. Teach client how to massage fundus as indicated by tone

E. Teach client about self-care information such as nutrition, signs of infection, breast care, elimination, activity, and rest

Postpartum Infections

INTRODUCTION

A. An infection accompanied by a temperature of 38°C (100.4°F) or higher after the first 24 hours after delivery
1. Temperature remains elevated on two or more occasions for longer than 24 hours
2. No other defined cause for the fever

B. Postpartum infection occurs after about 6% of births in the United States

C. Other perinatal events that can cause an elevated temperature
1. Dehydration from fluid loss during labor and delivery
2. Breast engorgement if temperature elevation occurs 48 to 72 hours after delivery
3. Postoperative elevation after a cesarean birth

D. The most common type of postpartum infection is endometritis, which occurs secondary to chorioamnionitis before birth

E. Cesarean section wound infection
1. Occurs after the third or fourth postoperative day
2. Can be masked by early postoperative fever

F. The most common causative agents of postpartum infections are the following
1. Anaerobic streptococcus
2. *Clostridia*
3. Beta-hemolytic streptococcus
4. *Escherichia coli*
5. *Klebsiella*

G. The three categories of postpartum infections are those involving
1. The reproductive or genital tract
2. The urinary tract
3. The breasts

CLINICAL PRACTICE

A. Assessment

1. History
   a. Long labor (longer than 24 hours, with fatigue and exhaustion that result in trauma or decrease the perception of the need to void)
   b. Anemia
   c. Traumatic delivery
   d. Postpartum hemorrhage
   e. Premature rupture of the membranes (PROM)
   f. Cesarean birth
   g. Malnutrition
   h. General debilitation
   i. Diabetes
   j. Intrauterine manipulation
   k. Many vaginal examinations during labor, especially after rupture of membranes (ROM)
   l. Hematoma
   m. Droplet infection from personnel
   n. Breaks in aseptic technique
   o. Frequent catheterization

    p. Poor personal care of client

    q. Laceration (third or fourth degree)

  2. Physical findings

    a. Genital tract infections involving the perineum, vulva, vagina, or cervix

      (1) Temperature: low grade 38 to 38.5°C (100.4 to 101°F)

      (2) Site of infection is red and warm to the touch

      (3) Drainage may or may not be present

      (4) Dysuria (burning on urination)

      (5) Pain

      (6) Edema

    b. Genital tract infections involving the muscle of the uterus (metritis) at the placental site (endometritis), or pelvic connective tissue (parametritis)

      (1) Temperature: 38.5 to 39.5°C (101 to 103°F)

      (2) Large, tender uterus and fundus is +1 on third postpartum day (subinvolution)

      (3) Malaise

      (4) Chills

      (5) Headache

      (6) Backache

      (7) Increased pulse rate (100 to 140 BPM)

      (8) Foul-smelling lochia that can be decreased or increased in amount

      (9) Diaphoresis

    c. Urinary tract infections and cystitis

      (1) Small voiding volume or inability to void

      (2) Pain with urination

      (3) Low-grade fever 38.5°C (101°F)

      (4) Hematuria

    d. Infections of the breast: mastitis

      (1) Temperature elevated to 40°C (104.1°F)

      (2) Chills

      (3) Malaise

      (4) Hard, red, and tender irregular mass in one or both breasts

      (5) Severe to acute pain and tenderness in one or both breasts

      (6) Cracked nipples

    e. Wound infections from cesarean section or dehiscence

      (1) Elevated temperature on third or fourth postpartum day

      (2) Drainage of pus or blood from the wound

      (3) Red and inflamed appearance of repaired edges

      (4) Presence of cellulitis

      (5) Wound opened and abdominal contents exposed to air

  3. Psychosocial findings

    a. Anxiety

    b. Stress

    c. Pain

  4. Diagnostic procedures

    a. Urinalysis

    b. Culture and sensitivity tests, as necessary, for lochia, urine, breast milk, blood, wound, vagina, and vulva; obtain cultures before starting antibiotic therapy

    c. Blood count: WBC count and hemoglobin and hematocrit

B. Nursing Diagnoses

1. Alteration in comfort related to infectious process
2. High risk for infection: genital, urinary, or breast, or wound dehiscence related to bacterial invasion
3. Alteration in body temperature related to perineal or wound infections

4. High risk for alteration in support related to extended hospitalization for perineal or wound infection
5. High risk for delay in attachment to newborn and maternal role development related to postpartum infection

C. **Interventions/Evaluations**

1. Alteration in comfort related to infectious process
    a. Interventions: provide the following (see Chapter 19 for a complete discussion of mastitis and lactation)
       (1) Adequate nutrition
       (2) Adequate fluids
       (3) Adequate rest and sleep
       (4) Frequent linen change
       (5) Breast and perineal care
       (6) Breast binder or brassiere
       (7) Administration of analgesics
       (8) Heat or cold treatment
       (9) Breasts kept empty
       (10) Facilitation of complete bladder emptying
       (11) Bed bath with back rub
    b. Evaluations
       (1) Client is comfortable
       (2) Client is free of pain
       (3) Client has no complaints
       (4) Client is resting well
2. High risk for infection: genital, urinary, or breast, or wound dehiscence related to bacterial invasion
    a. Interventions
       (1) Do culture and sensitivity tests
       (2) Provide antibiotics
       (3) Administer antipyretics
       (4) Ensure isolation
       (5) Use aseptic technique
       (6) Use good handwashing
       (7) Use semi-Fowler's position to facilitate drainage
       (8) Assess fundus for involution
       (9) Assess vital signs
       (10) Assess pain symptoms and administer medications on time
       (11) Monitor and record I&O
       (12) Provide frequent rest periods
       (13) Measure and record amount of redness and drainage
       (14) Maintain wound intact
       (15) If wound opens
           (a) Pack and repack the wound so it can heal by secondary intention
           (b) If dehiscence occurs, apply normal saline solution to sterile cloth, cover the protruding organs, and return client to operating room
    b. Evaluations
       (1) Infection does not result in more serious complications
       (2) Signs and symptoms of infection are recognized promptly with treatment protocols followed
       (3) No dehiscence occurs
3. Alteration in body temperature related to perineal or wound infections
    a. Interventions
       (1) Assess vital signs every 4 hours
       (2) Change bed linen when damp
       (3) Offer client bed bath or shower

        (4) Administer antipyretics
        (5) Force 2000 ml of fluid per shift
        (6) Record I&O
        (7) Offer client back rub or application of cool cloth to forehead
        (8) Change client's gown frequently
    b. Evaluation: body temperature remains normal for longer than 24 hours
  4. High risk for alteration in support related to extended hospitalization for perineal or wound infection
    a. Interventions
        (1) Allow client's family and friends to visit or telephone if client has sufficient energy
        (2) Keep client's family informed at all times
        (3) Have same nurse care for client whenever possible
        (4) Explain care measures to client
        (5) Allow client time to discuss feelings and concerns
    b. Evaluations
        (1) Client has support and maintains family contact
        (2) Client and family feel informed of client's condition
        (3) Client discusses problems with nurse
  5. High risk for delay in attachment to newborn and maternal role development related to postpartum infection
    a. Interventions
        (1) Arrange for adequate rest and sleep
        (2) Bring baby to client after she is rested
        (3) Allow client to offer care and comfort to her baby if she has the energy to do so
        (4) Explain positive aspects of baby to client
        (5) Give client positive reinforcement for tasks achieved
        (6) Allow other caregivers to care for the baby so client can rest and recover
        (7) Encourage client to take care of herself first before she takes care of her baby
    b. Evaluations
        (1) Client has minimal delay in bonding with baby
        (2) Client expresses positive feelings toward baby
        (3) Client feels comfortable with new skills learned to care for her baby's needs
        (4) Client is able to care for baby after she is well rested
        (5) Client allows others to care for baby
        (6) Client has help when she goes home so she can focus on getting to know her baby

HEALTH EDUCATION

A. Teach client about perineal care and how to wipe after voiding and defecation

B. Teach client about transmission of infection and ways to prevent complications and further infections

C. Arrange for household help for client, if necessary

D. Teach client about importance of rest, nutrition, and fluids

Thrombophlebitis

INTRODUCTION

A. Thrombophlebitis is an infection of the lining of a vessel in which a clot attaches to the vessel wall

B. Condition may involve the veins in the legs or the pelvis

C. Condition occurs in less than 1% of all postpartum women
1. Early ambulation after delivery decreases incidence
2. Still remains a concern because of the increased blood clotting factors in the postpartum period

D. Onset is usually between the 10th and 20th postpartum days

E. Thrombophlebitis puts the new mother at risk for a pulmonary embolism and death related to obstruction of the circulation to the lung

F. Superficial thrombophlebitis
1. Involves the saphenous (surface) venous system
2. May be caused in some women by the lithotomy position during delivery

G. Deep vein thrombophlebitis
1. Changes that take place in the deep veins of the calf, thighs, or pelvis predispose postpartum women to deep vein thrombophlebitis
2. One cause may be pressure from the fetal head during delivery, which traumatizes the pelvic veins
3. Increased risk of embolism

CLINICAL PRACTICE

A. Assessment
1. History
    a. Use of oral contraceptives before pregnancy
    b. Employment that requires prolonged sitting
    c. Obesity
    d. Hemorrhage
    e. Operative delivery
    f. Heart disease
    g. Anemia
    h. Long labor
    i. Postdelivery pelvic infection
    j. Increased parity
    k. Advanced age
    l. Noted between 10th and 20th postpartum day
    m. Past history of thrombophlebitis
2. Physical findings
    a. Positive Homans' sign: extend leg, support it under the knee, apply pressure to the foot (forced dorsiflexion); pain is experienced behind calf or in calf when thrombosis is present
    b. Elevated body temperature up to 40.5°C (105°F)
    c. Chills
    d. Pain experienced in leg
    e. Leg hot to touch
    f. Swelling and tenderness in leg
    g. Redness along vein affected in leg
    h. Pain in groin
    i. Leg may look white or pale in color in light skinned women
    j. Elevated pulse rate
    k. Hypotension
    l. Pain experienced in leg when walking
3. Psychosocial findings
    a. Change in pain perception
    b. Anxiety
    c. Inability to care for baby

   d. Discouragement
   e. Unwell feeling
4. Diagnostic procedures
   a. Hemoglobin level and hematocrit values
   b. Phlebography

B. Nursing Diagnoses

1. Altered peripheral tissue perfusion related to thrombophlebitis
2. Alteration in comfort related to pain of thrombophlebitis
3. Anxiety related to changes in activities of daily living, inability to care for newborn, and thrombophlebitis

C. Interventions/Evaluations

1. Altered peripheral tissue perfusion related to thrombophlebitis
   a. Interventions
      (1) Ensure bed rest at all times
      (2) Administer anticoagulants: administration of heparin and warfarin to prevent embolus
      (3) Elevate legs at all times
      (4) Administer oxygen, as necessary
      (5) Administer sedatives, as necessary
      (6) Force fluids each shift (2000 ml)
      (7) Provide elastic bandages to mid-thigh or elastic stockings
      (8) Observe for signs and symptoms of embolism
      (9) Administer antibiotics if infectious process persists
      (10) Ensure frequent rest periods
      (11) Assess infection site for pain, tenderness, temperature, and swelling
      (12) Assess vital signs at each shift
      (13) Instruct client to avoid oral contraceptives because of the inceased risk of clot formation
   b. Evaluations
      (1) Bed rest maintained with legs elevated
      (2) No signs or symptoms of embolism are noted
      (3) Vital signs remain stable
2. Alteration in comfort related to pain of thrombophlebitis
   a. Interventions
      (1) Apply continuous, moist heat to extremity
      (2) Explain importance of treatment
      (3) Avoid pillows behind knees or raising the knee gatch of the bed
      (4) Teach relaxation or distraction techniques
      (5) Elevate extremities on pillows for relief of venous aching
      (6) Avoid crossing of legs
      (7) Change position whenever necessary
      (8) Administer sedatives as necessary
      (9) Use a bed cradle to keep linens and blankets off of extremities
      (10) Administer pain relief medication, as needed
   b. Evaluations
      (1) Decreased pain reported by client
      (2) Effective use of relaxation techniques reported by client
3. Anxiety related to changes in activities of daily living, inability to care for newborn, and thrombophlebitis
   a. Interventions
      (1) Provide emotional support, as necessary
      (2) Stay with the client when she is anxious
      (3) Provide occupational therapy/diversion
      (4) Assure client that baby has appropriate care
      (5) Allow baby's siblings to visit client

(6) Explain thrombophlebitis to the family

(7) Refer client to social worker, if necessary

b. Evaluations

(1) Client is free to discuss concerns with nursing staff

(2) Nurse provides time with client to offer reassurance, explain procedures, or talk

(3) Baby is well cared for by a caregiver of the client's choice

(4) Client has a low level of anxiety

HEALTH EDUCATION

A. Teach client to avoid dehydration in warm weather

B. Teach client to wear warm clothes during cold weather to maintain adequate circulation

C. Teach client to avoid foods high in fat and cholesterol

D. Teach client to avoid periods of prolonged sitting at work, while traveling, or while watching television; getting up to walk around every half-hour or every hour prevents venous pooling in the legs by increasing circulatory return to the heart

E. Teach client to avoid pressure under the knees when propping up legs with pillows

F. Teach client to elevate the foot of the bed to promote venous drainage

G. Teach client to avoid crossing the legs while seated, which decreases circulation to the legs because of pressure on the popliteal space behind the knee

H. Teach client to elevate the legs when sitting, whenever possible

I. Teach client to reduce gastric distress caused by daily dose of anticoagulant by dividing it or taking with food

J. Teach client to avoid possible sodium warfarin (Coumadin) interaction with over-the-counter preparations, such as those containing acetylsalicylic acid formulations (aspirin-based products), and check with physician about the interactive effects of other prescribed drugs

K. Teach client to use an electric razor to avoid nicks or scrapes, or depilatories

L. Client should begin an exercise or daily walking program

M. Client should avoid garters and knee-high stockings

N. Client should practice relaxation techniques

O. Discuss with client risks of oral contraceptive use related to thrombophlebitis

Depression

INTRODUCTION

A. Postpartum depression and psychosis are maladaptations to the stress and conflicts of the postpartal period

B. "Baby blues"

1. Is the mildest form of postpartum depression
2. Occurs on the third to eighth postpartum day
3. Has an incidence of between 50 to 80% of all postpartum women
4. Symptoms disappear by the second postpartum week

C. Depression

1. Has an incidence of approximately 10% of all postpartum women
2. Depressed postpartum women are tearful and despondent, have feelings of inadequacy, and feel unable to cope
3. Is disabling
4. Can last up to 3 years postpartum

D. Postpartum psychosis

1. Includes hallucinations, delusions, and phobias
2. Has an incidence of 0.2% or 1 to 2/1000 postpartum women
3. Onset usually occurs immediately after delivery
4. Etiological theories
    a. Personal history
    b. Social and environmental factors
    c. Hormonal fluctuation during pregnancy and throughout the menstrual cycle
5. Predominant characteristics of a woman with this disorder
    a. Has a favorable attitude toward pregnancy
       (1) Welcomes pregnancy
       (2) Is elated during pregnancy
       (3) Is free from discomforts of pregnancy
       (4) Is eager to breastfeed and usually quite successful at breastfeeding
    b. Has labile emotions
       (1) Initially anxious
       (2) Elated during later pregnancy
       (3) Depressed during postpartum period
6. Hormonal basis
    a. A high level of elation is noted during pregnancy when the placental steroid levels are at high levels
    b. Subsequent depression is noted during the postpartum period when there is a sudden loss of the placental steroid output
    c. Controversy exists in the literature about the effects of the high prolactin levels in breastfeeding women, which inhibit progesterone release, and their relation to an increased risk for postpartum depression

CLINICAL PRACTICE

A. Assessment

1. History: symptoms include
    a. Previous psychological problems
    b. Diagnosis of neurosis or psychosis (schizophrenia)
    c. Poor coping skills
    d. Low self-esteem
    e. Sleep disturbances
    f. Mood swings and emotional distress
    g. Irritability
    h. Restlessness
    i. Tearfulness
    j. Extreme anxiety about baby's feeding, sleeping, or crying
    k. Guilt
    l. Anorexia
    m. Helplessness
    n. Inability to complete activities of daily living
    o. Family history of psychiatric disorders
    p. Many life stressors
    q. Substance abuse

      r. Metabolic disorders
      s. Sexually transmitted diseases (if not treated can manifest as signs and symptoms of depression and psychosis)
  2. Physical findings
      a. Serious hormonal disorders
      b. Dehydration related to inadequate intake of nutrition and fluids
      c. Fatigue and exhaustion
      d. Anxiety behaviors
      e. Speech and behavior may not make sense
      f. Trouble concentrating or maintaining attention
      g. May be breastfeeding
      h. Difficulty in breathing
      i. Heart palpitations
      j. Tremors
  3. Psychosocial findings
      a. Mood changes
      b. Poor self-esteem
      c. Poor social support networks
      d. Expression of concern about difficult labor and delivery
      e. Single, separated, or divorced status
      f. Marital problems
      g. Unplanned pregnancy
      h. Unwanted pregnancy
      i. Feelings of being unloved
      j. Poor relationship with mother
      k. Detachment from reality
      l. Disturbances in thinking, feeling, and behavior
      m. Poor interactions with baby, family, and staff
      n. Inability to relax
      o. Poor coping skills
  4. Diagnostic procedures
      a. Hormonal level determinations
      b. Blood tests for drugs and alcohol
      c. Psychological profile

B. Nursing Diagnoses

1. Impaired adjustment related to postpartum depression
2. High risk of maternal harm to newborn related to maternal depression

C. Interventions/Evaluations

1. Impaired adjustment related to postpartum depression
    a. Interventions
      (1) Observe client with baby, by herself, and with family and friends
      (2) Discuss client's plans for her baby and for herself
      (3) Assess sleeping, eating, resting, and coping behaviors
      (4) Assess skin turgor, lips, mucous membranes, and urinary output for symptoms of dehydration
      (5) Provide psychological support for depression
      (6) Initiate psychiatric consultation, which may result in
         (a) Administration of tranquilizers, if necessary
         (b) Transfer to psychiatric inpatient service
         (c) Psychotherapy
    b. Evaluations
      (1) Client uses appropriate coping strategies to care for self and baby
      (2) Client has realistic expectations for self and baby
      (3) Client perceives that she is receiving the support she needs
2. High risk of maternal harm to newborn related to maternal depression

a. Interventions
   (1) Assess psychosocial factors, mood, and support systems
   (2) Determine when significant others can be present to learn about infant's needs and infant care
   (3) Teach significant others signs and symptoms of depression
   (4) Allow client time for self and encourage her to have time away from baby
   (5) If client is breastfeeding, consider suggesting bottlefeeding to lower prolactin levels
   (6) Reinforce client's self-care activities
   (7) Encourage mothering behaviors and maternal role
   (8) Assist client with learning parenting skills
   (9) Arrange for social worker to visit client
   (10) Praise client's positive actions of mothering
   (11) Arrange for someone to be at home to help client
   (12) Allow client to ventilate her feelings
   (13) Accept client's feelings
   (14) Provide reality orientation
   (15) Listen to family's concerns and take very seriously
   (16) Follow through with resources to help family
   (17) Explain psychological changes during the postpartum period
   (18) Document client's learning needs
   (19) Assist family in crisis
   (20) Keep environment safe
   (21) Remove potentially harmful objects and weapons
   (22) Watch behavior of client: transfer to psychiatric inpatient service may be necessary
   (23) Ensure client takes her medication
   (24) Facilitate parental attachment
   (25) Encourage family support for client
   (26) Be aware that clients with depression or psychosis may harm their babies or commit suicide: take all client's behaviors seriously
b. Evaluations
   (1) Home is a safe environment for client and baby
   (2) Client has support to handle depressive episodes
   (3) Client and family share feelings and concerns openly
   (4) Baby is safe
   (5) Appropriate bonding is observed

HEALTH EDUCATION

A. Instruct family about how to provide safe and secure environment for client and baby

B. Discuss benefits of contraception during the period of depression

C. Instruct client about how to avoid crisis situations and develop coping skills

D. Instruct client in stress reduction techniques

E. Promote family awareness that postpartum depression and psychosis are not normal

---

CASE STUDIES AND STUDY QUESTIONS

P.H. is a 34-year-old woman who is a gravida 5, para 5 (G5P5) who has been delivered of a healthy boy weighing 4800 g (10 lb, 9.5 oz) after 16 hours of labor. She is breastfeeding her baby in the recovery room when she is assigned to your care. Her vital signs are stable. Her lochia is bright red and heavy, and has a clot about 2 cm (.79 inches) in diameter.

1. Which of the following is the most important assessment that needs to be performed?

   a. Checking her vital signs every 5 to 15 minutes for the first hour after delivery.

   b. Checking location and firmness of the fundus.

   c. Charting the amount and saturation of menstrual pads every hour.

   d. Continuing to support her breastfeeding efforts.

2. P.H. is considered to be at high risk for uterine atony because of which of the following?

   a. She is a grand multipara.

   b. Of the size of her baby.

   c. Of the length of her labor.

   d. All of the above.

3. You notice that P.H. has saturated four menstrual pads with bright red blood during a 1-hour period. Her vital signs are stable. You assess her bleeding to be which of the following?

   a. Subinvolution related to retained placental fragments.

   b. Related to a ruptured hematoma.

   c. Uterine atony.

   d. Related to a lacerated cervix.

4. The first nursing action you perform is to do which of the following?

   a. Chart your findings.

   b. Open the IV to increase her level of oxytocin.

   c. Turn P.H. on her left side.

   d. Massage the fundus.

5. The main cause of early postpartum hemorrhage is which of the following?

   a. Uterine atony.

   b. DIC.

   c. Retained placental fragments.

   d. Hematomas and lacerations.

6. The main cause of late postpartum hemorrhage is which of the following?

   a. Uterine atony.

   b. DIC.

   c. Retained placental fragments.

   d. Hematomas and lacerations.

7. The nursing actions to control bleeding and stabilize a mother's condition in hemorrhage related to atony are to do which of the following?

   a. Massage the fundus.

   b. Perform bimanual compression of the uterus if a physician is not available.

   c. Prepare an IV infusion of oxytocin.

   d. All of the above.

8. A hematoma is a collection of blood in the pelvic tissue due to damage to a vessel wall without laceration of the tissue. This trauma to the vessel can be a result of which of the following?

   a. Forceps manipulation.

   b. Pressure of the presenting part on pelvic structures.

   c. Excessive fundal pressure on the uterus.

   d. All of the above.

M.P. is a 24-year-old woman who is a gravida 1, para 1 (G1, P1). She was in labor for 28 hours. A cesarean section was performed because of failure to progress. She was delivered of a 3629 g (8 lb) boy in good health. After delivery, her vital signs were stable and lochia was slight, red color with no clots. She has had a Foley catheter inserted to straight drainage. Her dressing is clean and dry. Forty-eight hours after delivery, her temperature is 38°C (100.4°F) and continues to rise.

9. Which type of puerperal infection is it likely that M.P. has?

   a. Breast.

b. Bladder.

c. Vaginal.

d. Uterine.

10. What factors have predisposed her to a postpartum infection?

    (1) Age.   a. 1, 4.

    (2) Length of labor.   b. 2, 4.

    (3) Parity.   c. 3, 4.

    (4) Type of delivery.   d. 1, 2.

11. On a home visit, M.P. complains of severe breast pain; you assess for mastitis and find which of the following?

    a. Blisters on one of her nipples.

    b. A soft, regular mass.

    c. That she is afebrile.

    d. A hard, red, tender and irregular mass.

12. M.P. is concerned about breastfeeding and taking antibiotics for mastitis in her right breast. You advise her to do which of the following?

    a. Stop breastfeeding.

    b. Use only the left breast to feed the baby.

    c. Pump her breasts, discard the milk, and feed the baby with formula.

    d. Continue to breastfeed on both breasts because only a small amount of antibiotics pass in the milk.

13. Daily inspection of the perineum may reveal problems with the episiotomy such as which of the following?

    a. Hematoma.

    b. Infection.

    c. Edema.

    d. All of the above.

14. To promote healing of an episiotomy and prevent infection, the nurse should do which of the following?

    a. Teach the mother perineal care.

    b. Teach the mother about how infections are transmitted.

    c. Teach the mother about the importance of rest, nutrition, and fluid intake.

    d. All of the above.

L.G. is a 27-year-old overweight woman who is a gravida 3, para 3 (G3, P3) who was delivered of a girl weighing 2800 g (6 lb, 3 oz) by cesarean section. She had a prolonged labor of 27 hours.

15. What factor predisposes L.G. to thrombophlebitis?

    a. Obesity.

    b. Parity.

    c. Length of labor.

    d. Weight of baby.

16. L.G. is prescribed warfarin for thrombophlebitis; you advise her to avoid which of the following?

    a. Aspirin.

    b. Massage of extremities.

    c. Oral contraceptives.

    d. All of the above.

17. L.G. asks if her children can come to see her in the hospital; you respond that

    a. Her condition is very serious and she needs to rest right now.

    b. Only children over the age of 14 years can visit the unit.

    c. Her children may visit when she wants.

    d. You will call the social worker and the children can be cared for so she does not have to worry about them.

18. As part of your daily assessment for thrombophlebitis, you look for all except which of the following?

    a. Generalized pallor.

    b. Dyspnea.

    c. Tachycardia.

    d. Positive Homans' sign.

19. The physiological changes during pregnancy in the veins of the thighs or pelvis predispose a postpartum woman to which

of the following?

a. Deep vein thrombophlebitis.

b. Ecchymosis.

c. Inflammation.

d. Edema.

20. In taking a history for thrombophlebitis, you assess for which of the following?

a. Contraceptive use.

b. Obesity.

c. Postpartum pelvic infection.

d. All of the above.

M.Q. is a 21-year-old female who is a gravida 1, para 1 (G1, P1). At 39 weeks' gestation, she was vaginally delivered of a baby girl in good health. M.Q. was excited about being pregnant and felt well throughout her pregnancy. She is eager to breastfeed but feels anxious about being a new mother. You enter her room and she is crying because her husband cannot come to visit because he must work overtime.

21. Your nursing diagnosis is high risk for impaired adjustment related to "baby blues." Which of the following is correct?

a. This is a wrong diagnosis since the blues occur later in the postpartum period.

b. She is suffering from depression based on her pregnancy course.

c. She is suffering from psychosis because she has phobias.

d. She is severely depressed based on social and personal history.

22. Puerperal depression appears predominantly in women with labile emotions who are which of the following?

a. Initially anxious during pregnancy.

b. Elated during pregnancy.

c. Depressed during puerperium.

d. All of the above.

23. A controversy in the literature exists about women who severely harm or kill their babies during the postpartum period. This controversy centers on mothers who

a. Are usually depressed.

b. Breastfeed and have high levels of prolactin.

c. Have a crisis in their family.

d. All of the above.

24. Severe depressive episodes are considered to be which of the following?

a. More common today than in the past.

b. Rare.

c. Manic in nature.

d. None of the above.

25. Treatment for postpartum depression includes which of the following?

a. Active empathic listening.

b. Psychiatric care.

c. Antidepressive agents.

d. All of the above.

26. Postpartum psychosis includes the following symptom

a. Fear.

b. Tearfulness.

c. Delusions.

d. Elation.

27. When taking a history for depression, it is important to assess for

a. Low self-esteem.

b. Guilt.

c. Substance use.

d. All of the above.

Answers to Study Questions

1. b	2. d	3. c
4. d	5. a	6. c
7. d	8. d	9. d
10. b	11. d	12. d
13. d	14. d	15. a
16. d	17. c	18. a
19. a	20. d	21. a
22. d	23. b	24. b
25. d	26. c	27. d

REFERENCES

Adler, E.M., & Cox, J.L. (1983). Breastfeeding and postnatal depression. *Journal of Psychosomatic Research, 27*(2), 139–144.

Affonso, D.D. (1984). Postpartum depression: A review. *Birth, 11*(4), 231–235.

Auerbach, K., & Jacobi, A. (1990). Postpartum depression in the breastfeeding mother. *NAACOG's Clincial Issues in Perinatal and Women's Health Nursing, 1*(3), 375–384.

Brockington, I., & Kumar, R. (Eds.) (1982). *Motherhood and mental illness*. London, England: Academic.

Buesching, D., Glasser, M., & Frate, D. (1986). Progression of depression in the prenatal and postpartum periods. *Women and Health, 11*(2), 61–78.

Cantanzarite, V. (1986). Prostaglandin: Life-saving drugs for postpartum uterine atony [Letter to the editor]. *Western Journal of Medicine, 144*(4), 477.

Clough, D.H., & Higgins, P.G. (1981). Discrepancies in estimating blood loss. *American Journal of Nursing, 81*(2), 331–333.

Cruikshank, S.H., & Stoelk, E.M. (1985). Surgical control of pelvic hemorrhage. *Southern Medical Journal, 78*(5) 539–543.

Dalton, K. (1980). *Depression after childbirth*. London, England: Oxford.

Errante, J. (1985). Sleep deprivation or postpartum blues? *Topics in Clinical Nursing, 7*(2), 9–18.

Gennero, S. (1988, March/April). Postpartal anxiety and depression in mothers of term and preterm infants. *Nursing Research, 2*(2), 82–85.

Handford, P. (1985). Postpartum depression: What is it that helps? *The Canadian Nurse, 81*(1), 30–33.

Hayashi, R.H. (1986). Hemorrhagic shock in obstetrics. *Critical Care in Obstetrics, 13*(4), 755–763.

Kleiner, G.J. (1986). Depression in pregnancy. *Patient Care, 6*, 101–114.

Lucas, W.E. (1980). Postpartum hemorrhage. *Clinical Obstetrics and Gynecology 27*(1), 139–147.

Martell, L.K. (1990, March/April). Postpartum depression as a family problem. *MCN: American Journal of Maternal Child Nursing, 15*, 90–93.

Mayberry, L., & Forte, A. (1985). Related DIC. *MCN: American Journal of Maternal Child Nursing 10*(3), 168–173.

Metz, A., Sichel, D.A. & Goff, D.C. (1988, July). Postpartum panic disorder. *Journal of Clinical Psychiatry, 49*(7), 278–279.

Nisewander, K. (Ed.) (1988). *Manual of obstetrics: Diagnosis and therapy* (3rd ed.). Boston: Little, Brown.

Oxnick, K.J., & Yarbrough, M. (Eds.) (1984). *Infection control: An integrated approach*. St. Louis: Mosby.

Reed, M.D. (1988). Postpartum hemorrhage. *American Family Physician, 37*(3), 111–120.

Vestal, K.W., & McKenzie, C.A. (Eds.). (1983). *High-risk perinatal nursing*. Philadelphia: Saunders.

COMPLICATIONS OF THE NEWBORN

Susan Mattson, Bonnie Christoff, and Ksenia Zukowsky

CHAPTER

36

Risks Associated with Gestational Age and Birth Weight

Objectives

1. Describe physical characteristics of preterm, post-term, small-for-gestational-age (SGA), and large-for-gestational-age (LGA) infants

2. Recognize potential problems related to preterm, post-term, SGA, and LGA infants

3. Identify maternal risk factors that may contribute to prematurity, postmaturity, and SGA and LGA infants

4. Select appropriate nursing diagnoses for preterm, post-term, SGA, and LGA infants

5. Describe appropriate nursing interventions for preterm, post-term, SGA, and LGA infants

Small-for-Gestational-Age Infants

Introduction

A. The SGA infant is one whose length, weight, and head circumference are below the 10th percentile when compared with other infants of the same gestational age

B. The SGA infant can be preterm, term, or post-term

C. Conditions associated with SGA babies

1. Chronic hypertension or pregnancy-induced hypertension (PIH) in the mother
2. Maternal cardiac or renal disease
3. Maternal diabetes mellitus
4. Poor maternal nutritional state
5. Maternal use of alcohol, tobacco, or illegal drugs
6. Maternal age
7. Multiple gestation
8. Placental insufficiency
9. Placental and fetal abnormalities
10. Pregnancy occurring at high altitudes

D. The malnutrition or insult that occurs affects the fetus differently depending on the stage of fetal development

1. All organs are affected by intrauterine growth retardation (IUGR)
2. Early gestation is a time of rapid cell proliferation (hyperplasia)
   a. An insult at this time results in organs that contain cells that are normal size but fewer in number
   b. Infants are symmetrical but their organs are smaller
   c. Generally, these infants have a poor prognosis and may never catch up
3. Later in gestation, growth results from an increase in cell size (hypertrophy)
   a. An insult at this stage results in organs with a normal number of cells but that are smaller in size
   b. The brain and heart are larger in proportion to the reduced body weight, whereas the liver, spleen, adrenals, thymus, and placenta are small (asymmetrical IUGR)
   c. The infants have appropriate-sized heads and are of appropriate length, but their overall body weights and organ sizes are diminished
   d. Infants who have an insult later in gestation generally have a better prognosis that those with an earlier insult
   e. Because the number of cells is not decreased, the infant can catch up through adequate postnatal nutrition

E. The SGA infant may present with problems in the initial transitional period after birth

1. There is less reserve to tolerate the rigors of labor and delivery
   a. A small placenta may have diminished ability to exchange gases
   b. There is a higher incidence of perinatal asphyxia because of placental insufficiency, which may lead to the passage of meconium in utero
   c. A decrease in cardiac glycogen stores may result in bradycardia
2. Decreased glycogen stores increase the potential for hypoglycemia and hypothermia
3. Polycythemia is frequent and is probably a response to chronic fetal hypoxia

F. Congenital anomalies may be seen in as many as 35% of SGA infants (Lubchenco & Koops, 1987) and are more frequently associated with intrauterine insult early in gestation during cell multiplication and organogenesis

G. SGA fetuses have often been exposed to intrauterine infections such as rubella, cytomegalovirus (CMV), or toxoplasmosis

Clinical Practice

A. Assessment

1. History
   a. Antenatal findings
      (1) Weight gain
      (2) Age and socioeconomic status
      (3) Maternal illnesses
         (a) Renal disease
         (b) Cardiac problems
         (c) Hypertension
      (4) Maternal substance use
         (a) Alcohol
         (b) Illicit drugs
         (c) Tobacco
      (5) Elevated TORCH titer or other signs of infection
      (6) Documented oligohydramnios
   b. Intranatal findings

      (1) Color, consistency, and amount of amniotic fluid
      (2) Fetal heart rate (FHR) signs of distress
  2. Physical findings
    a. Soft tissue wasting and dysmaturity
      (1) Decreased amount of breast tissue
      (2) Diminished amount of skin folds; the skin is often loose, dry, and scaling (Sherwen, Scoloveno, & Weingarten, 1991)
      (3) Decreased amount of adipose tissue
    b. Smaller-than-average length, weight, and/or head circumference
      (1) A symmetrical SGA neonate is smaller in all three parameters
      (2) An asymmetrical SGA neonate has smaller-than-average weight and an average head circumference and length
        (a) Large head/body ratio is seen
        (b) Insult has occurred later in gestation with the brain being spared
        (c) Prognosis is better
        (d) Head control is often poor
    c. Muscle mass is diminished, especially in extremities
    d. Facial expression is wide eyed and alert
    e. Infant often appears hungry
  3. Diagnostic procedures
    a. Length, weight, and head circumference
    b. Gestational age assessment
    c. Assess for infections
      (1) Complete blood count (CBC) with differential and platelets (also assess for polycythemia)
      (2) Viral studies: TORCH titer
      (3) Possible spinal tap
      (4) Possible check of bilirubin level
      (5) Urine testing for CMV titer and culture
    d. Chromosome analysis if congenital anomalies are present
    e. Drug screen on urine if indicated by maternal history
    f. Ultrasound examination of head to rule out hydrocephaly
    g. Computer-assisted tomography (CT) scan to rule out hydrocephaly, microcephaly, or calcification

B. Nursing Diagnoses

1. High risk for altered nutrition: less than body requirements related to high metabolic rate seen in SGA neonate
2. High risk for infection if exposed to intrauterine infection
3. High risk for alteration in body temperature: hypothermia related to decreased glycogen stores and subcutaneous tissue
4. High risk for alteration in tissue perfusion related to polycythemia and/or hypothermia

C. Interventions/Evaluations

1. High risk for altered nutrition: less than body requirements related to high metabolic rate seen in SGA neonate
    a. Interventions
      (1) Provide a high-calorie formula: more than 20 kcal/oz (30 ml)
      (2) Decrease metabolic requirements, when possible
        (a) Feed by gavage
        (b) Provide neutral thermal environment
        (c) Decrease iatrogenic stimuli
          (i) Swaddle infant
          (ii) Offer pacifier
          (iii) Cluster nursing and other care
        (d) Ensure frequent and adequate rest for the infant

(3) Provide adequate nutrition to prevent hypoglycemia
  (a) Check Dextrostix or other bedside screening as needed
  (b) Offer frequent feedings (every 2 to 3 hours)
  (c) Offer early feeding (before 4 hours of age if not contraindicated)
  (d) Administer parenteral nutrition by hyperalimentation and intralipid infusion if oral route is not sufficient to sustain infant
(4) Administer IV dextrose infusions (usually 10%) at 4 to 8 mg/kg/min if extremely hypoglycemic (dextrose strength depends on infant's condition and serum glucose level)

b. Evaluations
  (1) Infant shows steady weight gain of approximately 15 to 30 g/day (0.5 to 1 oz)
  (2) Serum laboratory values remain within normal limits
  (3) Dextrostix values remain within normal ranges (usually above 40 mg/dl)
  (4) Growth plotted on charts shows a normal growth rate

2. High risk for infection if exposed to intrauterine infection
  a. Interventions
    (1) Provide care for the neonate using isolation precautions when congenital infections are suspected
    (2) Administer antibiotics as determined by appropriate cultures and physician's orders, for example:
      (a) Ampicillin, 100 mg/kg/day every 12 hours
      (b) Gentamycin, 2.5 mg/kg/day every 12 to 24 hours
      (c) Vancomycin, 15 mg/kg/day IV every 12 hours
      (d) Penicillin G, 250,000 IU IV every 12 hours
    (3) Use aseptic techniques and good handwashing
    (4) Analyze laboratory values to determine trends
      (a) CBC with differential
      (b) Platelet count
      (c) Cultures
      (d) Antibody titers
    (5) Assess infant's activity level: infant may be lethargic
    (6) Monitor infant's temperature for elevation or signs of hypothermia (above 37.2°C [99.6°F] or below 36.1°C [97°F] axillary)
  b. Evaluations
    (1) Neonate's blood culture is normal
    (2) Temperature remains within normal limits
    (3) Serum antibiotic levels are therapeutic
    (4) Activity level and tone remain normal or return to normal
    (5) Aseptic technique is maintained, preventing spread of infection (see Chap. 39 for further discussion of sepsis in the newborn)

3. High risk for alteration in body temperature: hypothermia related to decreased glycogen stores and subcutaneous tissue
  a. Interventions
    (1) Monitor incubator or warmer bed temperature and heater output: be concerned if there is constant heater output
    (2) Monitor infant's body temperature: axillary should be in range of 36.4° to 37°C (97.6° to 98.6°F)
    (3) Prevent unnecessary heat loss (to prevent cold stress)—for example, by avoiding use of cold scales and exposure of infant to drafts
  b. Evaluations
    (1) Normal body temperature is maintained
    (2) Neutral thermal environment is maintained
    (3) Infant shows no signs of cold stress, for example
      (a) Increased oxygen consumption
      (b) Hypoglycemia
      (c) Respiratory distress

4. High risk for alteration in tissue perfusion related to polycythemia and/or hypothermia
   a. Interventions
      (1) Obtain serum hemoglobin (normal, 15 to 21.5 g/dl) and hematocrit (normal, 45% to 65%) levels
      (2) Observe for signs and symptoms of polycythemia
         (a) Ruddy appearance
         (b) Cyanosis; may be more pronounced with activity and/or crying
         (c) Jaundice
         (d) Apnea
      (3) Provide adequate hydration (90 to 100 cc/kg/day) to prevent hyperviscosity of blood
      (4) Consider partial exchange transfusion if central hematocrit is greater than 70% or greater than 60 to 65% with a symptomatic infant
         (a) To prevent capillary congestion
         (b) To relieve hyperviscosity of blood
   b. Evaluations
      (1) Serum hematocrit maintained below 65%
      (2) Signs of polycythemia are absent
      (3) Neonate's intake and output (I&O) are adequate to achieve a urine output greater than 1.5 cc/kg/hr

Preterm Infants

Introduction

A. A preterm infant is one who is born before the end of 37 weeks' gestation

B. There are three categories of prematurity

1. Borderline
   a. Infants born between 37 and 38 weeks' gestation
   b. Usually weigh between 2500 and 3250 g (5 lb 8 oz to 7 lb 3 oz) at birth
   c. Account for 16% of all live births
2. Moderate
   a. Infants born between 31 and 36 weeks' gestation
   b. Usually weigh between 1500 and 2500 g (3 lb 5 oz to 5 lb 8 oz) at birth
   c. Account for 6 to 7% of all live births
3. Extreme
   a. Infants born between 24 and 30 weeks' gestation
   b. Usually weigh between 450 and 1500 g (1 lb to 3 lb 5 oz) at birth
   c. Account for 0.9% of live births
   d. Account for 84% of all neonatal deaths among infants of all gestational ages
   e. As many as 50% of survivors may be handicapped

C. Physical problems are directly associated with the degree of organ maturity; prematurity is not a disease but a lack of organ maturity

1. Without full development, the organs are usually not capable of functioning at the level needed to maintain extrauterine homeostasis
2. The more immature, or the lower the gestational age, the greater the risk of complications and system failure

D. The respiratory system is one of the last to mature; therefore, the preterm infant is at potential risk for numerous respiratory problems (see Chap. 37 for a complete discussion of neonatal respiratory distress)

1. Respiratory distress syndrome due to immature lungs and inadequate surfactant production
2. Decreased muscle mass in respiratory muscles

3. Apnea due to immaturity of respiratory center
4. An immature neonate's chest wall is very compliant; the infant may not be able to generate enough inspiratory pressure, resulting in inadequate respiratory effect
5. Other causes of respiratory problems
   a. Meconium aspiration
   b. Pulmonary hypoplasia
   c. Pulmonary hemorrhage
   d. Complications resulting from extrapulmonary disorders of vascular, metabolic, and neuromuscular origin

E. The cardiovascular system is also immature

1. Transition from fetal to neonatal circulation is in part a response to the increased level of oxygen in the circulation after the first breath; if oxygen levels remain low, fetal circulation may persist
   a. Preterm infants have a high incidence of patent ductus arteriosus (lack of closure or reopening of shunt allowing blood to bypass lungs)
   b. Foramen ovale can also reopen if pulmonary resistance is high
2. Preterm infants also have impaired regulation of blood pressure
   a. Fluctuations in cerebral blood flow are often seen
   b. These fluctuations predispose the fragile blood vessels in the brain to rupture, causing intraventricular hemorrhage (IVH)

F. The immune system is both immature and inexperienced, making the preterm infant susceptible to infections

1. Immunological ability depends in part on immunoglobulins (Ig), such as IgG, IgM, and IgA
2. Preterm infants often have a deficiency of IgG because transplacental transfer occurs around 34 weeks' gestation
3. IgA (the primary immunoglobulin in colostrum) is not available to the preterm infant if he or she does not receive breast milk or colostrum

G. The immature liver may be highly inefficient in conjugating bilirubin, leading to hyperbilirubinemia (see Chap. 38)

H. The preterm infant has great difficulty maintaining body temperature

1. This is primarily because of excessive heat loss due to the following
   a. Decreased or inadequate subcutaneous fat
   b. Large head/body ratio
   c. Lack of tone and flexion
2. Brown fat is often not available or is inadequate to generate heat, since sufficient stores are not available for use until approximately 30 weeks' gestation
3. Cold stress quickly depletes what brown fat and glycogen stores are present, resulting in the following
   a. Increased metabolic needs
   b. Increased oxygen consumption
   c. Consequences
      (1) Metabolic acidosis
      (2) Hypoxemia
      (3) Hypoglycemia

I. The preterm renal system is immature, resulting in the following

1. Decreased ability to concentrate urine
2. Lack of selectiveness in filtration
3. Decreased glomerular filtration rate (GFR)
   a. Decreased drug clearance
   b. Increased likelihood of retaining fluids

J. **Periventricular-intraventricular hemorrhage is of particular significance in the preterm infant**

1. The incidence increases with decreasing gestational age so that half of all infants born between 23 and 31 weeks' gestation have such hemorrhages (Usher, 1987)
2. An intracranial hemorrhage occurs when blood leaks into the cranial cavity from the vascular system in the brain
3. These neonates are susceptible because of several factors related to their developmental immaturity
   a. The germinal matrix in the periventricular area is perfused by abundant but fragile capillaries that rupture easily
   b. Rupture can have a number of causes
      (1) Abrupt increase in blood pressure secondary to the following
         (a) Resuscitation efforts
         (b) Infusion of hyperosmolar solutions
      (2) Abrupt change in cerebral blood flow (from hypoxia and rapid reinfusion)
      (3) Increased venous pressure from
         (a) Mechanical ventilation
         (b) Pneumothorax (which impedes venous return)
4. The more severe the hemorrhage, the poorer the outcome
   a. Severity is determined by the extent of the bleed and structures involved
   b. Many result in the development of some degree of hydrocephalus

K. **Gastrointestinal functioning is often compromised in preterm infants**

1. Necrotizing enterocolitis (NEC) is a serious and potentially life-threatening disease seen in sick preterm newborns
   a. Two most consistent factors in its development are the following
      (1) Ischemic injury to the immature intestinal mucosa
      (2) Presence of bacteria (usually resulting from enteral feedings)
   b. Symptoms are severe and may occur suddenly
      (1) Abdominal distension
      (2) Paralytic ileus or decrease in bowel peristalsis
      (3) Stools positive for occult blood
      (4) Temperature instability
      (5) Apnea and bradycardia
   c. Infants should be cared for in a neonatal intensive care unit (NICU)
2. Problems with nutritional intake often occur as a result of the following
   a. Immature gastrointestinal functioning
   b. Immature suck-and-swallow reflexes
   c. Compromised respiratory status
   d. Temperature instability

L. **Hypocalcemia occurs in 30 to 90% of preterm infants (Koo & Tsang, 1987)**

1. During pregnancy, calcium is actively transported across the placenta from mother to fetus, resulting in elevated serum calcium levels
2. At birth, this calcium supply is withdrawn, at which time the normal newborn increases his or her own levels of parathyroid hormone (PTH) to meet the resultant deficiency
3. In preterm infants (and infants of diabetic mothers [IDMs]), parathyroid adaptation to lower serum calcium levels appears to be blunted, leaving the infant susceptible to hypocalcemia

M. **Hypoglycemia is a common occurrence (see section on SGA infants for further discussion)**

Clinical Practice

A. Assessment

1. History: maternal risk factors
   a. Premature labor treated with bed rest and tocolytics
   b. Multiple gestation
   c. Infections
      (1) *Neisseria gonorrhoeae*
      (2) *Chlamydia*
      (3) Trichomonas
      (4) Group B beta streptococcus
      (5) Pyelonephritis
      (6) CMV
      (7) Hepatitis A and B
   d. Antepartum bleeding
   e. PIH
   f. Premature rupture of membranes
   g. Cervical insufficiency or incompetence
   h. Psychosocial stress or maternal behavior that promotes catecholamine release, leading to decreased uterine blood flow and uterine irritability
   i. No prenatal care
   j. Poor nutrition
   k. Use of illicit drugs
2. Physical findings
   a. Neurological: hypotonic resting posture (lack of flexion in arms and legs)
   b. Head
      (1) Is larger in proportion to body than with term infant
      (2) Skull bones are soft and spongy, especially along suture lines
      (3) Fontanelles are wide and soft, with overriding sutures
      (4) Ears are flat and shapeless, with an incurving of the upper pinna beginning at 34 weeks' gestation
      (5) Scalp hair is matted and somewhat woolly
   c. Skin
      (1) Edematous
      (2) Transparent and thin, but ruddy in color
      (3) Abundant lanugo
      (4) Minimal vernix caseosa at 28 weeks, but it increases with age
      (5) Susceptible to breakdown because of decreased cohesion between the dermis and epidermis
   d. Nipples are flat, with areolae appearing around 34 weeks' gestation; breast tissue is not usually palpable until 35 weeks
   e. Minimal sole creases on feet, progressively increasing with length of gestation
   f. Genitalia
      (1) Testes descend to the external inguinal ring at 30 weeks; there are few rugae in the scrotum
      (2) Labia minora and majora are widely separated, with a prominently exposed clitoris in very immature infants
   g. Thermal instability (at risk for heat loss) due to the following
      (1) Larger surface/weight ratio
      (2) Immature tone
      (3) Diminished stores of white and brown fat
         (a) White insulator fat is almost nonexistent
            (i) Infant has a scrawny appearance
            (ii) Lack of insulation allows for a more rapid transfer of heat from infant's core to the environment
         (b) Lack of brown fat (deposited about 30 to 36 weeks' gestation around

the scapula and kidneys) prevents nonshivering thermogenesis (the usual method of heat production in newborns)

h. An immature respiratory center is manifested in periods of apnea
   (1) Apnea is an absence of respiration lasting more than 20 seconds
   (2) A serious bradycardia can occur from apnea, with the heart rate decreasing to the 80s or lower, and with resultant cyanosis, hypotonia, and metabolic acidosis

i. Respiratory distress syndrome (RDS; hyaline membrane disease) may be present because of a deficiency of surfactant
   (1) Surfactant decreases the force of surface tension in the alveoli, preventing their collapse
   (2) Manifestations of RDS (see Chapter 37 for more information)
       (a) Retractions: supraclavicular, intercostal, and substernal
       (b) Tachypnea greater than 60/min
       (c) Central cyanosis
       (d) Nasal flaring
       (e) Expiratory grunting
       (f) Diminished air exchange

j. Hypoglycemia may be present because of a lack of glycogen stores necessary to meet the preterm infant's metabolic demands (see section on hypoglycemia in SGA infants for further discussion) manifested by
   (1) Lethargy
   (2) Tachycardia
   (3) Increased respiratory effort
   (4) Jitteriness

k. Presence of a soft cardiac murmur (often caused by a patent ductus arteriosus), which may be intermittent, evidenced by the following
   (1) Desaturation on pulse oximetry
   (2) Subtle color changes, often seen as duskiness

l. Signs and symptoms of infection may be present
   (1) Increase or decrease in WBC count with a shift to the left
   (2) Decrease in activity level; lethargy
   (3) Acute change in oxygen requirements or an increase needed in ventilatory settings; episodes of apnea
   (4) Feeding intolerance
   (5) Temperature instability (usually subnormal)
   (6) Color changes
       (a) Cyanosis
       (b) Ashen coloring
       (c) Mottled complexion

m. Evidence of intracranial hemorrhage
   (1) Usually occurs at 16 to 48 hours of age
   (2) Symptoms
       (a) Change in respiratory status (episodes of apnea)
       (b) Decreased hematocrit level that fails to rise after transfusion
       (c) Full and bulging fontanelles
       (d) Change in activity level
           (i) Diminished sucking reflex
           (ii) Myoclonic movements
           (iii) Lethargy
           (iv) Seizures
           (v) Decreased muscle tone

3. Diagnostic procedures
   a. Heart and respiratory rates
   b. Axillary, skin, and rectal temperatures
   c. Oxygen saturation levels by pulse oximetry and arterial blood gas assays
      (1) Oxygen saturation should be 85 to 95%

(2) Normal PaO_2 should be in high 40s to low 60s
d. Blood
  (1) Glucose
  (2) CBC with differential
  (3) Electrolyte values, including calcium
  (4) Blood urea nitrogen (BUN) and serum creatinine
  (5) Bilirubin concentrations
  (6) Cultures
e. Urine
  (1) Output (normal, 1 to 3 ml/kg/hr)
  (2) Specific gravity (normal, 1.002 to 1.010)
f. Chest x-rays
g. Head and abdominal circumferences
h. Daily weights
i. Feeding residuals
j. Ultrasound testing (especially after intracranial bleeds)
  (1) Confirms bleed
  (2) Rules out or documents hydrocephalus

B. Nursing Diagnoses

1. Ineffective thermoregulation related to large surface/body ratio and lack of fat stores
2. High risk for alteration in nutrition: less than body requirements related to diminished sucking reflex due to gestational immaturity
3. Impairment of skin integrity related to skin immaturity
4. Elimination processes: altered urinary elimination and retention related to renal immaturity
5. High risk for alteration in circulation processes: altered tissue perfusion related to impaired gas exchange
6. High risk for alteration in respiratory function related to respiratory immaturity
7. High risk for infection related to immature immune system and lack of normal flora

C. Interventions/Evaluations

1. Ineffective thermoregulation related to large surface/body ratio and lack of fat stores
   a. Interventions
     (1) Monitor neonate's temperature
       (a) Place on servo control mode under radiant warmer or in isolette to achieve a neutral thermal environment
       (b) Measure skin, axillary, and core temperatures if necessary
     (2) Prevent heat loss from evaporative, conductive, convective, and radiant means (see Chap. 23 for further discussion)
       (a) Do not bathe neonate without evaluating the consequences of cold stress
       (b) Place neonate on prewarmed surfaces or warm blankets
       (c) Place hat on neonate
       (d) Do not place neonate under air conditioning vents or near cold walls or windows
   b. Evaluations
     (1) Neonate's temperature is maintained within normal limits
       (a) Core (rectal), 35.5° to 37.5°C (96° to 99.5°F)
       (b) Abdominal (skin), 36.5°C (97.7°F)
     (2) Optimal equipment to maintain thermal neutrality for infant is provided
     (3) No signs of cold stress are observed

2. High risk for alteration in nutrition: less than body requirements related to diminished sucking reflex because of gestational immaturity
   a. Interventions
      (1) Generally, 90 to 120 kcal/kg/day is suitable for most infants; fluid volume requirements range from 80 to 120 ml/kg/day during the first week of life
      (2) Offer feedings via oral gavage until the neonate's suck-and-swallow reflex is established or coordinated, at about 34 weeks of gestation
         (a) Forty to 45% of the newborn's calories should come from carbohydrates
         (b) Feeding can be intermittent (most common) or continuous
            (i) Intermittent boluses are usually given every 1 to 4 hours
            (ii) Determine tolerance for feedings
               • Note amount and frequency of the following
                  □ Vomiting and regurgitation
                  □ Abdominal distension
                  □ Stools
               • Aspirate residue left in stomach before next intermittent feeding
         (c) While the infant is being fed by gavage, provide opportunity for non-nutritive sucking with pacifier
      (3) Feedings may be delivered by total parenteral nutrition (TPN) when the infant is unable to receive them enterally
         (a) TPN may be administered by either a central or peripheral route
         (b) Protein is supplied in the form of amino acids
         (c) Dextrose is the primary energy source
         (d) Fats are supplied as a lipid emulsion
         (e) Vitamins and minerals are added
      (4) Monitor daily weight gain and growth
         (a) Measure length and head circumference weekly
         (b) Plot measurements on standard growth chart
   b. Evaluations
      (1) The neonate gains 15 to 30 g (0.5 to 1 oz) of weight daily
      (2) Acceptable head circumference growth is approximately 0.5 to 1 cm/wk (⅜ in)
      (3) The neonate is able to self-console by non-nutritive sucking on a pacifier
      (4) The infant does not exhibit signs or symptoms of hypoglycemia
3. Impairment of skin integrity related to skin immaturity
   a. Interventions
      (1) Place only as much tape on the infant's skin as is necessary
      (2) Keep skin clean, dry, and free from abrasions
         (a) Avoid use of caustic solutions or alkaline-based soap, which destroys the acid mantle that is a barrier to growth of normal skin flora
         (b) Lotions and creams are not necessary for immature skin
      (3) The premature infant absorbs substances easily through skin up to the first 2 weeks of life, leading to a greater risk of toxicity
      (4) Place neonate under clear wrap or use double-walled isolettes to prevent excessive insensible water loss
      (5) Minimize friction to skin
   b. Evaluations
      (1) The neonate maintains good skin integrity as evidenced by lack of abrasions or other breakdown
      (2) The neonate does not have excessive insensible water loss
4. Elimination processes: altered urinary elimination and retention related to renal immaturity
   a. Interventions
      (1) Monitor urine output

(2) Monitor urine specific gravity

(3) Use dipstick for protein testing (lowered renal threshold)

(4) Weigh infant for signs of fluid deficit or excess evidenced by weight loss or gain

(5) Observe for signs of dehydration

    (a) Poor skin turgor

    (b) Sunken fontanelles

(6) Observe for signs of fluid overload

    (a) Edema

    (b) Bounding pulses or increased blood pressure

(7) Estimate insensible water loss, which is increased in the following situations

    (a) Infant is under radiant warmer

    (b) Infant receives phototherapy

    (c) Infant suffers skin breakdown

    (d) Infant is in respiratory distress

  b. Evaluations

    (1) Urine output is greater than 2 ml/hr

    (2) Specific gravity ranges between 1.002 and 1.010

    (3) Protein is not found in urine

    (4) Insensible water loss is minimized or accurately replaced

    (5) Signs of dehydration or fluid overload are not seen

5. High risk for alteration in circulatory processes: altered tissue perfusion related to impaired gas exchange

  a. Interventions

    (1) Auscultate heart for character, rate, and presence or absence of murmur

    (2) Palpate radial, brachial, femoral, and pedal pulses

    (3) Assess for dramatic or subtle color changes indicative of left-to-right shunting (from duskiness, circumoral cyanosis to mottling, and generalized cyanosis)

    (4) Monitor blood pressure

    (5) Assess capillary refill

  b. Evaluations

    (1) Heart sounds are normal; appropriate interventions are provided for variations from normal

    (2) Neonate is not cyanotic

    (3) Blood pressure remains between 48 and 70 mm Hg systolic and 25 to 48 mm Hg diastolic

    (4) Capillary refill will be normal (within 3 seconds)

6. High risk for alteration in respiratory function related to respiratory immaturity

  a. Interventions

    (1) Assess the neonate's respiratory effort in regard to rate, character, effort, and signs of respiratory distress (see Chapter 37)

    (2) Chest x-ray film may be required to determine if respiratory embarrassment is due to an aspiration pneumonia, respiratory distress syndrome, or both

    (3) Monitor to determine whether supplemental oxygen may be needed to maintain optimal oxygen saturation levels

      (a) Pulse oximetry

      (b) Arterial blood gas assay

  b. Evaluations

    (1) Neonate has a respiratory rate within normal limits (40 to 60 breaths/min)

    (2) Optimal oxygenation is maintained

    (3) Color remains normal

7. High risk for infection related to immature immune system and lack of normal flora (see Chap. 39 for complete discussion of sepsis in the newborn)

Large-for Gestational-Age Infants

Introduction

A. The large-for-gestational-age (LGA) infant is one whose weight, length, and head circumference is above the 90th percentile

1. LGA babies may be preterm, term, or post-term
2. Birth weight over 4000 g (8 lb, 14 ½ oz) often reflects a genetic predisposition, except for the infant of a diabetic mother (IDM)
   a. Large parents have large babies
   b. Some Native Americans are more likely to have LGA infants

B. Large size may necessitate a greater number of cesarean births among these infants

C. If an LGA baby is born vaginally, a high incidence of birth trauma may be seen

1. Fracture of the clavicle
2. Brachial plexus palsies
3. Depressed skull fractures
4. Cephalhematomas

D. LGA infants often experience fetal distress during a prolonged and difficult second stage

1. Shoulder dystocia may occur
2. Passage of meconium in utero may occur, with risk of aspiration

E. LGA infants are at risk for hypoglycemia related to early depletion of glycogen stores (see Chap. 41 on IDM for complete discussion)

Clinical Practice

A. Assessment

1. History
   a. Maternal
      (1) Previous birth of LGA infant
      (2) Large weight gain during pregnancy
      (3) Diabetes (classes A to C) during the pregnancy
      (4) Prolonged or difficult labor and birth, particularly a long second stage
      (5) Ultrasonography that confirms LGA infant
      (6) Ethnic background
   b. Infant
      (1) Ultrasonography that confirms LGA infant
      (2) Infant's weight, length, and head circumference plot out above the 90th percentile
      (3) Type of delivery
         (a) Cesarean birth
         (b) Vaginal delivery with possible shoulder dystocia
      (4) Apgar scores at 1 and 5 minutes suggestive of intrapartal hypoxia
      (5) Consistency, color, and amount of amniotic fluid
      (6) FHR patterns (especially in second stage of labor) suggestive of distress
2. Physical findings
   a. Weight greater than 4000 g (8 lbs, 14½ oz)
   b. Presence of caput succedaneum on the head
   c. Presence of cephalhematoma on head
      (1) May see skull fracture with resultant subdural or subarachnoid hemorrhage

(2) May have intracranial hemorrhage
d. May see facial nerve damage
  (1) Drooping mouth or eyelid on affected side
  (2) Asymmetrical movement of mouth
e. Evidence of brachial plexus palsies
  (1) Erb's palsy (affected by C-5 and C-6 nerve root damage)
    (a) Paralysis of muscles of upper arm
    (b) Affected arm hangs limp, abducted, and internally rotated at the shoulder
    (c) Affected arm is pronated at the elbow, and wrist is flexed
    (d) Deep tendon reflexes are absent
    (e) Moro response is one-sided
  (2) Klumpke's palsy (affected by damage to C-8 to T-1 nerve roots)
    (a) Affects the muscles of the hand
    (b) Hand appears claw shaped
    (c) Is rarely seen as an isolated entity
  (3) Brachial palsy affects the entire arm (entire plexus from C-5 to T-1 has been damaged)
    (a) Arm lies motionless
    (b) Arm is usually devoid of sweat and sensation
    (c) Hand becomes small, dry, and atrophic
f. Evidence of clavicle fracture
  (1) Decreased movement of affected arm; may be seen when startle reflex is elicited
  (2) Infant may cry or show other signs of distress when arm on affected side is moved
  (3) X-ray film confirms diagnosis
g. Evidence of hypoglycemia
  (1) Jitteriness
  (2) Lethargy
  (3) Dextrostix less than 40
    (a) Serum glucose below 35 mg/dl
    (b) Serum glucose below 25 mg/dl in preterm infants
h. Evidence of hypocalcemia, often due to birth asphyxia
  (1) Serum calcium below 7 mg/dl
  (2) Condition seen within first 2 days or at 6 to 10 days of life
    (a) At birth, PTH, vitamin D, and calcitonin levels are low
    (b) Levels rise slowly during the first few days of life to correct the deficiency
  (3) Affects 50% of IDMs
  (4) Symptoms include jitteriness, twitching, and convulsions
i. Signs of respiratory distress
  (1) Effort, character, and rate of respirations (labored, greater than 60 breaths/min)
  (2) Retractions: supraclavicular, intercostal, and substernal
  (3) Nasal flaring
  (4) Grunting
j. Quality of breath sounds assessed by auscultation
k. Possible barrel chest
3. Diagnostic procedures
a. Serum glucose
b. X-ray film to confirm or rule out birth injury
c. Ultrasound or CT scan for possible head injuries if cephalhematoma or depressed skull fracture is noted
d. Arterial blood gas assays if respirations are severely compromised

B. Nursing Diagnoses

1. High risk for alteration in nutrition: less than body requirements related to hypoglycemia

2. High risk for alteration in respiratory function related to aspiration of meconium

3. High risk for birth injury related to large size

C. Interventions/Evaluations

1. High risk for alteration in nutrition: less than body requirements related to hypoglycemia
    a. Interventions
        (1) Monitor Dextrostix at bedside or serum glucose levels if below 40 at bedside
        (2) If Dextrostix is below 40, offer 10% dextrose feeding immediately, if not contraindicated
            (a) Continue to administer frequent (every 2 to 3 hours) feedings
            (b) Deliver feedings by gavage in the following cases
                (i) Neonate has weak suck-and-swallow reflex
                (ii) Respiratory rate is greater than 60 breaths/min
            (c) Administer glucose parenterally if necessary
        (3) Monitor weight daily
        (4) Monitor intake and output
        (5) Observe for signs of hypoglycemia
    b. Evaluations
        (1) Serum glucose level is maintained above 40 mg/dl
        (2) Adequate urine output (greater than 1.5 cc/kg/hr) is seen
        (3) Adequate weight gain (30 to 50 g/day (1 to 2 oz) is seen
2. High risk for alteration in respiratory function related to aspiration of meconium (see also Chapter 37)
    a. Interventions
        (1) Prepare for delivery with appropriate resuscitation equipment and health care professional skilled at neonatal resuscitation
            (a) Nasal and oral suctioning while neonate's head is on the perineum
            (b) Endotracheal suctioning for meconium observed below the vocal cords
            (c) Chest physiotherapy as needed to assist with respirations
        (2) Provide appropriate follow-up respiratory support as needed
            (a) Endotracheal intubation
            (b) Positive-pressure ventilation
            (c) Supplemental oxygen
            (d) Chest physiotherapy
        (3) Provide alternate means of nutrition if increased respiratory rate (over 60/min) prevents oral feeding
        (4) Maintain infant in neutral thermal environment to prevent increased oxygen consumption related to cold stress
    b. Evaluations
        (1) Neonate shows no signs of aspiration, and airway remains patent
        (2) Clear breath sounds are auscultated
        (3) Neonate's color remains normal, without central cyanosis
        (4) Respirations are regular in rate and rhythm
3. High risk for birth injury related to large size
    a. Interventions
        (1) On physical examination, note the following
            (a) Size and position of cephalhematoma or caput succedaneum
            (b) Evidence of skull or clavicle fracture
            (c) Evidence of facial nerve or brachial plexus injury
        (2) Observe for jaundice secondary to bruising and trauma
            (a) Follow serum bilirubin levels (see also Chapter 38 for further discussion on hyperbilirubinemia)
            (b) Place infant under phototherapy lights if necessary
        (3) Provide treatment for any incidence of palsy

(a) Immobilize the affected arm for 7 to 10 days
(b) Provide gentle range of motion to extremity during the immobilization when indicated
(4) Provide treatment for fractured clavicle
(a) Obtain x-ray film for confirmation
(b) Immobilize affected arm and shoulder
(c) Provide comfort measures and pain medication as needed
b. Evaluations
(1) Effects of the trauma are minimized
(2) Discomfort due to fracture is minimized or improved
(3) Bilirubin levels remain within normal range or return to normal if phototherapy is instituted

Post-term Infants

Introduction

A. **A post-term pregnancy is one that extends past 42 weeks' gestation**

B. **Post-term infants may be LGA, appropriate for gestational age, SGA, or dysmature, depending on placental function**

1. If the placenta functions well, the fetus will continue to grow, which results in an LGA infant, who may have certain problems
   a. Birth trauma
   b. Hypoglycemia
2. If the placental functions decrease, the fetus may not receive adequate nutrition, and a wasting of subcutaneous fat occurs, resulting in fetal dysmaturity syndrome
   a. Occurs as a result of the inability of the placenta to continue to nourish the fetus adequately
   b. Occurs in three forms
      (1) Chronic placental insufficiency
         (a) No meconium staining
         (b) Infant appears malnourished with skin changes
         (c) Infant has an apprehensive look, reflecting hypoxia
      (2) Acute placental insufficiency
         (a) Infant has malnourished and apprehensive appearance
         (b) Green meconium staining of the skin, umbilical cord, and placental membrane occurs
      (3) Subacute placental insufficiency
         (a) Skin and nails are stained a bright yellow (from breakdown of green bile meconium stain)
         (b) Umbilical cord, placenta, and placental membrane may be greenish brown

C. **Because of the incidence of placental degeneration, post-term infants are susceptible to perinatal asphyxia**

1. Prenatal asphyxia often results in meconium passage in utero; Usher, Boyd, McLean, and Kramer (1988) found that meconium release occurs two times and meconium aspiration syndrome eight times as frequently in post-term neonates as in others (see also Chapter 37)
   a. Infants born through amniotic fluid containing meconium are at risk of aspirating the meconium
   b. Once meconium is noted in fluid, the neonatal team should be notified and plans made for suctioning and resuscitation at birth
      (1) Once the infant's head is delivered, the mouth and nose should be suctioned while still on the perineum

(2) Once the whole body is delivered, the infant should be placed under a radiant warmer and visualization of the cords accomplished with a laryngoscope

  (a) If meconium is visualized below the cords, endotracheal suctioning should be performed

  (b) The infant can be extubated once tracheal suction is no longer needed, and when he or she has adequate respirations

2. Intrauterine hypoxia may trigger increased red blood cell (RBC) production leading to polycythemia, which results in the following

 a. Sluggish perfusion and hyperviscosity

 b. Hyperbilirubinemia due to neonatal breakdown of RBCs

D. **Post-term infants are susceptible to hypoglycemia because of the rapid use of glycogen stores**

E. **Post-term infants often appear macerated because of shedding of the top three layers of skin**

1. Lotions and powders are not recommended

2. Subcutaneous fat deficiency is caused by skin wasting and predisposes the infant to hypothermia

F. **Amniotic fluid is often decreased, leading to potential distress in labor**

1. May see less than 300 ml of fluid

2. Decreased amniotic fluid places the infant at increased risk of asphyxia and aspiration by making the meconium less dilute (thicker)

3. In a neonate with no congenital anomalies, oligohydramnios confirms postmaturity and has been linked to FHR decelerations and bradycardia

Clinical Practice

A. Assessment

1. History

 a. Estimated date of confinement (EDC)

 b. Color, consistency, and amount of amniotic fluid

 c. Gestational age determined by ultrasonography if available

 d. Placental grading, if available (see also Chap. 11)

  (1) Grades II and III are mature

  (2) Grades are based on deposits of calcium in placenta that may interfere with adequate transfer of nutrients and oxygen to fetus

 e. FHR patterns seen in labor

  (1) Variable decelerations, which are often due to decreased amniotic fluid

  (2) Late decelerations, which are indicative of fetal distress

  (3) Bradycardia

 f. Apgar scores

2. Physical findings

 a. Neonate's skin is leathery, wrinkled, cracked, and peeling, with long fingernails

 b. Absence of lanugo

 c. Creases on the entire soles of the feet

 d. Breast tissue is large (greater than 1 cm), and the areolae are full and raised

 e. Cartilage on the ear is thick and firm

 f. Skin may be meconium stained

 g. Post-term SGA babies have a wide-eyed, alert appearance

  (1) Frequently appear hungry

  (2) Exhibit behaviors such as fist sucking and frantic rooting

 h. Post-term LGA infants may be lethargic and have poor sucking ability

 i. Observe for signs of respiratory distress

j. Observe for signs of birth trauma in large infants
3. Diagnostic procedures
    a. Gestational age assessment plotted on curve
    b. Chest x-ray film if needed to evaluate possible aspiration
    c. Glucose levels
    d. If respiratory distress present, monitor oxygenation
        (1) Pulse oximetry
        (2) Arterial blood gas assay

B. Nursing Diagnoses

1. High risk for alteration in respiratory function related to meconium aspiration
2. High risk for alteration in nutrition: less than body requirements related to hypoglycemia
3. High risk for alteration in skin integrity related to absence of protective vernix and prolonged exposure to amniotic fluid

C. Interventions/Evaluations

1. High risk for alteration in respiratory function related to meconium aspiration
    a. Interventions
        (1) Perform direct tracheal suctioning on the perineum, before first breath or once the infant is placed under a radiant warmer
        (2) Perform chest physiotherapy and postural draining with suctioning as needed to remove excessive meconium and secretions from oropharynx
        (3) Maintain a patent airway
        (4) Maintain neutral thermal environment by drying baby off once meconium and oral secretions are removed
        (5) Auscultate breath sounds
        (6) Offer supplemental oxygen via free flow, mask, or endotracheal tube as needed
        (7) Position infant's head to maintain proper airway alignment to reduce respiratory effort
        (8) Offer nutrition via gavage if respiratory distress prevents nipple feedings
        (9) Provide non-nutritive sucking
        (10) Monitor oxygenation via pulse oximetry or blood gas assay
    b. Evaluations
        (1) Aspiration syndrome is prevented or minimized as evidenced by the following
            (a) Clear breath sounds
            (b) Good air entry
            (c) No respiratory distress
        (2) Adequate nutrition is maintained
        (3) Oxygenation is maintained
2. High risk for alteration in nutrition: less than body requirements related to hypoglycemia—see same diagnosis in section on LGA infants
3. High risk for impaired skin integrity related to absence of protective vernix and prolonged exposure to amniotic fluid
    a. Interventions
        (1) Practice good handwashing between handling infants
        (2) Keep skin clean and dry
        (3) Avoid use of powders, creams, and oils
        (4) Avoid use of tape unless necessary
        (5) Repositioning frequently
            (a) These infants are often active and agitated
            (b) Prevents abrasions of elbows and knees
            (c) Decreases chance of infection due to breaks in skin

b. Evaluations
   (1) Skin integrity is maintained
   (2) Infection is prevented
   (3) No lesions or wounds are noted on neonate's skin

Health Education

Small-for-Gestational-Age Infants

A. Parents must be informed of possible causes of IUGR

B. Parents may need assistance with guilt if chronic illness is a factor or if mother used substances known to compromise fetal growth

C. Make parents aware of goal weight for infant to go home

D. Parents need instruction on managing infant at home

1. Preparation of higher caloric formula or frequent breastfeeding
2. Performance of gavage feedings if necessary
3. Use of developmental therapist to screen for milestones in development and help with achievement as child becomes older

Large-for-Gestational-Age Infants

A. Parents of an LGA infant may need to be reminded of the infant's immaturity and fragility, despite its large size

B. If the delivery was traumatic for the mother, she needs extra recovery time before assuming total responsibility for the infant's care

C. The large neonate may be difficult to position and lift, and the mother may need assistance with positioning the baby while feeding, especially if breastfeeding

D. Parents need education and reassurance about the presence and implications of caput succedaneum and cephalhematoma

1. Usually no treatment is required
2. Head shape returns to normal within a few weeks

E. Infants with birth traumas such as palsies and fractures need special care

1. Parents need to know how to handle damaged extremity and maintain alignment
2. Parents need instruction in range-of-motion exercises
3. Physical therapy may be required

F. Provide information about the possible causes of macrosomia

G. Provide appropriate feeding guidelines to prevent potential overfeeding or underfeeding

Preterm Infants

A. Parents of preterm infants may need to grieve the loss of the so-called perfect child and attach to one that was born too early

B. If the baby has respiratory sequelae, special instructions may be needed

1. Parents may have to perform suctioning on the infant as needed
2. Feeding schedules may have to be modified to accommodate the baby's limited abilities and tolerance
3. Chest physiotherapy may have to be continued
4. Home apnea monitoring may be required

C. Preterm babies may need high-calorie formulas or supplementation to breastfeeding to ensure adequate weight gain and growth

D. Inform parents of the extent, outcome, and prognosis after intracranial hemorrhages; they may need referrals for persistent neurodevelopmental delays

Post-term Infants

A. Parents of a post-term infant need to be informed if resuscitation was performed at delivery

1. How the infant tolerated the resuscitation
2. Any anticipated sequelae such as prolonged hypoxia

B. Describe any birth trauma that may have occurred and the possible treatment required

C. Discuss the infant's need for nutritional support

1. Explain the problems associated with hypoglycemia
2. Teach the parents to do gavage feedings if necessary
3. Explain that post-term infants may need to feed more frequently (i.e., every 2 or 3 hours)

CASE STUDIES AND STUDY QUESTIONS

A 2300-g (5 lb, 1 ½ oz) baby girl is born to a 25-year-old gravida 1, para 0 (G1,P0) woman by spontaneous vaginal delivery. The baby's length is 44 cm (17.5 in), and her head circumference is 30.5 cm (12 in). No physical abnormalities are noted on physical examination. Maternal history and a gestational age assessment reveal the neonate to be at approximately 38 weeks' gestation, and she is small for that gestational age.

1. What might you expect to find in the mother's history?

   a. Positive culture for gonorrhea.

   b. Weight gain of 15. 9 kg (35 lb).

   c. A history of smoking one pack of cigarettes per day.

   d. Documented class A diabetes.

2. What implications do the infant's measurements have?

   a. The insult occurred late in gestation, during the hypertrophy phase.

   b. The insult occurred early in gestation during the hyperplasia phase.

   c. The insult occurred during labor and delivery.

   d. The infant can catch up in weight with adequate nutrition.

3. To which of the following should the nurse be alert when caring for this infant?

   a. Projectile vomiting.

   b. Possible skull fracture.

   c. Positive drug screen.

   d. Hypothermia.

A 4100-g (9 lb, 1 ½ oz) boy is born after a difficult forceps delivery. The prenatal history reveals an uncomplicated pregnancy of 40 weeks' gestation. The baby's length is 53.3 cm (21 in), and his head circumference is 37 cm (14.6 in). On gestational age assessment, the infant is determined to be large for gestational age.

4. On physical examination, what might you expect to find with this infant?

   a. Club feet.

   b. Brachial plexus palsy.

   c. Thin and transparent skin.

   d. Diminished Babinski's reflex.

5. In actuality, the nurse finds that the baby probably has a fractured clavicle. This is confirmed by x-ray film. What may have led her to this conclusion?

   a. Asymmetrical startle reflex.

b. Drooping left eyelid.

c. Extreme jitteriness.

d. History of forceps delivery.

6. What should the nurse be alert for when caring for this infant?

   a. Hypothermia.

   b. Congenital anomalies.

   c. Respiratory distress.

   d. Hypoglycemia.

An 18-year-old gravida 1, para 0 (G1,P0) woman is delivered of a 2000-g (4 lb, 6 ½ oz) boy by cesarean section. The infant is assessed to be appropriate for his gestational age of 34 weeks. No abnormalities are noted on physical examination.

7. This infant is at risk for which of the following conditions?

   a. Hyperglycemia.

   b. Premature closure of the ductus arteriosus.

   c. Respiratory distress syndrome.

   d. Imperforate anus.

8. What might the nurse expect to find in the mother's history?

   a. Premature labor treated with tocolytics.

   b. Gestational diabetes.

   c. Previous infant with Down's syndrome.

   d. Exposure to rubella in the first trimester.

9. What might be detected in this infant during the first few days of life?

   a. Congenital syphilis.

   b. Renal agenesis.

   c. Cephalhematoma.

   d. Hyperbilirubinemia.

A 32-year-old gravida 3, para 2 (G3,P2) delivers a 3250-g (7 lb, 3 oz) girl through meconium-stained amniotic fluid at 42 weeks' gestation. The infant's initial presentation is

that she is limp, cyanotic, with minimal respirations and a heart rate below 100. Her oropharynx was suctioned while the head was on the perineum, and her cords were visualized by the neonatal team. Although she was suctioned through the endotracheal tube, no meconium was seen below the cords. With oxygen and stimulation, her Apgar scores at 5 and 10 minutes were 8 and 9, respectively.

10. What is the most serious consequence that could happen as a result of this delivery?

    a. Patent ductus arteriosus.

    b. Meconium aspiration.

    c. Hyaline membrane disease.

    d. Depressed skull fracture.

11. What would the nurse expect to see on examination of this infant?

    a. Abundant lanugo.

    b. Absence of sole creases.

    c. Leathery, cracked, and wrinkled skin.

    d. Large caput succedaneum.

12. What should the nurse do to protect this baby's skin from further trauma?

    a. Use powders and oils frequently.

    b. Restrain the baby so she will not scrape her knees and elbows.

    c. Wear gloves when handling the infant.

    d. Avoid the use of tape except when absolutely necessary.

13. Why is hyperbilirubinemia of special concern in preterm infants?

    a. Immature liver function.

    b. Poor vascular system.

    c. Decreased respiratory function.

    d. Immature endocrine system.

14. Which of the following physiological factors contributes to greater risk for alteration in skin integrity in preterm infants?

    a. Immature immunological system.

    b. Malfunctioning of regulatory organs such as the kidneys and respiratory tract.

c. Increased frequency of regurgitation.

d. Decreased cohesion between the dermis and epidermis.

15. Gavage feedings are frequently needed to meet the nutritional needs of preterm infants because:

a. Lactose enzyme activity is not adequate.

b. Suck-and-swallow reflexes are uncoordinated.

c. Renal solute load must be considered.

d. Hyperbilirubinemia is likely.

16. A 42-week post-term neonate was born with greenish discoloration of the nails and skin and greenish secretions in the nasal passages. Why might the infant be transferred to a level 3 nursery?

a. To determine the reason for the postmaturity.

b. To observe more closely for skin color changes.

c. To manage severe respiratory problems that could develop.

d. To manage the pulmonary hypotension that is likely to develop.

17. Factors that contribute to impaired fetal growth include:

a. Maternal obesity.

b. Class A to C maternal diabetes mellitus.

c. Grade III placenta.

d. Multiple births.

18. The LGA infant may experience which of the following problems?

a. Patent ductus arteriosus.

b. Facial nerve damage.

c. Hypercalcemia.

d. Poor suck-and-swallow coordination.

19. Which characteristic best describes an SGA infant?

a. Lack of movement of upper extremities.

b. Long fingernails that extend over the end of the fingers.

c. Prone to meconium aspiration syndrome.

d. Wasted and thin at birth, with loose and scaling skin.

Answers to Study Questions

1. c	2. b	3. d
4. b	5. a	6. d
7. c	8. a	9. d
10. b	11. c	12. d
13. a	14. d	15. b
16. c	17. d	18. b
19. d		

REFERENCES

Avery, G. (Ed.). (1987). *Neonatology: Pathophysiology and management of the newborn* (3rd ed.). Philadelphia: Lippincott.

Bell, E., & Oh, W. (1987). Fluid and electrolyte management. In G. Avery (Ed.), *Neonatology: Pathophysiology and management of the newborn* (3rd ed., pp. 775–794). Philadelphia: Lippincott.

Boyd, M., Usher, R., McLean, F., & Kramer, M. (1988). Obstetric consequences of postmaturity. *American Journal of Obstetrics and Gynecology, 158*(2), 334–338.

Cassady, G., & Strange, M. (1987). The small-for-gestational-age (SGA) infant. In G. Avery (Ed.), *Neonatology: Pathophysiology and management of the newborn* (pp. 299–378). Philadelphia: Lippincott.

Cohen, S., Kenner, C., & Hollingsworth, A. (1991). *Maternal, neonatal, and women's health nursing.* Springhouse, PA: Springhouse.

Eng, G. (1987). Neuromuscular diseases. In G. Avery (Ed.), *Neonatology: Pathophysiology and management of the newborn* (pp. 1158–1172). Philadelphia: Lippincott.

Foster, R., Hunsberger, M., & Anderson, J. (1989). *Family-centered nursing care of children.* Philadelphia: Saunders.

Kaempf, J., Bonnabel, C., & Hay, W. (1989). Neonatal nutrition. In G. Merenstein & S. Gardner (Eds.), *Handbook of neonatal intensive care* (pp. 177–203). St. Louis: Mosby.

Koo, W., & Tsang, R. (1987). Calcium and magnesium homeostasis in the newborn. In G. Avery (Ed.), *Neonatology: Pathophysiology and management of the newborn* (pp. 710–723). Philadelphia: Lippincott.

Korones, S. (1986). *High-risk newborn infant.* St. Louis: Mosby.

Lubchenco, L., & Koops, B. (1987). Assessment of weight and gestational age. In G. Avery (Ed.), *Neonatology: Pathophysiology and management of the newborn* (pp. 235–257). Philadelphia: Lippincott.

Merenstein, G., & Gardner, S. (1989). *Handbook of neonatal intensive care.* St. Louis: Mosby.

Reeder, S., & Martin, L. (1987). *Maternity nursing: Family, newborn, and women's health care* (16th ed.). Philadelphia: Lippincott.

Sherwen, L., Scoloveno, M., & Weingarten, C. (1991). *Nursing care of the childbearing family.* Norwalk, CT: Appleton & Lange.

Usher, R. (1987). Extreme prematurity. In G. Avery (Ed.), *Neonatology: Pathophysiology and management of the newborn* (pp. 264–298). Philadelphia: Lippincott.

Usher, R., Boyd, M., McLean, F., & Kramer, M. (1988). Assessment of fetal risk in postdate pregnancies. *American Journal of Obstetrics and Gynecology 158*(1), 259–264.

Phyllis Muchmore

Respiratory Distress

Objectives

1. Identify infants at risk for developing respiratory distress

2. Explain the pathophysiology of respiratory distress syndrome (RDS)

3. Identify risk factors and the maternal and fetal history predictive of RDS

4. Recognize signs and symptoms of RDS

5. Describe specific nursing interventions appropriate for the infant with RDS

6. Explain the pathophysiology of transient tachypnea of the newborn (TTNB)

7. Identify risk factors and the maternal and fetal history predictive of TTNB

8. Recognize signs and symptoms of TTNB

9. Describe specific nursing interventions that are appropriate for the infant with TTNB

10. Explain the pathophysiology of meconium aspiration syndrome (MAS)

11. Identify risk factors and the maternal and fetal history predictive of MAS

12. Recognize signs and symptoms of MAS

13. Describe specific nursing interventions that are appropriate for MAS

Introduction

There are five major systemic malfunctions that can cause respiratory distress during the neonatal period. Although it is important to recognize signs and symptoms and to provide the appropriate treatment related to the cause, this chapter will focus on the more common causes that directly involve the respiratory tract itself.

A. Cardiac diseases

1. Congenital heart disease (CHD)
2. Congestive heart failure (CHF)
3. Patent ductus arteriosus (PDA)

4. Arrhythmias, such as supraventricular tachycardia (SVT)
5. Heart failure, such as that related to arteriovenous malformation

B. Hematological disorders

1. Anemia
2. Hemorrhage
3. Polycythemia

C. Metabolic disorders

1. Acidosis
2. Hypoglycemia
3. Hyperglycemia
4. Hypocalcemia
5. Hypothermia
6. Hyperthermia
7. Hypermagnesemia
8. Congenital hyperthyroidism

D. Central nervous system disorders

1. Hemorrhage
   a. Intracranial
   b. Intraventricular/periventricular (IVH/PVH)
   c. Subdural (SDH)
   d. Subarachnoid (SAH)
2. Infection
3. Depression related to maternal drugs given during labor
   a. Magnesium sulfate
   b. Analgesics
4. Neonatal substance withdrawal syndrome
5. Malformations
   a. Anencephaly
   b. Porencephaly
6. Asphyxia
7. Neuromuscular involvement
   a. Spinal cord trauma
   b. Muscular dystrophies

E. Respiratory disorders

1. Most common conditions
   a. RDS
   b. TTNB
   c. Aspiration syndromes
      (1) MAS
      (2) Blood aspiration
      (3) Amniotic fluid aspiration
   d. Persistent pulmonary hypertension of the newborn (PPHN)
   e. Pneumonia
2. Less common conditions
   a. Pulmonary hemorrhage
   b. Pulmonary air leak syndrome (PALS)
      (1) Pneumothorax ([PTX] spontaneously occurs in 1 to 2% of all term neonates [Oellrich, 1985])
      (2) Pneumomediastinum
      (3) Pneumopericardium
      (4) Pulmonary interstitial emphysema (PIE)
3. Rare conditions
   a. Upper airway obstruction
      (1) Choanal atresia

(2) Pierre Robin syndrome
  b. Space-occupying lesions
    (1) Congenital diaphragmatic hernia (CDH)
    (2) Esophageal atresia (with or without tracheoesophageal fistula [TEF])

Clinical Practice

RESPIRATORY DISTRESS SYNDROME

A. Introduction: RDS is the major cause of respiratory distress in the newborn and prematurity is the single most important risk factor (Naglie 1991)

1. RDS (old nomenclature is hyaline membrane disease [HMD]) accounts for approximately 20 to 30% of all neonatal deaths and approximately 50 to 70% of all premature deaths (Naglie, 1991)
2. Pathophysiology: surfactant deficiency
   a. Surfactant is a complex mixture of phospholipids and proteins that forms a coat over the inner surface of the alveoli and decreases their natural tendency to collapse at the end of expiration (Naglie, 1991)
   b. Alveolar development occurs between 24 and 28 weeks gestation, which results in the following
     (1) Increase in pulmonary vascularization
     (2) Development of ability for gas exchange
     (3) Development and proliferation of type II respiratory cells responsible for surfactant production and synthesis
   c. Surfactant deficiency results in the following
     (1) Increased surface tension, leading to alveolar collapse
     (2) Diffuse atelectasis
     (3) Decreased lung compliance
     (4) Right-to-left intrapulmonary shunting with increased pulmonary vascular resistance (PVR)
3. Complications of RDS include the following
   a. PDA (patent ductus arteriosus) incidence increases with decreasing gestational age (see Chapter 42 for a complete discussion of PDA)
   b. Air leak syndromes (e.g., pneumothorax, pneumomediastinum, pneumopericardium) occur in 5 to 30% of infants with RDS (Naglie, 1991)
   c. IVH occurs in approximately 50% of infants weighing less than 1500 g (3 lb, 5 oz) (Naglie, 1991)
   d. Bronchopulmonary dysplasia (BPD) occurs in approximately 20% of infants with RDS (Naglie, 1991)
   e. Retinopathy of prematurity (ROP) occurs in 5 to 10% of the cases (Naglie, 1991)
   f. Necrotizing enterocolitis (NEC) occurs in approximately 2% of infants with RDS (Naglie, 1991)
   g. Pulmonary interstitial emphysema (PIE)
   h. Oxygen toxicity

B. Assessment

1. History (risk factors) (Naglie, 1991)
   a. At less than 28 weeks' gestation, 60% of neonates demonstrate clinical signs of RDS
   b. At 28 to 32 weeks' gestation, 50% of neonates demonstrate clinical signs of RDS
   c. At 37 weeks' gestation and older, 3 to 5% of neonates demonstrate clinical signs of RDS
   d. At birth, 10 to 15% of infants who weigh less than 2500 g (5 lb, 8 oz) demonstrate RDS; the highest incidence occurs among the group with the lowest birth weight (Naglie, 1991)

  e. RDS is increased
    (1) In males versus females (1.5 times higher incidence)
    (2) Among whites versus nonwhites
    (3) In infants of diabetic mothers (IDM); insulin is antagonistic to surfactant production
    (4) In the presence of asphyxia, regardless of gestational age
    (5) When birth is by cesarean section, especially in the absence of labor, related to the lack of a thoracic squeeze
    (6) In the second-born of twins: this may be related to the second-born's longer stay in the birth canal, with the second twin receiving an excess of amniotic fluid with the birth of the first twin
    (7) When prenatal maternal hypotension is present, with or without maternal hemorrhage
    (8) In the presence of rhesus (Rh) factor incompatibility, which will retard surfactant production
  f. RDS is decreased with
    (1) Prolonged, premature rupture of membranes (PROM)
    (2) Intrauterine growth retardation (IUGR)
    (3) Pregnancy-induced hypertension (PIH)
    (4) Maternal heroin addiction
    (5) Prenatal corticosteroids
2. Physical findings: symptoms of RDS occur within 4 to 24 hours after delivery; symptoms are usually apparent in the delivery room; typically, the clinical course of RDS worsens during the first 48 hours after birth and respiratory function generally begins to improve within 72 hours
  a. Intercostal, subclavicular, and substernal retractions occur due to the compliant chest wall of the preterm infant in addition to relatively noncompliant lungs
    (1) The preterm newborn's compliant chest wall decreases the range of expansion of the lung so that, with severe retractions, the infant must use the diaphragm as the primary means of ventilation
    (2) This condition gives rise to the "see-saw" respirations, in which the chest flattens and the abdomen bulges with inspiration
  b. Expiratory grunting, heard as a result of partial vocal cord closure, increases transpulmonary pressures in an attempt to improve lung volume capacity
  c. Nasal flaring is often present as the infant attempts to decrease nasal airway resistance
  d. Tachypnea with a respiratory rate of greater than 60 breaths/min is frequently seen
  e. Decreased breath sounds or unequal breath sounds are present
  f. Poor air entry is heard on auscultation
  g. Fine rales may be heard bilaterally or unilaterally
  h. Generalized cyanosis may be seen because of impaired ventilation and intrapulmonary and intracardiac shunting
    (1) Peripheral cyanosis alone is commonly seen in newborns and is usually not significant
    (2) The degree of cyanosis is dependent on the following
      (a) Hemoglobin concentration
      (b) Status of the peripheral circulation
      (c) Available light to visualize the cyanosis
      (d) Color perception of the observer (Huxtable, 1990)
  i. Tachycardia with a heart rate of 150 to 180 beats/min may be seen
  j. Hypothermia may occur despite a neutral thermal environment (NTE)
  k. Hypoglycemia with a glucose level of less than 20 mg/dl in the preterm infant may be noted
  l. Hypotension is seen
  m. Hypotonia results in a limp and flaccid infant

n. Apnea occurs
3. Diagnostic procedures
   a. Apgar scores may not reflect the severity of RDS
   b. Maturity assessment
      (1) Lecithin/sphingomyelin (L/S) ratio of greater than 2:1 indicates mature lungs
         (a) Lecithin and sphingomyelin are two of the phospholipids of which surfactant is composed
         (b) Lecithin is present by 27 weeks' gestation and its concentration rises sharply at 35 weeks' gestation
         (c) Sphingomyelin remains at a relatively constant level throughout pregnancy
      (2) The presence of phosphatidylglycerol (PG) confirms maturity and is especially important in the presence of maternal conditions such as diabetes to ascertain lung maturity
         (a) Is present at 37 weeks' gestation and levels rise to term
         (b) If greater than 1%, indicates mature lungs
      (3) Shake test or foam stability index (FSI) may be performed on amniotic fluid at the maternal bedside to quickly determine the presence of surfactant
   c. Chest x-ray film initially may appear better than the clinical course would suggest; the classic chest x-ray film findings include the following
      (1) Reticulogranular (ground-glass) pattern
      (2) Air bronchograms that demonstrate diffuse alveolar collapse surrounding open bronchi
      (3) Decreased lung volumes
      (4) Possible cardiomegaly
   d. Pulmonary function studies demonstrate
      (1) Decreased compliance of the lungs
      (2) Increased work of breathing
      (3) Normal airway resistance
   e. Arterial blood gas (ABG) assays show hypoxemia and hypercapnia; although values may vary between institutions, suggested ranges are
      (1) A pH of less than 7.26 (normal acceptable range is between 7.26 and 7.35) (Naglie, 1991)
      (2) Arterial partial pressure of carbon dioxide ($PaCO_2$) of less than 40 mm Hg (normal range is between 40 and middle 50s mm Hg) (Naglie, 1991)
      (3) Arterial partial pressure of oxygen (PaO_2) of less than high 40s mm Hg (normal range is high 40s to low 60s mm Hg, with pulse oximetry values of 85 to 95%) (Naglie, 1991)
      (4) Base deficit should not be allowed to become more acidotic than minus 3 or 4 (Naglie, 1991)

C. Nursing Diagnoses

1. Alteration in ventilation and oxygenation in response to inadequate respiratory effort secondary to prematurity
2. Impaired gas exchange related to decreased alveolar ventilation and/or decreased pulmonary perfusion secondary to lung immaturity
3. Altered tissue perfusion related to cardiorespiratory immaturity secondary to prematurity
4. High risk for alteration in respiratory function related to immobility of secretions
5. Activity intolerance related to insufficient cardiorespiratory function secondary to prematurity
6. Altered nutrition: less than body requirements related to respiratory distress
7. Alteration in fluid balance: related to a potential for fluid overload related to respiratory distress (Lapido, 1989)

D. Interventions/Evaluations

1. Alteration in ventilation and oxygenation in response to inadequate respiratory effort secondary to prematurity
   a. Interventions
      (1) Provide appropriate maternal and early neonatal care to prevent RDS
         (a) Improved prenatal care has been shown to decrease the incidence of preterm delivery
         (b) Administration of tocolytic agents delays or prevents preterm delivery
         (c) Administration of corticosteroids to mother may induce fetal lung maturity and prevent RDS; optimal time of administration is at 28 to 32 weeks' gestation
         (d) Early and effective resuscitation may improve infant outcome (see Chapter 21 for a discussion of neonatal resuscitation)
            (i) Avoid asphyxia
            (ii) Avoid hypothermia
            (iii) Avoid shock
            (iv) Avoid acidosis
      (2) Provide appropriate supportive measures for the neonate to offer optimal respiratory support
         (a) Intubate with the appropriate size of endotracheal tube (ETT). Choice of tube size is determined by the neonate's weight, as follows (American Heart Association, 1987):
            (i) Less than 1001 g: 2.5 mm
            (ii) 1001 to 2000 g: 3.0 mm
            (iii) 2001 to 3000 g: 3.5 mm
            (iv) Above 3001 g: 4.0 mm
         (b) Transfer infant to the neonatal intensive care unit (NICU) for possible mechanical ventilation
         (c) Place infant in appropriate concentration of oxygen via oxygen hood or nasal cannula as determined by an ABG assay if mechanical ventilation is not needed
            (i) Oxygen should always be warmed and humidified to prevent infant heat loss and drying of mucous membranes
            (ii) Oxygen concentrations should be monitored continuously and documented per facility protocol
      (3) Provide continuous monitoring of infant's condition
         (a) All infants should be connected to continuous cardiorespiratory monitors to detect abnormalities in heart rate and rhythm as well as apnea and bradycardia
         (b) Blood pressure should be monitored in all infants with RDS
         (c) An ABG assay should be performed, as needed, or every 4 hours (see normal values as stated earlier)
         (d) Ongoing infant respiratory status should be assessed every 1 to 4 hours
            (i) Ausculation of breath sounds
            (ii) Quality of air entry
            (iii) Respiratory effort and spontaneous respiratory rate
         (e) Serial chest x-ray films should be obtained as appropriate, to assess disease progression
      (4) Administer or provide the following as ordered by physician and per facility protocol
         (a) Exogenous surfactant therapy may be administered to the infant to support lung function until the infant's own supply is produced
            (i) Replacement protocol is dependent upon the following
               • Human versus artificial surfactant
               • Mode of delivery may be aerosol or direct instillation

- Optimal time of initial treatment is controversial
- Frequency of dosing is controversial
        (ii) The incidences of PDA, IVH, retinopathy of prematurity, and bronchopulmonary dysplasia have not decreased subsequent to the use of exogenous surfactants (Naglie, 1991)
    (b) Continuous positive airway pressure (CPAP) may be administered to infants who do not need mechanical ventilation
        (i) May be administered via ETT or nasal prongs
        (ii) CPAP is ineffective in resolving atelectasis but may decrease intrapulmonary shunting and improve ventilation to alveoli already open
            - Decreases functional residual capacity (FRC), thereby decreasing dead space
            - Decreases the work of breathing
            - Stabilizes chest wall
    (c) High-frequency ventilation may be used in infants for whom conventional ventilation is inadequate
        (i) Infants who fail to oxygenate
        (ii) Infants with PIE
  b. Evaluations
    (1) The neonate is appropriately and adequately resuscitated in the delivery room; there is minimal asphyxia, hypothermia, shock, and acidosis
    (2) The infant receives the appropriate ventilatory support
        (a) The appropriate size of ETT is used, based on weight
        (b) Mechanical ventilation versus CPAP
    (3) The infant receives the appropriate concentration of oxygen as evidenced by ABG assay
    (4) The infant's vital signs are within normal limits
        (a) Heart rate: less than 180 beats/min
        (b) Respiratory rate: less than 60 breaths/min
        (c) Blood pressure: within normal limits for size and gestational age
    (5) The neonate demonstrates minimal respiratory distress
        (a) Bilateral breath sounds
        (b) Good air entry
        (c) Consistent respiratory effort with spontaneous respirations
        (d) Minimal retractions
        (e) Absence of grunting and nasal flaring
        (f) Absence of central or generalized cyanosis
2. Impaired gas exchange related to decreased alveolar ventilation, and/or decreased pulmonary perfusion secondary to lung immaturity (see next nursing diagnosis for interventions and evaluations)
3. Altered tissue perfusion related to cardiorespiratory immaturity secondary to prematurity
  a. Interventions
    (1) Provide adequate ventilation and oxygenation
        (a) To decrease alveolar collapse
        (b) To decrease the work of breathing
        (c) To increase gas exchange at the alveolar level
        (d) To increase perfusion to vital organs and tissues of the body
    (2) Provide for adequate pulmonary perfusion to allow gas exchange to occur
        (a) With RDS, the ductus arteriosus and foramen ovale may fail to close and blood will be shunted past the lungs into the systemic circulation
        (b) Without adequate blood flow, PVR remains high and the lungs are unable to exchange oxygen and carbon dioxide (CO_2), thus further compromising the preterm infant
        (c) High PVR and hypoperfusion of the lungs and systemic circulation results in the following

(i) Hypoxemia

(ii) Tissue hypoxia

(iii) Metabolic acidosis (pH of less than 7.26)

(iv) Increased transudation of fluid into the lungs

(d) Prevent and treat factors related to decreased pulmonary perfusion, tissue perfusion, or both

   (i) Inadequate lung expansion
   - Inadequate thoracic squeeze to expel fetal lung fluid
   - Inability of the preterm infant to generate adequate alveolar opening pressures during the first few breaths

   (ii) Hypoxemia stimulates pulmonary vasoconstriction and continued flow across the ductus arteriosus
   - Principal stimulus for pulmonary vasodilation within the infant's first few breaths is an increase in PaO_2
   - With a rise in PaO_2, the ductus ateriosus closes, providing increased blood flow to the lungs

   (iii) Systemic hypotension results in pulmonary and systemic vasoconstriction
   - Normal blood pressure varies with size and gestational age (Korones, 1986)
     □ 1000 to 2000 g (2 lb, 3 1/2 oz to 4 lb, 6 1/2 oz) mean arterial blood pressure (MABP) = 30 mm Hg
     □ 2000 to 3000 g (4 lb, 6 1/2 oz to 6 lb, 10 oz) = 35 mm Hg
     □ 3000 to 4000 g (6 lb 10 oz to 8 lb, 13 oz) = 43 mm Hg
     □ Systolic blood pressure in infants less than 2500 g (5 lb, 8 oz) = 50 mm Hg
     □ Systolic blood pressure in infants more than 2500 g (5 lb, 8 oz) = 60 mm Hg
   - Prevention and treatment includes
     □ Administration of fluids to prevent or treat hypovolemia, such as 5% albumin, packed red blood cells (PRBC), and dextrose solutions
     □ Administration of pressor agents, such as dopamine, dobutamine, and epinephrine

   (iv) Hypothermia causes cold stress in the neonate, which results in vasoconstriction and subsequent lowering of PaO_2
   - Neutral thermal environment is defined as the condition under which the amount of heat produced is equal to the least amount of heat lost to the environment, with the least metabolic stress
   - Maintain a warm and humidified oxygen level
   - Do not place infants on cold surface or in drafts
   - Keep infant dry to prevent evaporative heat loss

   (v) Metabolic acidosis causes constriction of pulmonary vessels and decreased lung perfusion
   - Administer IV fluids, as indicated
   - Prevent excessive water loss
   - Administer buffer agents, as indicated
     □ Sodium bicarbonate ($NaHCO_2$)
     □ Tromethamine (THAM)

   (vi) Anemia is defined as a central venous hemoglobin level of less than 13 g/dl (hematocrit, 39%) or a capillary venous hemoglobin level less than 14.5 g/dl (hematocrit 43.5%)
   - Replacement of losses in excess of 10% blood volume, with total volume calculated using 85 mg/kg as a guide (Korones, 1987)
   - Blood transfusions to maintain a central venous hematocrit of at least 40% (hemoglobin value, 13.3 g/dl)

b. Evaluations
(1) The infant is adequately ventilated and oxygenated (see evaluations listed earlier for nursing diagnosis number 1)
(2) The neonate demonstrates the following signs of adequate pulmonary and tissue perfusion
(a) Well oxygenated, with normal PaO_2
(b) Absence of metabolic acidosis
(c) Normal systemic blood pressure
(d) Absence of hypothermia
(e) Normal hematocrit and hemoglobin level
4. High risk for alteration in respiratory function related to immobility of secretions
a. Interventions
(1) Provide airway patency by the removal of secretions, using accepted guidelines per facility protocol (Hodge, 1991)
(a) Use a catheter of appropriate size (a 5- or 6-mm catheter is recommended if possible, to pass infant's airway)
(b) Set the vacuum gauge at 50 to 80 cm of water pressure
(c) Suction only as needed; assess need to suction by the following
(i) Breath sounds
(ii) Tolerance to procedure
(iii) Type and amount of secretions
(iv) Clinical status
(d) Have two people perform the procedure whenever possible
(e) Preoxygenate and hyperinflate before suctioning
(i) Begin 1 minute before suctioning
(ii) Continue during and after procedure until the infant reaches presuctioning heart rate and oxygen saturation baseline (Hodge, 1991)
(f) Carefully pass the suction catheter only to the end of the ETT (or to measured length; this will prevent damage to the bronchial mucosa)
(g) Avoid repeated passes of the catheter, if possible
(h) Use irrigants (normal saline) only if secretions are thick and difficult to suction out of the ETT
(2) To minimize the risks of endotracheal suctioning, continuously monitor the infant's tolerance of the suctioning procedure, by observing for the signs and symptoms of
(a) Hypoxia resulting from reduced lung volume and alveolar volume which results in decreased oxygen saturation
(b) IVH as the result of increased cerebral blood flow velocity and increased intracranial pressure
(c) Bradycardia, dysrhythmias, or both
(d) Altered pulmonary functions as a result of a decrease in lung compliance
(e) Destruction of mucociliary transport secondary to repeated suctioning
(f) Mucosal ulceration and hemorrhage secondary to the trauma of repeated suctioning
(g) Perforation of the mucosa, pneumothorax, and pneumomediastinum
b. Evaluations
(1) The infant demonstrates improved respiratory function as indicated by the following
(a) Minimal signs of respiratory distress
(b) ABG assay within normal limits
(c) Vital signs within normal limits
(2) The infant demonstrates minimal negative side effects from the suctioning procedure

(a) The infant remains well oxygenated

(b) The infant's heart rate remains above 100 beats/min with no observable dysrhythmias

(c) The infant does not exhibit the following outcomes associated with repeated suctioning attempts

(i) Mucosal ulceration, hemorrhage, or both

(ii) Mucosal and tracheal perforation

(iii) Air leaks

5. Activity intolerance related to insufficient cardiorespiratory function secondary to prematurity

a. Interventions

(1) Provide for adequate oxygenation (see interventions listed earlier for nursing diagnosis number 1)

(2) Provide for minimal stimulation with appropriate sedation (if needed) to conserve energy stores

(a) Caretaking activities should be clustered to provide adequate periods of rest

(b) Minimal handling should be observed by all personnel; unnecessary touching should be avoided to provide a maximum opportunity for the parents for bonding (see Health Education section)

(c) Infant should be handled gently, with slow, purposeful movements rather than abrupt, jerky movements

(d) Sedation may be ordered for infants whose spontaneous activity level compromises effective ventilation, oxygenation, and caloric use (see interventions listed for nursing diagnosis number 6)

b. Evaluations

(1) The infant maintains adequate oxygenation

(2) The infant receives minimal tactile stimulation

(a) Caretaking activities are grouped together

(b) The infant is not touched except to provide necessary care

(c) Parents demonstrate knowledge of their infant's activity tolerance by minimizing stress during bonding activities

(d) The infant is handled gently and carefully

(e) Sedation is given to those infants who demonstrate excess activity, resulting in the following

(i) Failure to adequately ventilate

(ii) Failure to adequately oxygenate

(iii) Caloric expenditure in excess of caloric intake

6. Altered nutrition: less than body requirements related to respiratory distress

a. Interventions

(1) Provide sufficient calories to obtain optimal recovery as well as growth and development

(a) Infants less than 33 weeks' gestation should not be fed by nipple. Alternatives include

(i) Gavage feedings

(ii) Continuous nasogastric feedings

(iii) Transpyloric feedings

(b) Infants on ventilatory support should be kept fasting by using IV therapy

(c) Tachypneic infants may be fed carefully by gavage with or without supplementary IV therapy

(d) Hypoxemia precludes enteral feedings, which necessitates IV therapy

(e) Preferred treatment in the face of intolerance to enteral feedings is nutrition via IV

(2) Provide minimal stimulation with appropriate sedation (if needed) to conserve energy stores; in infants whose caloric intake is insufficient,

control of caloric expenditure may help to balance the infant's use of available calories

b. Evaluations
  (1) The infant demonstrates intake of sufficient calories
    (a) Range is 90 to 130 kcal/kg/day
    (b) Sufficient caloric intake is indicated by
      (i) Weight gain of 15 to 30 g/day (0.5 to 1.0 oz/day)
      (ii) Spontaneous activity level that does not compromise weight gain
  (2) The infant is maintained on enteral feedings, as tolerated
  (3) If an infant is unable to tolerate enteral feedings, appropriate IV nutrition is established and maintained
  (4) Minimal stimulation occurs with all infants with RDS to prevent excessive caloric expenditure
7. Alteration in fluid balance: related to potential for fluid overload because of respiratory distress
  a. Interventions
    (1) Provide appropriate supportive measures for the neonate to offer optimal respiratory support (see interventions listed earlier for nursing diagnosis number 1)
    (2) Provide for adequate hydration and observe for signs of fluid overload
      (a) Edema
      (b) Excessive weight gain
      (c) Bulging anterior fontanelle
    (3) Provide for adequate monitoring of fluid and electrolyte balance to prevent overhydration
      (a) Daily weight
        (i) Parameter that is the most important to monitor
        (ii) Weight gain of more than 15 to 30 g/day is excessive
      (b) Serum glucose level
        (i) Bedside monitoring (Chemstix, Dextrostix) every 4 hours and as needed to maintain serum glucose at 50 to 100 mg/dl
        (ii) Infants with RDS may experience erratic serum glucose levels and may need frequent changes in IV solution
      (c) Daily serum electrolyte values
        (i) Sodium = 130 to 145 mg/dl
        (ii) Potassium = 4 to 6 mg/dl
        (iii) Chloride = 95 to 106 mg/dl
        (iv) Calcium = 8 to 10 mg/dl (preterm may be adequate at 7 to 10 mg/dl)
      (d) Strict input and output: urine output (ml/kg/hr) should be calculated every 12 to 24 hours
      (e) Specific gravity of the urine may not be helpful if the infant is excreting large molecules such as protein and blood
  b. Evaluations
    (1) The infant is appropriately supported to minimize respiratory distress (see evaluations listed earlier for nursing diagnosis number 1)
    (2) The infant demonstrates signs and symptoms of adequate hydration but fluid overload is avoided as evidenced by
      (a) Decrease in ventilatory support
      (b) Urine output between 1 and 2 ml/kg/hr
      (c) Electrolyte values within normal limits
      (d) Weight loss in the first few days of life followed by a weight gain of 15 to 30 g/day (0.5 to 1.0 oz/day)
      (e) Absence of excessive generalized edema
    (3) Infants who weigh less than 1500 g (3 lb 5 oz) at birth, as well as those unable to meet caloric needs via enteral fluids, have an IV line established and maintained

(4) Fluid and electrolyte levels are monitored on a daily basis
    (a) Daily weight
    (b) Bedside monitoring of serum glucose level
    (c) Serum electrolyte values
    (d) Physical examination to determine hydration status

TRANSIENT TACHYPNEA OF THE NEWBORN

A. Introduction: TTNB is also referred to as wet lung syndrome, retained lung fluid (RLF) and RDS, type II

1. Pathophysiology: excess fluid in the lungs, failure to clear normal fetal lung fluid, or both
  a. Fluid accumulates in the peribronchial lymphatics and bronchovascular spaces
  b. Excess fluid may be related to the following
    (1) Aspiration
      (a) Amniotic fluid
      (b) Secretions
      (c) Tracheal fluid
    (2) Factors that promote the formation of interstitial lung fluid
      (a) Decreased plasma colloid osmotic pressure (hypoalbuminemia)
      (b) Increased interstitial colloid osmotic pressure (transudation of plasma proteins)
      (c) Increased capillary hydrostatic pressure
  c. Fetal lung fluid is normally cleared via the following
    (1) Expulsion during delivery
    (2) Absorption after delivery
      (a) Pulmonary circulation
      (b) Lymphatic drainage
  d. Failure to clear fetal lung fluid is usually due to the lack of a "thoracic squeeze" to expel the fluid during delivery; this may occur in
    (1) Cesarean section
    (2) Breech birth
    (3) Second-born of twins
    (4) Small-for-gestational-age infant
    (5) Rapid labor and delivery
2. There is no known residual pulmonary dysfunction
  a. Spontaneous pneumothorax may be seen
  b. Severe complications are rare

B. Assessment

1. History (risk factors)
  a. TTNB infants tend to be term or near term (36 weeks' and longer gestation) with mature lungs, as indicated by L/S ratio
  b. TTNB is increased
    (1) In large infants with a birth weight of more than 4000 g (8 lb 13 ½ oz)
    (2) In infants born by cesarean section
    (3) In breech births
    (4) In the second-born of twins
    (5) When labor and delivery are rapid and preclude the opportunity for an effective thoracic squeeze (especially in the small infant)
    (6) With a maternal history of heavy sedation
    (7) In infants with polycythemia, delayed cord clamping, or both; hyperviscosity of blood leads to sluggish circulation in the pulmonary vessels
    (8) In infants suffering from hypothermia at or shortly before birth
      (a) Hypothermia causes pulmonary vasoconstriction

(b) Vasoconstriction causes the infant to experience hypoxemia and increased oxygen consumption, which produces respiratory distress

2. Physical findings: symptoms of TTNB are usually present within the first hours of life (most often within 30 minutes); typically, the clinical course of TTNB occurs during the first 12 to 72 hours of life and the disease is self-limiting

   a. Transient tachypnea with a respiratory rate of 60 to 140 breaths/min (rarely lasts longer than 48 to 96 hours)
   b. Grunting
   c. Mild intercostal retractions
   d. Possible mild cyanosis
   e. Breath sounds that may be slightly decreased because of reduced air entry
   f. Absence of rales
   g. Nasal flaring
   h. Chest that may appear hyperexpanded or barrel shaped

3. Diagnostic procedures: TTNB is a diagnosis of exclusion

   a. A diagnosis of TTNB can be ascertained only after resolution of symptoms within the first 4 days
   b. Chest x-ray film reveals the following
      (1) Increased lung fluid, with fluid in the interlobar tissues
      (2) Prominent vascular marking (so-called hairy heart)
      (3) Flat diaphragm, with increased lung volume
      (4) Mild pleural effusions may be demonstrated
      (5) Presence of occasional mild cardiomegaly
      (6) Possible appearance of initial chest x-ray film as identical to RDS in the first 3 hours of life
   c. ABG assay
      (1) Mild hypoxemia
      (2) $PaCO_2$: normal to mildly elevated (less than 50 mm Hg)
      (3) pH: usually normal

C. **Nursing Diagnoses**

1. Alteration in oxygenation in response to inadequate respiratory effort secondary to retained lung fluid
2. Altered nutrition: less than body requirements related to respiratory distress

D. **Interventions/Evaluations**

1. Alteration in oxygenation in response to inadequate respiratory effort secondary to retained lung fluid
   a. Interventions
      (1) Be aware that assisted ventilation is seldom required
      (2) Provide appropriate oxygen therapy to maintain ABG values within normal levels
         (a) Normal ABG assays for the term infant
            (i) pH = 7.35 to 7.45
            (ii) $PaCO_2$ = 35 to 45 mm Hg
            (iii) PaO_2 = 50 to 70 mm Hg
         (b) Be aware that TTNB infants rarely require more than 70% fraction of inspired oxygen (FIO_2) (usually 35 to 40%)
         (c) Providing CPAP for the first few hours with severe pulmonary involvement may be useful
   b. Evaluations
      (1) The infant receives the appropriate concentration of oxygen
      (2) The infant's ABG values are within normal limits
      (3) The infant demonstrates minimal respiratory distress
         (a) Respiratory rate of less than 60 breaths/min
         (b) Minimal retractions

      (c) Bilateral breath sounds with good air entry
      (d) Absence of grunting and nasal flaring
      (e) Absence of generalized cyanosis
  2. Altered nutrition: less than body requirements related to respiratory distress
      a. Interventions
          (1) Care for TTNB is largely supportive
          (2) Enteral feedings may be established as the disease resolves
              (a) Respiratory rate of less than 60 breaths/min
              (b) Resolution of grunting and retractions
              (c) Adequate respiratory functioning with supplemental oxygen
      b. Evaluation: enteral feedings are initiated for the infant, with an intake of sufficient calories to promote optimal growth and development

MECONIUM ASPIRATION SYNDROME

A. Introduction

  1. Meconium aspiration is the most common of the aspiration syndromes
  2. Pathophysiology: there are two overlapping phenomena that occur with MAS
      a. Pneumonitis and pneumonia with or without air leak
          (1) Bile salts and pancreatic enzymes and other particles in the meconium cause a chemical pneumonitis
          (2) Meconium occludes the distal airways and acts as a ball valve mechanism that allows air in but obstructs air outflow during expiration; this leads to air trapping and air leak (pneumothorax and pneumomediastinum)
      b. Three general mechanisms in the fetus result in passage of meconium
          (1) Direct hypoxic bowel stimulation
              (a) Passage of meconium into the amniotic fluid may be the result of some intrauterine insult that causes fetal distress
              (b) Hypoxia and acidosis may result in relaxation of the anal sphincter and passage of meconium
          (2) Spontaneous gastrointestinal (GI) motility: there may be spontaneous normal physiological defecation in the term or post-term infant
          (3) Vagal stimulation with or without specific cause (is often due to cord compression)
      c. After the passage of meconium into the amniotic fluid, the fetus may swallow or aspirate the meconium into the mouth, pharynx, and trachea
          (1) With hypoxia, the fetus demonstrates normal or irregular respiratory movements
          (2) There can be intrauterine aspiration in overwhelming distress
          (3) The greatest risk for aspiration is at delivery, if there is meconium-stained fluid in the mouth and pharynx when the infant draws the first breath
      d. In addition to the mechanical damage done by the meconium itself, asphyxia is by far the most damaging aspect of MAS (MAS infants without asphyxia do better clinically) (Sills, 1991)
          (1) Meconium aspiration may be the only presenting event because there may be prolonged fetal asphyxia before and after the meconium aspiration
          (2) Asphyxia may lead to the following conditions
              (a) Edema of the airways
              (b) Necrosis of the airways
              (c) Vascular collapse of the alveoli
              (d) Pulmonary hemorrhage
  3. Incidence of MAS
      a. Ten to 15% of all births include the presence of meconium-stained amniotic fluid (Naglie, 1991)

b. Meconium may be aspirated from the trachea in approximately 56% of those infants born with 3+ or 4+ meconium (Naglie, 1991)

c. Approximately one-third of infants with meconium below the vocal cords become ill and require intensive care (Naglie, 1991)

d. With better obstetrical and pediatric management at birth, the incidence is decreasing

4. Complications of MAS include

a. Air leak syndrome (e.g., pneumothorax and pneumomediastinum) occurs in 20 to 30% of cases (Naglie, 1991)

b. Pulmonary interstitial emphysema

c. Pulmonary hemorrhage

d. Persistent pulmonary hypertension of the newborn

e. Pneumonia

f. Severe asphyxia

g. Infection

h. Thrombocytopenia

B. Assessment

1. History

a. MAS infants tend to be primarily term, post-term, or small for gestational age (SGA)

b. Perinatal factors associated with or predisposing to MAS include

(1) Prolonged labor

(2) Fetal bradycardia and distress

(3) Breech presentation

(4) Presence of meconium-stained amniotic fluid

(5) Delivery by cesarean section

(6) Low Apgar scores (less than 6)

(7) Absence of suctioning at the time of delivery

(8) IUGR

(9) Decreased fetal movements

(10) Maternal PIH, which leads to placental dysfunction

(11) Prolapsed umbilical cord or placental abruption

2. Physical findings

a. Severity of MAS correlates with

(1) Consistency of meconium

(a) Early in the labor, heavy "pea soup" consistency

(b) Late in the labor, passage of large particles

(2) Amount of meconium

(a) More than 2 ml in pharynx

(b) More than 2 ml in trachea

(3) Degree of consolidation on chest x-ray film

b. Meconium staining of skin, umbilical cord, and nails

c. Hyperexpansion of the chest (barrel shaped)

d. The following signs of respiratory distress occur in as many as 50% of MAS infants

(1) Grunting

(2) Retractions

(3) Nasal flaring

(4) Tachypnea

(5) Generalized cyanosis

(6) Irregular or gasping respirations, or both

(7) Coarse, bronchial breath sounds, with audible rales heard on auscultation

e. Clinical signs of congestive heart failure

3. Diagnostic procedures

a. ABG assays show hypoxemia with respiratory or metabolic acidosis, or both

b. Chest x-ray film
   (1) Hyperinflated lungs (9 to 11 ribs expanded) appear in 20 to 30% of cases (Pisanos, 1985)
   (2) Nonuniform, coarse, and patchy infiltrates radiate from one hilum into the peripheral lung fields
   (3) Infiltrates associated with focal areas of irregular aeration are present; some appear atelectatic or consolidated, and others appear emphysematous (air trapping)
   (4) Pleural fluid may be seen in 20 to 30% of the cases (Pisanos, 1985)

C. Nursing diagnoses

1. Alteration in ventilation and oxygenation in response to inadequate respiratory effort secondary to MAS
2. High risk for alteration in respiratory function related to immobility of secretions

D. Interventions/Evaluations

1. Alteration in ventilation and oxygenation in response to inadequate respiratory effort secondary to MAS
   a. Interventions
      (1) Provide appropriate delivery room care to prevent aspiration of any meconium found in the mouth and pharynx
         (a) Before delivery of the thorax
             (i) Suction mouth and hypopharynx
             (ii) Suction oropharynx and nares
         (b) At birth, the vocal cords should be visualized with a laryngoscope and the trachea should be suctioned
      (2) Provide appropriate supportive measures for the neonate to offer optimal respiratory support
         (a) Ventilatory support, if needed
             (i) Low peak inspiratory pressures (PIP) are preferred to prevent air leaks
             (ii) Infants who need support tend to do better with rapid ventilator rates and shorter inspiratory times
         (b) Provide for high oxygenation (PaO_2 of 75 to 90 mm Hg) to prevent vasoconstriction
         (c) Provide the following pharmacological assistance to achieve desired ventilation and oxygenation of the infant
             (i) Sedation to prevent "fighting the ventilator"
             (ii) Vasodilators to increase pulmonary blood flow to allow for adequate oxygenation
      (3) Provide continuous evaluation of infant's condition
         (a) Cardiorespiratory monitoring
         (b) Transcutaneous and oximetry monitoring
         (c) ABG assay
         (d) Ongoing respiratory status evaluations
         (e) Serial chest x-ray films
      (4) Prevent and treat conditions occurring secondary to inadequate ventilation and oxygenation
         (a) Systemic hypotension: treat with the following
             (i) Additional fluids
             (ii) Vasopressors
         (b) Persistent metabolic acidosis: treat with the following
             (i) Additional fluids
             (ii) Buffer agents as needed, to maintain a pH between 7.45 and 7.50
         (c) Anemia: transfuse with blood products, as indicated
         (d) Infection

(i) Meconium is an excellent growth medium for bacteria

(ii) Administration of prophylactic antibiotics may be indicated

b. Evaluations

(1) The infant receives adequate delivery room care to prevent MAS

(a) Suctioned on the perineum before delivery of the thorax

(b) Intubation and tracheal suctioning after birth

(2) The infant is appropriately ventilated

(a) Mechanical ventilation, as needed

(b) CPAP

(3) The infant is adequately oxygenated as evidenced by

(a) PaO_2 75 to 90 mm Hg

(b) The infant does not progress to or demonstrate signs of the severe consequences of MAS (persistent pulmonary hypertension, pneumonia, or air leaks)

(4) The infant receives pharmacological support, as needed, to achieve adequate ventilation and oxygenation

(5) The infant is continuously monitored

(6) The infant does not demonstrate the following conditions secondary to inadequate ventilation and oxygenation

(a) Hypotension

(b) Metabolic acidosis

(c) Anemia

(d) Infection

2. High risk for alteration in respiratory function related to immobility of secretions

a. Interventions

(1) Provide adequate chest physiotherapy: no value has been seen in tracheal lavage in the delivery room unless meconium is thick and particulate and unable to be removed (Naglie, 1991)

(2) Maintain intubation status until secretions are clear

b. Evaluations

(1) The infant is adequately suctioned in the delivery room as evidenced by minimal aspiration

(2) The infant receives adequate chest physiotherapy, as needed

(3) The infant demonstrates improved respiratory function evidenced by

(a) Resolution of respiratory distress

(b) Improving ABG assay values

(c) Vital signs within normal limits

Health Education

A. **The technological advances made in newborn care during the last 30 years have markedly decreased morbidity and mortality in this group of high-risk infants**

1. Technological advances have brought a heightened sensitivity to the psychological and emotional impact felt by the family of a sick neonate

2. This awareness has introduced the need for a family-centered approach to newborn care

3. In addition to the physiological care of the sick neonate, health care workers need to address the psychological needs of family members during this experience

4. Parental attachment to the infant with respiratory distress is especially difficult

a. The infant may be premature

b. Normal interaction may be severely curtailed

c. An infant who is sick enough to be on a ventilator or oxygen support may not give cues adequate to arouse parental attachment

B. The birth of a newborn who is sick represents a unique crisis for the family and perinatal health care team

1. The family must simultaneously adjust to the immediate situation and begin the normal developmental process of parenthood (Siegel, 1985)
2. Situational factors, such as the following, have an important bearing on the family's ability to cope with this present crisis and can affect the overall outcome
   a. The behavior and attitude of the hospital staff
   b. The sensitivity used in the transfer process, either to another facility or the NICU
   c. The flexibility in unit visitation and extended family involvement
   d. The instruction received by the family related to their infant's unique characteristics and behavior
   e. The staff's sensitivity to the family's responses and adaptation to crisis
   f. The use of emotionally supportive intervention programs in the nursery
   g. The development of appropriate discharge planning to provide adequate follow-up for the family

C. Discharge planning for the infant with respiratory distress may include the following

1. Family education
   a. Use of equipment needed in the care of the infant (e.g., oxygen and suctioning devices)
   b. When and how to perform chest physiotherapy
   c. Dosage, route of administration, side effects, and planned duration of use of all medications
   d. Nutritional information to maintain adequate calorie and fluid balance
      (1) Type of formula
      (2) How and when to feed the infant
      (3) Possible alternative feeding methods
      (4) If and when to provide oxygen during the feedings
   e. The use of home monitoring, if needed
   f. Infant cardiopulmonary resuscitation (CPR)
   g. Recognition of signs and symptoms of illness in the newborn
   h. Normal newborn care
2. Acquisition of specialized equipment, as well as the sources and mode of delivery on a continuing basis, of the following
   a. Ventilatory supplies
   b. Oxygen delivery equipment
   c. Suction machine and supplies
   d. Home monitoring equipment
3. All information and education given to the family should be in written form, if possible; in addition, whenever possible, demonstrations by the family, in return, reinforce learning

D. Long-term follow-up of the infant with respiratory distress is essential

1. Parents must have telephone numbers of the medical facility and personnel to call 24 hours a day in case of problems or equipment failure
2. Before hospital discharge, parents need to have information regarding follow-up appointments and referrals for long-term care

---

CASE STUDIES AND STUDY QUESTIONS

1. Which of the following prenatal factors predispose the neonate to development of respiratory distress?

   (1) Maternal diabetes.

   (2) Breech presentation.

   (3) Fetal scalp pH of 7.20.

   (4) 43 weeks' gestation.

a. a, c.

b. b, d.

c. a, b, c.

d. a, b, c, d.

2. Surfactant production for an infant with RDS will be inhibited owing to which of the following?

a. Prematurity.

b. Hypoxia.

c. Acidosis.

d. Drugs given to the mother.

e. All except d.

3. The *best* indicator of an infant's need for oxygen is which of the following?

a. Respiratory rate.

b. Skin color.

c. Arterial PaO_2.

d. Pulse rate.

4. Which of the following is characteristic of neonates with RDS?

a. Have a deficiency of pulmonary surfactant.

b. Are postmature.

c. Have sternal excursions.

d. Demonstrate tachypnea and expiratory grunting.

e. a and d.

5. Which of the following statement(s) is/are true about RDS?

a. It is characterized by atelectasis.

b. Acidosis perpetuates the decreased production of surfactant.

c. It may be induced by hypothermia in a preterm infant.

d. With adequate supportive care, it is self-resolving in approximately 72 hours.

e. a, b, c, d.

6. In RDS, blood may not be oxygenated because of which of the following?

a. A patent ductus arteriosus.

b. Failure of the foramen ovale to close.

c. Atelectasis of the alveoli.

d. Alkalosis.

e. a, b, c.

7. True or false: acidosis and hypothermia may lead to decreased pulmonary blood flow, which perpetuates decreased production of surfactant and may cause RDS.

a. True

b. False

8. A condition that usually occurs in term infants and cesarean section deliveries, that is manifested by tachypnea and is due to retained lung fluid, is called which of the following?

a. Pneumonia.

b. Transient tachypnea of the newborn.

c. Pulmonary hemorrhage.

d. Meconium aspiration.

9. When suctioning the neonate born through meconium-stained amniotic fluid, which of the following is suctioned first?

a. Both nares.

b. Stomach.

c. Trachea.

d. Oropharynx and nasopharynx (before the infant's body is delivered.

Answers to Study Questions

1. d	2. e	3. c
4. e	5. e	6. e
7. a	8. b	9. d

REFERENCES

1. Bloom, R.S., & Cropley, C. (1987). *Textbook of neonatal resuscitation.* Los Angeles, CA: American Heart Association.

2. Boynton, B.R. (1986). High-frequency ventilation in newborn infants. *Respiratory Care, 31,*(6) 340–345.
3. Cornish, J.D. (1991). Extracorpeal membrane oxygenation (ECMO): Indications and outcomes. In *Critical care of the neonate: Nursing care of the newborn in intensive care* (pp. 354–364). Irvine, CA: University of California.
4. Cunningham, D. (1991, March). *Anemia.* Paper presented at the University of California Irvine Medical Center, Neonatal Intensive Care Unit review course, Orange, CA.
5. Huxtable, R.F., Hicks, D.A., & Peduzi, M.C. (1990). Respiratory conditions of the newborn. In *Optimal care of the newborn: An introduction to neonatal nursing* (pp. 135–154) Irvine, CA: University of California.
6. Hodge, D. (1991). Endotracheal suctioning and the infant: A nursing care protocol to decrease complications. *Neonatal Network, 9*(5), 7–15.
7. Jobe, A. (1986). Surfactant treatment for respiratory distress syndrome. *Respiratory Care, 31*(6).
8. Kezler, M. (1990). Persistent pulmonary hypertension of the newborn. In *Critical care of the neonate: Nursing care of the newborn in intensive care* (pp. 266–270). Irvine, CA: University of California.
9. Korones, S.B. (1986). *High-risk newborn infants* (2nd ed.) (pp. 131–179). Saint Louis: Mosby.
10. Lapido, M. (1989). Respiratory distress revisited. *Neonatal Network, 8*(3), 9–14.
11. Miller, E.P., & Armstrong, C.L. (1990). Surfactant replacement therapy: Innovative care of the premature infant. *Journal of Obstetric, Gynecologic, and Neonatal Nursing, 19*(1), 14–17.
12. Naglie, R. (1991, March). *Neonatal respiratory distress.* Paper presented at the University of California Irvine Medical Center, Neonatal Intensive Care Unit Review Course, Orange, CA.
13. Oellrich, R.G. (1985). Pneumothorax, chest tubes, and the neonate. *MCN: American Journal of Maternal Child Nursing, 10*(1), 29–35.
14. Parry, W.H., Baldy, M.A., & Gardner, S.C. (1985). Respiratory diseases. In G.B. Merenstein & S.C. Gardner (Eds.), *Handbook of neonatal intensive care* (pp. 301–344). St. Louis: Mosby.
15. Pisanos, D., & Honeyfield, M.E. (1985). *Neonatal respiratory distress: Causes and management.* Unpublished manuscript.
16. Pramanik, A.K. (1991). New synthetic surfactant helps infants breathe more easily. *Neonatal Intensive Care, 4*(1), 32–33, 45–46.
17. Siegel, R., Gardner, S.L., & Merenstein, G.B. (1985). Families in crisis: Theoretical and practical considerations. In G.B. Merenstein & S.L. Gardner (Eds.), *Handbook of neonatal intensive care* (pp. 421–448). St. Louis: Mosby.
18. Sills, J. (1991, February). *Management of meconium aspiration in the delivery room.* Paper presented at the Mortality and Morbidity Conference, Newport Beach, CA.
19. University of California, Irvine, Department of Obstetrics and Gynecology (1990). An introduction to bedside measurement of lung function in infants. In *Critical care of the neonate: Nursing care of the newborn in intensive care* (pp. 296–305). Irvine, CA: University of California.
20. University of California, Irvine, Department of Obstetrics and Gynecology (1990). Neonatal respiratory distress: Differential diagnosis. In *Critical care of the neonate: Nursing care of the newborn in intensive care* (pp. 259–265). Irvine, CA: University of California.

38

Ksenia Zukowsky,
Judy E. Smith,
and Bonnie Christoff

Hyperbilirubinemia

Objectives

1. Describe the physiological process of the production, conjugation, and elimination of bilirubin in the neonate

2. Define the differences between conjugated and unconjugated bilirubin

3. Identify the neonatal complications that interfere with normal bilirubin conjugation in the neonate

4. Describe the maternal and neonatal factors that contribute to jaundice in the neonate

5. Identify the physical signs of hyperbilirubinemia in the neonate

6. Specify nursing interventions that are effective in providing nursing care to neonates with hyperbilirubinemia

7. Analyze the total, direct, and indirect values of bilirubin levels to determine their potential significance on the neonate's physical condition

8. Distinguish the differences between the various causal factors and related outcomes of jaundice in the neonate

9. Discuss the complications related to an interruption in the bilirubin conjugation process and identify the strategies that would either eliminate or alter the interruption in the process

Introduction

Physiologic jaundice is a condition that is commonly seen in the term neonate during the second or third day of life (second to ninth day in preterm neonates) and is not considered to be pathological unless bilirubin levels exceed the normal physiological limitations of a healthy neonate. Pathologic hyperbilirubinemia, which cannot be defined only by serum concentrations of unconjugated bilirubin, has diverse etiologies that are frequently, but not always, interlinked. Jaundice is a manifestation of bilirubin accumulation in extravascular tissues.

A. Bilirubin production and conjugation

1. Bilirubin has two forms

      a. Unconjugated or indirect
         (1) Fat soluble
         (2) Toxic to tissues
      b. Conjugated or direct
         (1) Water soluble
         (2) Nontoxic to tissues

2. The majority of bilirubin comes from the destruction of hemoglobin
      a. Catabolism of 1 g of hemoglobin results in the production of 34 mg of bilirubin (Oski, p. 749, 1991)
      b. Destruction of circulating erythrocytes accounts for approximately 75% of the daily bilirubin production in the normal term neonate (Oski, 1991, p. 749)
         (1) The neonate has a large red cell mass per kilogram of body weight. The neonate's red blood cells have a life span that is only two-thirds that of an adult's red blood cells. (Oski, p. 749, 1991)
         (2) The shortened life span of the neonate's RBCs accounts for the increased breakdown and subsequent increased production of bilirubin
      c. The remaining 25% of the daily bilirubin production in the newborn originates from the following other sources
         (1) Destruction of heme proteins
         (2) Free heme from liver
         (3) Destruction of the RBC precursor in bone marrow

3. Process of bilirubin conjugation (Fig. 38–1)
      a. Within the circulatory system, unconjugated bilirubin tightly bound to albumin is transported to the liver, where the conjugation process takes place

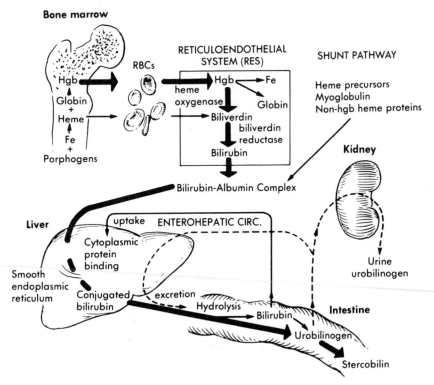

Figure 38–1
Process of bilirubin conjugation. (Reprinted with permission from Gartner, L.M., in N.S. Assali (Ed.), Disorders of bilirubin metabolism. In *Pathophysiology of gestation.* (Vol. 2, p. 457) New York: Academic Press, 1972.)

b. Bilirubin is then released from the albumin binding site and undergoes the following
  (1) Transfer across the hepatocyte membrane
  (2) Cytoplasmic protein binding
      (a) Within the liver, bilirubin is bound to ligandin and other hepatic proteins
      (b) This binding helps to prevent a back-up of bilirubin into the general circulation
  (3) Transport (while bound to protein)
      (a) Smooth endoplasmic reticulum is the site of conjugation process
      (b) Process of conjugation transforms the poorly soluble, unconjugated bilirubin into a water-soluble form that can be excreted by the neonate; this process
          (i) Requires oxygen
          (ii) Requires glucose
  (4) Excretion (after conjugation) into the bile, into the intestine, and finally mainly into the neonate's stool as stercobilin
      (a) Some bilirubin is excreted through the kidneys as urobilinogen
      (b) In the intestine, the enzyme glucuronidase may break the ester linkage of the bilirubin, causing it to become unconjugated
          (i) Can occur in the sterile (uncolonized) intestine
          (ii) Can be catalyzed if normal bacterial colonization has occurred
      (c) The newly unconjugated bilirubin may be reabsorbed into the neonate's circulation, necessitating a repetition of the entire conjugation process
4. Neonatal hyperbilirubinemia can occur from the following
  a. An increased load of circulating bilirubin, resulting from the following
      (1) Polycythemia
      (2) Isoimmune hemolytic disease
      (3) Structural and enzyme defects of RBCs
      (4) Drug toxicity (chemical hemolysis)
      (5) Extravascular hemolysis
          (a) Enclosed hemorrhage, as in cephalhematoma
          (b) Ecchymosis
  b. Impaired hepatic function (e.g., defective uptake, conjugation, or excretion)
      (1) Deficient glucuronyl transferase activity
      (2) Biliary obstruction or biliary atresia
      (3) Infection
      (4) Metabolic problems, such as
          (a) Galactosemia
          (b) Breast milk jaundice
          (c) Hypothyroidism
  c. Perinatal complications, because of
      (1) Asphyxia
      (2) Hypothermia
      (3) Hypoglycemia
  d. Decreased albumin binding sites, because of
      (1) Preterm birth
      (2) Competition with drugs having an affinity for the binding sites
      (3) Acidosis
  e. Delayed meconium passage
      (1) Meconium contains 0.5 to 1 mg of bilirubin per gram
      (2) Delayed meconium passage increases the amount of bilirubin that returns to the unconjugated state and then is reabsorbed across the intestinal mucosa (Korones, 1986, p. 320)
5. Rate of bilirubin level increase

a. Must exceed 4 to 6 mg/dl before it is visible as jaundice
b. In physiologic jaundice
  (1) Bilirubin level increase first appears after 24 hours of age in term neonates and after 48 hours of age in preterm neonates
    (a) Reaches peak at day 3 or 4 and disappears by end of day 7 in term neonates
    (b) Reaches peak at day 5 or 6 and disappears by the end of day 9 or 10 in preterm neonates
  (2) Indirect bilirubin value does not usually exceed 12 mg/dl
  (3) Direct bilirubin value does not usually exceed 1 to 1.5 mg/dl
  (4) Daily increases of bilirubin do not usually exceed 5 mg/dl
c. In pathologic jaundice, bilirubin level increase
  (1) Appears within the first 24 hours of life
  (2) Persists beyond the age for disappearance in term and preterm neonates
  (3) Has no specific serum level that can be used for diagnosis
d. Kernicterus
  (1) Bilirubin encephalopathy is the most serious complication of hyperbilirubinemia
  (2) Yellow staining of brain tissue occurs and creates morphological changes in brain cells, which results in irreversible damage
  (3) Approximately half of affected neonates do not survive
  (4) Condition is generally thought to occur at bilirubin levels in excess of 20 mg/dl in full-term neonates (Korones, 1986, p. 328)

B. Phototherapy

1. Treatment is widely used to manage and control rising bilirubin levels
2. Mechanism of phototherapy action is not fully understood
  a. Treatment is thought to reduce serum bilirubin levels by facilitating biliary excretion of unconjugated bilirubin
  b. Treatment causes the formation of photoisomers, which are more water soluble and, therefore, more easily excreted in stool and urine
    (1) Unconjugated bilirubin is rapidly converted to photobilirubin and lumirubin (Oski, 1991, p. 756)
    (2) Photobilirubin and lumirubin are rapidly taken up by the liver and transported into the bile (Gartner, 1987, p. 962)
    (3) Process occurs independent of hepatic conjugation of bilirubin
  c. White, daylight, cool blue, and special blue are among the various types of phototherapy lights available
    (1) Lights with high-energy output, ranging between 420 and 450 nm in the blue spectrum, are the most effective (Gartner, 1987, p. 926)
    (2) Optimal-energy-output-light levels should be monitored to ensure that levels are maintained to achieve maximal efficiency
  d. Home monitoring and treatment
    (1) Bilirubin levels can be accurately determined during a home visit by using a bilirubinometer (Brucker & MacMullen, 1987)
    (2) Home phototherapy provided by home health care services can prevent a readmission of neonate to the hospital and separation of neonate from parents

Clinical Practice

A. Assessment

1. History
  a. Maternal
    (1) Mother's blood type can have an impact on neonate's bilirubin levels by causing intravascular hemolysis via an antigen-antibody reaction

          (a) Rh disease

          (b) ABO incompatibility

          (c) Positive Coombs's test

      (2) Insulin-dependent diabetic mother

          (a) Neonate has an increased RBC mass at birth

          (b) Breakdown of a high number of aged RBCs results in excessive amounts of bilirubin in the neonate

      (3) Maternal and paternal ethnicity

          (a) Japanese, Chinese, Korean, Greek, and Native American neonates have a higher incidence of hyperbilirubinemia

          (b) Mean serum levels of unconjugated bilirubin in Japanese, Chinese, Korean, Greek, and Native American neonates are higher than the mean levels for neonates of other ethnic origins (Jones, 1990)

             (i) Mean serum levels of unconjugated bilirubin for the former are 10 to 14 mg/dl

             (ii) This mean is approximately double that of neonates of other ethnic origins

          (c) Afro-American neonates tend to have lower mean levels of bilirubin when compared with control populations (Jones, 1990)

      (4) Maternal drugs used during the last 3 months of pregnancy

          (a) The following drugs interfere with the binding of bilirubin to albumin in neonates

             (i) Sulfonamides

             (ii) Salicylates

          (b) Oxytocin (pitocin) is associated with a higher incidence of neonatal jaundice (Korones, 1986, p. 323)

      (5) A previous infant with diagnosed breast milk jaundice: there is a 70% possibility of recurrence in subsequent siblings of an infant diagnosed with breast milk jaundice (Korones, 1986, p. 326)

          (a) Breast milk jaundice occurs in 1 to 5% of breastfed term neonates

          (b) Affected breast milk contains substances that inhibit the activity of glucuronyl transferase in the neonatal liver

          (c) Bilirubin levels continue to rise on the fourth and fifth days, when physiologic jaundice should be subsiding

             (i) Rise to peak concentrations of between 10 and 27 mg/dl between 10 to 15 days of age

             (ii) Gradually decrease from peak levels to normal levels between 3 and 12 weeks of age (Korones, 1986, p. 326)

  b. Labor and delivery history

      (1) Drug use of the following

          (a) Oxytocin

          (b) Diazepam

          (c) Bupivacaine (in epidural anesthesia)

      (2) Delayed umbilical cord clamping

          (a) Allows an excessive amount of blood to be transfused from the placenta to the neonate

          (b) Increase in quantity of RBCs results in the following

             (i) Sequestration of greater numbers of aged RBCs

             (ii) Excessive amounts of bilirubin from breakdown of aged RBCs (Korones, 1986, p. 321)

      (3) Operative delivery: ecchymosis and extravascular hemolysis may be increased by use of forceps or vacuum extractor

  c. Perinatal complications

      (1) Cephalhematoma

      (2) Cerebral hemorrhage

      (3) Pulmonary hemorrhage

      (4) Any occult bleeding

(5) Maternal and fetal transfusion

(6) Hypoxia: causes increase in free fatty acids, which compete with bilirubin for albumin binding sites

(7) Infection (bacterial, viral, or protozoal)

    (a) Hemolysis

    (b) Hemolytic anemia

(8) Low Apgar scores at 1 minute and at 5 minutes may indicate a potential complication

d. Postnatal complications

    (1) Caloric deprivation, causing weight loss, results from

        (a) Infrequent feedings

        (b) Poor suck-and-swallow reflex

        (c) Decrease in gastric motility and enzymatic activity

    (2) Glucose-6-phosphate dehydrogenase (G-6-PD) deficiency

        (a) Is enzymatic deficiency

        (b) Disrupts erythrocyte metabolism and causes hemolysis

        (c) Occurs primarily among Afro-Americans, Filipinos, Sephardic Jews, Sardinians, Greeks, and Arabs (Korones, 1986, p. 298)

        (d) Manifests as jaundice on the second or third day of life and jaundice persists into the second or third week of life (Gartner, 1987, p. 945)

2. Physical findings

a. Visible jaundice progresses in a cephalocaudal direction and can be seen first in facial skin, sclera, and gums, and later, in the torso and lower extremities

b. Bilirubin levels

    (1) Elevated umbilical cord blood bilirubin level

    (2) Pattern of jaundice onset, length, and duration

c. Small-for-gestational-age condition that is associated with infection

d. Small head circumference (microcephaly) that is associated with infection

e. Cephalhematoma, ecchymosis, and abrasions are indicative of a traumatic delivery process

f. Pallor that is suggestive of hemolytic anemia

g. Petechiae that is suggestive of the following

    (1) Congenital infection

    (2) Overwhelming sepsis

    (3) Severe hemolytic disease

h. Plethora that is associated with polycythemia

i. Vomiting that is suggestive of the following

    (1) Sepsis

    (2) Pyloric stenosis

j. Hepatosplenomegaly that is suggestive of the following

    (1) Chronic intrauterine infection

    (2) Hemolytic anemia

k. Congenital anomalies: increased incidence of jaundice is associated with infants with trisomies (Korones, 1986, p. 324)

3. Diagnostic procedures

a. Maternal blood group and indirect Coombs's test to rule out possibilty of ABO or Rh incompatibility

b. Serological assays to rule out congenital syphilis

c. Hemoglobin to rule out the following

    (1) Anemia

    (2) Polycythemia: hemoglobin concentration higher than 22 g/dl (Korones, 1986, p. 324)

d. Complete blood count (CBC) with differential

    (1) Elevated reticulocyte count suggests hemolytic disease

    (2) RBC morphology

        (a) Spherocytes suggest ABO incompatibility

(b) RBC fragmentation suggests disseminated intravascular coagulopathy (DIC)

(3) WBC count

(a) Less than 5000/mm^3 suggests infection (Korones, 1986, p. 324)

(b) Increase in bands to more than 2000/mm^3 suggests infection

(4) Platelets: thrombocytopenia suggests infection

(5) Sedimentation rate values in excess of 5 mm^3 during first 48 hours is suggestive of infection or ABO incompatibility

(6) Elevated direct bilirubin (conjugated) level suggests infection or severe Rh incompatibility (Korones, 1986, p. 324)

B. Nursing Diagnoses

1. High risk for impairment of neonatal skin integrity related to diarrhea, urinary excretions of bilirubin, and exposure to phototherapy lights
2. High risk for injury of the neonatal cornea related to phototherapy light exposure and continuous wearing of protective eye shields
3. High risk for neonatal fluid volume deficit related to phototherapy light exposure
4. Ineffective neonatal thermoregulation related to phototherapy light exposure
5. High risk for alteration in parenting related to parent-infant separation secondary to phototherapy treatments

C. Interventions/Evaluations

1. High risk for impairment of neonatal skin integrity related to diarrhea, urinary excretions of bilirubin, and exposure to phototherapy lights
   a. Interventions
      (1) Diapering of neonate may be accomplished by using a paper face mask with the metal strip removed
         (a) Allows maximal skin exposure for phototherapy lights
            (i) Provides protection for genitals and bedding
            (ii) Shields a minimum of jaundiced skin
         (b) Typical for stools to be loose, greenish, frequent, and expelled with force
      (2) Important to protect neonate's skin from excoriation by thoroughly removing urine and feces with each diaper change
      (3) Important to change diapers frequently
      (4) Important to keep neonate's skin clean and dry by frequently checking bedding for dampness or stool soiling
   b. Evaluations
      (1) Neonate's skin remains clean and dry while under phototherapy lights
      (2) There are no signs of redness or excoriation on neonate's skin
2. High risk for injury of the neonatal cornea related to phototherapy light exposure and continuous wearing of protective eye shields
   a. Interventions
      (1) Protect neonate's eyes from phototherapy lights by eye shields to prevent eye damage
      (2) Secure placement of the eye shield headband tightly enough to prevent slippage and accidental eye exposure but not so tightly that constraint and excessive pressure are placed on the neonate's eyes
      (3) Remove eye shields when neonate is not under phototherapy lights
         (a) For feedings
         (b) For procedures not performed under phototherapy lights
      (4) Make sure the neonate's eyes are closed when applying the eye shields
      (5) Change eye shields frequently and watch for signs of conjunctivitis, such as the following
         (a) Purulent discharge
         (b) Edema

   b. Evaluations
     (1) Neonate wears protective eye shields at all times while under phototherapy lights
     (2) There are no signs of excessive eye shield pressure on neonate's skin around the eyes
     (3) There are no signs of conjunctivitis in neonate
3. High risk for neonatal fluid volume deficit related to phototherapy light exposure
   a. Interventions
     (1) Increase fluid intake to offset the following
       (a) Increase in metabolic rate caused by phototherapy
       (b) Significant increase in water loss through the skin
       (c) Increase in water content and frequency of stools
       (d) Water loss caused by hyperthermia
     (2) Offer neonate frequent feedings
       (a) Feed as often as tolerates (approximately every 2 hours)
       (b) Increase calories to offset rapid intestinal transit time (frequent stooling) and decreased intestinal absorption of milk
   b. Evaluations
     (1) Fluid intake is increased
     (2) Neonate remains well hydrated while under phototherapy lights
4. Ineffective neonatal thermoregulation related to phototherapy light exposure
   a. Interventions
     (1) Maintain a thermal homeostasis while neonate is under phototherapy lights by using a servo control mechanism, such as the following
       (a) Isolette
       (b) Radiant warmer
     (2) Offer neonate fluids frequently and maintain dry bedding
       (a) Hypothermia stimulates the release of free fatty acids, which compete for albumin binding sites
       (b) Hyperthermia increases the neonate's metabolic rate
   b. Evaluations
     (1) Neonate maintains a normal temperature while under phototherapy lights
     (2) Neonate's bedding is clean and dry
     (3) Neonate is covered and kept warm when not under phototherapy lights (i.e., for feedings and other procedures)
5. High risk for alteration in parenting related to separation of mother and father from neonate secondary to phototherapy treatments
   a. Interventions
     (1) Encourage parents to participate in the caretaking responsibilities of their neonate
     (2) Encourage parents to hold their neonate for short periods
     (3) Encourage parents to provide gentle stroking and touching of the neonate while she or he is under phototherapy lights
   b. Evaluations
     (1) Parents actively participate in caretaking activities with their neonate
     (2) Parents provide soothing tactile stimulation to their neonate while he or she is under phototherapy lights

Health Education

A. Provide nontechnical information to parents about serum bilirubin levels while the neonate is being monitored, and encourage their questions and concerns about their neonate's condition

B. Support mother's or father's attempts to feed the neonate and encourage frequent feedings to provide neonate with adequate hydration and increased calories

C. Mother may be discharged from the hospital and have to leave her neonate at the hospital for phototherapy treatments

1. Parents require a great deal of support during the temporary separation from their neonate
2. Parents need to be provided with accurate and appropriate information about their neonate's condition
3. Parents need to be reinforced by praising their caretaking activities when they come to visit their neonate

D. Parents should be instructed about signs, symptoms, and treatment of hyperbilirubinemia that may occur at home as a result of early discharge programs

1. Monitoring of neonate's behaviors indicative of increasing bilirubin levels
2. Blanching of neonate's skin to determine degree of jaundice
3. Placing of neonate's bassinet or cradle near a window during the daytime to take advantage of sunlight
4. Maintaining of sufficient hydration level in neonate
5. Advising of when to bring the neonate to the health care provider for evaluation of increasing bilirubin levels

---

CASE STUDIES AND STUDY QUESTIONS

Baby M. was delivered after a 16-hour induced labor. Maternal membranes were artificially ruptured, fluid was clear, and an oxytocin infusion was initiated. The mother was afebrile throughout the labor. The second stage of labor was 2 hours, 45 minutes. Review of the mother's prenatal and labor history yielded the following information: blood type, A+; VDRL, nonreactive; alpha-fetoprotein (AFP) levels, normal; average blood pressure, 116–124/76–82; total weight gain, 12.25 kg (27 lb); medications, prenatal vitamins, iron, and aspirin for stress headaches; gestational age = 40 4/7 weeks; non-stress test, reactive. Baby M. had the umbilical cord wound twice around her neck, required stimulation to initiate breathing and administration of oxygen by face mask. Apgar scores were 7 at 1 minute and 8 at 5 minutes.

1. From the above information, which of the following factors place Baby M. at increased risk for hyperbilirubinemia?

   a. Ruptured maternal membranes for 16 hours.

   b. Postmaturity.

   c. Mother's blood type is A+.

   d. Induced labor using oxytocin.

2. All of the following factors indicate that Baby M. is at greater risk for hyperbilirubinemia except

   a. The 1-minute Apgar score.

   b. Gestational age of 40 4/7 weeks.

   c. The aspirin mother took for her headaches.

   d. Respirations had to be stimulated and oxygen administered.

On her second day of life, Baby M. required phototherapy treatment. Her mother was being discharged from the hospital and came to the nursery to breastfeed her baby before leaving. Baby M.'s mother was crying and did not want to go home without her baby; Baby M.'s father was trying to comfort her.

3. While Baby M. is under phototherapy lights, it is important to do which of the following?

   a. Keep the baby under the lights continuously so that there will be maximal effectiveness in the shortest period.

   b. Limit any unnecessary touch stimulation because Baby M.'s metabolism is already high and touch could further increase it.

c. Discontinue Baby M.'s breastfeeding because the fluid content of breast milk is deficient for a neonate undergoing phototherapy.

d. Prevent hypothermia, hyperthermia, or both in Baby M.

4. Baby M.'s mother is crying, expresses fear about her infant's health, and does not want to leave. Which intervention would be the *least* effective?

a. Encourage the mother to come in to feed her baby as often as possible.

b. Emphasize the temporary nature of hyperbilirubinemia and explain the monitoring of Baby M.'s bilirubin levels.

c. Remind the mother that newborns require demanding care, which is very fatiguing to a new mother, and that she should take this added opportunity to rest and recover.

Answers to Study Questions

1. d	2. b	3. d
4. c		

REFERENCES

Bobak, I., Jensen, M., & Zalar, M. (Eds.). (1989). *Maternity and gynecologic care* (4th ed.) (pp. 526–530, 996–1003). St. Louis: Mosby.

Brooten, D. (1985). Breast milk jaundice. *Journal of Obstetric, Gynecologic, and Neonatal Nursing, 14*(3), 220–223.

Brucker, M., & MacMullen, N. (1987). Neonatal jaundice in the home: Assessment with a noninvasive device. *Journal of Obstetric, Gynecologic, and Neonatal Nursing, 16*(5), 355–358.

Carpenito, L. (1989). *Handbook of nursing diagnosis*. Philadelphia: Lippincott.

Gartner, L. (1987). Jaundice and liver disease. In *Neonatal–perinatal medicine diseases of the fetus and infant* (4th ed.) (pp. 946–947). St. Louis: Mosby.

Jones, M. (1990). A physiologic approach to identifying neonates at risk for kernicterus. *Journal of Obstetric, Gynecologic, and Neonatal Nursing, 19*(4), 313–318.

Korones, S. (1986). *High-risk newborn infants* (4th ed.) (pp. 317–334). St. Louis: Mosby.

Maisels, M. (1988). Jaundice in the healthy newborn infant: A new approach to an old problem. *Pediatrics, 81*(4), 505–510.

Maisels, M. (Ed.). (1987). Neonatal jaundice. In *Neonatology, pathophysiology, and management of the newborn* (3rd ed.). Philadelphia: Lippincott.

Maisels, M. (1982). Jaundice in the newborn. *Pediatrics in Review, 3*(10), 305–319.

Merinstein, G., & Gardner, S. (1989). *Handbook of neonatal intensive care* (2nd ed.). St. Louis: Mosby.

Olds, S., London, M., & Ladewig, P. (1988). *Maternal-newborn nursing* (3rd ed.) (pp. 1040–1044). Menlo Park, CA: Addison-Wesley.

Oski, F. (1991). Disorders of bilirubin metabolism. In S. Shaffer & G. Avery (Eds.), *Diseases of the newborn* (6th ed.) (pp. 749–757). Philadelphia: Saunders.

Wilkerson, N. (1988). A comprehensive look at hyperbilirubinemia. *MCN: American Journal of Maternal Child Nursing, 13*, 360–364.

Other

NAACOG (1986, July). Phototherapy and nursing care of the newborn with hyperbilirubinemia. *OGN Nursing Practice Resource*.

Phyllis Muchmore

Sepsis in the Newborn

Objectives

1. List the three primary sources of infection in the neonate

2. Describe the mechanisms that provide the major defenses against infection in the neonate

3. List the infections included in the TORCHS (toxoplasmosis, other [hepatitis B], rubella, cytomegalovirus, herpes simplex, and syphilis) syndrome and describe the primary signs and symptoms of each

4. Describe at least three diagnostic procedures helpful in differentiating the TORCHS syndrome from other possible conditions in the newborn

5. Describe signs and symptoms common to infants with a postnatally acquired infection

6. Recognize infants at risk for developing septicemia

7. List the diagnostic procedures that are the most helpful in determining the etiology of sepsis in the newborn

8. List and describe the medical treatment for newborn septicemia

9. List the most important nursing responsibilities in caring for the septic newborn

Introduction

A. **Pathophysiology: contact between a susceptible host and a potentially pathogenic organism**

1. Infection may be acquired in the following ways
   a. Transplacentally
   b. Via the ascending birth canal
   c. Postnatally in the nursery, from caregivers, or from the following
      (1) Equipment for resuscitation
      (2) Contamination at the time of umbilical cord clamping
      (3) Oxygen and suction lines
      (4) Incubators
      (5) Cleaning procedures for various equipment

(6) Disposable equipment
(7) Inadequate handwashing
(8) Invasive procedures
(9) Indwelling lines
(10) Open wounds
(11) Postoperative incision sites
2. Etiology of infection
   a. Bacterial agents
      (1) These cause three major clinical diseases (Korones, 1986)
         (a) Pneumonia
         (b) Septicemia
         (c) Meningitis
      (2) Gram-negative rods produce 75 to 85% of bacterial infections (Korones, 1986)
         (a) *Escherichia coli*
         (b) *Pseudomonas aeruginosa*
         (c) *Klebsiella pneumoniae*
         (d) *Serratia marcescens*
      (3) Gram-positive cocci produce the remaining 15 to 25% of major neonatal infections
         (a) Group B streptococci
         (b) Staphylococcci
   b. Viral agents are less frequent causes but can cause morbidity and mortality
      (1) Cytomegalovirus (CMV)
      (2) Rubella virus
      (3) Herpes simplex virus (HSV)
      (4) Hepatitis viruses
      (5) Enteroviruses (poliovirus, coxsackieviruses, and echoviruses)
      (6) Varicella-zoster (VZ) virus
   c. Protozoan agent (*Toxoplasma gondii*) causes toxoplasmosis

B. **Neonatal defense mechanisms against invasion by infectious agents are interdependent and multiple but immature and result in a limited ability to fight infection**

1. Nonspecific factors are active against any organism that is encountered
   a. Surface protection is provided by the skin and mucous membranes
   b. Systemic protection is also provided by the inflammatory response
2. Specific factors involve the production of antibodies (which counteract only a single organism)
   a. Antibody: a protein synthesized by specific types of cells in response to antigenic stimulation (Korones, 1976, p. 370)
   b. Antigen: any substance that stimulates the production of antibodies (Korones, 1976, p. 290)
   c. Immunoglobulin (Ig): one of three types of antibodies that circulate in plasma
      (1) IgG
         (a) Crosses the placenta to the fetus
         (b) Is antibody to the majority of bacterial and viral organisms previously encountered by the mother
         (c) Increases in levels with increasing gestational age
         (d) Is depleted by 3 months of age if maternally acquired (the preterm neonate's supply is limited and, therefore, depleted much sooner)
         (e) Does not contain antibodies against enteric gram-negative rods
      (2) IgM
         (a) Does not cross the placenta
         (b) A low level of production begins in fetus at 20 weeks' gestation

(c) Increases in the presence of intrauterine infections (may be helpful marker of intrauterine exposure to infection)

(d) In fetus, tends to be nonspecific because any infectious agent stimulates production in the fetus

(e) In adult, IgM contains antibodies specific to gram-negative organisms

(3) IgA

(a) Does not cross the placenta

(b) Is produced by the fetus in negligible amounts at birth

(c) Is unclear what role is; is found over surfaces of intestine, respiratory mucosa, and renal epithelial surfaces (secretory IgA)

(d) Is found in breast milk, thereby imparting immunity to mucosal surfaces of the neonate's intestine

C. **Incidence of infection is believed to be approximately 4 to 10/1000 live births, with a mortality rate of 13 to 45% (Bell, 1991)**

D. **Complications of infection**

1. Fetal abnormality or stillbirth
2. Because of the neonate's inability to localize infection, systemic septicemia, meningitis, or both, may occur after any type of invasion by an organism
   a. Adjacent tissues and organs are easily penetrated
   b. Blood-brain barrier is ineffective, which leads to meningitis in approximately 30% of septic newborns (Korones, 1986)
3. Long-term sequelae in survivors depend on type and source of infection
   a. Developmental abnormalities
   b. Neurological sequelae
   c. Motor and sensory abnormalities
   d. Physical and growth impairments

Clinical Practice

INTRAUTERINE-ACQUIRED INFECTION

The most common intrauterine infections comprise the TORCHS (toxoplasmosis, other [hepatitis B], rubella, cytomegalovirus, herpes simplex, and syphilis) syndrome. With the exception of herpes simplex, these infections are usually transmitted via the placenta to the fetus before birth; with the exception of toxoplasmosis, neonates with TORCHS are all potentially infectious to their caretakers (see Chapter 27 for a complete discussion of maternal infections).

A. **Assessment**

1. Toxoplasmosis (Bruhn & Jones, 1985)
   a. History of maternal infection
      (1) Influenza like illness
      (2) Posterior cervical adenitis
      (3) Chorioretinitis
      (4) Exposure to feline feces or ingestion of raw meat
   b. Physical findings in newborn
      (1) Prematurity
      (2) Intrauterine growth retardation (IUGR)
      (3) Hydrocephalus
      (4) Chorioretinitis
      (5) Seizures
      (6) Hepatosplenomegaly
      (7) Thrombocytopenia

        (8) Jaundice
        (9) Generalized lymphadenopathy
      (10) Rash
  c. Diagnosis
        (1) Organism is rarely isolated
        (2) Occasional cysts are found in placenta or tissues of fetus or newborn
        (3) Sabin-Feldman dye test titer is higher than 1 : 1000 at birth
        (4) Calcifications appear on skull x-ray film in some cases

2. Rubella (Bruhn & Jones, 1985)
  a. History of maternal infection
        (1) Mother may be relatively symptom free
        (2) Mother may have mild respiratory illness with or without rash
  b. Physical findings in newborn
        (1) IUGR
        (2) Sensorineural deafness
        (3) Cataracts
        (4) Jaundice
        (5) Purpura
        (6) Hepatosplenomegaly
        (7) Microcephaly
        (8) Chronic encephalitis
        (9) Chorioretinitis
      (10) Cardiac defects
  c. Diagnosis
        (1) Virus is isolated from throat, blood, urine, and cerebrospinal fluid (CSF)
        (2) A fourfold titer rise occurs in an indirect hemagglutination (IHA) test or a fluorescent antibody absorption (FTA-ABS) test

3. CMV (Bruhn & Jones, 1985)
  a. History of maternal infection: usually asymptomatic
  b. Physical findings in newborn
        (1) IUGR
        (2) Jaundice
        (3) Purpura
        (4) Hepatosplenomegaly
        (5) Microcephaly
        (6) Brain damage
        (7) Intracerebral calcification
        (8) Chorioretinitis
        (9) Progressive sensorineural hearing loss
  c. Diagnosis
        (1) Virus is isolated from urine, pharyngeal secretions, and peripheral leukocytes
        (2) Demonstration of characteristic nuclear inclusions in urine, certain tissues, or both, may be helpful
        (3) Calcification is seen on skull and bone x-ray films in some cases

4. Herpes simplex is most often acquired during delivery via the birth canal; can also be acquired as an ascending infection when rupture of membranes occurs more than 4 hours before delivery (Bruhn & Jones, 1985)
  a. History of maternal infection
        (1) May be asymptomatic
        (2) May demonstrate lesions
  b. Physical findings in newborn
        (1) May have localized skin lesions
        (2) May have generalized illness involving the liver, lungs, and central nervous system (CNS)
  c. Diagnosis

    (1) Virus is isolated from tissue of the neonatal respiratory and maternal genital tracts, blood, urine, and CSF

    (2) Virus is identified by fluorescent tests

    (3) Serological tests (complement fixation test [CF], enzyme-linked inmunosorbent assay [ELISA], and neutralization) are performed

5. Syphilis (Bruhn & Jones, 1985)

    a. History of maternal infection

        (1) Evidence of a multisystem illness

        (2) Evidence of a primary syphilitic chancre on the cervix or rectal mucosa

    b. Physical findings in newborn

        (1) May be asymptomatic

        (2) Hepatitis

        (3) Pneumonitis

        (4) Bone marrow failure

        (5) Myocarditis

        (6) Meningitis

        (7) Nephrotic syndrome

        (8) Rash on the palms and soles

    c. Diagnosis

        (1) Identification of the spirochetes from nonoral lesions by examination with a darkfield microscope

        (2) An increase or absence of decrease in values of laboratory tests such as venereal disease research laboratory and rapid plasma reagin (RPR)

        (3) Periostitis on long-bone x-ray examination

        (4) Positive VDRL result on CSF specimen

        (5) Calcifications on bone x-ray films

POSTNATALLY ACQUIRED INFECTION

The most common etiology of neonatal infection is bacteria acquired either at delivery, in the hospital nursery, or from the home environment.

A. Assessment

1. History: increased susceptibility to development of neonatal sepsis

    a. Infants with a history of

        (1) Rupture of fetal membranes longer than 24 hours

        (2) Birth after prolonged or difficult labor

        (3) Maternal history of infection

            (a) Fever

            (b) Amnionitis

            (c) Foul-smelling amniotic fluid

            (d) Urinary tract infection (UTI)

        (4) Fetal distress with or without meconium in the amniotic fluid

        (5) Signs of infection developing within 24 hours after birth

    b. Postnatal symptoms and contributory factors

        (1) Prematurity

        (2) Low birth weight (small for gestational age [SGA])

        (3) Asphyxia

        (4) Born out of asepsis (BOA)

        (5) Invasive procedures (e.g., central IV lines)

        (6) Ventilatory support and oxygen therapy

        (7) Presence of congenital malformation (e.g., omphalocele and meningomyelocele)

        (8) Surgical procedures

        (9) Breaks in skin integrity (from fetal monitoring)

      (10) Multiple gestation

   (11) Aspiration by the neonate
  c. Environmental factors
   (1) Overcrowded nursery
   (2) Poor handwashing
   (3) Poor aseptic technique
   (4) Poor isolation precautions
2. Physical findings of sepsis in newborn: most often subtle, nonspecific, or may be indicative of metabolic problems or intracranial hemorrhage
  a. Vital signs
   (1) Temperature instability (especially hypothermia)
   (2) Apnea or irregular respirations with or without signs of respiratory distress, which may initially improve with oxygen therapy (demonstrated in 20 to 30% of septic newborns) (Korones, 1986)
   (3) Tachypnea
   (4) Hypotension
   (5) Tachycardia
   (6) Bradycardia
   (7) Pale, dusky, and shocklike appearance (late sign)
  b. Feeding problems
   (1) Failure to digest feedings (determined by aspirating stomach contents before feeding)
   (2) Poor feeding
   (3) Vomiting and diarrhea (in approximately 30% of septic newborns [Korones, 1986])
   (4) Abdominal distension
  c. Metabolic problems
   (1) Hypoglycemia
   (2) Hyperglycemia: more common than hypoglycemia in infants weighing less than 1000 g (2 lbs, 3 ½ oz)
   (3) Glucosuria with no change in IV concentration or rate
   (4) Hyperbilirubinemia with hepatosplenomegaly
  d. Activity: described as any change from previous behavior
   (1) Lethargy or hypotonia
   (2) Irritability
   (3) Seizures with or without raised anterior fontanel and jitteriness (late signs)
  e. Bleeding problems: may reflect coagulation disturbances such as the following
   (1) Petechiae
   (2) Purpura
   (3) Blood in stool
   (4) Blood in stomach aspirate
  f. Local infections
   (1) Skin
    (a) Pustules
    (b) Draining lesions
    (c) Rash
   (2) Eyes
    (a) Infected conjunctivae
    (b) Purulent drainage
    (c) Erythema
    (d) Pustules
   (3) Umbilicus
    (a) Omphalitis
    (b) Erythema
    (c) Drainage
    (d) Odor

        (4) Joints
           (a) Decreased movement
           (b) Edema
           (c) Erythema

3. Diagnostic procedures
   a. Cultures: the most valid method of establishing a diagnosis of bacterial sepsis (Bruhn & Jones, 1985)
      (1) Blood
      (2) CSF: Gram's stain, glucose and protein content, and cell count
      (3) Gastric aspirate: obtain in delivery room, if possible, for Gram's stain and culture (may indicate only colonization)
      (4) Urine culture: results are most accurate when obtained by suprapubic aspiration
      (5) Surface cultures: ear and nasopharyngeal (may indicate only colonization)
      (6) Maternal cultures
      (7) Tracheal aspirate
      (8) Site culture for local infection
      (9) Rectal swab: performed if history of amnionitis or diarrhea known
   b. Hematology (Bell, 1991)
      (1) White blood cell (WBC) count, with an absolute neutrophil count (ANC) less than 1000 mm^3 and immature forms/total neutrophils more than 0.25
      (2) Platelet count of less than 100,000 mm^3
      (3) Erythrocyte sedimentation rate (ESR) of more than 15 mm/hr on first day of life
   c. Other procedures
      (1) Chest x-ray film
      (2) Blood gas assays may indicate metabolic acidosis (pH of less than 7.20 and base deficit of more than 10)
      (3) Analysis of umbilical cord section for inflammatory changes is performed if omphalitis is suspected
      (4) Metabolic laboratory studies for associated problems and differential diagnosis, such as glucose, electrolytes, and calcium, are performed
      (5) Antigen detection tests: are available for group B streptococci, *Neisseria meningitidis, Haemophilus influenzae,* and *Streptococcus pneumoniae*

B. **Nursing Diagnoses**

1. High risk for sepsis related to prenatal exposure to infectious organisms
2. High risk for infection related to environmental hazards, such as personnel, equipment, and other newborns
3. High risk for infection related to vulnerability of infant's immature immunological system (or inadequate secondary defenses)
4. High risk for developing respiratory distress secondary to septicemia
5. High risk for developing severe fluid and electrolyte imbalances secondary to systemic infection
6. High risk for altered body temperature related to the body's response to pathogens
7. High risk for altered glucose metabolism related to septicemia
8. High risk for developing anemia related to an increased turnover of red blood cells secondary to systemic infection
9. High risk for altered bilirubin excretion secondary to septicemia

C. **Interventions/Evaluations**

1. High risk for sepsis related to prenatal exposure to infectious organisms
   a. Interventions
      (1) Review the maternal, delivery, and neonatal history for high-risk factors (see section on history)

(2) Provide continuous monitoring for infants with a suggestive history
   (a) Evaluate for clinical signs (see section on physical findings)
   (b) Perform appropriate laboratory studies (see section on diagnostic procedures)
   (c) Provide cardiorespiratory monitoring if indicated
   (d) Provide transcutaneous monitoring (TCM) and oximetry if signs of respiratory involvement
   (e) Obtain serial chest x-ray film studies to detect early lung involvement (e.g., pneumonia)
   (f) Inspect all breaks in the skin (e.g., from fetal monitoring) frequently for signs of infection
      (i) Irritation
      (ii) Rash
      (iii) Redness
      (iv) Infiltration
(3) Report suspicious findings immediately to provide early treatment and decreased morbidity and mortality
   (a) Clinical manifestations of neonatal sepsis are so-called soft signs that may be related to other problems; the nurse or the parent may be the first person to notice these subtle changes
   (b) Infection may develop so quickly that any delay in treatment may be catastrophic (Amlie, 1990)
b. Evaluations
   (1) Neonate's cardiorespiratory status remains stable
   (2) Continuous monitoring immediately detects any subtle changes or soft signs in the neonate
2. High risk for infection related to environmental hazards, such as personnel, equipment, and other newborns
a. Interventions
   (1) Prevent exposure to infection in the delivery room
      (a) Protect neonate from contact with maternal feces
      (b) Use sterile technique when cutting umbilical cord
      (c) Instill local eye treatment to protect neonate from gonococcal infection
   (2) Minimize contact between infants to prevent spread of infective organisms
      (a) Follow the American Academy of Pediatrics recommendation of a minimum area of 20 sq ft per infant in the regular nursery and a minimum area of 40 sq ft per infant in an intermediate nursery (Amlie, 1990)
      (b) Observe appropriate isolation procedures per facility protocol for infants known to be infected or to have been exposed to communicable diseases (e.g., rubella)
      (c) Cohorting infants may be used during outbreaks of infection within the nursery; the object of cohorting is to limit the number of contacts of each infant with other infants and personnel (Amlie, 1990)
   (3) Proper handling of medical devices helps to prevent the infant's exposure to infective organisms
      (a) Adhere to sterilization procedures
      (b) Discard disposable equipment after use
      (c) Change IV solutions and all tubing every 24 to 48 hours (Amlie, 1990)
      (d) Change all respiratory and suctioning equipment frequently and ensure that there has been proper cleaning and sterilization before each use
   (4) Ensure that all invasive procedures are performed aseptically
   (5) Prevent infant exposure to infected personnel
      (a) Strictly enforce handwashing
      (b) Do not allow infected personnel into the nursery

        (c) Personnel should wear disposable gowns when handling infants
   b. Evaluations
      (1) The infant is protected from nosocomial infection in the delivery room
      (2) The infant is protected from contact with other infants
      (3) All medical equipment used is appropriately handled to prevent contamination of the infant
      (4) Aseptic technique is observed to prevent the introduction of infectious organisms
3. High risk for infection related to vulnerability of infant's immature immunological system (or inadequate secondary defenses)
   a. Interventions
      (1) Provide antibiotic therapy per orders to eliminate infectious organisms
         (a) After cultures have been obtained, double antibiotic therapy is initiated to treat both gram-positive and gram-negative organisms (The following example is one that may vary among facilities)
           (i) For gram-positive organisms: administer ampicillin or penicillin
           (ii) For gram-negative organisms: administer gentamicin or kanamycin
         (b) When the specific organism has been identified, the most specific antibiotic should be administered, for example (may vary among facilities)
           (i) Streptococci: ampicillin plus an aminoglycoside
           (ii) *Staphylococcus aureus:* methicillin
           (iii) *Pseudomonas* organisms: carbenicillin
           (iv) Systemic fungal infections: amphotericin B or fluorocytosine (5-FC)
         (c) If the cultures are negative and the infant is healthy, antibiotics may be discontinued after 3 days
         (d) Treatment time for positive cultures follows (Bruhn & Jones, 1985)
           (i) Blood: 14 to 21 days
           (ii) CSF: 14 days for gram-positive organisms; 14 to 21 days for gram-negative organisms
           (iii) Urinary tract infection: 10 days
           (iv) Endocarditis: 6 weeks
      (2) Prevent or treat side effects of antibiotic therapy
         (a) Avoid indiscriminate or inappropriate use of systemic antibiotics, which may
           (i) Cause undesirable side effects
           (ii) Favor the emergence of resistant strains of organisms
           (iii) Alter the normal flora of the newborn
         (b) Apply the following rule of thumb: the most appropriate and least toxic antibiotic or antibiotic combination should be continued for an appropriate period by a suitable route (Bruhn & Jones, 1985)
         (c) Monitor side effects of antibiotic therapy with the following
           (i) Serum drug levels
           (ii) Blood urea nitrogen (BUN) and creatinine levels to indicate renal toxicity
           (iii) Frequent electrolyte panels to assist in monitoring electrolyte disturbances that may be caused by certain antibiotics
           (iv) Long-term follow-up, such as eye and hearing evaluations, to alert the health care team to possible problems (e.g., aminoglycosides may be ototoxic in some infants)
         (d) Observe for clinical signs and symptoms of adverse antibiotic interactions
           (i) Skin flushing
           (ii) Hypotension
           (iii) Decreased urine output

(iv) Tachycardia

(3) Use appropriate skin care to protect the infant's primary barrier against organisms (Amlie, 1991)

(a) Delay cleansing of skin until infant has been adequately warmed after delivery

(b) Use cotton sponges (not gauze) soaked with sterile water to remove blood from the face and head, and meconium from the perianal area

(i) A nonmedicated soap may be used, if needed

(ii) Multi-use bar and liquid soaps should not be used because they may be contaminated with bacteria

(c) Avoid cleansing the remainder of the skin unless grossly soiled

(d) Cleanse buttocks and perianal areas with water with or without a mild soap with each diaper change

(e) Be aware of umbilical cord care alternatives

(i) Alcohol

(ii) Triple dye

(iii) Antimicrobial agents

(f) To further protect the newborn's skin, avoid the use of lotions and adhesive tapes (Poulsen, 1990)

(4) Provide therapy to assist the newborn's immature immunological system in fighting infection

(a) Transfusions of adult blood or fresh frozen plasma may provide complement and other immune factors

(b) Exchange transfusion may be performed in cases of overwhelming sepsis to give complement and immune factors as well as to reduce the load of bacterial endotoxin

(c) Granulocyte transfusions in ill infants with neutropenia have been successful, although there remain potential complications such as graft-versus-host reactions and transmission of other infections (e.g., CMV infection)

(d) The majority of Ig transfusion preparations on the market today contain 95 to 98% IgG, which raises the level of circulating antibody and improves the function of the immune system; most infants tolerate these transfusions well, and studies indicate that a single transfusion produces adequate IgG levels for 3 to 4 weeks (Bell, 1991)

(5) Provide for minimal handling, with sedation if needed, to facilitate the infant's immunological system in fighting the infection

(a) Group care activities together to allow for adequate periods of sleep and rest

(b) Assist parents in recognizing their infant's needs for rest and quiet

b. Evaluations

(1) The infant has appropriate cultures performed and begins to receive antibiotic therapy specific to the particular infection

(2) The infant is monitored for possible side effects of the antibiotic therapy, as indicated by the following

(a) Appropriate serum drug level

(b) BUN and serum creatinine levels within normal limits

(c) Electrolyte values within normal limits

(d) Absence of clinical evidence of adverse drug reactions

(3) The infant receives the appropriate skin care to prevent contact with infectious organisms

(4) The infant receives supplementary treatment to assist the immune system, as needed

(5) The infant is handled only as necessary to provide infant with maximal periods of rest

4. High risk for developing respiratory distress secondary to septicemia

a. Interventions

          (1) Provide appropriate respiratory care, as needed
             (a) Intubate if severe apnea is present or as indicated by arterial blood gas (ABG) levels
             (b) Provide oxygen, as needed
             (c) Monitor respiratory distress with blood gas assays, transcutaneous monitoring, and oximetry
          (2) Prevent and correct metabolic acidosis, as needed
       b. Evaluations
          (1) The infant receives the appropriate respiratory care
          (2) Metabolic acidosis is prevented or treated
   5. High risk for developing severe fluid and electrolyte imbalances secondary to systemic infection
       a. Interventions
          (1) Maintain adequate fluid and electrolyte balance
             (a) Monitor serum electrolyte values and correct imbalances, as needed
             (b) Assess intake and output (I&O) accurately
             (c) Assess appropriateness of enteral feedings and supplement with IV therapy, as needed
          (2) Maintain cardiovascular integrity
             (a) Monitor vital signs frequently, including blood pressure
             (b) Provide volume expanders (5% albumin) and blood transfusions, as indicated
             (c) Monitor urine output carefully
       b. Evaluations
          (1) Fluid and electrolyte balance is monitored and maintained
          (2) Cardiovascular integrity is assessed and maintained
   6. High risk for altered body temperature related to the body's response to pathogens
       a. Interventions
          (1) Maintain the infant in a neutral thermal environment (NTE)
          (2) Monitor both infant temperature and environmental temperature
       b. Evaluation: the infant's temperature remains within normal limits
   7. High risk for altered glucose metabolism related to septicemia
       a. Interventions
          (1) Monitor serum glucose level every 4 hours or as needed (may use bedside monitoring such as Chemstix)
          (2) Ensure adequate glucose intake
       b. Evaluation: the infant's blood glucose level is within normal limits (more than 40 mg/dl)
   8. High risk for developing anemia related to an increased turnover of RBCs secondary to systemic infection
       a. Interventions
          (1) Monitor hemoglobin and hematocrit values daily
          (2) Transfuse blood, as needed
       b. Evaluation: the infant's hemoglobin and hematocrit values are within normal limits
   9. High risk for altered bilirubin excretion secondary to septicemia
       a. Interventions
          (1) Monitor serum bilirubin levels daily
          (2) Treatment may include phototherapy, increased fluid intake, or both
       b. Evaluation: the infant's bilirubin level is maintained within normal limits or decreases in response to treatment

Health Education

The diagnosis of neonatal sepsis may be a major crisis for the parents of either an otherwise well or a previously ill newborn. The family of the septic infant may need support in accepting a possibly impaired infant, support in weathering this crisis, or both.

A. The family is an important link in preventing infection

1. Instruct in strict handwashing and proper gowning technique
2. The family must stay at their infant's bedside, thus preventing the possible spread of infection to other infants
3. With proper precautions, there is no evidence to support the necessity for restriction of sibling visitation (Bruhn & Jones, 1985)
   a. Screening for possible illness in siblings
      (1) Respiratory symptoms (cough, runny nose, and sore throat)
      (2) Gastrointestinal symptoms (nausea, vomiting, and diarrhea)
      (3) Presence of skin lesions
   b. Recent sibling exposure to childhood illnesses
      (1) Rubella
      (2) Mumps
      (3) Chickenpox (varicella-zoster virus)

B. Isolation of the infant from the family should be minimized

1. Isolation may be necessary because of the infant's condition
2. Isolation often is related to overly strict nursery policy or protocol
3. Isolation may produce feelings by the family of helplessness as well as of guilt and fear

C. The following information about the infant's condition should be given to the family to allay fears and reduce anxiety and guilt

1. The infant's general condition and course of treatment
   a. Probable source of infection
   b. Treatment recommended
   c. Short-term effects of the illness and treatment, as well as any long-term sequelae, need to be explained
2. IV therapy can be frightening to the family
   a. Scalp IV lines may be of particular concern
      (1) The hair must be shaved (saving the baby's hair to offer to the parents for the baby book may be helpful)
      (2) It is a common misperception that the needle is piercing the baby's brain
   b. The septic infant may not tolerate oral feedings and may need an IV line for fluid management as well as medication
      (1) The infant's inability to use a nipple creates anxiety in the family
      (2) The family needs to be taught how to touch and hold the infant without disturbing the IV line
      (3) The family needs to be taught the importance of saving all diapers and emesis for the nurse to see, weigh, and test
3. If the infant is ill enough to require continuous monitoring, the equipment's function should be explained to the family
   a. Monitoring equipment may preclude the family's holding the infant
   b. Monitor alarms can be frightening; their meaning and the availability of staff to assist the infant should be explained

D. The infant's daily care should be explained and demonstrated to the family, with return demonstrations by the family when possible, of the following

1. Infant bathing
2. Umbilical cord care
3. Temperature maintenance and reading of a thermometer
4. Feeding
5. Infant resuscitation and actions to take in an emergency
6. Signs and symptoms of illness in the newborn

CASE STUDIES AND STUDY QUESTIONS

Marcia Gates, a 24-year-old gravida 2, para 2 (G2,P2), was delivered of a 3000-g (6 lb, 10 oz) boy at 38 weeks' gestation after a 36-hour period of spontaneously ruptured membranes. Marcia was afebrile at the time of delivery. The delivery was uncomplicated and the infant's Apgar scores were 6 at 1 minute and 9 at 5 minutes. The infant went to the term nursery. At 2 hours of age, he developed respiratory distress with a respiratory rate of 70 and grunting in room air.

1. Sources of neonatal infection include which of the following?

   a. Transplacental transfer.

   b. The birth canal.

   c. Caregivers and nursery equipment.

   d. a, b, c.

   e. a and b.

2. The most likely diagnosis of Baby Gates is which of the following?

   a. Congenital anomalies.

   b. Sepsis.

   c. Apnea.

   d. Fetal alcohol syndrome.

3. The most significant factor(s) predisposing Baby Gates to septicemia is (are) which of the following?

   a. Prematurity.

   b. Prolonged rupture of fetal membranes.

   c. Exposure to potential organisms in the environment.

   d. Immature immunological system.

   e. a, b, c, d.

   f. All except c.

4. Which of the following immunoglobulins crosses the placenta during intrauterine life, thus affording the newborn limited protection?

   a. IgG.

   b. IgA.

   c. IgM.

   d. None of the above.

5. Signs and symptoms of infection that Baby Gates may demonstrate include all except which of the following?

   a. Temperature instability.

   b. Tachycardia.

   c. Respiratory distress.

   d. Feeding well.

   e. Apnea.

6. Aids to a diagnosis of sepsis may include which of the following?

   a. Blood cultures.

   b. Complete blood count.

   c. Chest x-ray film.

   d. Blood gas assays.

   e. All of the above.

7. Treatment of Baby Gates's sepsis may include which of the following?

   a. Antibiotics.

   b. Transfusions of Igs, blood, and granulocytes.

   c. Transfer to a level III (tertiary) facility.

   d. All of the above.

8. Nursing responsibilities in caring for the septic infant include which of the following?

   a. Maintenance of appropriate isolation.

   b. Continuous monitoring of infant.

   c. Establishment and maintenance of IV patency, as needed.

   d. Ordering laboratory work, as indicated.

   e. a, b, c.

   f. a, b, c, d.

9. Long-term effects of congenital infections include which of the following?

   a. Developmental disabilities.

   b. Motor and sensory abnormalities.

   c. Growth retardation.

   d. a, b, c.

10. The septic infant may demonstrate which

of the following sequelae to the illness, treatment, or both?

a. Hypoglycemia.

b. Polycythemia.

c. Metabolic alkalosis.

d. Protein deficiency.

Answers to Study Questions

1. e	2. b	3. b
4. a	5. d	6. e
7. d	8. e	9. d
10. a		

REFERENCES

Amlie, R.N. (1991). Neonatal infection. In *Critical care of the neonate: Nursing care of the newborn in intensive care* (pp. 365–374). Irvine: University of California.

Bell, S.G. (1991). Intravenous immunoglobulin therapy in neonatal sepsis. *Neonatal Network, 9*(6), 9–14.

Bruhn, F.W., & Jones, B. (1985). Infection in the neonate. In G.B. Merenstein & S.L. Gardner (Eds.), *Handbook of neonatal intensive care* (pp. 279–297). St. Louis: Mosby.

Carey, B.E. (1989). Major complications of central lines in neonates. *Neonatal Network, 7*(6), 17–28.

Johnstone, H.A., & Marcinak, J.F. (1990). Candidiasis in neonatal sepsis. *Neonatal Network, 9*(6), 9–14.

Korones, S.B. (1986). *High-risk newborn infants* (4th ed.) (pp. 214–235). St. Louis: Mosby.

Poulsen, N. (1990). Candidiasis in the premature infant. *Neonatal Network, 8*(4), 9–14.

Ramirez, A. (1989). The neonate's unique response to drugs: Unraveling the cause of drug iatrogenesis. *Neonatal Network, 7*(5), 45–49.

Rosenberg, A.L. (1991). The return of congenital syphilis. *Neonatal Network, 9*(5), 17–22.

Thigpen, J.L. (1991). Responding to research: Realistic use of scrub clothes and cover gowns. *Neonatal Network 9*(5), 41–44.

Wenneberg, R.P., & Goetzman, B.W. (1985). *Neonatal intensive care manual* (pp. 56–92). Chicago: Year Book.

Woleske, M. (1989). Antenatal HIV screening. *Neonatal Network, 8*(2), 7–13.

Judy E. Smith

The Drug-Dependent Neonate

Objectives

1. Discuss the incidence of illegal drug use among women of childbearing age

2. Discuss placental transfer of illegal drugs from maternal circulation to fetal circulation

3. Describe the highlights of fetal metabolism of illegal drugs

4. Describe the signs and symptoms of the neonatal abstinence syndrome

5. Identify and describe the effects of prenatal marijuana exposure on the neonate

6. Identify and discuss the effects of prenatal cocaine exposure on the neonate

7. Identify and discuss the effects of prenatal heroin exposure on the neonate

8. Identify and describe the effects of prenatal methadone exposure on the neonate

9. Identify the effects of prenatal exposure to nonopiate drugs and phencyclidine piperidine (PCP) on the neonate

10. Select and explain specific nursing interventions that are effective with neonates who have been prenatally exposed to illegal drugs

11. Develop effective teaching strategies for parents or caregivers for an infant prenatally exposed to illegal drugs

Introduction

A. **Exposure to an illegal drug during gestation has been reported to occur in as many as 11% of all newborns**

1. The use of illegal drugs includes all racial and socioeconomic groups
2. Most illegal drugs have been shown to freely cross the placenta to the fetus
   a. Drugs that affect the nervous system are typically lipophilic and have low molecular weights that facilitate placental crossing
   b. Distribution of a drug between maternal and fetal circulations frequently occurs
      (1) There is rapid equilibration of the drug between the circulations of the mother and fetus

(2) Exact distribution has not been determined, but significant levels are found in fetuses of mothers who use drugs (Chasnoff, 1991)

B. Fetal metabolism of illegal drugs is compromised

1. The fetal liver, even at term, is immature and not fully functional
2. The fetal liver can metabolize some drugs
   a. The resulting metabolites are frequently water soluble
   b. Water solubility hinders the passage of the metabolite back across the placenta and into the maternal circulation, where it can be excreted
3. The majority of drugs have a longer half-life in the fetus than in the adult

C. Illegal drug exposure can create the following problems in fetal and neonatal development

1. Congenital abnormalities
2. Fetal growth retardation
3. Neonatal growth retardation
4. Neurobehavioral developmental problems

D. Drug withdrawal

1. The fetus can experience in utero withdrawal when the drug-dependent pregnant woman abstains from drug use
2. Neonatal abstinence syndrome can occur after birth, which forces the withdrawal of specific drugs from the neonate
   a. Signs and symptoms in the neonate mimic those seen in adults experiencing withdrawal
   b. The most significant signs and symptoms of withdrawal in the neonate are the following
      (1) High-pitched or shrill cry
      (2) Gastrointestinal disturbances
         (a) Vomiting
         (b) Diarrhea
         (c) Excessive sucking
      (3) Tremulousness
      (4) Excoriation of knees and elbows related to increased restlessness and sleeplessness
      (5) Respiratory disturbances
         (a) Tachypnea
         (b) Nasal congestion
         (c) Frequent yawning
         (d) Sneezing
      (6) Seizure activity (Chasnoff, 1986, p. 53)
   c. Many of the signs of drug withdrawal in the neonate are similar to those of other neonatal problems, such as sepsis, hypoglycemia, and central nervous system disorders; therefore, testing to rule out these conditions should be considered in addition to drug screening

E. Marijuana

1. Marijuana is the most commonly used illegal drug among childbearing age women in the United States
   a. Use is similar among women of various racial and ethnic groups in the United States
   b. Prevalence of use is regional
      (1) Women in the western part of the United States report a higher use than do women in other regions
      (2) Women in the southern part of the United States report the lowest use (Day & Richardson, 1991)

c. The constituents, including the psychoactive component, can cross the placenta and be stored in the amniotic fluid (Fried, 1986)
d. May be present in breast milk of mothers who use the drug
2. Neonatal effects of prenatal marijuana exposure include the following
   a. Intrauterine growth
      (1) Whether or not prenatal marijuana exposure has an effect on neonatal size at birth is controversial
      (2) There is a possible link to a slightly decreased neonatal length at birth (Day & Richardson, 1991)
   b. Length of gestation
      (1) Incidence of preterm labor and birth may be increased
      (2) Studies conflict: some have found an increase in premature birth and others have found no effects
   c. There has been no significant increase in the incidence of minor or major physical anomalies reported in neonates known to be prenatally exposed to marijuana
   d. Neurobehavioral effects of prenatal marijuana exposure
      (1) All findings are debatable
      (2) Possible altered visual responsiveness
      (3) Possible increased incidence of tremors and startle responses
      (4) Possible decreased total quiet sleep time (Day & Richardson, 1991)

F. Cocaine

1. Women of childbearing age constitute 15 to 17% of the regular users of cocaine (Peters & Theorell, 1991)
2. Cocaine is most often used in combination with marijuana but is also used in combination with other illegal drugs
3. Cocaine readily crosses the placenta to the fetus because it is lipophilic and has a low molecular weight
4. Cocaine is present in the breast milk of mothers who use the drug
5. Neonatal effects of prenatal cocaine exposure include the following
   a. It is currently thought that many of the effects are due to an interruption of blood flow to developing or previously developed fetal structures, such as the following conditions
      (1) Intrauterine growth retardation caused by decreased uterine blood flow
         (a) Low birth weight
         (b) Smaller-than-normal head circumference
         (c) Decreased body length
      (2) Prematurity caused by uterine hypertension and hyperirritability
      (3) Intracranial hemorrhage caused by in utero fetal hypertension
      (4) Nonduodenal intestinal atresia caused by superior mesenteric artery insufficiency
      (5) Limb reduction defects caused by brachial artery insufficiency (Jones, 1991)
   b. Urinary tract anomalies
      (1) Urethral obstruction malformation (prune-belly syndrome)
      (2) Hydronephrosis
      (3) Hypospadias
   c. Problems in neurodevelopmental behaviors can last 4 to 6 months or longer in neonate
      (1) Depressed interactive behaviors, such as gaze aversion
      (2) Poor organizational response to environmental stimuli
         (a) Poor consolability
         (b) Difficulty in shutting out intrusive stimuli
         (c) Increased irritability
         (d) Tremulousness
         (e) Frequent startle responses

    (3) Increased muscle tone
      (a) Muscular rigidity
      (b) Difficulty in bringing the arms to midline
    (4) Poor feeding tolerance
    (5) Irregular sleeping patterns
    (6) Abnormal breathing patterns
      (a) Cocaine-exposed neonates have a 15% (a 5 to 10 times increased risk) incidence of sudden infant death syndrome (SIDS)
      (b) Abnormal breathing occurs, particularly during sleep

G. Heroin

1. Heroin continues to be a highly used illegal drug
2. Heroin is not generally thought to be a teratogen capable of producing congenital malformation
   a. Easily crosses the placenta via simple diffusion from an area of high maternal concentration to an area of low fetal concentration (Flandermeyer, 1987)
   b. The hazards of heroin to the fetus are thought to be the direct effects of the drug on the fetus and the maternal lifestyle associated with heroin use
    (1) The mother typically does not seek early prenatal care related to fear of detection of heroin use and to an absence or irregularity of menses caused by heroin that makes amenorrhea a norm in her life
    (2) There is an increased maternal and fetal exposure to serious infection, such as the following
      (a) Sexually transmitted diseases
      (b) Hepatitis
      (c) Acquired immunodeficiency syndrome (AIDS)
    (3) The heroin-using mother is frequently malnourished
3. Heroin causes vasoconstriction, which results in reduced blood flow to the uterus and subsequent fetal hypoxia (Flandermeyer, 1987)
4. Small amounts are present in breast milk of mothers who use heroin
5. Neonates who have been prenatally exposed to heroin have increased perinatal morbidity and mortality rates compared with nonexposed neonates
6. Neonatal effects of prenatal heroin exposure include the following
   a. Neonatal abstinence syndrome
    (1) Causes severe neonatal withdrawal symptoms
    (2) Has an average onset of symptoms between 6 and 12 hours after birth
    (3) Has an average peak of symptoms between 48 and 72 hours
   b. Withdrawal symptoms possibly persisting in a subacute form for 4 to 6 months after birth
   c. Increased incidence of meconium aspiration at birth
   d. Increased incidence of neonatal sepsis
   e. Intrauterine growth retardation
    (1) Low birth weight
    (2) Decreased length
    (3) Small head circumference
   f. Neurodevelopmental behavioral problems
    (1) Tremulousness and irritability
    (2) Poor organizational responses to environmental stimuli
    (3) Poor motor control
    (4) Difficult to console
    (5) Poor suck-and-swallow coordination, which leads to poor feeding tolerance
   g. Decreased incidence of respiratory distress syndrome
    (1) Heroin is thought to enhance pulmonary surfactant production
    (2) The red blood cells of heroin-exposed neonates have a heightened ability to carry oxygen (Flandermeyer, 1987)
   h. Reduced incidence of hyperbilirubinemia

(1) Liver cell exposure to heroin causes an increase in glucuronyl transferase activity, a vital component in the bilirubin conjugation process
(2) Bilirubin is conjugated and excreted more efficiently

H. Methadone

1. Used as a heroin substitute in carefully controlled programs to reduce or eliminate the use of heroin
   a. Administered orally instead of parenterally (as is heroin)
   b. Eliminates the problems of unknown contaminants and variable purity of heroin that is sold on the street
   c. Initially administered in a higher dose to stabilize the mother; dosage is then decreased to produce a smooth withdrawal to the lowest possible maintenance level to avoid withdrawal signs and symptoms and to minimize adverse fetal effects
2. High levels of methadone can produce a more severe and prolonged abstinence syndrome for the newborn than does heroin
3. Neonatal effects of prenatal methadone exposure include the following
   a. Intrauterine growth retardation
      (1) Low birth weight
      (2) Small head circumference
      (3) Decreased length
   b. Neonatal abstinence syndrome
      (1) Onset of symptoms is between 36 and 72 hours
      (2) Peak of symptoms is at 6 days
      (3) Subacute symptoms last up to 4 to 6 months
   c. Neurodevelopmental behavioral problems are similar to those caused by heroin

I. Non-narcotic substances: sedatives, stimulants, and phencyclidine piperidine (PCP)

1. No evidence of neonatal abstinence syndrome
2. Neonatal effects of exposure include the following
   a. Intrauterine growth does not seem to be influenced by these substances
   b. Neurodevelopmental behavior is characterized by the following
      (1) Decreased interactive ability
      (2) Decreased state control and increased state lability
      (3) Poor consolability

Clinical Practice

A. Assessment

1. History
   a. Maternal report of illegal drug use during pregnancy
   b. Evidence of maternal illegal drug use before birth
   c. Positive maternal urine drug screen
   d. Absence of prenatal care or late prenatal care
   e. Maternal malnutrition
   f. Maternal infection
   g. Amount, route, and time of last maternal drug dose before birth
   h. Specific street drug(s) used by mother
   i. Pattern of maternal drug abuse: chronic or sporadic
   j. Labor and delivery complications
   k. Neonate's Apgar scores at 1 minute and at 5 minutes
   l. Delivery room resuscitative efforts
   m. Preterm labor and delivery

2. Physical neonatal findings
   a. Small-for-gestational-age size
   b. Congenital anomalies
   c. Microcephaly
   d. Presence of fever
   e. Diaphoresis
   f. Tremors
   g. High-pitched cry
   h. Hyperactive reflexes
   i. Excessive mouthing of fists and sucking
   j. Restlessness
   k. Irritability and sleeplessness
   l. Muscular rigidity
   m. Tachypnea, apnea, or both
   n. Vomiting
   o. Diarrhea
   p. Excoriation of knees and elbows
   q. Nasal stuffiness
   r. Sneezing
   s. Frequent yawning
   t. Seizure activity
   u. Prematurity
3. Diagnostic procedures
   a. Urine drug screen
   b. Sepsis: protocol for specimen collection and testing

B. Nursing Diagnoses

1. Alteration in nutrition and fluids: less than body requirements related to vomiting and diarrhea, uncoordinated suck-and-swallow reflex, and hypertonia secondary to drug withdrawal
2. Impaired skin integrity related to excoriation of face, knees, elbows, and perianal area secondary to constant activity and frequent loose stools
3. Sleep pattern disturbance related to drug withdrawal
4. Alteration in parenting related to hyperirritability and poor consolability of the neonate

C. Interventions/Evaluations

1. Alteration in nutrition and fluids: less than body requirements related to vomiting and diarrhea, uncoordinated suck-and-swallow reflex, and hypertonia secondary to drug withdrawal
   a. Interventions
      (1) Provide small and frequent feedings with high-calorie formula
         (a) Decrease volume while increasing calories
         (b) Avoid misperception of irritability for hunger, which can lead to overfeeding and exacerbate the problem
         (c) Minimize handling infant after feeding to discourage vomiting
         (d) Elevate the head of the infant's bed to discourage vomiting
      (2) Feed by gavage
         (a) Ensures adequate caloric intake
         (b) Avoids the uncoordinated suck-and-swallow reflex problem
         (c) Allows feeding via an indwelling nasogastric tube to avoid disturbing infant's sleep
      (3) Pacifier used to meet infant's sucking needs
      (4) Intravenous therapy used as needed, per orders
   b. Evaluations
      (1) Neonate shows signs of adequate hydration

(2) Neonate gains adequate daily weight after initial normal birth weight loss

(3) Incidence of vomiting and diarrhea is minimal or absent

2. Impaired skin integrity related to excoriation of face, knees, elbows, and perianal area secondary to constant activity and frequent loose stools

a. Interventions

(1) Keep all bedding clean and dry

(2) Keep the skin clean and dry

(a) Leave buttocks open to air

(b) Use a paper face mask with ties as a diaper to allow air circulation and deflect loose stools

(3) Use soft bed linens, such as sheepskin, especially for the face

(4) Position neonate to avoid pressure on excoriated areas

(5) Apply an Op-Site dressing on abraded knees and elbows, as needed

(6) Monitor excoriated areas for signs of secondary infection

b. Evaluations

(1) Excoriations show signs of healing

(2) No new sites of excoriation or abrasion appear

(3) No signs of secondary infection at existing excoriated sites appear

3. Sleep pattern disturbance related to drug withdrawal

a. Interventions

(1) Swaddle the infant

(a) To promote rest

(b) To reduce the self-stimulation that is produced by flailing

(2) Offer pacifier to help infant self-console by sucking

(3) Minimize environmental stimuli

(a) Move infant to a quiet or private area of the nursery

(b) Reduce incoming light by shielding part of the isolette or crib, dimming the nursery lights (if possible), or both

(4) Administer medications as needed and per protocol; those most frequently prescribed are the following

(a) Phenobarbital

(b) Paregoric

(c) Diazepam

(d) Chlorpromazine

b. Evaluations

(1) The neonate has uninterrupted sleep cycles throughout a 24-hour period

(2) Withdrawal signs and symptoms are minimized to allow neonate uninterrupted sleep cycles

4. Alteration in parenting related to hyperirritability and poor consolability of the neonate

a. Interventions

(1) Encourage parental visits and telephone calls

(2) During visits, encourage parents' active participation in the infant's care

(3) Develop and implement a teaching strategy that gives parents anticipatory guidance, knowledge, and specific techniques for dealing with a drug-exposed infant (see section on health education)

(4) Give parents counseling about available resources and necessary follow-up care for the infant

b. Evaluations

(1) Parents demonstrate effective ways of handling and feeding the neonate

(2) Parents demonstrate effective ways of comforting the neonate

(3) Parents express and cope with frustrations about their infant and begin to use outside resources as sources of support

(4) Parents freely express any feelings of guilt about their contribution to the infant's physical withdrawal and distress

Health Education

A. Health education should focus primarily on the parents' (or the foster parents') acquisition of knowledge and skill about the special needs of an infant who was exposed to an illegal drug during pregnancy

B. Health education should also focus on anticipatory guidance to help parents anticipate and effectively deal with their infant's behavior

1. Parameters of so-called normal behavior should be explored with parents and techniques to cope with the behavior must be explained and demonstrated
   a. Swaddling
   b. Importance of non-nutritive sucking
   c. Avoidance of overfeeding
   d. Avoidance of overstimulation
2. The mother may view infant irritability as the infant's dislike of her or as manipulative behavior on the part of the neonate
   a. Explain that the infant experiences discomfort and is reacting to internal sensations by being irritable
   b. Explain that the neonate does not possess the cognitive abilities to be manipulative
   c. Instruct the mother about how to give soothing care to the neonate and the importance of responding to the infant's cry for assistance

C. Provide instruction about the following

1. Effective feeding techniques
2. Effective holding techniques
3. Effective comforting techniques
4. Administration of medications (when to medicate, and what to expect from the medications)

CASE STUDIES AND STUDY QUESTIONS

Baby M. was born after a 37-week pregnancy. She was small for gestational age, had microcephaly, and appeared constantly agitated. She tolerated her formula feedings poorly and yet always seemed hungry. Her mother denied any drug use during pregnancy. Baby M.'s urine screen was positive for heroin.

1. Baby M. will most likely
   a. Have development of respiratory distress syndrome because she is preterm and small for gestational age.
   b. Have development of hyperbilirubinemia because she is preterm and feeding poorly.
   c. Have a need for more frequent feedings in larger amounts because she is small for gestational age and always appears to be hungry.
   d. Have a need for relocation to a quieter area of the nursery and for shielding of the top of her crib from light.

2. Baby M.'s umbilical cord and nails are meconium stained. This was most likely caused by which of the following?
   a. Hypoxia during labor because she is a preterm infant.
   b. Hypoxia caused by heroin's effect on the uteroplacental blood flow.
   c. Inaccurate dating of the pregnancy because heroin causes amenorrhea and the mother does not know when she conceived.
   d. A probable heart defect from heroin exposure, which caused intrauterine hypoxia.

3. Baby M. should be closely monitored for which of the following additional signs and symptoms of drug withdrawal?
   a. Progressive lethargy.
   b. Seizure activity.

c. Generalized, flat, macular rash.

d. Subconjunctival hemorrhages.

4. Baby M. is jittery, fussy, and constantly moving her legs in a crawling motion. Her knees are abraded and her cheeks are fiery red. Which of the following is the *best* intervention?

 a. Position her to avoid pressure on her excoriated areas, make sure her skin is clean and dry, and swaddle her.

 b. Feed her by gavage and administer medication to decrease her constant activity.

 c. Have her mother cuddle and hold her so that she can be consoled and mother-infant attachment is encouraged.

 d. Clean the excoriated areas with an antiseptic soap to prevent secondary infection, position her off of the excoriated areas, and loosely wrap to allow air to circulate.

5. For which period can Baby M. be expected to exhibit withdrawal signs and symptoms?

 a. The next 48 hours.

 b. Seventy-two hours, with the peak effects occurring at 48 hours.

 c. Up to 4 to 6 months after birth.

 d. Up to 6 to 12 hours after birth.

Baby J. was born by emergency cesarean section at 36 weeks' gestation. His mother arrived in the emergency room with bleeding and severe noncyclical abdominal pain. She stated that she had had a few strong contractions preceding the bleeding followed by constant pain. The diagnosis was abruptio placentae. The mother admitted to occasional recreational use of cocaine. She had recently been given 3 g of cocaine and just before arriving at the emergency room, she and her husband had "done a line" together. Baby J. is small for gestational age and examination reveals that he has hypospadias.

6. Which other physical finding might an examination of Baby J. reveal?

 a. Hepatosplenomegaly.

b. Imperforate anus.

c. Petechiae.

d. Small head circumference.

7. In the nursery, Baby J. cries frequently and cannot seem to settle down like the rest of the babies. Noises startle him. He becomes overly agitated and jittery when his diapers are changed. He is reacting this way for which of the following reasons?

 a. He is preterm and cannot coordinate his movements as well as term babies.

 b. He is having difficulty in shutting out intrusive stimuli because of prenatal cocaine exposure.

 c. His nervous system is too immature at 36 weeks' gestation.

 d. He needs more frequent feedings to counteract the hypoglycemia caused by prenatal cocaine exposure.

8. Baby J.'s mother has planned to breastfeed him and says she wants to get started right away. Which of the following information does this mother need?

 a. Babies who have had prenatal cocaine exposure should take nothing by mouth until all diagnostic test results have been thoroughly examined.

 b. Baby J. is preterm, is small for gestational age, and will have cocaine-related feeding problems that can best be managed by giving him high-calorie formula.

 c. The mother should not have any problems breastfeeding Baby J. because the effect of prenatal cocaine exposure on the fetus accelerates maturation.

 d. Cocaine can appear in breast milk and she will continue to expose Baby J. to cocaine if she uses the drug while lactating.

9. Baby J.'s father wants to know for how long Baby J. will have the shakes and be so hard to console when he cries. Which of the following is the correct reply?

 a. For 4 to 6 months.

 b. For 2 weeks.

c. For 4 weeks.

d. For 5 to 7 days.

10. Baby J. is discharged from the hospital. His parents are instructed about the importance and use of an apnea monitor at home for which of the following reasons?

a. Preterm babies are prone to late-onset respiratory distress syndrome; therefore, Baby J. should be monitored.

b. Babies exposed to cocaine in utero have a higher incidence of bronchopulmonary dysplasia.

c. Small-for-gestational-age babies frequently have respiratory problems that are unnoticed.

d. The risk for sudden infant death syndrome (SIDS) in babies prenatally exposed to cocaine is 5 to 10 times higher than that of normal babies.

Answers to Study Questions

1. d	2. b	3. b
4. a	5. c	6. d
7. b	8. d	9. a
10. d		

REFERENCES

Chasnoff, I. (1986). Perinatal addiction. Consequences of intrauterine exposure to opiate and non-opiate drugs. In I. Chasnoff (Ed.), *Drug use in pregnancy* (pp. 52–63). Lancaster, England: MTP.

Chasnoff, I. (1988). Newborn infants with drug withdrawal symptoms. *Pediatrics in Review, 9*(9), 273.

Chasnoff, I. (1991). Chemical dependency and pregnancy. *Clinics in Perinatology, 18*(1), ix–x.

Chasnoff, I., Burns, K., Burns, W., & Schnoll, S. (1986). Prenatal drug exposure: Effects on neonatal and infant growth and development. *Neurobehavioral Toxicology and Teratology, 8,* 357–362.

Chasnoff, I., Hatcher, R., & Burns, W. (1980). Early growth patterns of methadone-addicted infants. *American Journal of Diseases of Children, 134,* 1049–1051.

Chasnoff, I., Lewis, D., & Squires, L. (1987). Cocaine intoxication in a breast-fed infant. *Pediatrics, 80*(6), 836–838.

Day, N., & Richardson, G. (1991). Prenatal mariajuana use: Epidemiology, methodologic issues, and infant outcomes. *Clinics in Perinatology, 18*(1), 77–91.

Flandermeyer, A. (1987, December). A comparison of the effects of heroin and cocaine abuse upon the neonate. *Neonatal Network,* 42–47.

Free, T., Russell, F., Mills, B., & Hathaway, D. (1990). A descriptive study of infants and toddlers exposed prenatally to substance abuse. *MCN: American Journal of Maternal Child Nursing, 15,* 245–249.

Fried, P. (1986). Marijuana and human pregnancy. In I. Chasnoff (Ed.), *Drug use in pregnancy* (pp. 64–74). Lancaster, England: MTP.

Hoegerman, G., Wilson, C., Thurmond, E., & Schnoll, S. (1990). Drug-exposed neonates. *Western Journal of Medicine, 152,* 559–564.

Jones, K. (1991). Developmental pathogenesis of defects associated with prenatal cocaine exposure: Fetal vascular disruption. *Clinics in Perinatology, 18*(1), 139–146.

Kennard, M. (1990). Cocaine use during pregnancy: Fetal and neonatal effects. *Journal of Perinatal and Neonatal Nursing, 3*(4), 53–63.

Lewis, K., Bennett, B., & Schmeder, N. (1989). The care of infants menaced by cocaine abuse. *MCN: American Journal of Maternal Child Nursing, 14,* 324–329.

Merker, L., Higgins, P., & Kinnard, E. (1985, May/June). Assessing narcotic addiction in neonates. *Pediatric Nursing,* 177–182.

Olds, S., London, M., & Ladewig, P. (1988). *Maternal newborn nursing* (3rd ed.) (pp. 983–985). Menlo Park, CA: Addison-Wesley.

Peters, H., & Theorell, C. (1991). Fetal and neonatal effects of maternal cocaine use. *Journal of Obstetric, Gynecologic, and Neonatal Nursing, 20*(2), 121–126.

Petitti, D., & Coleman, C. (1990). Cocaine and the risk of low birth weight. *American Journal of Public Health, 80*(1), 25–27.

Regan, D., Ehrlich, S., & Finnegan, L. (1987). Infants of drug addicts. At risk for child abuse, neglect, and placement in foster care. *Neurotoxicology and Teratology, 9*(4), 315–319.

Smith, J. (1988). The dangers of prenatal cocaine use. *MCN: American Journal of Maternal Child Nursing, 13*(3), 174–179.

Smith, J., & Deitch, K. (1987). Cocaine: A maternal, fetal, and neonatal risk. *Journal of Pediatric Health Care, 1*(3), 120–124.

Sweet, A. (1982). Narcotic withdrawal syndrome in the newborn. *Pediatrics in Review, 3*(9), 285–291.

41

Bonnie Christoff
and Ksenia Zukowsky

Infant of a Diabetic Mother

Objectives

1. Describe the appearance of an infant of a diabetic mother (IDM)

2. Identify risk factors associated with an IDM

3. Identify manifestations of the following risks in the newborn: hypoglycemia, respiratory distress, hypocalcemia, macrosomia, and hyperbilirubinemia

4. Formulate appropriate nursing diagnoses for these infants from assessment data

5. Implement a plan of care based on the diagnoses

Introduction

A. Insulin-dependent diabetes mellitus occurs in 0.5% of all pregnancies

1. Gestational diabetes is found in as many as one in 20 (3 to 8%) pregnancies
2. In women over 35 years of age, gestational diabetes is discovered in one in six pregnancies (Moore, 1991)

B. Reducing the risks from maternal diabetes to the infant begins with careful prenatal care so that maternal glucose levels are safely maintained (see Chapter 29 for a complete discussion of the diabetic client)

C. Maternal diabetes places the infant at risk for pre- and postnatal complications

1. The alteration in glucose metabolism in a diabetic mother affects the infant in utero and immediately after birth
   a. Glucose molecules readily cross the placenta, resulting in fetal blood sugar levels that are 80% of maternal levels
   b. The fetus responds by producing large quantities of insulin, leading to a state of hyperinsulinemia
   c. The increased amount of glucose present is reserved as glycogen stores and results in macrosomia from accelerated cellular development (Peller et al., 1985)
   d. Insulin acts as a growth hormone in the fetus; hyperinsulinemia also produces macrosomia from increased hepatic glycogen and total body fat stores

e. After delivery, the supply of glucose rapidly diminishes, yet the level of insulin remains constant
  (1) Hypoglycemia is found in more than 50% of IDMs; only a small number, however, are symptomatic (Avery, 1987)
  (2) The outcome and incidence of neurological developmental abnormalities from the hypoglycemia are related to the duration and severity of the hypoglycemic episode(s)
2. The alteration in growth physiology of the fetus usually results in growth acceleration
  a. Sixteen to 40% of babies are large for gestational age (LGA) (Jovanoc, 1983)
    (1) Infants born to diabetics in classes A through C are often LGA
    (2) Because of an interruption of uterine blood flow from vascular involvement, infants born to women in classes D through R are often small for gestational age (SGA) or growth retarded (IUGR); these infants require special consideration related to their low birth weight and compromised metabolic status (see Chapter 36 for a further discussion of IUGR babies)
  b. LGA babies are at risk for birth injury
    (1) Unlike other LGA neonates, IDMs characteristically have increased subcutaneous fat deposits rather than increased length and head size (Korones, 1986)
    (2) A cesarean section may be warranted if the fetus is estimated to be over 4200 to 4300 g (9 lb, 4½ oz to 9 lb, 8 oz) to avoid traumatic injury from a vaginal birth
3. IDMs are at increased risk for respiratory distress because of delay in surfactant production (see Chapter 37 for a complete discussion of respiratory distress)
  a. Excess insulin produced by the fetus's pancreas results in delayed surfactant production, probably by interfering with the lung's ability to use phospholipids by blocking receptor sites
    (1) This delay in surfactant production is found primarily in class A through C diabetics
    (2) Class D through R diabetics may have normal maturation because the incidence of respiratory distress syndrome (RDS) is less in the presence of IUGR, pregnancy-induced hypertension (PIH), and other sources of intrauterine stress often found with class D through R diabetics
  b. To avoid iatrogenic RDS, it is suggested that the usual parameters of fetal lung maturity be adjusted for IDMs
    (1) The lecithin/sphingomyelin (L/S) ratio should be 2.5:1 to 3:1 (depending on clinician and/or institution preference)
    (2) Phosphatidylglycerol (PG) should be greater than 3% (a value that reflects its presence); RDS may still occur if PG is present in trace amounts (Moore, 1991)
4. IDMs frequently demonstrate hyperbilirubinemia (see Chapter 38 for a complete discussion)
  a. Polycythemia is seen in 15 to 30% of IDMs
    (1) Polycythemia is diagnosed by a hemoglobin (Hgb) level above 22 g/dl and a hematocrit (Hct) above 65%
    (2) It may be related to the following
      (a) Increased viscosity of blood as a result of maternal diabetes
      (b) Chronic fetal hypoxia, which causes increased red blood cell (RBC) production (Sherwen, Scoloveno, & Weingarten, 1991)
  b. The subsequent neonatal breakdown of RBCs predisposes the IDM to hyperbilirubinemia because of the increased number of cells present
  c. Birth injuries may sequester blood; when RBCs are broken down at a later time, hyperbilirubinemia may result
  d. Impairment of hepatic function by neonatal hypoglycemia also interferes with bilirubin conjugation
5. IDMs are also prone to hypocalcemia

a. Defined as serum calcium below 7 mg/dl
b. Found in about 50% of IDMs (Reeder & Martin, 1987)
c. Usually manifested in the first 2 to 3 days of life
d. Several factors may be involved in its development
  (1) During pregnancy, a maternal hyperparathyroid state exists to meet the increased calcium needs of both mother and fetus
    (a) After delivery, the large supplies of calcium are withdrawn
    (b) If the fetus's reserves are low (or, in the case of the IDM, whose needs are great), decreased calcium is found
    (c) In the IDM, parathyroid hormone production to lowered calcium levels is blunted
  (2) Hypocalcemia may occur as a result of birth asphyxia
  (3) It may also be related to a decreased magnesium level, which suppresses parathyroid hormone production, thus decreasing calcium levels
6. Congenital anomalies occur in 4.5 to 6% of diabetic pregnancies (which is a three- to fourfold increased rate over that seen in the general pregnant population) (see Chap. 42 for further discussion of congenital anomalies)
a. Common defects seen include
  (1) Cardiac
    (a) Transposition of the great vessels
    (b) Ventricular septal defects
    (c) Atrial septal defects
    (d) Approximately 50% of IDMs also have cardiomegaly (Peller, Tsang, Meyer, & Braun, 1985), which may decrease cardiac output from the impaired ventricular contractility (Wallter, 1985)
  (2) Central nervous system (CNS)
    (a) Anencephaly
    (b) Meningomyelocele
    (c) Hydrocephalus
    (d) Spina bifida
  (3) Gastrointestinal: imperforate anus
  (4) Musculoskeletal
    (a) Limb reduction defects
    (b) Caudal regression (a defect specific to IDMs, since caudal regression is a result of hyperglycemia [Moore, 1991])
b. Increasing evidence exists that preconceptual and prenatal (especially in the first trimester) control of maternal blood glucose will directly affect the incidence of anomalies
  (1) It is hypothesized that hyperglycemia causes an alteration in cell division during embryogenesis (Mills, 1982)
  (2) The incidence of anomalies can be correlated with glycosylated hemoglobin (Hb A1c) levels in the mother
    (a) Levels below 8.5% result in a 3 to 4% anomaly rate (which is consistent with nondiabetic occurrence rates)
    (b) Levels over 8.5% yield a 22.4% occurrence rate
    (c) It is suggested that levels be kept below 7% to avoid anomalies due to hyperglycemia (Moore, 1991)

Clinical Practice

A. Assessment

1. History
a. Maternal diabetes classification
  (1) Insulin use and dose
  (2) Serum glucose levels and trends (especially Hb A1c)
  (3) Episodes of ketoacidosis

     b. Perinatal asphyxia
       (1) Evidence of distress on fetal monitor record
       (2) Meconium in amniotic fluid
       (3) Apgar score less than 5 at 1 minute or less than 7 at 5 minutes
     c. Type of delivery
       (1) Cesarean section
       (2) Vaginal
         (a) Length of second stage
         (b) Shoulder dystocia
         (c) Use of forceps or vacuum extractor
2. Physical findings
     a. LGA infant (macrosomia)
       (1) Weight above the 90th percentile
       (2) "Fat" baby with round face
     b. Plethora related to polycythemia
     c. Signs of hypoglycemia
       (1) Glucose levels
         (a) Bedside glucose screening below 40
         (b) Blood glucose values less than 40 mg/dl (Polk, 1991, p. 969)
       (2) Jitteriness and tremors
       (3) Lethargy
       (4) High-pitched cry
       (5) Tachypnea (greater than 60 breaths/min)
     d. Jaundice caused by hyperbilirubinemia: serum bilirubin values above 12 mg in term infant and above 15 mg in preterm infant
     e. Respiratory distress
       (1) Tachypnea (greater than 60 breaths/min)
       (2) Nasal flaring
       (3) Retractions: supraclavicular, intercostal, and substernal
       (4) Expiratory grunting
       (5) Color changes: pale, dusky, and cyanotic
     f. Signs of hypocalcemia (many infants are asymptomatic)
       (1) Serum level below 7 mg/dl
       (2) Tremors and jitteriness
       (3) Prolonged Q-T interval on electrocardiogram (ECG)
       (4) High-pitched cry
       (5) Cyanosis
       (6) Feeding intolerance, including vomiting
     g. Congenital anomalies (see Chapter 42 for complete discussion)
       (1) Congenital heart disease
       (2) Musculoskeletal defects such as caudal regression may be evident
       (3) CNS anomalies: neural tube defects
     h. Birth injuries (see Chapter 36 for a complete discussion)
       (1) Brachial plexus injuries
       (2) Facial paralysis
       (3) Clavicular fracture
       (4) Cephalhematoma and depressed skull fracture
3. Diagnostic procedures
     a. Vital signs, including blood pressures on all four extremities
     b. Infant's weight, length, and head circumference plotted against gestational age chart
     c. Blood glucose levels
     d. Complete blood count (CBC) with differential for polycythemia
     e. Serum bilirubin values
     f. Chest x-ray film and arterial blood gas assay if evidence of respiratory distress
     g. Echocardiogram and ECG if evidence of cardiac anomalies

h. Serum calcium and magnesium if evidence of hypocalcemia
i. Genetic consultation if evidence of congenital abnormalities

B. Nursing Diagnoses

1. Alteration in metabolism related to hyperinsulinemia secondary to maternal diabetes
2. High risk for alteration in respiratory effort related to inadequate surfactant production
3. High risk for trauma or birth injury related to large size
4. High risk for alteration in metabolism related to hyperbilirubinemia
5. High risk for alteration in metabolism related to hypocalcemia

C. Interventions/Evaluations

1. Alteration in metabolism related to hyperinsulinemia secondary to maternal diabetes
   a. Interventions
      (1) Monitor glucose levels
         (a) At birth
         (b) Every 2 hours for first 8 hours
         (c) Every 4 hours for 24 hours or until stable
      (2) Offer glucose, breast milk, or formula before 4 hours of age
         (a) If Dextrostix below 40, immediately provide infant with 10% glucose solution via nipple; gavage if
            (i) Respiratory rate over 60 breaths/min
            (ii) Suck-and-swallow reflex weak or uncoordinated
         (b) Administer IV glucose infusion, if necessary, at 4 to 8 mg/kg/min
      (3) Observe for signs and symptoms of hypoglycemia
         (a) Jitteriness and tremors
         (b) Lethargy
         (c) High-pitched cry
         (d) Tachypnea
      (4) Provide neutral thermal environment (NTE) to avoid cold stress, which increases glucose metabolism
      (5) Monitor infant's weight for adequate weight gain
   b. Evaluations
      (1) Glucose levels within normal limits
         (a) Dextrostix above 40
         (b) Serum glucose levels above 40 mg/dl
      (2) No signs or symptoms of hypoglycemia seen
      (3) NTE maintained as evidenced by axillary temperature remaining between 97.6° and 98°F (36.4° to 36.7°C)
      (4) Infant gains appropriate weight of 15 to 30 g (0.5 to 1 oz)/day
         (a) Caloric intake: 90 to 120 cal/kg/day
         (b) Fluid intake: 100 to 160 cc/kg/day
         (c) Urine output: above 2 cc/kg/hr
2. High risk for alteration in respiratory effort related to inadequate surfactant production (see Chapter 37)
3. High risk for trauma or birth injury related to large size (see Chapter 36)
4. High risk for alteration in metabolism related to hyperbilirubinemia (see Chapter 38)
5. High risk for alteration in metabolism related to hypocalcemia
   a. Interventions
      (1) Obtain serum calcium and magnesium levels
      (2) Observe for signs and symptoms of hypocalcemia
         (a) Muscle twitching and jitteriness
         (b) Increased muscle tone

(c) High-pitched cry

(d) Cyanosis

(e) Feeding intolerance, including vomiting

(3) Add calcium supplements to IV fluids if hypocalcemia documented by laboratory studies

    (a) 24 to 35 mg/kg/24 hr is commonly used dose (Klaus & Fanaroff, 1986)

    (b) If neonate seizes, IV calcium may be given as a bolus; exercise extreme caution because it may result in bradycardia or asystole (Avery, 1987)

(4) Administer magnesium if hypomagnesemia documented by laboratory studies

    (a) If below 1.2 mg/dl, give 50% magnesium sulfate solution 0.2 ml/kg IM

    (b) If 1.2 to 1.5 mg/dl (with less severe symptoms), oral magnesium may be given with feedings at 20 to 40 mg/kg/day (Behrman, 1987; Klaus & Fanaroff, 1986)

b. Evaluations

(1) No signs or symptoms of hypocalcemia observed

(2) Serum calcium levels remain 8 to 10 mg/dl

(3) Serum magnesium levels remain 1.5 to 2.0 mg/dl

Health Education

A. Preconceptual counseling is extremely important so that the client understands the importance of maintaining a euglycemic state before and during the pregnancy (especially in the first trimester)

B. The client needs to be informed about the disease and its influence on pregnancy and the fetus and neonate

1. Causes of macrosomia
2. Possibility of congenital anomalies
   a. Possible need for immediate intervention
   b. Future prognosis
   c. Genetic counseling
3. Possible interventions required for respiratory distress, hypoglycemia, or both
4. Possible need for the infant to be cared for in a neonatal intensive care unit, which may be located separately from the mother's caretaking institution

C. The parents may need information and assistance regarding care for an LGA infant

1. The baby is still fragile, although large
2. The infant may need more frequent feedings, which may be a strain for the nursing mother
3. The mother may need assistance in handling the infant because of its large size, especially if she was delivered of the infant by cesarean section
4. Instruct the parents in appropriate feeding guidelines to prevent over- or underfeeding

D. The parents may require education and reassurance about birth injuries

1. Cephalhematoma resolves in 4 to 6 weeks
2. Palsies and fractures
   a. Parents need to know how to handle the infant
   b. Parents may need to perform range of motion exercises
   c. Infant may require physical therapy

CASE STUDIES AND STUDY QUESTIONS

A 4200-g (9 lb, 4 oz) boy was born via cesarean section at 39 weeks' gestation to a 25-year-old gravida 1, para 0 (G1,P0) class C diabetic woman. His 1-minute Apgar score was 6 (2 points off for color and 1 each off for tone and irritability), and his 5-minute Apgar score was 8 (1 each off for color and tone). On admission to the nursery, the following information was established: length 50.2 cm (19¾ in); Dextrostix, 40; heart rate, 142; respiration, 55, with slight nasal flaring; 37 weeks by Dubowitz scale for gestational age.

1. The anticipated problems that you might see in this neonate include

   a. Hypoglycemia

   b. Hypocalcemia

   c. RDS

   d. Jaundice

   e. All of the above

2. At 30 minutes of age, the infant is jittery and tachypneic (respirations of 65 breaths/min), and his Dextrostix is below 40. What would be the expected serum glucose level?

   a. 60 mg/dl

   b. 25 mg/dl

   c. Zero

   d. Same as the Dextrostix

3. What is an appropriate intervention to perform while awaiting the serum glucose report?

   a. Start an IV and give a bolus of 8 mg of glucose to the infant.

   b. Feed the infant a 10% glucose solution orally via nipple.

   c. Gavage the infant with a 10% glucose solution.

   d. Feed the infant 1 to 2 oz (30 to 60 ml) of formula.

4. The infant's respiratory distress appears more evident with increased nasal flaring and substernal retractions. His respiratory rate remains elevated. What is the most likely explanation for this?

   a. Hypoglycemia decreases the need for oxygen.

   b. LGA infants frequently show signs of RDS.

   c. Infants with 5-minute Apgar scores of 8 often develop RDS.

   d. Hyperinsulinemia may delay surfactant production.

5. Congenital anomalies are seen with increased frequency in IDMs. Answer as true or false.

6. Common congenital anomalies that are seen include which of the following?

   (1) Transposition of the great vessels.

   (2) Caudal regression.

   (3) Prune-belly syndrome.

   (4) Cleft lip or palate.

   (5) Polydactyly.

   a. 1

   b. 1, 2

   c. 1, 3

   d. 1, 2, 5

   e. 2, 4

Answers to Study Questions

1. e	2. b	3. c
4. d	5. True	6. b

REFERENCES

Avery, G. (1987). *Neonatology: Pathophysiology and management of the newborn* (3rd ed.). Philadelphia: Lippincott.

Behrman, R. (Ed.) (1987). *Nelson textbook of pediatrics* (13th ed.). Philadelphia: Saunders.

Black, V. (1982). Neonatal polycythemia and hyperviscosity. *Pediatric Clinics of North America, 29,* 1137–1182.

Carpenito, L. (1989). *Handbook of nursing diagnosis.* Philadelphia: Lippincott.

Faranoff, A. (1987). *Neonatal perinatal medicine.* St. Louis: Mosby.

Haymond, M. (1979). Glucose homeostasis in children with severe congenital heart disease. *Journal of Pediatrics, 95,* 220–225.

Hollingsworth, D. (1983). Endocrine and metabolic homeostasis in diabetic pregnancy. *Clinics in Perinatology, 10*(3), 593–614.

Jovanoc, L. (1983). Pump therapy offers convenience for insulin-dependent women. *Infusion, 1*(2), 15–17.

Klaus, M., & Fanaroff, A. (1986). *Care of the high risk neonate.* Philadelphia: Saunders.

Korones, S. (1986). *The high-risk newborn infant.* St. Louis: Mosby.

Merinstein, G., & Gardner, S. (1989). *Handbook of neonatal intensive care.* St. Louis: Mosby.

Mills, J. (1982). Malformations in infants of diabetic mothers. *Teratology, 24,* 385–391.

Moore, T. (1991, April). Management of diabetes in pregnancy. Paper presented at the southern California section, NAACOG spring conference. San Diego, CA.

Pederson, L. (1977). Problems and management. *In* L. Pederson (Ed.), *The pregnant diabetic and her newborn.* Baltimore: Williams & Wilkins.

Peller, M., Tsang, R., Meyer, R., & Braun, C. (1985). Relationship of prospective diabetes control in pregnancy to neonatal cardiorespiratory function. *Journal of Pediatrics, 106,* 86–97.

Pieny, K. (1980). Hyperbilirubinemia in infants of diabetic mothers. *Pediatrics, 6,* 417–423.

Polk, D. (1991). Disorders of carbohydrate metabolism. *In* H. Tausch, R. Ballard, & M. Avery (Eds.), *Schaffer and Avery's Diseases of the Newborn* (p. 969). Philadelphia: Saunders.

Reeder, S., & Martin, L. (1987). *Maternity nursing* (16th ed.). Philadelphia: Lippincott.

Sherwen, L., Scoloveno, M., & Weingarten, C. (1991). *Nursing care of the childbearing family.* Norwalk, CT: Appleton & Lange.

Smith, B., Gerard, G., & Robert, M. (1987). Insulin antagonism of cortisol action: Synthesis by cultured fetal lungs. *Journal of Pediatrics, 87,* 955–970.

Tsang, R. (1972). Hypocalcemia in infants of diabetic mothers. *Journal of Pediatrics, 80,* 384–389.

Wallter, F. (1985). Cardiac output of insulin dependent mothers. *Journal of Pediatrics, 107,* 109–118.

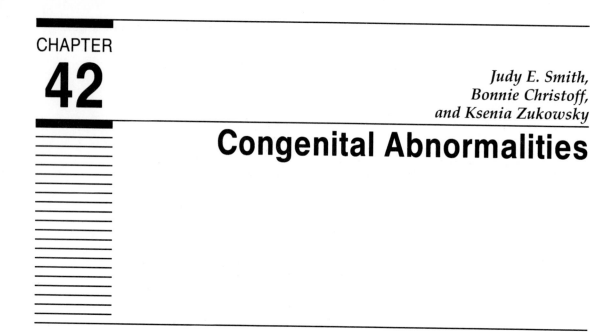

Judy E. Smith,
Bonnie Christoff,
and Ksenia Zukowsky

Congenital Abnormalities

Objectives

1. Identify the incidence, risk factors, anatomy, pathophysiology, signs, and associated complications of the following congenital heart defects: patent ductus arteriosus, ventricular septal defects, atrial septal defects, coarctation of the aorta, tetralogy of Fallot, complete transposition of the great vessels, hypoplastic left heart, and aortic stenosis

2. Describe specific nursing interventions that are appropriate for each type of congenital heart defect

3. Design health education to meet the needs of parents and family of a neonate with congenital heart disease

4. Identify the incidence, risk factors, anatomy, pathophysiology, signs, and associated complications of the following gastrointestinal congenital anomalies: pyloric stenosis; cleft lip and palate; imperforate anus, anal agenesis, and rectal atresia; omphalocele and gastroschisis; and espohageal atresia and tracheoesophageal fistula

5. Describe specific nursing interventions that are appropriate for each type of gastrointestinal anomaly

6. Design health education to meet the specific needs of parents and family of a neonate with a congenital gastrointestinal anomaly

7. Identify the incidence, types, risk factors, anatomy, pathophysiology, signs, and associated complications of hydrocephalus and spina bifida

8. Describe specific nursing interventions that are appropriate for the initial care of a neonate with spina bifida, or hydrocephalus, or both

9. Design health education to meet the initial needs of parents and family of a neonate born with spina bifida, hydrocephalus, or both

10. Identify the incidence, imminent danger, anatomy, pathophysiology, signs, survival rate, and associated complications of congenital diaphragmatic hernia in the neonate

11. Describe specific emergency nursing interventions that are appropriate to perform in the delivery room when a neonate is born with congenital diaphragmatic hernia

12. Identify immediate health educational needs of parents and family of a neonate born with congenital diaphragmatic hernia

Congenital Heart Disease

INTRODUCTION

A. The neonate's circulatory system undergoes several physiological changes after birth

1. The termination of fetal circulation and the initiation of adult circulation involve the closure of the three fetal shunts: the foramen ovale, the ductus arteriosus, and the ductus venosus
2. The physiological changes create a decrease in pulmonary vascular resistance and a concomitant rise in systemic pressure
3. There is an increase in oxygenation, causing vascular dilation in the pulmonary circulation
   a. Increased oxygenation stimulates the constriction of the ductus arteriosus
   b. Increased pressure in the pulmonary tree changes the gradient between the aorta and the pulmonary artery to functionally stop flow through the ductus arteriosus
   c. Pulmonary vascular dilation and equalization of the pressure gradient between the atria force closure of the foramen ovale

B. Cardiac defects or lesions are categorized as

1. Acyanotic, left-to-right shunts
2. Cyanotic, right-to-left shunts

C. Cardiac lesions can be divided into four groups

1. Lesions that increase pulmonary blood flow
2. Lesions that decrease pulmonary blood flow
3. Lesions that create obstruction
4. Lesions that create directional shunts

D. The incidence of congenital heart disease in neonates is 1% of all live births (Wolfe & Wiggins, 1991, p. 427)

E. The etiology of congenital heart defects is often unknown, with only 8% known to be associated with a single mutant gene or chromosomal abnormalities (Wolfe & Wiggins, 1991, p. 427)

1. At least 90% are believed to be because of multifactorial inheritance and a complex interaction between genetic and environmental factors
2. Teratogens are associated with a small percentage of congenital defects; however, very few have been shown to cause congenital heart disease (Hazinski, 1984, p. 166) (see Chapter 13 for complete discussion of teratogens)
3. Maternal rubella during the first 8 weeks of gestation is associated with a 50% chance that the neonate will have congenital rubella syndrome, which includes cardiac defects (Hazinski, 1984, p. 166) (see Chapter 27 for complete discussion of the effects of maternal rubella and Chapter 39 for discussion of congenital infections in the neonate)
4. Approximately 10% of infants of diabetic mothers who are insulin-dependent may have congenital heart disease (Hazinski, 1984, p. 166) (see Chapter 41 for complete discussion of infants of diabetic mothers)
5. Up to 50% of infants with fetal alcohol syndrome have associated congenital heart disease (Hazinski, 1984, p. 166) (see Chapter 32 for discussion of fetal alcohol syndrome)
6. Chromosomal anomalies or syndromes are associated with cardiac defects; approximately 30 to 40% of neonates with trisomy 21 (Down's syndrome) have cardiac anomalies (Hazinski, 1984, p. 166) (see Chapter 3 for discussion of chromosomal anomalies)

CLINICAL PRACTICE

Patent Ductus Arteriosus

A. Introduction

1. Patent ductus arteriosus (PDA) occurs in 5 to 10% of all congenital heart disease in neonates, excluding preterm infants (Parks, 1984, p. 134)
2. In preterm neonates, the incidence of PDA is 20 to 60% among infants weighing less than 1500 g (3 lb, 5 oz) (Wolfe & Wiggins, 1991, p. 432)
3. PDA is common in neonates whose mothers had rubella during the first trimester (Wolfe & Wiggins, 1991, p. 432)
4. PDA is twice as common in females as in males (Wolfe & Wiggins, 1991, p. 432)
5. An anatomical and functionally open shunt exists connecting the pulmonary artery and the aorta (Fig. 42–1)

B. Assessment

1. Physical findings
   a. A harsh murmur heard at the second left intercostal space, at the left sternal border, and inferior to the left clavicle (Wolfe & Wiggins, 1991, p. 432)
      (1) The murmur is systolic and then becomes continuous
      (2) Thrill over the suprasternal notch and along the upper left and right sternal borders (Hazinski, 1984, p. 167); many times, this thrill can be visualized as active precordium
      (3) Bounding femoral pulses
      (4) Pulse pressure is widened; greater than half the systolic pressure (Wolfe & Wiggins, 1991, p. 432)
      (5) Signs in preterm neonates are those associated with respiratory distress
         (a) Tachypnea
         (b) Retractions
         (c) Hypoxemia
         (d) Hypercapnia
      (6) An early sign signifying the presence of a significant left-to-right shunt with concomitant congestive heart failure is an increasing dependence on oxygen and respiratory support (Wolfe & Wiggins, 1991, p. 433)
      (7) Cardiomegaly
         (a) If the shunt is large, there is both left atrial and left ventricular enlargement
         (b) If the shunt is small or moderate in size, the heart is not enlarged (Wolfe & Wiggins, 1991, p. 433)
2. Diagnostic procedures
   a. Electrocardiogram: may be normal or may show left ventricular hypertrophy
   b. Echocardiogram: enlargement of left atrium indicates congestive heart failure
   c. Chest x-ray film: detects heart enlargement

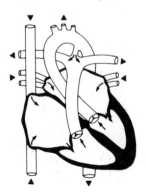

Figure 42–1
Patent ductus arteriosus. (Reprinted with permission of Ross Laboratories, Columbus, OH 43216, from Clinical Education Aid. © Ross Laboratories.)

Ventricular Septal Defect

A. Introduction

1. A ventricular septal defect (VSD) is an opening in the septum between the right and left ventricles that results from imperfect ventricular formation during early fetal development (Fig. 42–2)
   a. Varies in size
   b. May involve either the membranous or muscular portion of the ventricular septum
   c. A shunting of blood from the left to the right ventricle occurs during systole because of higher pressures in the left ventricle
   d. If pulmonary hypertension is present, the blood shunts from the right to the left ventricle, causing cyanosis
2. VSD is the most commonly occurring form of congenital heart disease, with an incidence of 20 to 25% among neonates with cardiac defects (Parks, 1984, p. 128)
3. VSD frequently occurs in association with other congenital heart disease
4. VSD is more common in males than in females (Fink, 1985, p. 26)

B. Assessment

1. Physical findings
   a. Small VSDs
      (1) Neonate usually shows no signs other than a soft murmur
      (2) Normal growth patterns
      (3) One-third close spontaneously (Hazinski, 1984, p. 172)
   b. Large VSDs
      (1) Murmur is usually holosystolic and frequently accompanied by a thrill (Hazinski, 1984, p. 173)
      (2) Tend to become smaller with advancing age (Parks, 1984, p. 132)
   c. Signs of VSD
      (1) Tachypnea
      (2) Poor feeding tolerance
      (3) Diaphoresis
      (4) Signs associated with congestive heart failure related to left-to-right shunt increasing pulmonary blood flow
2. Diagnostic procedures
   a. Chest x-ray film
      (1) Cardiomegaly
      (2) Left and right ventricular hypertrophy
   b. Echocardiogram
      (1) Defects of 4 mm or larger can be visualized
      (2) Can pinpoint anatomical location of lesion in 65 to 75% of cases (Wolfe & Wiggins, 1991, p. 430)

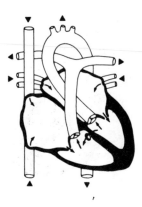

Figure 42–2
Ventricular septal defects. (Reprinted with permission of Ross Laboratories, Columbus, OH 43216, from Clinical Education Aid. © Ross Laboratories.)

Atrial Septal Defects

A. Introduction

1. An atrial septal defect (ASD) is an opening in the atrial septum that occurs as a result of improper septal formation in early fetal cardiac development (Fig. 42–3)
   a. Permits shunting of blood between the two atria
   b. An incompetent or malformed foramen ovale is the most common defect
2. This type of defect occurs in 10% of infants with congenital heart disease (Wolfe & Wiggins, 1991, p. 428)
   a. Twice as common in females as in males (Wolfe & Wiggins, 1991, p. 428)
   b. Up to 40% spontaneously close within the first 5 years of life (Parks, 1984, p. 126)
3. Three major types
   a. Ostium secundum
      (1) Most common
      (2) Located in the area of the foramen ovale or in an intermediate position on the atrial septum
      (3) May be associated with mitral valve prolapse (Hazinski, 1984, p. 169)
   b. Sinus venosus
      (1) Positioned high in the atrial septum
      (2) Least common
      (3) Frequently associated with partial anomalous venous return (Wolfe & Wiggins, 1991, p. 428)
      (4) May be associated with mitral valve prolapse (Parks, 1984, p. 125)
   c. Ostium primum
      (1) Positioned low in the atrial septum
      (2) Classified as a type of atrial septal defect
      (3) Results from incomplete fusion of the embryonic endocardial cushions, which help to form the lower portion of the atrial septum
      (4) Accounts for approximately 4% of all cases of congenital heart disease
      (5) Incidence is 20% in Down's syndrome (Wolfe & Wiggins, 1991, p. 431)

B. Assessment

1. Physical findings
   a. Many neonates with this defect are asymptomatic
   b. S_2 widely split
   c. Grade I through III/IV ejection systolic murmur at the pulmonary area
   d. Widely radiating systolic murmur
   e. Diastolic flow murmur at lower left sternal border in large shunts
   f. Congestive heart failure (Wolfe & Wiggins, 1991, p. 428)
2. Diagnostic procedures
   a. Chest x-ray film

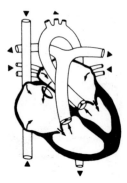

Figure 42–3
Atrial septal defects. (Reprinted with permission of Ross Laboratories, Columbus, OH 43216, from Clinical Education Aid. © Ross Laboratories.)

      (1) Cardiomegaly
      (2) Main pulmonary artery may appear dilated
   b. Echocardiogram
      (1) Direct visualization of the defect
      (2) Left-to-right shunt
   c. Electrocardiogram
      (1) Bundle branch block
      (2) Right axis deviation

Coarctation of the Aorta

A. Introduction

1. Coarctation of the aorta is a narrowing of the aortic lumen within the area of the aortic arch (Fig. 42–4)
2. A common cardiac anomaly that accounts for 6% of all congenital heart disease (Wolfe & Wiggins, 1991, p. 437)
   a. Occurs in three times as many males as females
   b. Produces an obstruction to the flow of blood through the aorta
   c. Incidence is 30% in infants with Turner's syndrome (Parks, 1984, p. 152)
3. Coarctation of the aorta syndrome
   a. Infant is symptomatic
   b. Associated PDA, VSD, and bicuspid aortic valve
4. Defect may occur in one of three locations depending on the position of the obstruction in relation to the ductus arteriosus
   a. Preductal
      (1) Coarctation is proximal to the ductus arteriosus
      (2) Associated with other cardiac defects in approximately 40% of cases (Parks, 1984, p. 152)
   b. Postductal
      (1) Coarctation is distal to the ductus arteriosus
      (2) The neonate is usually asymptomatic
      (3) Not usually associated with other cardiac defects (Parks, 1984, p. 152)
   c. Juxtaductal
      (1) Most common location
      (2) In juxtaposition to the ductus arteriosus

B. Assessment

1. Physical findings
   a. Diminished or absent femoral pulses
   b. Blowing systolic murmur in left axilla
   c. Pulse lag in lower extremities
   d. Blood pressure is greater in upper extremities than in lower extremities (Wolfe & Wiggins, 1991, p. 437)

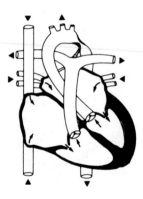

Figure 42–4
Coarctation of the aorta. (Reprinted with permission of Ross Laboratories, Columbus, OH 43216, from Clinical Education Aid. © Ross Laboratories.)

  e. Poor feeding tolerance
  f. Poor weight gain during the first 2 to 6 weeks of life
  g. Pallor
  h. Respiratory distress (Parks, 1984, pp. 154–155)
  i. Neonates can be asymptomatic
2. Diagnostic procedures
  a. Blood pressures from all four extremities may reveal discrepancies
  b. Electrocardiogram
    (1) May be normal
    (2) May show evidence of slight left ventricular hypertrophy
    (3) In symptomatic neonates, may show evidence of right ventricular hypertrophy
  c. Chest x-ray film may show possible cardiomegaly with prominent pulmonary venous congestion (Hazinski, 1984, p. 219)
  d. Echocardiogram may permit direct visualization of the coarctation

Tetralogy of Fallot

A. Introduction

1. Characterized by a combination of four defects (Fig. 42–5)
  a. Ventricular septal defect
  b. An overriding aorta: aorta overrides the septal defect
  c. Pulmonary stenosis
  d. Hypertrophy of the right ventricle
2. The most common type of cyanotic heart lesion; accounts for 10 to 15% of all congenital heart disease (Wolfe & Wiggins, 1991, p. 444)
3. Severity of symptoms depends on the degree of pulmonary stenosis, the magnitude of ventricular septal defect, and the degree to which the aorta overrides the septal defect

B. Assessment

1. Physical findings
  a. Respiratory distress
  b. Cyanosis: degree is directly related to the extent of pulmonary stenosis (Hazinski, 1984, p. 190)
    (1) If the ductus arteriosus is patent, the neonate may have minimal cyanosis
    (2) On constriction of the ductus arteriosus, the infant will frequently have cyanosis upon exertion (Hazinski, 1984, p. 190)
    (3) Crying or feeding increases cyanosis and respiratory distress
  c. Systolic ejection murmur located at the left upper sternal border (Wolfe & Wiggins, 1991, p. 444)

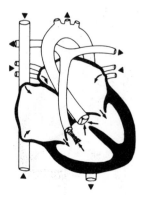

Figure 42–5
Tetralogy of Fallot. (Reprinted with permission of Ross Laboratories, Columbus, OH 43216, from Clinical Education Aid. © Ross Laboratories.)

2. Diagnostic procedures
   a. Chest x-ray film
      (1) May appear entirely normal
      (2) Right ventricle hypertrophy
      (3) Boot-shaped appearance of the heart secondary to the small pulmonary artery
   b. Laboratory findings
      (1) Hemoglobin values are mildly to markedly elevated
      (2) Hematocrit and red blood cell count are mildly to markedly elevated depending on the extent of arterial oxygen desaturation (Wolfe & Wiggins, 1991, p. 445)
   c. Echocardiogram
      (1) Right ventricular wall thickening visualized
      (2) Visualization of the overriding aorta and the ventricular septal defect (Wolfe & Wiggins, 1991, p. 445)

Complete Transposition of the Great Vessels

A. Introduction

1. The second most common type of cyanotic congenital heart disease is complete transposition of the great vessels
   a. Incidence: 16% of all cyanotic congenital heart disease
   b. More frequent in males than females, with a 3 : 1 ratio (Wolfe & Wiggins, 1991, p. 449)
2. Transposition is caused by an embryological abnormality in the spiral division of the truncus arteriosus (Wolfe & Wiggins, 1991, p. 449)
   a. There is a straight division without the normal spiraling
   b. As a result, the aorta originates from the right ventricle and the pulmonary artery originates from the left ventricle (Fig. 42–6)
3. Usually associated with other cardiac abnormalities
   a. Ventricular septal defects in 80%
   b. Pulmonary stenosis in 50% (Parks, 1984, p. 165)
4. Survival depends on early diagnosis and aggressive treatment
   a. An abnormal communication between the two separate circulations must be present to sustain life
   b. A PDA and a ventricular septal opening can sustain life until corrective surgery is done (duct-dependent lesion)
   c. Mortality rate is 10% (Wolfe & Wiggins, 1991, p. 451)

B. Assessment

1. Physical findings
   a. Cyanosis: most are cyanotic at birth
   b. Usually large birth weights at around 4 kg (9 lb)

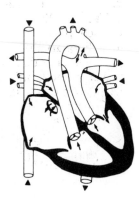

Figure 42–6
Complete transposition of great vessels. (Reprinted with permission of Ross Laboratories, Columbus, OH 43216, from Clinical Education Aid. © Ross Laboratories.)

    c. Possible pulmonic stenosis murmur (depending on the type of associated cardiac defects); however, many do not have murmurs

    d. Signs of congestive heart failure

        (1) If the ventricular septal defect is large

        (2) Develop at approximately 3 weeks of age because of enormous pulmonary blood flow (Wolfe & Wiggins, 1991, p. 450)

    e. Normal peripheral pulses (if congestive heart failure is absent)

2. Diagnostic procedures

    a. Chest x-ray film

        (1) Findings are usually nonspecific

        (2) Possible cardiomegaly (Parks, 1984, p. 167)

    b. Echocardiogram reveals abnormal relationship of the great vessels

    c. Cardiac catheterization gives the definitive diagnosis and is used to perform a septostomy between the two ventricles (Wolfe & Wiggins, 1991, p. 450)

Hypoplastic Left Heart

A. Introduction

1. Hypoplastic left heart syndrome includes various defects that are either valvular or vascular obstructive lesions on the left side of the heart

    a. There is severe obstruction in either the filling or the emptying of the left ventricle

    b. As a result of the obstruction during intrauterine life, there is a very small quantity of blood filling the left ventricle; subsequently hypoplasia develops (Wolfe & Wiggins, 1991, p. 449)

2. The most common obstructive lesions are mitral atresia and aortic atresia or both

    a. Aortic atresia will rapidly cause congestive heart failure, and death usually occurs within the first week of life

    b. Infants with mitral atresia and large communicating atrial and ventricular septal defects may live longer depending on when congestive heart failure develops

3. Hypoplastic left heart accounts for 2% of all congenital heart defects

4. This condition is the leading cause of death from cardiovascular disease within the first 2 weeks of life (Hazinski, 1984, p. 227)

5. The neonate is usually duct dependent; as the ductus arteriosus closes, the neonate's condition deteriorates

B. Assessment

1. Physical findings

    a. Generalized cyanosis

    b. Soft, systolic murmur just left of the sternum

    c. Diminished pulses

    d. Tachycardia

    e. Tachypnea

    f. Pulmonary rales

    g. Respiratory distress

    h. Pallor and mottling

2. Diagnostic procedures

    a. Chest x-ray film

        (1) May appear normal at birth

        (2) Followed by rapid and progressive cardiac enlargement and pulmonary venous congestion

    b. Electrocardiogram

        (1) Right atrial hypertrophy

        (2) Right ventricular hypertrophy

   c. Echocardiogram
     (1) Diminished aorta and left ventricle
     (2) Poorly defined mitral valve (Wolfe & Wiggins, 1991, p. 449)

Aortic Stenosis

A. Introduction

1. Aortic stenosis is an obstruction to the outflow from the left ventricle at or near the aortic valve (Wolfe & Wiggins, 1991, p. 438)
2. Accounts for approximately 5% of all congenital heart disease
3. Aortic stenosis is divided into four anatomical categories
   a. Valvular aortic stenosis
     (1) The most common form; accounts for 75% of all valvular aortic stenoses
     (2) Unicuspid is most common in neonate and is critical
     (3) More common in males than in females (Wolfe & Wiggins, 1991, p. 438)
   b. Subvalvular aortic stenosis
     (1) Membranous or fibrous ring just below the aortic valve
     (2) The ring forms a diaphragm with a hole
     (2) Accounts for 20% of all aortic stenoses
   c. Supravalvular aortic stenosis
     (1) Associated with a family history, abnormal facies, and mental retardation (Wolfe & Wiggins, 1991, p. 439)
     (2) The least common form of aortic stenosis
     (3) Constriction of the ascending aorta just above the coronary arteries
   d. Hypertrophic subaortic stenosis
     (1) Marked hypertrophy of the entire left ventricle and the ventricular septum
     (2) A family history is often present
4. Frequently associated with other congenital heart defects (Hazinski, 1984, p. 223)

B. Assessment

1. Physical findings
   a. Most are asymptomatic in infancy
   b. Systolic ejection murmur at upper right sternal border (Wolfe & Wiggins, 1991, p. 438)
   c. Thrill in carotid arteries
   d. Systolic click at the apex
   e. Congestive heart failure in severe aortic stenosis
     (1) Peripheral pulses are weak and thready
     (2) Tachypnea
     (3) Increased respiratory effort
     (4) Diaphoresis
     (5) Poor feeding
     (6) Poor weight gain (Hazinski, 1984, p. 224)
2. Diagnostic procedures
   a. Chest x-ray film
     (1) Usually indicates that heart is not enlarged
     (2) Left ventricle is slightly prominent (Wolfe & Wiggins, 1991, p. 439)
   b. Echocardiogram
     (1) Eccentric aortic valve closure
     (2) Moderate to severe aortic obstruction (Hazinski, 1984, p. 224)

C. Nursing Diagnoses (for immediate care)

1. Alteration in tissue perfusion related to decrease in circulating oxygen
2. High risk for alteration in nutrition: less than body requirements related to inadequate sucking, fatigue, and dyspnea

3. High risk for alteration in fluid volume: excess related to cardiac failure
4. Alteration in cardiac output: decrease related to cardiac failure
5. Alteration in respiratory function related to decreased cardiac output
6. Activity intolerance related to insufficient oxygenation secondary to cardiac defect

D. Interventions/Evaluations

1. Alteration in tissue perfusion related to decrease in circulating oxygen
   a. Interventions
      (1) Monitor blood pressure and maintain within normal limits (mean pressure, 30)
      (2) Administer vasopressor medications as per orders; example: dopamine, 5 to 20 mcg/kg/day
      (3) Assess capillary refill: 1 to 4 seconds
      (4) Assess for signs of shock
         (a) Pallor
         (b) Thready pulses
         (c) Hypotension
         (d) Tachycardia
         (e) Poor capillary refill
      (5) Monitor pulse oximetry
   b. Evaluations
      (1) Vital signs and blood pressure remain within normal range
      (2) The neonate remains free of any signs of shock
2. High risk for alteration in nutrition: less than body requirements related to inadequate sucking, fatigue, and dyspnea
   a. Interventions
      (1) Offer feedings frequently and in small amounts
      (2) Use soft nipple and offer frequent rest periods throughout feeding
      (3) Feed via gavage if tachypneic (rates greater than 60 breaths/min)
      (4) Increase calorie content of feeding
         (a) 24 cal/oz
         (b) 27 cal/oz
         (c) 30 cal/oz
   b. Evaluations
      (1) The neonate gains adequate daily weight: 10 to 30 g/day (10 to 15 g/day preterm; 20 to 30 g/day term)
      (2) The neonate does not show signs of fatigue during feeding
3. High risk for alteration in fluid volume: excess related to cardiac failure
   a. Interventions
      (1) Restrict fluids, as ordered
      (2) Monitor intake and output
      (3) Obtain daily weights
      (4) Monitor for signs of fluid overload
         (a) Edema around eyes
         (b) Edema of hands and feet
         (c) Hepatomegaly
         (d) Rales
         (e) Rhonchi
         (f) Cardiac enlargement
         (g) Excessive weight gain
      (5) Offer high-calorie feedings to minimize fluid intake
      (6) Administer diuretic medications per orders
      (7) Monitor electrolytes
   b. Evaluations
      (1) The neonate does not show any signs of fluid overload
      (2) The neonate gains appropriate daily weight while on fluid restriction or diuretic medications, or both

4. Alteration in cardiac output: decrease related to cardiac failure
   a. Interventions
      (1) Consolidate nursing care to minimize handling
      (2) Maintain neutral thermal environment to avoid cold stress
      (3) Minimize crying and agitation by using comfort measures
      (4) Feed by gavage if signs of respiratory distress are present
      (5) Administer medications (such as digitalis) to increase cardiac output per orders
   b. Evaluations
      (1) The neonate shows minimal agitation and crying
      (2) The neonate maintains vital signs and blood pressure within normal ranges
5. Alteration in respiratory function related to decreased cardiac output
   a. Interventions
      (1) Monitor blood gases, vital signs, and pulse oximetry
      (2) Administer oxygen as needed
      (3) Minimize agitation and crying by using comfort measures
      (4) Feed via gavage if signs of respiratory distress are present
   b. Evaluations
      (1) Vital signs and blood gases remain within normal ranges
      (2) The neonate shows minimal agitation and crying
      (3) The neonate does not show signs of respiratory distress
6. Activity intolerance related to insufficient oxygenation secondary to cardiac defect
   a. Interventions
      (1) In non–duct-dependent lesions, increase oxygen concentration when neonate is being suctioned or manipulated for a procedure
      (2) Avoid excessive stimulation; cluster interventions
      (3) Adapt feedings to minimize energy expenditure
         (a) Offer small, frequent feedings
         (b) Use soft nipples with large holes
         (c) Place infant in a position with the head elevated during gavage feeding
         (d) Allow frequent rest periods during feedings
   b. Evaluations
      (1) The neonate tolerates minimal activity without signs of stress
      (2) The neonate maintains a quiet, restful state during rest periods
      (3) The neonate does not become excessively fatigued during feedings and gains adequate weight daily

HEALTH EDUCATION

The parents of a neonate with congenital cardiac disease need education regarding:

A. Signs of cardiac deterioration

B. Any surgical procedures to be performed on their neonate as well as postoperative home care

C. Medication administration, signs of toxicity, and indications for use

D. Activity tolerance of their neonate; organization of care to minimize stress of the infant

E. Respiratory support measures

F. Use of various monitors

G. Sources in the community for emotional support

H. Feeding strategies and formula preparation (if appropriate)

Gastrointestinal Congenital Anomalies

INTRODUCTION

A. Gastrointestinal tract anomalies involve any part of the primitive tube from the hypopharynx to the anal dimple (Filston & Izant, 1986, p. 135)

B. The four most common lesions are

1. Atresia: a complete loss of luminal continuity
2. Stenosis: a narrowing of the bowel wall
3. Duplication: replication of any length of the gastrointestinal tube
4. Functional obstruction: lesions that are not associated with anatomical malformation
   a. Pyloric stenosis
   b. Meconium ileus

CLINICAL PRACTICE

Pyloric Stenosis

A. Introduction

1. Pyloric stenosis is a benign overgrowth of the pyloric musculature
2. Unknown etiology
3. Incidence is approximately 1 in 500 births (Sondheimer & Silverman, 1991, p. 540)
   a. Males are affected three to four times more frequently than females
   b. Incidence is greater in white infants than in Afro-American infants (Benson, 1986, p. 811)
   c. A coincidence of pyloric stenosis can exist in twins and in fathers and sons (Sondheimer & Silverman, 1991, p. 540)

B. Assessment

1. History
   a. Neonate's feeding behaviors
   b. Parent with pyloric stenosis as an infant
2. Physical findings
   a. Vomiting, usually with projectile force
      (1) Starts at birth in 10%
      (2) Usually begins at 2 to 4 weeks of age in 90%
      (3) Does not contain bile
      (4) May be blood streaked
   b. Poor weight gain or weight loss (after the initial birth weight loss of 5 to 10%)
      (1) Appears hungry
      (2) Nurses avidly
      (3) Fails to thrive
   c. Dehydration
   d. Fretfulness
   e. Apathy
   f. Palpable, olive-sized mass in the upper right quadrant (Sondheimer & Silverman, 1991, p. 540)
3. Diagnostic procedures
   a. Upper gastrointestinal barium series x-ray films
      (1) Delay in gastric emptying
      (2) Elongated narrowed pyloric channel ("string sign")
   b. Elevated unconjugated bilirubin level in 2 to 3% of neonates with pyloric stenosis
   c. Hypochloremic alkalosis with potassium depletion

d. Hemoconcentration as evidenced by increased hematocrit and hemoglobin values (Sondheimer & Silverman, 1991, p. 540)

C. Nursing Diagnoses (for immediate care)

1. Altered nutrition: less than body requirements related to vomiting
2. High risk for infection related to aspirational pneumonia secondary to fluid aspiration

D. Interventions/Evaluations

1. Altered nutrition: less than body requirements related to vomiting
   a. Interventions
      (1) Neonate is kept fasting preoperatively
         (a) Hydration is achieved by IV infusion of 80 to 100 cc/kg/day
         (b) Correction of electrolyte imbalance may be necessary
      (2) Postoperatively
         (a) Feedings started with glucose water
         (b) Glucose water feedings are followed by diluted formula feedings every 2 hours until full-strength feedings are instituted at 24 hours post surgery (Mulligan, 1986, p. 342)
   b. Evaluations
      (1) The neonate is adequately hydrated before surgery
      (2) Urine output is at least 2 cc/kg/hr
      (3) The neonate adequately gains weight postoperatively and discontinues projectile vomiting
2. High risk for infection related to aspirational pneumonia secondary to fluid aspiration
   a. Interventions
      (1) Place in side-lying position to facilitate drainage
      (2) Suction nasopharyngeal cavity as necessary
      (3) Monitor respiratory effort, character and quality of sounds bilaterally, and monitor vital signs (see Chapter 37 for a complete discussion of respiratory distress and Chapter 39 for a discussion of neonatal infection)
      (4) If necessary and ordered, administer antibiotic medication
   b. Evaluations
      (1) The neonate does not show any signs of respiratory infection or respiratory distress
      (2) The neonate's nasopharyngeal cavity is free of secretions and emesis

E. Health Education

1. Encourage parents to verbalize their frustrations regarding feeding their neonate and teach them about common feelings among new parents of neonates with anomalies
2. Explain to parents about preparations for surgical procedures and what to expect immediately after surgery
3. Teach parents how to initially feed their neonate following surgery and encourage their participation in the neonate's total presurgical and postsurgical care

Cleft Lip and Cleft Palate

A. Introduction

1. Cleft lip
   a. Can occur with or without cleft palate
   b. Is more common in males
   c. May be unilateral or bilateral (Figs. 42–7, 42–8, and 42–9)

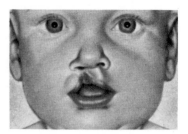

Figure 42–7
Cleft lip. Unilateral incomplete. (Reprinted with permission of Ross Laboratories, Columbus, OH 43216, from Clinical Education Aid. © Ross Laboratories.)

      (1) Complete
      (2) Incomplete
   d. Incidence is 1 in 1000 infants
      (1) With one affected child, the risk is 2 to 4% in the second child
      (2) With one affected parent, the risk is 2 to 4% in the first child
      (3) With two affected children, the risk is 10% in the third child
      (4) With one affected parent and one affected child, the risk is 10 to 20% in the second child (Manchester, Stewart, & Sujansky, 1991, p. 1034)
2. Cleft palate
   a. Isolated cleft palate occurs more frequently in females than in males
      (1) May involve just the soft palate (Fig. 42–10)
      (2) May involve both the soft and the hard palates (Figs. 42–11 and 42–12)
      (3) Can be V- or horseshoe-shaped
   b. Incidence is 1 in 2000 infants
      (1) With one affected child, the risk is 2% in the second child
      (2) With two affected children, the risk is 6 to 8% in the third child
      (3) With one affected parent, the risk is 4 to 6% in the child
      (4) With one affected parent and one affected child, the risk is 15 to 20% in the second child (Manchester, Stewart, & Sujansky, 1991, p. 1034)
3. The incidence of facial clefting has racial variations (Manchester, Stewart, & Sujansky, 1991, p. 1035)
   a. Asians: 1.61 per 1000 live births
   b. Whites: 0.9 per 1000 live births
   c. Afro-Americans: 0.31 per 1000 live births
4. Facial clefting is associated with an increased incidence of other abnormalities, such as congenital heart disease

B. Assessment

1. History
   a. Maternal use of anticonvulsants
   b. Fetal alcohol syndrome
   c. Amniotic band syndrome
   d. Chromosomal abnormalities
2. Physical findings
   a. Unilateral or bilateral visible defect
   b. Flattening or depression of midfacial contour in cleft lip

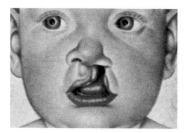

Figure 42–8
Cleft lip. Unilateral complete. (Reprinted with permission of Ross Laboratories, Columbus, OH 43216, from Clinical Education Aid. © Ross Laboratories.)

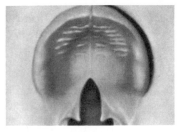

Figure 42–9
Cleft lip. Bilateral complete. (Reprinted with permission of Ross Laboratories, Columbus, OH 43216, from Clinical Education Aid. © Ross Laboratories.)

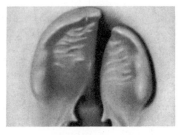

Figure 42–10
Cleft palate. Soft palate only. (Reprinted with permission of Ross Laboratories, Columbus, OH 43216, from Clinical Education Aid. © Ross Laboratories.)

Figure 42–11
Cleft palate. Unilateral complete. (Reprinted with permission of Ross Laboratories, Columbus, OH 43216, from Clinical Education Aid. © Ross Laboratories.)

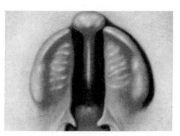

Figure 42–12
Cleft palate. Bilateral complete. (Reprinted with permission of Ross Laboratories, Columbus, OH 43216, from Clinical Education Aid. © Ross Laboratories.)

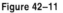

  c. Fissure connecting oral and nasal cavities in cleft palate
  d. Difficulty in sucking
  e. Expulsion of formula or breast milk through the nares
  f. Dehydration
  g. Poor weight gain or weight loss (following the initial birth weight loss of 5 to 10%)

C. Nursing Diagnoses (for immediate care)

1. Altered nutrition: less than body requirements related to inability to adequately suck and swallow
2. High risk for infection related to aspiration pneumonia secondary to fluid aspiration
3. High risk for alteration in parenting related to inadequate bonding secondary to failure to accept impaired infant

D. Interventions/Evaluations

1. Altered nutrition: less than body requirements related to inability to adequately suck and swallow
  a. Interventions
   (1) Feed with a special nipple and bottle set
   (2) Burp frequently
    (a) Tendency to swallow air
    (b) Increased tendency for reflex vomiting
   (3) Follow milk feedings with water to prevent milk crusting in cleft areas
   (4) Feed in upright position with head and chest tilted slightly back to aid swallowing and discourage aspiration
   (5) Feed high-calorie-per-ounce formula to increase caloric intake
   (6) Plot weight gain to determine if pattern indicates adequate caloric intake
   (7) Maintain meticulous oral hygiene
  b. Evaluations
   (1) Neonate is gaining weight appropriate to age
   (2) Neonate is not vomiting feedings
   (3) Neonate is not excessively fatigued after feeding
   (4) Neonate's hunger appears to have been satisfied following feeding
2. High risk for infection related to aspiration pneumonia secondary to fluid aspiration
  a. Interventions
   (1) Place in prone or side-lying position to facilitate drainage
   (2) Suction nasopharyngeal cavity as necessary
   (3) Monitor respiratory effort, character and quality of sounds bilaterally, and monitor vital signs (see Chapter 37 for a complete discussion of respiratory distress and Chapter 39 for a discussion of neonatal infection)
  b. Evaluations
   (1) The neonate does not show any signs of respiratory infection or respiratory distress
   (2) The neonate's nasopharyngeal cavity is free of secretions, emesis, and crusting
3. High risk for alteration in parenting related to inadequate bonding secondary to failure to accept impaired infant
  a. Interventions
   (1) Support parental coping and assist parents with grief over loss of idealized baby
   (2) Encourage parents to verbalize feelings about the defect and the feeding frustrations
   (3) Provide role modeling while interacting with the neonate so that parents can internalize positive interaction

(4) Refer parents to community agencies and support groups
b. Evaluations
(1) Parents are able to freely verbalize their feelings and frustrations about their infant
(2) Parents are involved in the neonate's care in the hospital and frequently seek information about the infant's progress
(3) Parents exhibit bonding behaviors with their infant

E. Health Education

1. Early parental recognition of upper respiratory infections and ways to decrease incidence
2. Use of specialized feeding equipment and appliances for infants with facial clefts
3. Feeding techniques to ensure adequate intake, decrease risks of aspiration, and increase retention of the feeding
4. Signs and symptoms of complications
5. Plans for follow-up care

Anorectal Anomalies

A. Introduction

1. Anorectal anomalies occur at the rate of 1 in 3000 to 4000 births (Sondheimer & Silverman, 1991, p. 549)
a. Incidence is not influenced by mother's age, parity, or race
b. No strong genetic predisposition
2. Anorectal anomalies are classified into six categories (Sondheimer & Silverman, 1991, p. 549)
a. Anterior displacement of anal opening
(1) More common in females than in males
(2) Usually associated with a posterior rectal shelf
b. Anal stenosis
(1) Anal aperture is extremely small
(2) Stools are ribbonlike
(3) Condition accounts for approximately 10% of all anorectal anomalies
c. Imperforate anal membrane
(1) Membrane completely covers the anal aperture
(2) Meconium cannot be passed
d. Anal agenesis
(1) Defective development of the anus
(2) Anal dimple is present
(3) May or may not be associated with a fistula
e. Rectal and anal agenesis
(1) Accounts for 75% of anorectal anomalies
(2) Is almost always associated with a fistula
(3) Is associated with other major congenital malformations
f. Rectal atresia
(1) Anal canal and lower rectum form a blind pouch
(2) Anus is separated by a distance from a blind upper rectal pouch (Sondheimer & Silverman, 1991, p. 549)
3. Most types are more common in males than in females
4. Associated anomalies
a. 10% have associated esophageal atresia and tracheoesophageal fistula
b. Congenital heart disease
c. Vertebral anomalies
d. Renal anomalies
e. Limb dysplasia (Mulligan, 1986, p. 335)

B. Assessment

1. Physical findings
   a. No passage of meconium
      (1) Imperforate anus
      (2) Anal agenesis
      (3) Rectal and anal atresia
   b. Complete absence of anal features
   c. Anal dimple without an opening
   d. Abdominal distension
   e. Constipation: anterior displacement and anal stenosis
   f. Ribbonlike stools
   g. Greenish, bulging membrane in anal area: imperforate anal membrane
   h. No puckering on stimulation of the perianal area
   i. Fistulas
      (1) Vestibular or vaginal in females
      (2) Rectovesical or rectourethral in males (Sondheimer & Silverman, 1991, p. 549)
2. Diagnostic procedures
   a. X-ray film to determine the extent of associated anomalies of the bowel and urogenital tract and any underlying cardiac anomalies
   b. Urine examined for presence of meconium
   c. Passage of a nasogastric tube tests for patency of the esophagus

C. Nursing Diagnoses (for immediate care)

1. Alteration in bowel elimination related to anorectal anomaly
2. High risk for alteration in urinary elimination related to fistulas
3. High risk for alteration in parenting related to inadequate bonding secondary to failure to accept impaired infant

D. Interventions/Evaluations

1. Alteration in bowel elimination related to anorectal anomaly
   a. Interventions
      (1) Monitor meconium passage: should occur within 24 hours after delivery
      (2) Stimulate perianal area to encourage meconium passage if anal aperture is present
      (3) Prepare neonate for surgical procedure if imperforate anal membrane or agenesis is medically diagnosed
         (a) Anal membrane excision for imperforate anal membrane
         (b) Colostomy for all cases of rectal agenesis without a communicating fistula
   b. Evaluations
      (1) Presence or absence of meconium passage is documented
      (2) Neonate with anal stenosis passes meconium with perianal stimulation
2. High risk for alteration in urinary elimination related to fistulas
   a. Interventions
      (1) Measure urinary output
      (2) Monitor urine for presence of meconium
      (3) Monitor for signs of urinary tract infection
   b. Evaluations
      (1) Urinary output is adequate
      (2) No meconium is present in the urine
      (3) The neonate does not have any signs of urinary tract infection
3. High risk for alteration in parenting related to inadequate bonding secondary to failure to accept impaired infant
   a. Interventions
      (1) Support parental coping and assist parents with grief over loss of idealized infant

(2) Encourage parents to verbalize feelings about the defect

(3) Provide role modeling while interacting with the neonate so that parents can internalize positive interaction

(4) Refer parents to community agencies and support groups for parents of infants with colostomies

(5) Praise all parental efforts to provide care for the neonate in the hospital

b. Evaluations

(1) Parents are able to freely verbalize their feelings about their infant

(2) Parents are involved in the neonate's care in the hospital and frequently seek information about the infant's progress

(3) Parents exhibit bonding behaviors with their infant

E. Health Education

1. Type of defect and procedures to correct the defect
2. Colostomy care
3. Community resources (such as supply companies)

Omphalocele and Gastroschisis

A. Introduction

1. Omphalocele is a herniation of the intestine and liver into the base of the umbilical cord that occurs between the 11th and 12th weeks of gestation when the alimentation tract should have withdrawn back into the fetal abdomen

   a. The smaller defects contain one or two loops of bowel

   b. The larger defects can contain the liver, spleen, and a major portion of the intestines (Coran, 1978, p. 190)

   c. Incidence is 1 in 10,000 births (Sondheimer & Silverman, 1991, p. 545)

   d. There is no defect of the abdominal wall

   e. Cardiac anomalies are associated with 20% of the neonates with omphalocele (Sondheimer & Silverman, 1991, p. 545)

2. Gastroschisis is a herniation of the bowel and other viscera through a defect in the abdominal wall

   a. There is no covering over the eviscerated organs

   b. The eviscerated bowel loops are dark red and edematous and covered with a gelatinous layer that is adherent

   c. All neonates with gastroschisis have associated malrotation and some degree of congenital shortening of the small bowel (Sondheimer & Silverman, 1991, p. 545)

   d. The incidence is 1 in 10,000 to 15,000 live births

   e. Intestinal atresias are frequently associated with gastroschisis

   f. Preterm birth occurs in 40% of neonates with gastroschisis

B. Assessment

1. History

   a. Polyhydramnios

   b. Visualization by ultrasonography

   c. Elevated maternal serum alpha-fetoprotein

   d. Preterm labor in the case of gastroschisis

2. Physical findings

   a. Visible defect over the abdominal area

   (1) Omphalocele is covered with a sac consisting of peritoneum and amniotic membrane (Schuster, 1986, p. 741)

   (2) Gastroschisis defect exposes viscera because of lack of any covering

   b. Intrauterine growth retardation (gastroschisis)

C. Nursing Diagnoses (for immediate care in the delivery room)

1. Impaired skin integrity related to congenital abdominal defect

2. High risk for fluid volume deficit because of lack of skin integrity and exposed abdominal contents
3. High risk for infection because of lack of skin integrity
4. High risk for alteration in body temperature because of evaporative loss

D. Interventions/Evaluations

1. Impaired skin integrity related to congenital abdominal defect
   a. Intervention (immediate): cover defect with warm, normal saline–moistened sterile gauze and place plastic wrap over dressing
   b. Evaluations
      (1) No further impairment of skin integrity occurs
      (2) Omphalocele sac remains intact
      (3) Herniated viscera remain normal in color and remain moist
2. High risk for fluid volume deficit related to lack of skin integrity and exposed abdominal contents
   a. Interventions (immediate)
      (1) IV fluids and albumin
      (2) Keep fasting
      (3) Keep the dressing moist
      (4) Monitor glucose levels and electrolytes
      (5) Insert nasogastric tube to decompress bowel
   b. Evaluations
      (1) Hydration is maintained
      (2) Loops of bowel protruding through the defect do not distend
3. High risk for infection because of lack of skin integrity
   a. Interventions (immediate)
      (1) Maintain sterility of dressing
      (2) Position neonate to prevent any trauma or pressure on the defect
      (3) Administer antibiotics per orders
   b. Evaluations
      (1) No evidence of further trauma to the defect
      (2) No signs or symptoms of infection
4. High risk for alteration in body temperature because of evaporative loss
   a. Interventions (immediate)
      (1) Place in isolette and maintain thermal neutral environment
      (2) Keep moistened dressings warm to prevent heat loss
      (3) Minimize neonate's exposure to moist bedding
   b. Evaluation: neonate's temperature remains within normal limits

E. Health Education

1. Parents are grieving the loss of an idealized perfect baby and need anticipatory guidance about the normal grief process
2. Parents need to know what to expect before birth, if at all possible
3. Parents need to know about treatment and procedures planned for their infant
4. Referral to community resources

Tracheoesophageal Fistula and Esophageal Atresia

A. Introduction

1. Tracheoesophageal fistula (TEF) and esophageal atresia are associated conditions that are characterized by a blind esophageal pouch and, possibly, a fistulous connection between the esophagus and the trachea
2. The defect occurs during the fourth to sixth gestational weeks
3. The incidence is 1 in 4425 live births (Coran, 1978, p. 46)
4. There are five variations of this defect
   a. Esophageal atresia with distal TEF is the most common form of the defect and occurs in 85% of neonates with esophageal atresia (Fig. 42–13)

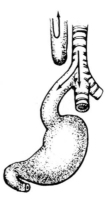

Figure 42–13
Esophageal atresia with distal tracheoesophageal fistula. (From Whaley, L.F., Wong, D.L. [1991]. *Nursing care of infants and children* [4th ed.] [p. 498.]. St. Louis, MO: Mosby–Year Book, Inc.)

    b. Esophageal atresia without a fistula and with an intact tracheobronchial tree occurs in 8% of neonates with the defect (Fig. 42–14)

    c. A third variation of TEF is characterized by an abnormal fistulous connection between an otherwise normal trachea and esophagus; this variation, also called an H-type fistula, occurs in 4% of neonates with the defect (Fig. 42–15)

    d. An esophageal atresia with a proximal TEF is a rare variation occurring in only 1% of neonates with the defect (Fig. 42–16)

    e. An esophageal atresia with a proximal TEF and a distal TEF is another rare variation and occurs in only 1% of neonates with the defect (Fig. 42–17)

5. Vertebral, cardiac, renal, and anal anomalies are associated with TEF
6. Pneumonia and actelectasis frequently occur in the right upper lobe
7. All forms of TEF and esophageal atresia must be surgically corrected

B. Assessment

1. History: polyhydramnios related to the high level of gastrointestinal obstruction
2. Physical findings
    a. Excessive, bubbling mucous secretions requiring urgent and frequent suctioning
    b. Continuous drooling
    c. Choking
    d. Abdominal distension beginning soon after birth because of inspired air entering the stomach
    e. Respiratory distress
        (1) Retractions
        (2) Nasal flaring
        (3) Expiratory grunt
        (4) Seesaw respirations

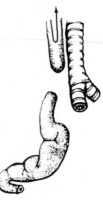

Figure 42–14
Esophageal atresia without a fistula and with an intact tracheobronchial tree. (From Whaley, L.F., Wong, D.L. [1991]. *Nursing care of infants and children* [4th ed.] [p. 498.]. St. Louis, MO: Mosby–Year Book, Inc.)

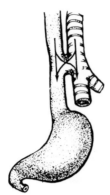

Figure 42–15
Tracheoesophageal fistula with abnormal fistulous connection between trachea and esophagus (H-type fistula). (From Whaley, L.F., Wong, D.L. [1991]. *Nursing care of infants and children* [4th ed.] [p. 498.]. St. Louis, MO: Mosby–Year Book, Inc.)

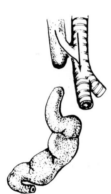

Figure 42–16
Esophageal atresia with proximal tracheoesophageal fistula. (From Whaley, L.F., Wong, D.L. [1991]. *Nursing care of infants and children* [4th ed.] [p. 498.]. St. Louis, MO: Mosby–Year Book, Inc.)

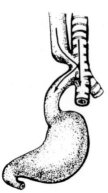

Figure 42–17
Esophageal atresia with proximal tracheoesophageal fistula and distal tracheoesophageal fistula. (From Whaley, L.F., Wong, D.L. [1991]. *Nursing care of infants and children* [4th ed.] [p. 498.]. St. Louis, MO: Mosby–Year Book, Inc.)

(5) Tachypnea

(6) Cyanosis: central and peripheral

(7) Diminished breath sounds bilaterally

(8) Rhonchi

  f. Immediate regurgitation of feedings

  g. Tachycardia

3. Diagnostic procedures

  a. Unsuccessful attempt to pass a nasogastric tube

  b. Chest x-ray film

    (1) Visualization of the blind pouch with nasogastric tube curled in it

    (2) Gas can be visualized in the abdomen if there is a distal TEF

C. Nursing Diagnoses (for immediate care)

1. Ineffective airway clearance because of immobility of secretions
2. Ineffective breathing pattern related to fistulous connection between trachea and esophagus
3. Alteration in nutrition: less than body requirements related to esophageal atresia
4. Fluid volume deficit secondary to esophageal drainage, frequent suctioning, and fasting status

D. Interventions/Evaluations

1. Ineffective airway clearance because of immobility of secretions

  a. Interventions

    (1) Place nasogastric tube and connect to low intermittent suction

    (2) Place in warmed isolette

    (3) Elevate the head of the bed 20° to 40° to prevent reflux of gastric contents

    (4) Keep fasting

    (5) Place the neonate on cardiac and respiratory monitors

  b. Evaluations

    (1) Excessive secretions are removed

    (2) Airway remains patent

    (3) Apnea or bradycardia or both are quickly detected and treated

2. Ineffective breathing pattern related to fistulous connection between trachea and esophagus

  a. Interventions

    (1) Keep neonate from crying because crying can cause air to pass through the fistula and distend the abdomen, causing greater respiratory distress

    (2) Keep fasting

    (3) Administer oxygen as needed

    (4) Monitor respiratory status and keep intubation equipment in a location that is close to the neonate

  b. Evaluations

    (1) Neonate cries only minimally and abdomen does not distend

    (2) Signs of respiratory distress are minimized

3. Alteration in nutrition: less than body requirements related to esophageal atresia

  a. Interventions

    (1) Establish IV to maintain hydration

    (2) Administer parenteral dextrose solution to maintain blood glucose levels within normal limits

    (3) Monitor intake and output

    (4) Monitor electrolyte and glucose levels

  b. Evaluations

    (1) Neonate shows signs of adequate hydration

    (2) Blood glucose levels remain within the normal limits of 45 to 90 mg/dl

    (3) Urine output is at least 2 cc/kg/hr

4. Fluid volume deficit secondary to espohageal drainage, frequent suctioning, and fasting status
   a. Interventions
      (1) IV fluids at the rate of 80 to 100 cc/kg/day
      (2) Warmed isolette to prevent insensible water loss
   b. Evaluations
      (1) Neonate shows signs of adequate hydration
      (2) Urine output is at least 2 cc/kg/hr

E. **Health Education**

1. Parents are grieving the loss of a perfect baby; they need anticipatory guidance about the normal grief process
2. Parents need to be kept informed by clarifying and reinforcing the physician's explanations about the malformation, surgical repair, preoperative and post-operative care of the infant, and the prognosis; parents' questions should be encouraged
3. Parents should be instructed on how to be involved in their infant's care while in the hospital
4. Explain to the parents staged repair, provision of a gastrostomy and ligation of the fistula, and repair of the atresia

Hydrocephalus

A. Introduction

A. Congenital hydrocephalus is characterized by a state of progressive ventricular enlargement in association with an increased volume of cerebrospinal fluid

B. In communicating hydrocephalus, the cerebrospinal fluid can circulate through the ventricular system and into the subarachnoid space unobstructed

C. In noncommunicating hydrocephalus, the cerebrospinal fluid is blocked by an obstruction in the ventricular system or the blockage occurs from the ventricular system into the subarachnoid space

D. The anomaly occurs at approximately the sixth week of gestation

E. The incidence of congenital hydrocephalus is 1 in 2000 births

1. Caused by congenital malformation
2. Associated with other anomalies
   a. Spina bifida
   b. Myelomeningocele
   c. Renal defects
   d. Cardiac defects
   e. Colon and anal agenesis
   f. Cleft lip and palate
   g. Chromosomal anomalies (Romero, 1988, p. 22)

Clinical Practice

A. Assessment

1. History
   a. Ultrasound test shows enlarged head
   b. Cephalopelvic disproportion
   c. Cesarean section delivery

2. Physical findings
   a. Head circumference greater than the 90th percentile for gestation
   b. Enlarged or full fontanelles
   c. Wide or split suture lines
   d. "Setting sun" eyes
   e. Excessive rate of head growth
   f. Impaired extraocular movement
   g. Hypertonia of the lower extremities
   h. Generalized hyper-reflexia
   i. Vomiting
3. Diagnostic procedures
   a. Computed tomographic (CT) scan
   b. Magnetic resonance imaging (MRI)
   c. Ultrasound test
   d. Plotting of the head circumference

B. Nursing Diagnoses (for immediate care)

1. Impaired physical mobility secondary to increased size and weight of the head
2. High risk for alteration in skin integrity secondary to increased size and weight of the head

C. Interventions/Evaluations

1. Impaired physical mobility secondary to increased size and weight of the head
   a. Interventions
      (1) Provide extra support of the neonate's head and neck while providing care and performing procedures
      (2) Change head position frequently (every 2 hours), maintaining proper alignment to ensure a patent airway
   b. Evaluations
      (1) The neonate has adequate support of the head
      (2) Airway remains patent and uncompromised by position
2. High risk for alteration in skin integrity secondary to increased size and weight of head
   a. Interventions
      (1) Clean and dry skin creases after feeding or vomiting
      (2) Use sheepskin under head or place infant on a waterbed or an egg crate mattress
      (3) Reposition neonate's head every 2 hours
      (4) Monitor any reddened areas, and position infant away from any questionable areas
   b. Evaluation: neonate's skin will remain intact and show no signs of beginning breakdown

Health Education

A. Parents need education regarding the shunting procedure

B. Parents need physician's explanations clarified and reinforced

C. Instruct parents about ways in which they can become involved in the infant's care while in the hospital

D. Encourage parents to ask questions and to express their concerns

E. Parents are grieving the loss of an idealized perfect baby; they need anticipatory guidance about the normal grief process (see Chapter 25 for a complete discussion of grief)

F. Referral to community resources and support groups

Spina Bifida

Introduction

A. Spina bifida is a malformation of the spine in which the posterior portion of the laminae of the vertebrae fails to close during the fourth week of gestation

B. The incidence is 1 in 1000 to 1200 births (Epstein, 1986, p. 1425)

1. Occurs more frequently in females than in males
2. Most commonly caused by multifactorial inheritance in which genes interact with environmental factors
3. Incidence varies according to geographic area and ethnic differences
   a. Occurs more frequently on the British Isles
   b. Occurs more frequently in whites

C. Spina bifida is the most common congenital malformation of the central nervous system

D. Spina bifida is divided into two categories: ventral defects and dorsal defects

1. Ventral defects
   a. Are extremely rare
   b. Involve the splitting of the vertebral body and the presence of a cyst that is neurenteric in origin (Romero, 1988, p. 37)
   c. The lesion is usually seen in the lower cervical and upper thoracic vertebrae
2. Dorsal defects
   a. Dorsal defects are the most common
   b. Dorsal defects are subdivided into two categories: spina bifida occulta and spina bifida aperta
      (1) Spina bifida occulta
         (a) The defect is limited to the vertebrae, with no visible external defect other than perhaps a tuft of hair (Fig. 42–18)
         (b) The spinal cord and meninges are normal; therefore there are usually no symptoms
         (c) It is the most common type of spina bifida and has been estimated to occur in close to 25% of all normal children (Peterson, 1986, p. 377)
      (2) Spina bifida aperta (Fig. 42–19)
         (a) Accounts for 85% of all visible dorsal defects
         (b) Meningocele
            (i) Cord membranes protrude through an opening in the vertebrae, forming a cyst filled with cerebrospinal fluid and covered with either a thin meningeal membrane or skin
            (ii) The cord and nerve roots are normal

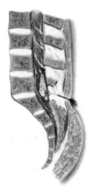

Figure 42–18
Dermal sinus tract with dermoid cyst. (Reprinted with permission of Ross Laboratories, Columbus, OH 43216, from Clinical Education Aid. © Ross Laboratories.)

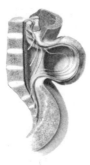

Figure 42–19
Myelomeningocele. (Reprinted with permission of Ross Laboratories, Columbus, OH 43216, from Clinical Education Aid. © Ross Laboratories.)

        (iii) Hydrocephalus is associated in 9% of neonates with this type of lesion (Peterson, 1986, p. 377)
    (c) Myelomeningocele (see Fig. 42–19)
        (i) Both spinal cord and membranes protrude through an opening in the vertebrae
        (ii) Poorly epithelialized, bluish sac with irregular dimpling
        (iii) The lesion often has a raw, ulcerated area overlying neural tissue
        (iv) Lesion usually occurs in the lumbar area
        (v) Function distal to the lesion is usually absent or severely compromised
        (vi) Hydrocephalus is associated with 75% of neonates with this type of lesion
        (vii) Other associated anomalies are
            • Arnold-Chiari malformation of the brain, in which there is an elongation and downward displacement of the cerebellar midline and midbrain deformity
            • Dislocation of the hips
            • Talipes equinovarus (clubfoot)
            • Congenital scoliosis (Peterson, 1986, p. 377)
        (viii) Only about 60% are operable (surgical reduction)

Clinical Practice

A. Assessment

1. History
   a. Elevated maternal serum alpha-fetoprotein levels
   b. Ultrasound visualization of the defect
   c. A parent or sibling with spina bifida (increases incidence)
   d. Hydrocephalic fetus
2. Physical findings
   a. Presence of a spinal lesion
   b. Tuft of hair over sinus tract in lumbar area (spina bifida occulta)
   c. Enlarged head circumference: hydrocephalus
   d. Lack of spontaneous movement of the lower extremities
   e. Hip clicks: congenital hip dislocation
   f. Clubfoot
   g. Scoliosis
   h. Flaccid or spastic muscles in the lower extremities
   i. Urine and stool leakage

B. Nursing Diagnoses (for immediate care in the delivery room)

1. High risk for infection related to rupture of the sac or open lesion secondary to spinal defect
2. Ineffective thermoregulation related to an open lesion secondary to spinal defect

C. Interventions/Evaluations

1. High risk for infection related to rupture of the sac or open lesion secondary to spinal defect
   a. Interventions
      (1) Place neonate only in prone or side-lying position
      (2) Cover the lesion with sterile, moist dressings
      (3) Keep meconium or urine away from lesion
      (4) Administer antibiotics per orders
   b. Evaluations
      (1) The membranous sac stays intact
      (2) Aseptic environment is maintained around and over the lesion
      (3) The neonate does not show any signs of infection
2. Ineffective thermoregulation related to an open lesion secondary to spinal defect
   a. Interventions
      (1) Immediately place neonate in a prone position in a thermal neutral environment
      (2) Provide sterile, warm, moist covering for lesion and cover with plastic wrap to prevent evaporative loss of heat
      (3) Minimize neonate's exposure to moist bedding
   b. Evaluation: neonate maintains body temperature within the range of normal limits

Health Education

A. Parents need education about realistic expectations for their infant and education about surgical reduction and shunting procedures, if applicable

B. Parents need the physician's explanations clarified and reinforced

C. Instruct parents about ways in which they can become involved in the infant's care while in the hospital

D. Encourage parents to ask questions and to express their concerns

E. Parents are grieving the loss of an idealized perfect baby and will need anticipatory guidance about the normal grieving process (see Chapter 25 for complete discussion about grief)

F. Referral to community resources, support groups, and developmental and medical follow-up

Congenital Diaphragmatic Hernia

Introduction

A. Congenital diaphragmatic hernia is a malformation that consists of herniation of abdominal organs into the thorax related to a defect in the diaphragm (Rosenberg & Battaglia, 1991, p. 89)

1. Defect occurs from incomplete embryonic formation of the diaphragm
2. The left side of the diaphragm is involved much more frequently (90%) than the right side (Reid, 1986, p. 477)
   a. In left-sided involvement, the intestines, stomach, and spleen compress the lung
   b. Compression during fetal life causes hypoplasia or dysplasia of the lung or both

B. Abdominal contents in the thorax cause a mediastinal shift, which can result in

1. Interference with venous return to the heart
2. Reduction in cardiac output
3. Metabolic acidosis

C. **Diaphragmatic hernia causes complete compromise of ventilation on the involved side and, if the defect is large, additional compromise on the unaffected side**

1. Severe and dramatic respiratory distress is usually seen immediately following birth
2. The most severely affected neonates will typically gasp a few times at birth but never really establish respiration
3. If the respiratory distress is only moderate at birth, it usually progresses at an alarming rate as the intestine in the chest cavity expands with the normal entry of swallowed air (Korones, 1986, p. 281)

D. **Diaphragmatic hernia occurs at the rate of 1 in 2200 to 8000 live births**

E. **Mortality rate for neonates with this anomaly is 50%, with survival dependent upon**

1. The degree of hypoplasia in the contralateral lung
2. Rapid diagnosis and immediate surgical intervention to repair the defect in the diaphragm
3. The degree of persistent pulmonary hypertension following defect repair

F. **Complications associated with diaphragmatic hernia are**

1. Malrotation of the gut
2. Opposite side pneumothorax
3. Persistent pulmonary hypertension

Clinical Practice

A. **Assessment**

1. History
   a. Term or post-term
   b. Polyhydramnios is present in more than 50% (Korones, 1986, p. 281)
2. Physical findings
   a. Large- or barrel-chested
   b. Scaphoid abdomen
   c. Respiratory distress (ranges from mild to life threatening)
      (1) Difficulty in initiating respiration
      (2) Gasping respirations
      (3) Retractions and nasal flaring
      (4) Cyanosis
      (5) Decreased or absent breath sounds on the side of the hernia
   d. Displacement of the cardiac impulse to one side of the chest
   e. Infrequent bowel sounds may be heard in the chest
   f. Asymmetrical chest expansion
3. Diagnostic procedures
   a. Chest x-ray film
      (1) Diaphragmatic margin is absent on the defective side
      (2) Presence of loops of intestine in the chest cavity, which may be gas filled, giving a multicystic appearance
      (3) Mediastinal shift to the opposite side
   b. Arterial blood gas assay
      (1) Hypoxemia
      (2) Respiratory acidosis
      (3) Metabolic acidosis

B. Nursing Diagnoses (for immediate care)

1. Impaired gas exchange related to decreased ventilation secondary to hypoplastic lung
2. Alteration in tissue perfusion related to cardiopulmonary dysfunction secondary to pulmonary hypertension

C. Interventions/Evaluations

1. Impaired gas exchange related to decreased ventilation secondary to hypoplastic lung
   a. Interventions
      (1) Delivery room resuscitation
         (a) Neonate must be immediately intubated; bag-and-mask ventilation must be avoided because air can be forced into the intestine, which will further compromise lung space in the chest
         (b) Mechanical ventilation pressures should be kept at a minimal level to avoid pneumothorax
         (c) Administer 100% oxygen to increase the PaO_2 and decrease persistent pulmonary hypertension
      (2) Gastric decompression should be initiated by inserting a large-bore nasogastric tube and advancing it as far as possible
      (3) Positioning
         (a) Place in high semi-Fowler's position so that gravity can help keep abdominal organ pressure off of the diaphragm
         (b) Turn the neonate onto the affected side to allow unaffected lung to expand
   b. Evaluation: the neonate's respiratory effort receives optimal support until emergency surgical intervention occurs
2. Alteration in tissue perfusion related to cardiopulmonary dysfunction secondary to pulmonary hypertension
   a. Interventions
      (1) Hyperoxygenate to minimize hypoxemia
      (2) Ventilate with small tidal volumes at a rapid respiratory rate to provide oxygenation and decrease risk of pneumothorax
   b. Evaluation: further respiratory compromise is minimized and tissue perfusion is maintained until emergency surgical intervention occurs

Health Education

A. Explain the nature of the defect to the parents calmly and in simple terms

1. Parents will be in an emotional state of shock, and simple terms will aid comprehension
2. Attitude of health professionals toward the neonate's crisis and defect will influence the parents' reactions

B. Once the infant has been stabilized and transferred to surgery, parents will need careful and complete explanations

1. Encourage parents and family to ask questions and express concerns about the crisis
2. Dispel any myths regarding the etiology of the defect and any guilt assumed by either parent

C. Parents will be simultaneously mourning the loss of a perfect newborn and coping with the threat of the infant's death

1. Family members and friends who are present to support the parents can be taught some simple crisis intervention techniques
2. Family members and friends can be taught the importance of "silent" presence and active listening to support the parents during the time of crisis

CASE STUDIES AND STUDY QUESTIONS

Baby J. is a 4-hour-old term neonate who was delivered via a spontaneous, vaginal delivery to a 28-year-old mother. The only problem throughout the pregnancy was polyhydramnios. His 1- and 5-minute Apgar scores were 8 and 9, respectively. In the term nursery he has a heart rate of 140 beats/min and a respiratory rate of 54. Baby J. has required frequent oral suctioning with a bulb syringe because of excessive bubbly secretions in his mouth.

1. Excessive bubbly secretions from Baby J.'s mouth are most indicative of

    a. A stressful labor and birth.

    b. A cardiac defect.

    c. Pyloric stenosis.

    d. Tracheoesophageal fistula.

2. Another assessment that supports the conclusion reached in question 1 is

    a. The 1-minute Apgar score.

    b. A history of polyhydramnios.

    c. His tachycardia.

    d. His tachypnea.

3. Based on the answer given in question 1, what other anomaly or problem is associated with Baby J.'s condition?

    a. Meconium aspiration syndrome.

    b. Polydactylism

    c. Renal anomaly.

    d. Intraventricular hemorrhage.

At delivery, it was discovered that Baby T., a term female, had a myelomeningocele. Her mother refused alpha-fetoprotein screening early in the pregnancy. She also didn't want to hear anything about the types of defects alpha-fetoprotein screening detects or anything about defects at all. She firmly felt that if a pregnant woman thinks about abnormalities in the baby that she is carrying, those abnormalities frequently occur.

4. Baby T.'s myelomeningocele

    a. Contains both spinal cord and meninges protruding through an open defect in her back.

    b. Contains only meninges protruding through an open defect in her back.

    c. Is most likely in the thoracic region of her back because that is the most common location of myelomeningocele.

    d. Would be classified as a type of spina bifida occulta that causes all function distal to the lesion to be absent.

5. Baby T. should be carefully assessed for the following associated anomaly

    a. Congenital hip dislocation.

    b. Pyloric stenosis.

    c. Tracheoesophageal atresia.

    d. Imperforate anus.

6. Baby T. is at high risk for associated hydrocephalus. With her type of lesion, what percentage of neonates have hydrocephaly?

    a. 45%

    b. 60%

    c. 75%

    d. 90%

7. Baby T.'s mother is extremely upset. Between her sobs, she wants to know how this could have happened to her baby. She says she was very careful not to think about abnormalities during her pregnancy, she did everything right, and her baby should be perfect just the way she dreamed her baby would be. The nurse's best response is based on the understanding that

    a. Baby T.'s mother did not have enough information about alpha-fetoprotein screening early in her pregnancy.

    b. Baby T.'s mother had dreamed about having the perfect baby, which indicates that had she known about the neural tube defect early in the pregnancy she would have electively aborted.

    c. Baby T.'s mother is extremely immature based upon the feeling that just because she did everything right her baby should be perfect.

    d. Mothers frequently fantasize during pregnancy about having a healthy, perfect baby, and when a baby with an anomaly is born, the mother must grieve the loss of her perfect baby.

Baby L. was delivered by cesarean section for nonprogressive labor at 38 weeks' gestation because of cephalopelvic disproportion. Her mother is an insulin-dependent diabetic. Baby L. is large for gestational age. Her Apgar scores were 9 at 1 minute and 9 at 5 minutes. She was admitted to the term nursery with orders to begin glucose feedings and monitor her serum glucose levels. By day 3, she became progressively intolerant of her feedings, becoming tachypneic with each feeding. Her color remains pink. Baby L.'s mother complains that it is taking her longer and longer to feed and that the baby seems to tire easily.

8. Based on Baby L.'s history, she is at a higher risk for and is showing signs of

    a. Transposition of the great vessels.

    b. Diaphragmatic hernia.

    c. Tetralogy of Fallot.

    d. A ventricular septal defect.

9. Based upon the answer to question 8, you would expect Baby L.'s chest x-ray to show

    a. Left and right ventricular hypertrophy.

    b. A boot-shaped appearance of the heart.

    c. Left atrial hypertrophy.

    d. Mediastinal shift to the opposite side of the defect.

Baby G. is a term neonate just delivered after a 13-hour labor without any complications. His Apgar scores are 9 and 9 at 1 and 5 minutes, respectively. On admission to the term nursery, the nurse performing the physical assessment discovers that Baby G. has an anal dimple but no anal aperture.

10. One of the first procedures done by the nurse is to insert a nasogastric tube in Baby G. The purpose of this is

    a. To obtain a gastric specimen for culture.

    b. To determine if Baby G. has an associated tracheoesophageal anomaly.

    c. To lavage Baby G.'s stomach.

    d. To remove the accumulation of amniotic fluid Baby G. swallowed during

the birth process because there is no outlet.

11. Another initial procedure that the nursery nurse performed was to place a urine collection bag on Baby G. Baby G. voided shortly after, and a urine specimen was obtained. It is important to examine the urine for

    a. The presence of bacteria.

    b. The presence of WBCs.

    c. The presence of meconium.

    d. The presence of bilirubin.

12. A term infant develops severe respiratory distress within minutes after birth. On physical examination, the chest is hyperexpanded and the point of maximal impulse (PMI) is shifted to the right. Which of the following is the most likely cause for this infant's respiratory distress?

    a. Diaphragmatic hernia.

    b. Congenital pneumonia.

    c. Right pneumothorax.

    d. Transposition of the great vessels.

13. Transposition of the great vessels

    a. Occurs more frequently in females than in males at a ratio of $3:1$.

    b. Is an embryonic abnormality in the spiral division of the truncus arteriosus.

    c. Is classified as an acyanotic congenital heart disease with a left-to-right shunt.

    d. Is usually associated with renal and musculoskeletal anomalies in the neonate.

14. Signs in the neonate that indicate a diaphragmatic hernia may include

    a. Respiratory distress.

    b. Decreased breath sounds on the affected side.

    c. Presence of a scaphoid abdomen.

    d. Bile-stained emesis.

    e. a and b.

    f. All except d.

Baby B. is a 3-day-old term infant born by cesarean section for fetal distress. His Apgar scores were 8 and 9 at 1 and 5 minutes, respectively. He is a fretful baby who frequently sucks his fist, nurses vigorously at the breast, and always seems hungry. His mother has reported that since her milk has "come in," Baby B. nurses quickly, gulps the milk, and then vomits almost all of it and seems immediately hungry again. She reports that he has done this for the last three consecutive feedings but had been nursing well before her milk came in.

15. In the absence of any other signs, Baby B.'s problems are most indicative of

   a. Tracheoesophageal fistula.

   b. Consumption of too much milk in too short a period of time.

   c. Pyloric stenosis.

   d. An uncoordinated suck-and-swallow reflex, which is causing him to gulp, then vomit.

16. Based upon the answer to question 15, when you ask Baby B.'s mother further about her baby's feeding problem you would not be surprised to hear the following additional information

   a. Baby B. chokes, sputters, and constantly dribbles milk while he is feeding.

   b. Baby B. has projectile vomiting.

   c. Baby B. becomes cyanotic during his vigorous feedings.

   d. Baby B.'s emesis has a greenish tinge because of bile staining.

17. All of the following statements about cleft lip and palate are true with the exception of

   a. The risk of incidence is increased if a parent, a sibling, or both have the defect.

   b. Cleft lip is more common than cleft palate.

   c. Isolated cleft palate occurs more frequently in females than in males.

   d. There are no variations of incidence in facial clefting, that can be solely attributed to race.

Baby O. was born at 36 weeks' gestation. On admission to the newborn nursery, the baby's respiratory rate was 80, her color was pink, and her cry was lusty. Two hours later, Baby O.'s respiratory rate was 78 and she had developed slight retractions. Auscultation of her heart revealed a harsh murmur that was best heard at a location that is high on the left sternal border, just under the left clavicle at the second intercostal space.

18. Baby O.'s signs are most indicative of

   a. A patent ductus arteriosus.

   b. An atrial septal defect.

   c. Coarctation of the aorta.

   d. Aortic stenosis.

19. Based upon your answer to question 18, you would expect the following finding on Baby O.'s chest x-ray

   a. Dilation of the main pulmonary artery.

   b. Prominent pulmonary venous congestion.

   c. Left ventricular enlargement.

   d. Normal heart size.

20. All of the following statements regarding gastroschisis are true with the exception of

   a. There is an increased incidence of preterm birth associated with gastroschisis.

   b. If the gastroschisis includes a defect in the abdominal wall, it is classified as an omphalocele.

   c. There is no skin covering the eviscerated organs.

   d. Intestinal atresias are frequently associated with gastroschisis.

Answers to Study Questions

1. d	2. b	3. c
4. a	5. a	6. c
7. d	8. d	9. a
10. b	11. c	12. a
13. b	14. f	15. c
16. b	17. d	18. a
19. d	20. b	

REFERENCES

Benson, C. (1986). Infantile hypertropic pyloric stenosis. In K. Welch (Ed.), *Pediatric surgery: Vol. 2* (4th ed.). Chicago: Year Book.

Coran, A. (1978). Omphalocele, gastroschisis and other anomalies of the abdominal wall. In *Surgery of the neonate* (pp. 196–202). Boston: Little, Brown.

Epstein, M. (1986). Spina bifida and hydrocephalus. In K. Welch (Ed.), *Pediatric surgery: Vol. 2* (4th ed.) (pp. 1436–1440). Chicago: Year Book.

Filston, H., & Izant, R. (1986). Congenital anomalies presenting with obstructive gastrointestinal symptoms. In M. Klaus & A. Fanaroff (Eds.), *Care of the high-risk neonate* (3rd ed.) (pp. 135–136). Philadelphia: Saunders.

Fink, B. (1985). *Congenital heart disease* (2nd ed.). Chicago: Year Book.

Hazinski, M. (1984). *Nursing care of the critically ill child* (pp. 63–250). St. Louis: Mosby.

Korones, S. (1986). *High-risk newborn infants* (4th ed.). St. Louis: Mosby.

Manchester, D., Stewart, J., & Sujansky, E. (1991). Genetics and dysmorphology. In W. Hathaway, J. Groothuis, W. Hay, & J. Paisley (Eds.), *Current pediatric diagnosis and treatment* (10th ed.) (pp. 1016–1049). Norwalk: Appleton & Lange.

Mulligan, K. (1986). Gastrointestinal disorders. In N. Streeter (Ed.), *High-risk neonatal care* (pp. 315–346). Rockville, MD: Aspen.

Olds, S., London, M., & Ladewig, P. (1988). *Maternal newborn nursing* (3rd ed.). Menlo Park: Addison-Wesley.

Parks, M. (1984). *Pediatric cardiology for practitioners* (2nd ed.) (pp. 123–193). Chicago: Year Book.

Peterson, P. (1986). Neurologic assessment in the neonate. In N. Streeter (Ed.), *High-risk neonatal care* (pp. 365–380). Rockville, MD: Aspen.

Reid, T. (1986). Transport of the high-risk neonate. In N. Streeter (Ed.), *High-risk neonatal care* (pp. 477–510). Rockville, MD: Aspen.

Romero, R. (1988). Central nervous system. In *Prenatal diagnosis of congenital anomalies* (pp. 46–53, 220–223). Norwalk: Appleton & Lange.

Rosenberg, A., & Battaglia, F. (1991). The newborn infant. In W. Hathaway, J. Groothuis, W. Hay, & J. Paisley (Eds.), *Current pediatric diagnosis and treatment* (10th ed.) (pp. 50–103). Norwalk: Appleton & Lange.

Schuster, S. (1986). Omphalocele and gastroschisis. In K. Welch (Ed.), *Pediatric surgery: Vol. 2* (4th ed.) (pp. 740–747). Chicago: Year Book.

Sondheimer, J., & Silverman, A. (1991). Gastrointestinal tract. In W. Hathaway, J. Groothuis, W. Hay, & J. Paisley (Eds.), *Current pediatric diagnosis and treatment* (10th ed.) (pp. 538–572). Norwalk: Appleton & Lange.

Wolfe, R., & Wiggins, J. (1991). Cardiovascular diseases. In W. Hathaway, J. Groothuis, W. Hay, & J. Paisley (Eds.), *Current pediatric diagnosis and treatment* (10th ed.) (pp. 412–469). Norwalk: Appleton & Lange.

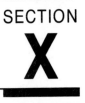

RESEARCH AND ETHICS

CHAPTER 43

Nancy Donaldson

Research and Ethical Issues

Objectives

1. Identify components of the investigative role of the nurse

2. Discuss the value of research conduct and utilization

3. Select and differentiate sources of nursing information

4. Describe steps in developing a single case study for presentation or publication

5. Describe the contribution of conceptual frameworks to the development and evaluation of a nursing research study

6. Describe the process for establishing organizational nursing research conduct and utilization programs in a clinical setting

7. Identify characteristics of a clinical trial

8. Describe ethical research principles and appropriate interventions when the rights of human research subjects are actually or potentially threatened

9. Analyze factors to consider in approaching the resolution of an ethical dilemma

10. Evaluate the scientific merit and clinical utility of a selected nursing research report

Introduction

A. This chapter presents concepts related to the investigative role of the clinical nurse and introduces strategies for conducting and using research in clinical practice

B. It is recognized that the educational backgrounds and research expertise of readers vary widely

C. This chapter is intended to engage all readers to consider their investigative role and to provide an opportunity for them to update and reinforce their knowledge and encounter new information

D. All readers are encouraged to pursue further study using the references included in the chapter

Clinical Practice: The Research Process

A. Investigative roles in nursing

1. Defining research and research utilization
   a. Research, a tool of science, is systematic inquiry used to answer a specific question through scientific methods; conducting a study
   b. Research utilization is using the products or processes of research or both as a basis for practice; putting new knowledge into practice
2. Investigative roles
   a. Each nurse is responsible for contributing, in appropriate ways, to the development of nursing science by participating, directly or indirectly, in nursing research conduct and utilization
   b. Investigative roles are related to educational preparation in nursing; coursework in research design and critique begins at the undergraduate level and is increasingly complex and advanced in graduate and doctoral studies
      (1) Nurses with an ADN have learned to
         (a) Be aware of nursing research
         (b) Identify clinical problems that need systematic investigation
         (c) Identify clinical concerns that might benefit from research utilization
      (2) Nurses with a BSN are prepared to
         (a) Read, interpret, and evaluate research for use in practice
         (b) Identify clinical problems and questions for investigation
         (c) Actively participate in conducting a research study
         (d) Participate in transforming research findings into practice
      (3) Nurses with an MSN are prepared to
         (a) Evaluate the scientific body of knowledge related to a specific clinical problem or question
         (b) Critically analyze factors affecting a specific clinical issue or problem
         (c) Collaboratively participate in designing, conducting, reporting, and evaluating research studies
         (d) Critically evaluate related nursing studies for application to practice
         (e) Initiate research utilization activities
      (4) Nurses with a doctoral degree are prepared to
         (a) Initiate descriptive and exploratory research studies
         (b) Design and conduct correlational and experimental studies
         (c) Apply a variety of methods to evaluate the effects of nursing actions on client outcomes
         (d) Collaborate on integrating the scientific body of knowledge
         (e) Disseminate and transform research results and processes into clinical nursing practice
3. Standards related to investigative roles
   a. At the individual level, the nurse is expected to actively pursue specified investigative role functions
   b. At the organizational level, nursing service organizations are expected to integrate research conduct and utilization activities into the organizational philosophy and strategic goals
4. The research utilization process is based on linking clinical practice problems to a cluster of research findings that are relevant and suitable as the basis for a proposed change in practice or as an innovation
   a. Establish organizational mechanisms to support research utilization activities
   b. Identify client care problems
   c. Identify and assess relevant research-based knowledge
   d. Design a research-based practice innovation
   e. Conduct a clinical trial and evaluation of the innovation

f. Determine whether to adopt, modify, or reject the innovation

g. Integrate, extend, and maintain the approved innovation

B. The spirit of inquiry

1. If nursing is to be scientifically based, then the products and processes of nursing research must be integrated into nursing practice
2. Nursing knowledge has been derived from many sources
   a. Tradition: knowledge derived from past practice
   b. Authority: knowledge derived from experts
   c. Trial and error: knowledge based on guessing
   d. Art: knowledge based on learned "how to"
   e. Ethics: knowledge derived from moral imperatives
   f. Intuition: knowledge derived from hunches
   g. Research: knowledge derived from scientific inquiry
3. A spirit of inquiry is expressed when nurses identify questions or problems that arise from practice and examine nursing and interdisciplinary literature that may be relevant
4. Activities that reflect a spirit of inquiry include
   a. Participation in journal clubs
   b. Regular reading of one or more nursing journals in a selected specialty
   c. Attending clinical conferences and grand rounds
   d. Attending regional and national clinical research conferences
   e. Communicating clinical questions and perspectives to nurse researchers
   f. Participating as a member of a nursing research project team
   g. Sharing results of an investigative project in a poster, publication, or presentation

C. Access to nursing information resources

1. Every year, 250,000 articles are published in over 20,000 biomedical journals
   a. Nursing knowledge exists in computer-based electronic data bases and bound books, journals, and reference sources
   b. Scientific knowledge doubles every 2 years
2. Nurses must regularly use nursing information resources to ensure that their practical knowledge is up-to-date
   a. Searching the literature
      (1) Provides information regarding a problem or question
      (2) Reveals prior research or opinion on a topic
      (3) Identifies sources of expertise
      (4) Provides background or perspective, clarifies issues, and generates ideas for problem solving
   b. Most current information is contained in recent journal articles, considered to be primary sources
   c. Textbooks are secondary sources that provide comprehensive information, although it is usually less current
   d. Pamphlets published by professional and health-related organizations are important sources of current nursing information
   e. Abstracts are capsule summaries of research reports and findings and are often available in a computer information data base
   f. Conference proceedings contain abstracts and summaries of program presentations and are often the most current source of new information
   g. Selected nursing-related data bases are available via computer and reference text searching
      (1) MEDLINE: available from National Library of Medicine; indexes 3200 biomedical journals
      (2) Cumulative Index of Nursing and Allied Health Literature (CINAHL): indexes 300 journals in nursing and allied health
      (3) Educational Resources Information Center (ERIC)

(4) HEALTH: Health planning and administration from the National Library of Medicine

(5) Social Sciences Citation Index (SOCIAL SCISEARCH): indexes 3700 journals in social and behavioral sciences, including nursing

3. Literature search strategies
   a. Identify key concepts and terms relevant to the topic
   b. Refer to data base reference to select subject headings that best fit the topic and concepts
   c. Combine subject headings with connecting words to construct a search strategy and produce the information desired
   d. Run the search and evaluate the fit between search findings and topic
   e. Consult with reference librarian, as needed, to refine search strategy to produce the best search outcome

D. **Establishing research conduct and utilization programs in clinical settings**

1. Gain organizational commitment
   a. Link the development of the research initiative to the institutional mission, organizational philosophy, and strategic plan
   b. Identify organizational benefits related to staff development, ensuring the scientific basis for practice and quality assurance monitoring
   c. Consider the potential benefits of participating in externally funded nursing systems, continuing education, and clinical evaluation special projects
2. Establish a nursing research committee
   a. Identify key clinical and administrative staff with a strong interest in developing the institution's nursing research program
   b. Identify community contacts with nursing research experts who would be interested in participating
   c. Collaboratively develop committee by-laws and a strategic plan to guide the first year
   d. Use internal and external resources to develop an educational program geared to strengthen the knowledge and skill of the committee related to research conduct and utilization in clinical settings
3. Inventory and develop resources
   a. Identify nursing staff members with advanced research education, experience, or both
   b. Evaluate institutional access to nursing information resources such as books and journals for literature searching
   c. Work with the institutional review board (IRB) to identify the organizational research review process
   d. Collaborate with nursing faculty in affiliated nursing programs
   e. Identify and collaborate with established researchers in other disciplines who may provide consultation, role modeling, and assistance
   f. Identify institutional, regional, and national public and private sources of funds to support nursing research conduct and utilization projects

E. **Clinical research approaches**

1. Theoretical and conceptual frameworks: through the looking glass
   a. Theoretical and conceptual frameworks provide the structural logic essential for organizing strong research
      (1) Theories describe, explain, or predict relationships among concepts
      (2) Concepts of the research problem, stated as a research question, suggest the theoretical perspective used in a particular study
      (3) While multiple theoretical perspectives may be relevant to any one study, the investigator selects the theoretical framework best suited to the project
      (4) The theoretical and conceptual framework
         (a) Guides the literature review

      (b) Influences the research design and procedure

      (c) Directs the selection of instruments

      (d) Gives meaning to the interpretation of the findings and conclusions

    (5) Research studies that lack a theoretical perspective lack internal logic and consistency and cannot be linked to prior research that may be related

  b. Characteristics of a strong and logical framework as the basis for conducting a research study

    (1) The theoretical framework is clearly identified, key concepts are specified, and the relationships among concepts that are supported by research are explicit

    (2) There is a logical, plausible link between the theoretical framework and the research problem or question being investigated

    (3) The rationale for the selection of the framework is presented clearly and substantiated

    (4) The research method and design are linked to the framework (for example, the timing and content of measurement)

    (5) Findings and conclusions can be explained in terms theoretically related to the framework

2. Single case studies

  a. Single case research has been the basis for some of health science's most influential inquiries; Freud and Piaget were classic case study researchers whose single case reports continue to be cited

  b. Case study investigations focus on a single unit of analysis, for example, one person, group, organization, or society

  c. Case studies are relevant to nursing in several ways

    (1) They examine and describe an individual's response to controlled interventions or naturally occurring events over time

    (2) They bridge the gap between research and practice

    (3) They provide potential integration of interdisciplinary view

    (4) They enable individual nurses to examine and cluster individual cases

  d. Factors to consider when selecting a client for a case study

    (1) Nature and specificity of the nursing plan of care

    (2) Access to multiple observations over time

    (3) Ability to measure and describe client responses to nursing therapy

    (4) Opportunity to repeat or replicate case and nursing treatment to validate findings

  e. Format for a single case study

    (1) Case problem and purpose

    (2) Relevant background information and literature

    (3) Introduction of the subject and setting

    (4) Review of the history, nursing assessment, diagnosis, and interventions

    (5) Sources of data and procedure for data collection

    (6) Presentation and analysis of findings

    (7) Conclusions and implications for research and practice

  f. Sharing findings from a single case study

    (1) Begin with a presentation in a familiar clinical setting; invite feedback and revise the report, as needed

    (2) Prepare a poster for presentation at a regional or national meeting

    (3) Prepare a written case study report and submit for publication

3. Clinical trials

  a. Purpose of the randomized controlled trial (RCT)

    (1) Comparatively tests the effects of a selected research treatment

    (2) Enables investigator to have maximum control over factors known to influence determination of experimental effects of a selected research treatment

  b. Characteristics of RCTs

(1) Randomization: subject sample is selected from population-at-large by chance and assigned to treatment or control group(s) by chance

(2) Control: investigator has the ability to control the administration of the experimental treatment and factors that might confound the effect(s) of the experiment

(3) Comparison: treatment effects are determined by comparing effects of treatment group with those of a control or nontreatment group to assess the extent to which the observed treatment outcomes are the result of the experiment versus chance

(4) Blinding: preventing the investigator assessing the treatment effects from knowing the subject's study group assignment

c. Contributions of RCTs to nursing practice research

(1) The RCT is the method of choice when the research question demands a design that can examine cause-and-effect relationships

(2) The RCT is the ultimate research design for assessing the effects of selected nursing actions on client outcomes

(3) The RCT design enables the investigator to compare and evaluate the clinical merit of well-developed nursing interventions by either withholding treatment from the control group or comparing a new and innovative treatment with current common practice to determine which intervention has the best treatment effect(s)

4. Evaluating the scientific merit and clinical utility of new knowledge in a research report

a. Critical appraisal of a research study is the essential first step in assessing the potential value of the findings for practice

b. General criteria for evaluating a research report (Table 43–1)

(1) A common approach to reviewing and evaluating the scientific merit and clinical usefulness of a published research report is to refer to an established set of review criteria that provide a systematic approach to analyzing the article and cue the reader to key points to consider

(2) In addition, the clinical expertise of the reader, based on personal, educational, and professional experience, is an invaluable source of insight when considering the merit and usefulness of research outcomes

c. Determining clinical utility or applicability of research outcomes integrates an evaluation of overall scientific merit with specific consideration of the clinical relevance, risks and benefits, feasibility, costs and benefits, and potential for clinical evaluation

d. The checklist questions in Table 43–1 are designed to provide a systematic guide to evaluating the clinical usefulness of nursing research findings

(1) Replication

(a) Is there scientific evidence of more than one study reporting similar findings

(b) Are these studies conceptually linked and scientifically sound

(2) Scientific merit

(a) Are the theoretical structure, research design, instrumentation, and sample characteristics and size logically linked and clinically valid

(b) Is the data analysis procedure appropriate

(c) Is the research question answered and are the findings thoroughly discussed, explained, and linked to the theoretical framework

(3) Risk and benefit: what is the degree of relative risk and benefit of any proposed nursing action change for the client, the individual nurse, the nursing service, and the institution

(4) Does the potential benefit of any nursing action innovation suggest changing practice before additional clinical evaluation, or does the degree of potential risk suggest the need to replicate the original study or undertake thorough clinical evaluation before changing practice

(5) Degree of clinical merit

Table 43–1
GENERAL CRITERIA FOR EVALUATING A RESEARCH REPORT

Step 1. Research problem
  1. Is the problem clearly and concisely stated?
  2. Is the problem adequately narrowed down into a researchable problem?
  3. Is the problem significant to nursing?
  4. Is the relationship of the identified problem to previous research clear?

Step 2. Literature review
  1. Is the literature review logically organized?
  2. Does the review provide a critique of the relevant studies?
  3. Are the gaps in knowledge about the research problem identified?
  4. Are important relevant references omitted?

Step 3. Theoretical or conceptual framework
  1. Is the theoretical framework easily linked with the problem, or does it seem forced?
  2. If a conceptual framework is used, are the concepts adequately defined and are the relationships among these concepts clearly identified?

Step 4. Research variables
  1. Are the independent and dependent variables operationally defined?
  2. Are any extraneous or intervening variables identified?

Step 5. Hypotheses
  1. Is a predicted relationship between two or more variables included in each hypothesis?
  2. Are the hypotheses clear, testable, and specific?
  3. Do the hypotheses logically flow from the theoretical or conceptual framework?

Step 6. Sampling
  1. Is the sample size adequate?
  2. Is the sample representative of the defined population?
  3. Is the method for selection of the sample appropriate?
  4. Are the sample criteria for inclusion into the study identified?
  5. Is there any sampling bias in the chosen method?

Step 7. Research design
  1. Is the research design adequately described?
  2. Is the design appropriate for the research problem?
  3. Does the research design control for threats to internal and external validity of the study?
  4. Are the data collection instruments described adequately?
  5. Are the reliability and validity of the measurement tools adequate?

Step 8. Data collection methods
  1. Are the data collection methods appropriate for study?
  2. Are the data collection instruments described adequately?
  3. Are the reliability and validity of the measurement tools adequate?

Step 9. Data analysis
  1. Is the results section clearly and logically organized?
  2. Is the type of analysis appropriate for the level of measurement for each variable?
  3. Are the tables and figures clear and understandable?
  4. Is the statistical test the correct one for answering the research question?

Step 10. Interpretation and discussion of the findings
  1. Are the interpretations based on the data obtained?
  2. Does the investigator clearly distinguish between actual findings and interpretations?
  3. Are the findings discussed in relation to previous research and to the conceptual/theoretical framework?
  4. Are unwarranted generalizations made beyond the study sample?
  5. Are the limitations of the results identified?
  6. Are implications of the results for clinical nursing practice discussed?
  7. Are recommendations for future research identified?
  8. Are the conclusions justified?

  (Beck, C. [1989]. The research critique. General criteria for evaluating a research report. *Journal of Obstetric, Gynecologic, and Neonatal Nursing, 19*[1], 18–22.)

          (a) Does the research report substantiate the importance of the clinical problem that is the focus of the research study

          (b) Does the research report examine the extent to which the findings may be useful

      (6) Clinical control: do nurses have direct or indirect control over the clinical factors that make possible successful implementation of the clinical innovation

      (7) Feasibility

          (a) Is it reasonable and realistic to undertake the changes in practice suggested by the research study

          (b) Are the necessary resources available or obtainable

          (c) What are the fiscal implications of the potential change

      (8) Evaluation

          (a) Is there methodological and clinical expertise available to support undertaking the clinical evaluation of the proposed change in practice

          (b) Do the evaluation outcomes support the original research findings and justify the proposed change in practice

  5. Ethical decision making

    a. Protecting the rights of human research subjects

      (1) Ethical research principles

          (a) Right to freedom from intrinsic risk of injury: potential risk to human research subject must be assessed, and subject must be fully advised of actual or potential risks of study participation and must voluntarily consent to participate

          (b) Right to privacy and dignity: requires full disclosure of alternative treatments and study procedure and requirements before induction of a human research subject and right to decline or withdraw participation without prejudice

          (c) Right to anonymity: requires every effort to ensure confidentiality of study information and findings and anonymity of subject with information and data

      (2) Role of the IRB

          (a) The human subjects review committee (or IRB) is an institutional mechanism to review and monitor the conduct of research that involves human research subjects to ensure that their rights are protected

          (b) Membership on the IRB is expected to represent all occupations and groups within a selected setting who may be directly or indirectly involved in research

          (c) Federal guidelines for human research subjects review designate three general categories of review

             (i) Exempt—no committee review required; administrative review

            (ii) Expedited—requires review by administrative/IRB representative(s)

            (iii) Full review—Requires review and approval by institutional IRB

            (iv) The review category is assigned based on

                • Nature of the study design and procedure

                • Actual or potential risk to the subjects

      (3) Informed consent and nursing accountability

          (a) Before administering any investigational drug or treatment, the nurse must ensure that the protocol has been reviewed by the IRB and that informed consent has been obtained and documented in the client's record

          (b) If a human research subject refuses an investigational drug or treatment, the subject may be exercising the right to withdraw from the study; the drug or treatment should be withheld and the investigator notified

(c) Nurses who formally or informally participate in a research study are advised to request a complete copy of the research proposal and are encouraged to review the proposal, examine any related clinical protocols, and initiate discussion with the principal investigator to answer any questions

(d) If the nurse becomes aware that the rights of human research subjects may be compromised, the nurse is expected to bring this information to the attention of the IRB

b. Resolving ethical dilemmas in obstetrical and gynecological nursing

(1) Contemporary obstetrical and gynecological nursing practice presents nurses with numerous ethical dilemmas that require moral reasoning to determine the best action to take and the moral rationale for that action

(2) In resolving ethical dilemmas, the nurse must consider personal, professional, and societal values; potential value conflict; and the limitations of personal and organizational moral development

(3) Knowledge of the professional code of ethics of nurses and the ability to apply the ethical principles of the code on a continuing basis are prerequisites to professional practice and ethical decision making (American Nurses' Association, 1985)

c. Guidelines for ethical decision making

(1) Identify the nature of the conflict, the issues, and the principle from the nurses' code that are at stake

(2) Consider which action reflects the greatest reverence for life and acceptance of death

(3) Decide which action reflects the greatest goodness and rightness; approaches for determining goodness and rightness include

(a) The principle of beneficence: requires the health-care provider to do good and implies balancing the benefit of a therapeutic action with the burden of that action

(b) The deontological perspective: requires appraisal of duty and the rightness or wrongness of an act, regardless of the outcome of the act

(c) The teleological perspective: focuses on the outcome of the act and defines right and wrong based on consequences

(d) The utilitarianism perspective: defines the concept of right as based on determining which action does the most good for the most people

(e) Paternalism: emphasizes beneficence over autonomy and implies that moral goodness of what is best supersedes the expressed will of the client

(4) Which alternative is most just or fair

(5) Seek consultation from objective experts, bioethicists, or both

(6) Convene a conference where all interested parties can share their values and concerns and participate in examining and determining the resolution to the ethical dilemma

STUDY QUESTIONS

1. Consider two nursing facts you use in clinical practice on a regular basis. Trace the source of knowledge for each fact and determine the basis for the knowledge. Is it based on tradition, authority, art, intuition, or research?

2. List four ways in which you express your investigative role.

3. Select a familiar clinical setting and explore research conduct and utilization resources available to staff nurses. For example, is there a staff person who is responsible for research in nursing? Is there a nursing research committee? Are there nursing research journals and books in the library? Is continuing education available for staff related to research? How would you rate the organization's overall spirit of inquiry? Is there an active IRB? Does a member of the nursing staff serve as a member of the IRB?

4. Select and state a clinical nursing problem or question arising from your practice.

5. Consider the clinical nursing problem or question you chose. Go to the library and initiate a preliminary literature search (focus on nursing research literature that has appeared within the last 5 years) and identify two research report articles that are relevant to your clinical problem or question. List the two article citations.

6. Read each of the two articles you selected thoroughly. For each article, answer the following questions.

   a. What was the problem the research addressed?

   b. What was the research question?

   c. What did the investigator do to answer the question?

   d. What was the theoretical perspective or framework the investigator chose to guide the study?

   e. Based on your clinical and educational background, list the strengths and limitations of the research.

   f. What are the clinical implications of each of the articles?

7. Select one of the articles and review that article using the criteria in Table 43–1 for a more thorough and systematic approach to a review of the article.

8. Identify three typical clinical situations that you consider to be actually or potentially ethically difficult. For each situation, what is the essence of the ethical dilemma?

9. For each situation, which three of the guidelines for ethical decision making would be most useful in resolving the ethical dilemma posed by the situation? Why?

REFERENCES

American Nurses' Association. (1985). *Code for nurses, with interpretive statements.* Kansas City, MO: Author.

American Nurses' Association Commission on Nursing Research (1981). *Guidelines for the investigative functions of nurses.* Kansas City, MO: Author.

Beck, C. (1990). The research critique: General criteria for evaluating a research report. *Journal of Obstetric, Gynecologic, and Neonatal Nursing, 19*(1), 18–22.

Brett, J. (1987). Use of nursing practice research findings. *Nursing Research, 36*(6), 344–349.

Burns, N., & Grove, S. (1987). Utilization of research in nursing practice (ch. 21). In *The practice of nursing research: Conduct, critique and utilization.* Philadelphia: Saunders.

Carper, B. (1978). Fundamental patterns of knowing in nursing. *Advances in Nursing Science, 1*(1), 13–23.

Cobb, A. (1987). Ten criteria for evaluating qualitative research proposals. *Journal of Nursing Education, 26*(4), 138–143.

Crane, J. (1985). Using research in practice: Research utilization nursing models. *Western Journal of Nursing Research, 7*(4), 494–497.

Crane, J. (1985). Using research in practice: Research utilization theoretical perspectives. *Western Journal of Nursing Research, 7*(2), 261–268.

Cronenwett, L. (1986). The research role of the clinical nurse specialist. *Journal of Nursing Administration, 16*(4), 10–11.

Cronenwett, L. (1987). Research utilization in a practice setting. *Journal of Nursing Administration, 17*(7, 8), 9–10.

Duffy, M. (1988). The research appraisal checklist: Appraising nursing research reports. In O. Strickland, & C. Waltz, (Eds.), *Measurement of nursing outcomes: Measuring nursing performance* (Vol. 2). New York: Springer.

Fawcett, J. (1982). Utilization of nursing research findings. *Image: Journal of Nursing Scholarship, 16*(2), 57–59.

Fawcett, J. (1984). Another look at utilization of nursing research. *Image: Journal of Nursing Scholarship, 16*(2), 59–62.

Fetter, M., Feetham, S., D'Apolito, K., Chaze, B., Fink, A., Frink, B., Hougart, M., & Rushton, C. (1989). Randomized clinical trials: Issues for researchers. *Nursing Research, 38*(2), 117–120.

Haller, K., & Reynolds, M. (1986). Using research in practice: A case for replication in nursing—Part 2. *Western Journal of Nursing Research, 8*(2), 249–252.

Holm, K. (1983). Single subject research. *Nursing Research, 32*(4), 253–255.

Holm, K., & Liewellyn, J. (1986). Research utilization. In K. Holm (Ed.), *Nursing research for nursing practice.* Philadelphia: Saunders.

Horsley, J. (1983). *Using research to improve nursing practice: A guide.* Orlando, FL: Grune & Stratton.

Horsley, J. (1985). Using research in practice: The current context. *Western Journal of Nursing Research,* 7(1), 135–139.

Horsley, J., Crane, J., & Bingle, J. (1978). Research utilization as an organizational process. *Journal of Nursing Administration, 8*(7), 4–6.

Jacox, A. (1978). Determining a study's relevance for clinical practice. *American Journal of Nursing, 78*(11), 1882–1889.

Kilby, S., Fishel, C., & Gupta, A. (1989). Access to nursing information resources. *Image: Journal of Nursing Scholarship, 21*(1), 26–30.

Krueger, J. (1977). Utilizing clinical nursing research findings in practice: A structured approach. In M. Batey (Ed.), *Communicating nursing research, Volume 9: Nursing in the bicentennial year.* Boulder, CO: Western Interstate Commission for Higher Education.

Krueger, J., Nelson, A., & Wolanin, M. (1978). Research utilization, Part III. In *Nursing research development, collaboration and utilization.* Germantown, MD: Aspen.

Larson, E., & Satterthwaite, R. (1989). Searching the literature: A professional imperative. *American Journal of Infection Control, 17*(6), 359–364.

Lindeman, C. (1984). Dissemination of nursing research. *Image: Journal of Nursing Scholarship, 16*(2), 57–59.

Loomis, M. (1985). Knowledge utilization and research utilization in nursing. *Image: Journal of Nursing Scholarship, 17*(2), 35–39.

Mateo, M., & Kirchhoff, K. (1991). *Conducting and using research in the clinical setting.* San Francisco, CA: Williams & Wilkins.

Meier, P., & Pugh, E. (1986). The case study: A viable approach to clinical research. *Research in Nursing & Health, 9,* 195–202.

NAACOG. (1990, December). Quality assurance. *OGN Nursing Practice Resource.*

Phillips, L. (1986). *A clinician's guide to the critique and utilization of nursing research.* Norwalk, CT: Appleton-Century-Crofts.

Stetler, C., & Marram, G. (1976). Evaluating research findings for applicability in practice. *American Journal of Nursing, 24*(9), 559–563.

Woods, N., & Catanzaro, M. (1988). *Nursing research: Theory and practice.* St. Louis, MO: Mosby.

ADDITIONAL REFERENCES

Barger, S. (1987). The potential for research and research use in academic nurse-managed centers. *Nurse Educator, 12*(6), 19–22.

Barnard, K. (1980). Knowledge for practice: Directions for the future. *Nursing Research, 29,* 208–212.

Batey, M. (1975). Research: Its dissemination and utilization in nursing practice. *Washington State Journal of Nursing,* Winter, 6–9.

Bergman, R. (1984). Omissions in nursing research. *International Nursing Review, 31*(2), 55–56.

Breu, C., and Dracup, K. (1976). Implementing nursing research in a critical care setting. *Journal of Nursing Administration, 6*(10), 14–17.

Brossard-Bryant, P. (1981). Problem solving via research. *Supervisor Nurse, 12,* 36–37.

Clark, N., & Lenburg, C. (1980). Knowledge-informed behavior and the nursing culture. *Nursing Research, 29*(4), 244–249.

Conway, M. (1978). Clinical research: Instrument for change. *Journal of Nursing Administration, 8*(12), 27–32.

Davis, M. (1981). Promoting nursing research in the clinical setting. *Journal of Nursing Administration, 11*(3), 22–27.

Fawcett, J. (1980). A declaration of nursing independence: The relation of theory and research to nursing practice. *Journal of Nursing Administration, 10*(6), 36–39.

Fine, R. (1980). Marketing nursing research. *Journal of Nursing Administration, 10*(11), 21–23.

Goode, C., Lovett, M., Hayes, J., & Butcher, L. (1987). Use of research based knowledge in clinical practice. *Journal of Nursing Administration, 17*(12), 11–18.

Hunt, J. (1981). Indicators for nursing practice: The use of research findings. *Journal of Advanced Nursing, 6,* 189–194.

King, D., Barnard, K., & Hoehn, R. (1981). Disseminating the results of nursing research. *Nursing Outlook, 24,* 164–169.

Miller, J., & Messenger, S. (1978). Obstacles to applying nursing research findings. *American Journal of Nursing, 78*(4), 632–634.

Rizzuto, C. (1988). Research in service settings: Part I—Consortium Project outcomes. *Journal of Nursing Administration, 18*(2), 32–37.

Sashkin, M., Morris, W., & Horst, L. (1973). A comparison of social and organizational change models. *Psychological Review, 80*(6), 510–526.

Stetler, C. (1985). Research utilization: Defining a concept. *Image: Journal of Nursing Scholarship, XVII*(2), 40–44.

Index